Principles and Practice of Photoprotection

Steven Q. Wang • Henry W. Lim
Editors

Principles and Practice of Photoprotection

Adis

Editors
Steven Q. Wang
Dermatology Service
Memorial Sloan-Kettering Cancer Center
Basking Ridge, NJ
USA

Henry W. Lim
Department of Dermatology
Henry Ford Medical Center - New Center One
Detroit, MI
USA

ISBN 978-3-319-29381-3 ISBN 978-3-319-29382-0 (eBook)
DOI 10.1007/978-3-319-29382-0

Library of Congress Control Number: 2016936370

Springer Cham Heidelberg New York Dordrecht London

Printed on acid-free paper

Adis is a brand of Springer

Springer International Publishing AG Switzerland is part of Springer Science+Business Media (www.springer.com)

Preface

Photoprotection captures the interest of physicians, academic researchers, industry scientists, law makers, marketers, general media, and consumers. It is a dynamic field where progresses and advancements often hinge on close collaboration of multidisciplinary teams. In the past decade, significant development has been made in the realm of sunscreens where novel UV filters and innovative formulation techniques have improved both the efficacy and aesthetic components of end products. To enhance protection from UV and even visible and infrared radiation, there has been active research exploring the application of antioxidants, nanotechnology, and DNA repair enzymes in photoprotection. Along the way, there has been a general trend towards global harmonization in guidelines for both testing and labeling claims in sunscreens. At the same time, recent clinical trials have demonstrated the benefits of sunscreen in protecting against skin cancer and photoaging. Continual research has shown the importance of photoprotection in preventing photodermatoses and photoaggravated autoimmune diseases. Despite these scientific and medical advances, there remain many myths and controversies, especially in the general media, surrounding the safety and efficacy of sunscreens and other photoprotective modalities. Continued education of the general public to practice proper photoprotective behaviors is needed.

This book aims to showcase all the rich facets and themes associated with photoprotection. Each chapter, which starts with a brief synopsis, is written by experts in their respective fields. The contributing authors have decades of clinical, research, or practical experience, and we are grateful to having enlisted this panel of experts to share their knowledge on this important topic. We sincerely hope the readers will find this book as an informative and practical guide.

Basking Ridge, NJ, USA — Steven Q. Wang
Detroit, MI, USA — Henry W. Lim

Acknowledgments

This book is dedicated to our families: Judy and Kevin and Mamie. We thank them for their patience and sacrifice throughout the course of this project.

Contents

Part I

Chapter 1
Clinical and Biological Relevance of Visible and Infrared Radiation

Kelsey Lawrence, Mohammed Al-Jamal, Indermeet Kohli, and Iltefat Hamzavi

Key Points

- Biologically, visible radiation has been shown to induce erythema, pigmentation, free radical production, and DNA damage, while infrared radiation has been shown to induce erythema, thermal pain, photoaging, cytotoxicity, DNA damage, and oxidative stress.
- Visible light has been shown to be an action spectrum in solar urticaria, chronic actinic dermatitis, and porphyrias; it is used for the treatment of hyperbilirubinemia. Infrared radiation can cause erythema ab igne and squamous cell carcinoma.
- Lasers with wavelengths in the visible and infrared spectrum can be used to treat vascular and pigmented lesions, keloids, etc. IPL, LLLT, and PDT are other light sources with wavelengths in the visible and infrared spectrum that are also used to treat numerous dermatologic conditions.
- New imaging techniques that use visible and infrared radiation have been recently developed. The data is promising and could greatly impact the field of dermatology in the future.
- Active research is ongoing on effective photoprotective measures against visible light and infrared radiation.

K. Lawrence, MD • M. Al-Jamal, MD • I. Kohli, PhD • I. Hamzavi, MD, FAAD (✉)
Department of Dermatology, Henry Ford Hospital,
3031 W. Grand Blvd., Suite 800, Detroit, MI 48202, USA
e-mail: klawrenc@med.wayne.edu; maljama1@hfhs.org;
ikohli1@hfhs.org; ihamzav1@hfhs.org

S.Q. Wang, H.W. Lim (eds.), *Principles and Practice of Photoprotection*,
DOI 10.1007/978-3-319-29382-0_1

1.1 Introduction

The sun emits electromagnetic radiation encompassing a wide range of wavelengths (Table 1.1). The wavelengths must be able to penetrate the ozone layer in order to reach the earth's surface. The radiation that reaches the earth is made up of 50 % visible light, 40 % infrared radiation (IR), and 9 % ultraviolet (UV) radiation [1]. It should be noted that in the UV spectrum, only UVB and UVA reach the surface of the earth; UVC is filtered out completely in the hemisphere. There has been extensive research into the effects of UV radiation on the skin, but until recently there has not been much research on the effects of visible and infrared radiation on the skin. This chapter will discuss the biological and clinical relevance of visible and infrared radiation.

Electromagnetic radiation is made up of photons, which have the properties of both waves and particles. When photons reach the surface of the skin, they can be reflected, scattered, absorbed, or transmitted. Reflection occurs at the skin surface and can be used for diagnostic purposes but is not useful therapeutically. Scattering is altering the direction of light transmission and also affects the depth of penetration. Most of the scattering of light is done by the collagen that is present in the dermis. However, scattering is also dependent on the wavelength, with shorter wavelengths undergoing more scattering compared to longer wavelengths [2].

In order for a photon to exert a clinical effect, it must be absorbed. Molecules in the skin that absorb photons are called chromophores. Absorption is dependent on the depth of penetration of the radiation and the wavelength absorbed by the chromophore. The depth of penetration into the skin varies with wavelength; the longer

Table 1.1 Electromagnetic spectrum and corresponding wavelengths

Light spectrum	Wavelength
Gamma ray	less than 0.01 nm
X-ray	0.01–10 nm
Ultraviolet	10–400 nm
UVC	200–290 nm
UVB	290–320 nm
UVA	320–400 nm
Visible	400–700 nm
Violet	400–450 nm
Blue	450–495 nm
Green	495–570 nm
Yellow	570–590 nm
Orange	590–620 nm
Red	620–700 nm
Infrared-A	700–1400 nm
Infrared-B	1400–3000 nm
Infrared-C	3000 nm – 1 mm
Microwave	1 mm–1 m
Radio	1 mm–100 km

wavelengths penetrate deeper than shorter wavelengths. Therefore, blue light, which is at the shorter end of the wavelength spectrum of visible light, can be used clinically for lesions contained in the epidermis, while red light, which has a longer wavelength, is useful for thick lesions or to target deeper structures [2, 3].

A variety of molecules can act as chromophores, some examples being amino acids, lipids, porphyrins, photosensitizing drugs, DNA, hemoglobin, bilirubin, melanin, and water. When a chromophore absorbs a photon, the chromophore transitions to an excited state, transiently. The chromophore releases energy, in the form of heat or light, when it returns to the ground state. The chromophore can then transfer this energy to another molecule or undergo chemical changes. Multiple photons are necessary to produce sufficient energy to cause cellular changes, which then leads to a clinical effect [2, 4]. The amount of absorption depends on the chromophores in the skin and the wavelength of light used. The energy absorbed is also known as the energy density, or fluence, and is measured in joules per square centimeter [5].

1.2 Visible Spectrum

Visible light is the portion of the electromagnetic radiation responsible for general illumination and is visible to the human eye. The wavelength of the visible radiation spectrum is from 400 to 700 nanometers (nm). Each color of light represents a different wavelength, with blue being at the shorter end of the spectrum and red at the longer end (Fig. 1.1). See Table 1.1 for more details on specific wavelengths.

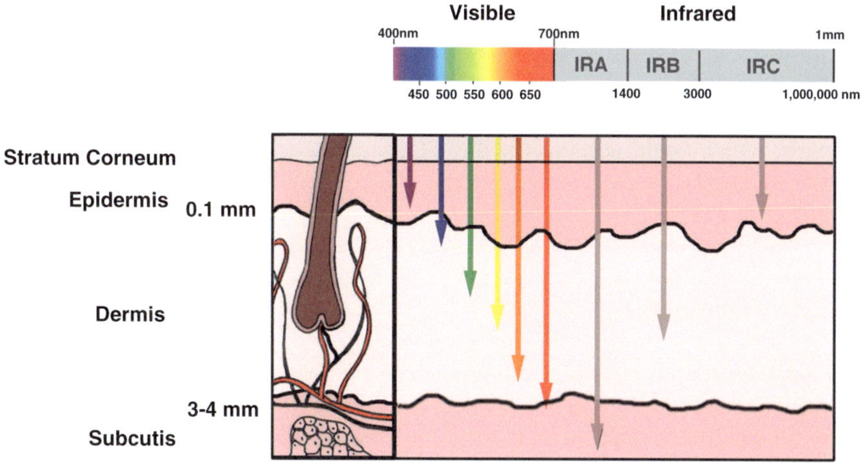

Fig. 1.1 The wavelengths and their corresponding depth of penetration in the skin of each band within the visible and infrared spectrum

1.2.1 Biological Effects

1.2.1.1 Erythema

Erythema is a cutaneous inflammatory reaction and can be associated with warmth and tenderness; blisters can form if severe. Erythema during or immediately after sun exposure can occur transiently in fair skin types. Delayed erythema occurs in all skin types, with a peak occurring between 6 and 24 h after exposure [6–8].

Erythema is mostly caused by UVB radiation. However, UVA radiation, primarily UVA2 (320–340 nm), can contribute to skin erythema, and visible light has been shown to induce transient erythema [9]. The minimal erythema dose (MED) is 1000-fold more for UVA when compared to UVB [10, 11]. It is thought that the erythema caused by visible radiation is caused through a different mechanism than UVB-induced erythema, due to the differing depths of penetration. Dilatation of the vessels of the subpapillary plexus is the suggested mechanism for skin erythema from visible light, while erythema from UV radiation is thought to be from dilation of upper dermis capillaries since UV radiation does not penetrate as deeply [12].

Skin type plays a role in the timing and intensity of erythema from visible radiation. Mahmoud et al., using a light source that emits 98.3 % visible light, found that visible light can induce erythema, in individuals with Fitzpatrick skin types IV–VI, immediately after exposure, surrounding the area of immediate pigment darkening. However, the erythema started to fade 30 min later and was completely gone in 2 h. Of note, they were unable to induce any erythema in skin type II individuals even at the highest dose tested, 480 J cm^{-2}. The authors proposed a possible thermal effect from the reaction within the chromophores causing vasodilation and therefore erythema. They also proposed that the increased melanin concentration, one of the chromophores with absorption in the visible light spectrum, in the darker skinned individuals could account for the increased heat production and therefore the increased erythema that occurred in darker skin types [9].

However, in the study done by Porges et al., erythema was induced in individuals with Fitzpatrick skin types II, III, and IV only but not V and VI. Although, of note, the filter that was used did allow part of the UVA spectrum (385–400 nm) to pass through, which could account for the differing results between the two studies. Porges et al. also proposed that thermal effects may account for the erythema response [6, 9, 13].

1.2.1.2 Pigmentation

Skin pigmentation is classified into immediate pigment darkening (IPD), persistent pigment darkening (PPD), and delayed tanning (DT). IPD appears immediately and fades within 20 min. PPD persists for 2–24 h. Both IPD and PPD are caused from oxidation and redistribution of preexisting melanin. DT occurs days later and is from synthesis of new melanin [7, 14]. Most research thus far regarding pigmentation is done on UV radiation.

Kollias and Baqer used a polychromatic light source with wavelength from 390 to 1700 nm, which consists of the visible spectrum and part of the spectrum of infrared radiation. They were able to induce pigmentary changes; however, they did not notice any erythema or thermal changes, even after 3 h of irradiation with a total dose of 270 W cm^{-2}. IPD was present, and pigmentation that lasted for 10 weeks was observed when doses greater than 720 J cm^{-2} were used [15]. Rosen et al. showed that visible radiation up to 470 nm can induce an IPD response; this study was performed by using a xenon-mercury arc lamp with grating holographic monochromator to select for wavelengths of 334, 365, 405, 435, or 549 nm and spectrophotometric analysis of skin reflectance [16]. Pathak et al. identified the peak IPD response to be between 380 and 500 nm using a fixed exposure of 45 J cm^{-2} [17].

Ramasubramaniam et al. used midday sunlight in Bangalore, India, with filters to determine the cutaneous effects of visible light (greater than 420 nm) and UV light (less than 400 nm) on pigmentation on Fitzpatrick skin types IV and V. They found there is not a significant difference in the IPD produced by UV and visible light. They identified similarly shaped action spectra for IPD and PPD when comparing UV and visible light. However, UV radiation is much more efficient in producing IPD, and the PPD response by visible light is much less intense. Since UV and visible light produced similar action spectra, though, they believe it is likely the same melanin precursor that UV and visible light are interacting with in order to induce these effects [18].

Mahmoud et al., using a light source that emits 98.3 % visible light, also found that visible radiation induced immediate pigmentation on volunteers with Fitzpatrick skin types IV–VI, with the lowest effective dose being 40 J cm^{-2} [9]. The pigment was darker as the dose was increased. They noted that the pigment was most intense in type V skin type volunteers. The pigmentation was still present at 2 weeks, the end point of their study, even at the lower doses. However, they found that no pigmentation was induced in skin type II individuals, using the same light source and doses. The pigmentation induced in this study was more intense and lasted longer than the pigmentation described by Ramasubramaniam et al. (ref). However, the light source in Mahmoud et al. was artificial, while natural sunlight was used in the study done by Ramasubramaniam et al., and the dose used was four times higher in the study by Mahmoud et al., which could account for the differences [9, 18]. Confocal microscopy used by Mahmoud et al. showed that visible radiation induced redistribution of melanin from the basal layer to the upper epidermis. Diffuse reflectance spectroscopy also showed increased melanin content directly related to the visible radiation dose [9].

Of note, Duteil et al. showed recently that not all wavelengths of visible light have the same effect on pigmentation. Healthy volunteers of skin types III and IV were irradiated with wavelengths from both ends of the visible spectrum and the results compared. Blue-violet light (415 nm) induced pronounced and longlasting pigmentation (up to 3 months) in both skin types, while red light (630 nm) did not induce pigmentation [19].

Porges et al. used a solar stimulator to expose individuals with Fitzpatrick skin types II, III, and IV to light from 385 to 690 nm and observed IPD and DT as well as erythema. The IPD and erythema faded over 24 h. The DT remained unchanged for 10 days. The threshold for PPD (greater than 80 J cm^{-2}) was slightly higher than that for IPD (between 40 and 80 J cm^{-2}), while the threshold for DT was higher than the threshold for IPD. Porges et al. were able to induce pigmentation in lighter skin types, while Mahmoud et al. were not. These differences could be due to the small amount of wavelengths outside the visible spectrum UV from 385 to 400 nm in the study done by Porges et al. or from the limited amount of infrared radiation in the light source in the study done by Mahmoud et al. [9, 13].

Visible light-induced pigmentation, especially in darker skin types, may be clinically relevant by potentially playing a role in pigmentation disorders. Melasma and post-inflammatory hyperpigmentation are much more prominent in darker skinned individuals. This is consistent with the clinical observation that sunscreens, which protect against UV but not visible radiation, do not fully protect the progression of these conditions [6].

1.2.1.3 Free Radical Production

Reactive oxygen species (ROS) are chemically reactive molecules containing oxygen. Free radicals are hazardous to living organisms and have been associated with many pathological processes by damaging most cellular components. ROS are continually generated as a byproduct of metabolism, and cells have antioxidants to protect themselves from the detrimental effects of ROS. Any increase in ROS production or decrease in defense against ROS can lead to oxidative damage. Free radicals are a type of ROS with unpaired valence electrons. An oxygenation product from ascorbate, the ascorbate free radical, is a marker of oxidative stress that can be easily measured with electron spin spectroscopy [20–22].

A study by Haywood observed ascorbate free radical production in ex vivo human skin using solar-simulated light. They used sunscreen (SPF 25, containing the UVA filter butylmethoxyldibenzoyl methane) to block UV radiation and were therefore able to determine that visible light is responsible for 33 % of the free radical production in the substratum corneum, while UV accounts for the rest [23, 24]. In addition, Liebel et al. showed that commercially available sunscreens had minimal effect on reducing visible light-induced ROS, proinflammatory cytokines, and MMP-1 expression. However, when pretreatment with a photostable UVA/UVB sunscreen that contained an antioxidant was applied before visible light radiation, the production of ROS, proinflammatory cytokines, and MMP-1 expression was significantly reduced [25]. This is important because current sunscreens do not offer protection against visible light and with this information that is clearly something to look into in the future.

1.2.1.4 DNA Damage

It has been well described that UVB is the predominant spectrum causing direct DNA damage, and indirect DNA damage through ROS is predominantly induced by UVA. Recently, the effects of visible light on DNA damage were studied. Edstrom et al. irradiated normal skin with 126 J cm^{-2} visible light which corresponds to about a half hour outside on a Sweden summer day. An Osram xenon arc lamp with two filters was used to block out all but the visible spectrum. This was done three times weekly for 4 weeks while taking intermittent punch biopsies. They found that visible light increased p53-positive cells as well as proliferation in the epidermis, although to a lesser extent than UVA1 (340–400 nm). p53 normally downregulates bcl-2, but interestingly they found a slight increase in bcl-2 in the epidermis, which could potentially mean the *p53* gene was mutated [26].

Kielbassa et al. used a xenon arc lamp with grid monochromator and/or cutoff filters (to make monochromatic radiation) to study the spectrum in which dimers and oxidative DNA modification occur in hamster cells. From UVA1 range into the visible light spectrum, oxidative DNA damage was observed, with a peak between 400 and 450 nm [27]. Hoffmann-Dorr et al. analyzed the effect of visible light on direct and indirect DNA damage on melanoma cells and human skin fibroblasts. Visible light induces ROS, which indirectly damages DNA. They concluded that the oxidative damage from 400 to 500 nm accounted for 10 % of the total indirect damage that occurs with sunlight exposure [28]. Liebel et al. showed that visible light radiation induced production of ROS, proinflammatory cytokines, and MMP-1 expression. However, neither thymine dimers are produced from visible light radiation nor TNF-alpha expression induced [25]. Now that visible light is being used more clinically, in lasers and photodynamic therapy (PDT), the long-term effects on DNA are becoming clinically relevant.

1.2.2 *Clinical Effects*

1.2.2.1 Solar Urticaria

Solar urticaria is an uncommon photosensitivity disorder, making up 0.4 % of all urticarial cases in a 30-year retrospective study [29]. It is a type I immediate hypersensitivity response, mediated by mast cells. Urticarial lesions occur within minutes of sun exposure and resolve within 2 h if exposure is discontinued. Action spectrum can be in the UVB, UVA, and visible light ranges [30–33]. Augmentation and inhibition spectrums have also been described outside of the activating spectrum, but vary by patient; the clinical relevance of this is not yet known [31, 33–35].

1.2.2.2 Chronic Actinic Dermatitis

Chronic actinic dermatitis (CAD) is a chronic eczematous, photodistributed eruption that is most commonly seen in elderly males. The action spectrum for CAD is typically UVB alone or UVB and UVA; however, visible light has been reported to precipitate CAD in a few cases. Visible light can induce CAD in patients who are also affected by UVB alone or UVB and UVA [36]. However, a few rare cases were reported to only react to visible light, 600 nm [37]. Phototest results are almost always abnormal in moderate to severe cases of CAD, so can be used to confirm the diagnosis [24, 37, 38].

1.2.2.3 Porphyrias

In cutaneous porphyrias, interaction of elevated levels of circulating porphyrins with sunlight (Soret band, 400–410 nm) causes cutaneous phototoxicity. Two types of cutaneous phototoxic lesions can occur, one caused by accumulation of water-soluble uroporphyrins and coproporphyrins and the other by accumulation of lipophilic protoporphyrin. The accumulation of water-soluble porphyrins leads to skin fragility and blister formation, exemplified by porphyria cutanea tarda, the most common type of cutaneous porphyria. The accumulation of lipophilic porphyrins leads to an immediate burning sensation in the skin after light exposure and can also be associated with swelling, redness, purpura, and erosions; these features are characteristics of erythropoietic protoporphyria [39].

1.2.2.4 Hyperbilirubinemia

Phototherapy is one of the methods used to treat hyperbilirubinemia in neonates. Blue to green light phototherapy lamps are the most effective ones in lowering serum bilirubin levels because these wavelengths penetrate the skin and are absorbed well by bilirubin [40]. Fluorescent tubes or light-emitting diodes (LEDs) can be used [41, 42]. Structural photoisomers of bilirubin are produced after phototherapy, which can then be excreted through bile and urine [43]. Two other less significant mechanisms by which phototherapy decreases serum bilirubin are through photooxidation or photooxygenation to biliverdin, maleimides, or propentdyopents and phototherapy-induced addition to protein-bound bilirubin [44, 45].

1.2.2.5 Acne Vulgaris Treatment

Acne lesions have been reported to decrease after exposure to blue, red, violet, or UV light. Some individuals report an improvement in their acne after sun exposure. The exact mechanism of action has not been completely elucidated; however, it is believed that the light works through anti-inflammatory and antibacterial mechanisms. Furthermore, it is known that porphyrins are produced by *Propionibacterium acnes*; therefore, exposure to Soret band results in the destruction of the bacteria. In fact, this is the rational for the use of photodynamic therapy in the treatment of acne vulgaris [5, 46–48].

1.3 Infrared Radiation (IR)

The wavelength of infrared radiation ranges from 700 nm to 1 millimeter (mm). It is further divided into infrared radiation A (IR-A), which ranges from 700 to 1400 nm; infrared radiation B (IR-B), which is from 1400 to 3000 nm; and infrared radiation C (IR-C) from 3000 nm to 1 mm (Fig. 1.1). Infrared radiation, especially IR-A, is perceived as heat. The portion of infrared radiation that reaches the Earth's surface is mostly IR-A radiation. IR-A and IR-B are able to penetrate the epidermis, dermis, and subcutaneous tissue. IR-C is almost completely absorbed by the water in the epidermis [49].

1.3.1 *Biological Effects*

1.3.1.1 Physical Effects

Erythema

IR can cause erythema, typically lasting less than 1 h, and is believed to be due to vasodilation secondary to a thermal effect. By 24 h, no erythema or pigmentation is observed [6]. The erythema observed has been used to determine standardized ways to measure IR doses. The minimal response dose and minimal heating dose have been described [50, 51].

Thermal Pain

Thermal pain caused by overwarming of tissues can occur in response to IR exposures. Even single overexposures can cause skin burns, *urticarial thermalis*, or collapse of the circulatory system [49].

Photoaging

Photoaging is a term used to describe the characteristic changes that occur to the skin after chronic exposure to sunlight, originally believed to be solely due to chronic UV radiation. Some common symptoms of photoaging include wrinkles, telangiectasias, solar lentigines, laxity, and a change of the texture to leathery. IR was first found to contribute to photoaging when it was shown in albino guinea pigs that UV plus IR exposure induced more photoaging than just UV radiation alone [52].

There are multiple mechanisms by which IR, mostly IR-A (760–1400 nm), is suggested to induce photoaging. Increased expression of MMP-1 is one of these mechanisms, which leads to increased degradation of collagen [53]. It has also been proposed that IR disturbs the electron flow in the mitochondria, which results in insufficient energy production in dermal fibroblasts. Different signaling pathways are then triggered, and alterations in functional and structural aspects of the skin occur [54]. Additionally, IR has been shown to cause decreased antioxidant enzyme activity, to stimulate angiogenesis, and to increase the number of mast cells, all of which have been found associated with photoaging [55, 56].

1.3.1.2 Molecular Effects

Cytotoxicity and DNA Damage

IR has not been found to induce DNA damage alone [6]. IR appears to have a protective effect on UV-induced cytotoxicity and DNA damage. Menezes et al. found a longlasting partial protection from UVA- and UVB-induced cytotoxic damage after prior radiation with IR light [57]. Jantschitsch et al. irradiated *in vivo* mouse skin with IR-A prior to UVB radiation and found decreased UVB-induced apoptosis and DNA damage compared to irradiation with UVB alone. Decreased UVB-induced DNA damage was seen in *in vitro* human skin fibroblasts after IR radiation [58].

Markers of Damage

Due to acute and chronic adverse effects described above that can occur from IR exposure, indicators are needed in order to better understand the tissue threshold for damage. The expression of matrix metalloproteinase (MMP)-1 has been proposed a useful marker of early IR damage at the cellular level. MMP-1 expression increases in response to over-warming of tissue, UV overexposure, or mechanical stress. Other markers that have been explored include heat shock proteins, ROS, and apoptosis-related proteins. However, results of these investigations are contradictory in many cases, so specific conclusions cannot be elucidated at this time [49].

Oxidative Stress

IR has been shown to induce oxidative stress both by increasing formation of free radicals and decreasing the antioxidant content in human skin. Zastrow et al. found that the amount of excess free radical formation was not only dependent on the dose of radiation but also on the skin temperature increase due to IR radiation (760–1600 nm). Using an *in vitro* human fibroblast model, Jung et al. showed that IR radiation at 37 °C did not induce excess free radical production, while at 39 °C or higher, production of excess free radicals was observed. Now that the detrimental effects of IR radiation have been well described, it is clear that protection from IR radiation is necessary and important and will be addressed further in the section on sunscreen [6, 53, 59, 60].

1.3.2 Clinical Effects

1.3.2.1 Erythema ab Igne and Squamous Cell Carcinoma

Erythema ab igne is an erythematous or hyperpigmented, reticulated dermatosis that is caused from chronic exposure to low levels of IR. Identified causes of *erythema ab igne* include laptop computers, heating pads, car heaters, electric space heaters, hot water bottles, and heated reclining chairs. Treatment is withdrawal of the heat source, and if done, patients have a good prognosis [61].

1.3.2.2 Acne Vulgaris Treatment

Acne vulgaris has recently been shown to be successfully treated with light in the visible range, as discussed above, but also with light sources in the infrared spectrum. Diode lasers have been used to reduce acne lesions. The 810 and 1450 nm diode lasers have been used successfully. The diode lasers work by inducing short-term thermal alteration of sebaceous glands. When the 810 nm diode laser was investigated, it was done following the administration of indocyanine green chromophore. The indocyanine green concentrated in the sebaceous glands and was subsequently targeted by the diode laser. The data for acne treatment with diode lasers is promising; however as with acne treatment with visible light sources, more research is necessary to elucidate the long-term efficacy and cost-effectiveness of these treatment options [5, 62, 63].

1.4 Treatment Modalities Utilizing Visible and IR Spectrum

1.4.1 Thermal Treatment Modalities

1.4.1.1 Lasers

Introduction to Lasers

Lasers can be classified by the wavelength they emit, as this is a very important property of the laser. Examples of lasers that emit wavelengths in the visible light spectrum are argon, KTP, copper bromide, APTD, krypton, PDL, ruby, and alexandrite lasers. Table 1.2 lists some of the common lasers with wavelength in the visible light spectrum and their respective wavelengths [5, 64].

There are many uses for lasers in dermatology. Some examples of what lasers emitting wavelengths in the visible spectrum are used for include vascular lesions, pigmented lesions, vitiligo, tattoo removal, hair removal, and keloids.

Lasers for Vascular Lesions

Common vascular lesions that have been successfully treated with lasers are port-wine stains, hemangiomas, and telangiectasia. Vascular lesions contain oxygenated hemoglobin, which is the molecule the laser targets for destruction when treating vascular lesions. Oxyhemoglobin absorbs light strongly at wavelengths of 418, 542, and 577 nm. PDL was specifically designed to treat vascular lesions based on the

Table 1.2 Lasers in the visible and IR light spectrum and their respective wavelength peaks

Laser	Wavelength peaks
Argon	488 and 514 nm
Potassium titanyl phosphate (KTP)	532 nm
Copper bromide	510 and 578 nm
Argon-pumped tunable dye (APTD)	577 and 585 nm
Krypton	568 nm
Pulsed dye laser (PDL)	585–595 nm
Helium-neon laser	632.8
Ruby	694 nm
Alexandrite	755 nm
Diode	800–810 nm
Nd:YAG	1064 nm
Nd:YAG (long pulsed)	1320 nm
Diode (long pulsed)	1450 nm
Erbium/glass	1540 nm
Erbium:YAG (pulsed)	2490 nm
Carbon dioxide	10,600 nm

selective photothermolysis theory and is currently the first-line treatment for vascular lesions [5, 64–66].

The Nd:YAG laser has also been used successfully for a variety of vascular lesions such as port-wine stains, hemangiomas, and facial telangiectasia. Also, the Nd:YAG and 800 nm diode lasers have been used successfully for varicose and spider veins; however, sclerotherapy remains the gold standard for these lesions [5, 67].

Pigmented Lesion Removal

Melanin has a broad absorption spectrum, from 504 to 750 nm. The wavelengths at the shorter end of the range are more effective at removing pigmented lesions. Longer wavelength lasers are useful for lesions with deeper pigment due to the increased tissue penetration. The response of the tattoo to specific lasers is very dependent on the color, depth, and nature of the tattoo pigment [5, 64, 68].

The pulsed lasers are also successful in removing tattoo pigment. The pigment is altered by the lasers and then subsequently removed by tissue macrophages. For black pigment, the Q-switched (QS) ruby, QS alexandrite, or QS Nd:YAG lasers are most effective because black pigment absorbs throughout the red and infrared spectrum. Blue and green pigments absorb best in the 600–800 nm range and therefore are best removed with ruby or alexandrite lasers. Yellow, orange, and red pigments are removed most effectively with green light, making the 510 nm PDL or 532 nm QS Nd:YAG laser the best options for these pigments [5, 64].

The Nd:YAG laser has been found to be useful for pigmented lesions when the pigment resides deeper in the dermis. Long-pulsed diode and long-pulsed Nd:YAG lasers have been especially effective at eradicating pigmented lesions with terminal hair growth, such as congenital melanocytic nevi and Becker's nevi [5, 64].

Laser Hair Removal

Light with wavelength between 600 and 1200 nm is best for hair removal because the light can penetrate to the appropriate depth in the dermis and is able to target the melanin in the hair shaft, hair follicle epithelium, and heavily pigmented matrix. The energy is absorbed by the melanin-rich matrix and hair shaft, which then undergoes a photothermal reaction and destroys the surrounding hair follicle [5, 64, 69].

Lasers currently approved for hair reduction include the long-pulsed ruby, long-pulsed alexandrite, pulsed diode, and long-pulsed Nd:YAG [5, 64, 70]. Of note, intense pulse light (IPL) with wavelength from 590 to 1200 nm can also be used for hair removal and will be discussed in further detail below.

Lasers for Keloids

PDL has recently been used for the treatment of keloids and hypertrophic scars. PDL has been shown to decrease erythema, increase pliability, and improve texture, bulk, and dysesthesias [5, 64, 71–73].

Ablative Lasers

Ablative lasers are used primarily for cutaneous facial resurfacing for severely photodamaged skin, photoinduced facial rhytides, dyschromias, and atrophic scars. High-energy, pulsed, and scanned CO_2 and erbium:YAG lasers are the main ablative lasers in use today, while the CO_2 laser is currently the gold standard for facial rejuvenation [5].

The short-pulsed erbium:YAG laser, 2940 nm, was designed to have the beneficial effects of the CO_2 laser while limiting the unwanted side effects. The erbium:YAG has milder improvement than the CO_2 laser but with also milder side effects and faster recovery time [5].

Additionally, there are numerous other uses for the CO_2 laser, which includes removing a variety of epidermal and dermal lesions, treating premalignant and malignant lesions, and excisional and incisional operations [5].

1.4.1.2 Intense Pulsed Light Therapy

Intense pulsed light (IPL) refers to a high-intensity polychromatic incoherent light with a wavelength range from 515 to 1200 nm; different filters can be used to obtain specific wavelengths within this range. Depending on the target structure, the right wavelength can be selected for heating and destruction [24]. The light is delivered in series of single, double, or triple pulse sequences. The filters that only allow shorter wavelengths through should only be used in fair-skinned individuals because shorter wavelength light interacts more readily with melanin in the epidermis, which can lead to hypopigmentation or dyspigmentation. IPL has been used to successfully treat a variety of vascular lesions and benign pigmented lesions and for hair removal. Longer pulse durations make it possible to slowly heat deeper structures, making this method very useful for thick port-wine stains and hemangiomas [5, 74].

1.4.2 Nonthermal Treatment Modalities

1.4.2.1 Low-Level Light Therapy

Low-level light therapy (LLLT) uses low-power light sources. LLLT can be performed with either coherent light sources (lasers) or noncoherent light sources (light-emitting diodes (LEDs)). LLLT is lower intensity and causes lower temperature changes and less discomfort than other types of laser, while still being effective [24].

LLLT works by absorption of red and near-infrared light by the protein components of the respiratory chain in the mitochondria, mostly cytochrome *c* oxidase. Absorption leads to dissociation of inhibitory nitric oxide from cytochrome *c* oxidase and then increased enzyme activity, electron transport, and ATP production. LLLT has also been shown to increase expression of genes related to cellular migration and proliferation and also alters expression of growth factors and cytokines [24].

Red LED LLLT has also been found to inhibit fibroblast proliferation in vitro without affecting viability. Therefore, red LED LLLT could be a possible treatment for scars or proliferative disorders in the future [75].

The helium-neon laser is a type of LLLT with wavelength of 632.8 nm. The helium-neon laser has recently been shown to be another therapeutic option for vitiligo, specifically segmental vitiligo. The mechanism by which this works is by inducing melanocyte proliferation through the interaction with type IV collagen via mitochondria-related pathways [76, 77].

The current uses of LLLT within the IR spectrum are to stimulate wound healing and hair growth and for the treatment of herpes simplex. It has been shown that LLLT stimulates wound healing by promoting contraction through the induction of fibroblast to myofibroblast transition [78]. Recently, LLLT using a 1072 nm LED light source has been found to be a potential treatment for herpes simplex labialis. Significantly reduced healing times were experienced in patients treated with LLLT [79].

1.4.2.2 Photodynamic Therapy

Photodynamic therapy (PDT) is a common way visible light is used clinically. PDT is approved for the treatment of actinic keratosis in the United States; however, there are many off-label uses which continue to expand [80]. PDT requires a photosensitizer, a light source, and oxygen [81, 82].

Light Source

Any light source can be used for PDT, as long as the wavelength of light coincides with the absorption spectrum of the photosensitizer, and the penetration depth of the light is equal to the depth of the target cells or target tissue. Protoporphyrin IX has important absorption peaks in the red and blue wavelength regions, from 404 to 420 nm and at 635 nm. Therefore, continuous red and blue light are very commonly used in PDT [81].

Clinical Uses of PDT

Aminolevulinic acid (ALA) is only approved in North America for the treatment of hypertrophic actinic keratosis on the face and scalp in combination with blue light. Methyl aminolevulinate (MAL) is approved for non-hyperkeratotic actinic keratosis of the face and scalp in the United States [81].

There are numerous off-label uses of PDT. PDT has been used to treat noninvasive, nonmelanoma skin cancers (NMSCs), mycosis fungoides, Kaposi's sarcoma, extramammary Paget's disease, cutaneous B-cell lymphoma, vascular malformations, acne vulgaris, rosacea, hidradenitis suppurativa, morphea, actinic cheilitis, cutaneous warts, condyloma acuminata, epidermodysplasia verruciformis, molluscum contagiosum, herpes simplex virus, onychomycosis, cutaneous leishmaniasis, erythrasma (*Corynebacterium minutissimum* infection), keloids, and hypertrophic scars [81]. PDT has also been used for photorejuvenation.

1.5 Photoprotection Against Visible and IR Spectrum

Currently available sunscreens protect against UV radiation but do not protect against the visible spectrum of light. Up to 50 % of free radicals formed during solar radiation are generated following exposure to visible and infrared spectra; therefore, it would be necessary to provide photoprotection in these spectra as well. Meinke et al. showed that antioxidants and inorganic, i.e., physical filters, along with organic UV filters, are necessary to provide protection from the entire solar spectrum [83].

Visible light photoprotection is relevant in several clinical situations. Some photodermatoses have action spectrum in the visible light range. Photofrin, used in systemic PDT, has an action spectrum in the visible light range [24]. Furthermore, visible light can induced persistent pigmentation in dark-skinned individuals, as described before [12].

At this time there is no organic filter for visible light. The only filters that are able to reflect and scattered visible light are optically opaque filters. Zinc oxide (ZnO) and titanium dioxide (TiO_2) are two inorganic sunscreen agents that protect against visible light in some forms. When visible light photons encounter non-micronized ZnO or TiO_2 particles, the light gets reflected into the direction of our eyes, therefore causing the ZnO and TiO_2 to appear white. The particle size determines the absorption range. ZnO and TiO_2 used in sunscreens are micronized (particle size of less than 100 nm in diameter) because they are then less visible on the skin and more cosmetically acceptable. Ferrous oxide, which is pigmented and opaque, has recently been used and found to be effective in offering sun protection in the visible light spectrum [84].

1.6 Diagnostic Imaging

Noninvasive, diagnostic imaging is a rapidly expanding field. Confocal scanning laser microscopy and optical coherence tomography are two ways noninvasive imaging is being used to image the skin. Confocal scanning microscopy uses a near-infrared light source and allows for imaging of tissue in vivo, in real time, with the same resolution as conventional histology. The epidermis, microvascular blood flow, and inflammatory cells can be identified. Possible uses of this imaging technique include potentially diagnosing lesions without biopsy and detecting tumor margins [5, 85–87].

Optical coherence tomography uses low-coherence interferometry and provides two-dimensional images up to 1.5 mm deep. The architecture of the epidermis and papillary dermis can be visualized. However, individual cells cannot be visualized. This imaging technique can potentially be used to diagnose skin tumors and bullous diseases without biopsies [5, 88, 89].

There are numerous other, new imaging applications using the infrared spectrum. Near-infrared fluorescence has been shown to accurately assist in sentinel lymph node mapping intraoperatively [90]. Recently, infrared images of individuals' faces have been used to determine acne severity and monitor acne treatment efficacy [91]. Most of these imaging techniques are still in the early stages of development. However, the data is promising and could greatly impact the field of dermatology in the future.

References

1. Brenner M, Hearing VJ (2008) The protective role of melanin against UV damage in human skin. Photochem Photobiol 84(3):539–549
2. Baron ED, Suggs AK (2014) Introduction to photobiology. Dermatol Clin 32(3):255–266, vii
3. Barolet D (2008) Light-emitting diodes (LEDs) in dermatology. Semin Cutan Med Surg 27(4):227–238
4. Rabe JH et al (2006) Photoaging: mechanisms and repair. J Am Acad Dermatol 55(1):1–19
5. Tanzi EL, Lupton JR, Alster TS (2003) Lasers in dermatology: four decades of progress. J Am Acad Dermatol 49(1):1–31; quiz 31–34
6. Sklar LR et al (2013) Effects of ultraviolet radiation, visible light, and infrared radiation on erythema and pigmentation: a review. Photochem Photobiol Sci 12(1):54–64
7. Honigsmann H (2002) Erythema and pigmentation. Photodermatol Photoimmunol Photomed 18(2):75–81

8. Schmalwieser AW, Wallisch S, Diffey B (2012) A library of action spectra for erythema and pigmentation. Photochem Photobiol Sci 11(2):251–268
9. Mahmoud BH et al (2010) Impact of long-wavelength UVA and visible light on melanocompetent skin. J Invest Dermatol 130(8):2092–2097
10. Parrish JA, Zaynoun S, Anderson RR (1981) Cumulative effects of repeated subthreshold doses of ultraviolet radiation. J Invest Dermatol 76(5):356–358
11. Harmful effects of ultraviolet radiation. Council on Scientific Affairs (1989) JAMA 262(3):380–384
12. Rottier PB, Van Der Leun JC (1960) Hyperaemia of the deeper cutaneous vessels after irradiation of human skin with large doses of ultra-violet and visible light. Br J Dermatol 72: 256–260
13. Porges SB, Kaidbey KH, Grove GL (1988) Quantification of visible light-induced melanogenesis in human skin. Photodermatol 5(5):197–200
14. Lim HW, Honigsmann H, Hawk JLM (2007) Photodermatology. Informa Healthcare USA, Inc., New York, pp 75–89
15. Kollias N, Baqer A (1984) An experimental study of the changes in pigmentation in human skin in vivo with visible and near infrared light. Photochem Photobiol 39(5):651–659
16. Rosen CF et al (1990) Immediate pigment darkening: visual and reflectance spectrophotometric analysis of action spectrum. Photochem Photobiol 51(5):583–588
17. Pathak MA, Riley FC, Fitzpatrick TB (1962) Melanogenesis in human skin following exposure to long-wave ultraviolet and visible light. J Invest Dermatol 39:435–443
18. Ramasubramaniam R et al (2011) Are there mechanistic differences between ultraviolet and visible radiation induced skin pigmentation? Photochem Photobiol Sci 10(12):1887–1893
19. Duteil L et al (2014) Differences in visible light-induced pigmentation according to wavelengths: a clinical and histological study in comparison with UVB exposure. Pigment Cell Melanoma Res 27(5):822–826
20. Loertzer H et al (2006) Formation of ascorbate radicals as a measure of oxidative stress: an in vitro electron spin resonance-study using 2,2-Azobis (2-amidinopropane) dihydrochloride as a radical generator. Transplant Proc 38(3):674–678
21. Halliwell B, Whiteman M (2004) Measuring reactive species and oxidative damage in vivo and in cell culture: how should you do it and what do the results mean? Br J Pharmacol 142(2):231–255
22. Buettner GR, Jurkiewicz BA (1993) Ascorbate free radical as a marker of oxidative stress: an EPR study. Free Radic Biol Med 14(1):49–55
23. Haywood R (2006) Relevance of sunscreen application method, visible light and sunlight intensity to free-radical protection: a study of ex vivo human skin. Photochem Photobiol 82(4):1123–1131
24. Mahmoud BH et al (2008) Effects of visible light on the skin. Photochem Photobiol 84(2):450–462
25. Liebel F et al (2012) Irradiation of skin with visible light induces reactive oxygen species and matrix-degrading enzymes. J Invest Dermatol 132(7):1901–1907
26. Edstrom DW, Porwit A, Ros AM (2001) Effects on human skin of repetitive ultraviolet-A1 (UVA1) irradiation and visible light. Photodermatol Photoimmunol Photomed 17(2):66–70
27. Kielbassa C, Roza L, Epe B (1997) Wavelength dependence of oxidative DNA damage induced by UV and visible light. Carcinogenesis 18(4):811–816
28. Hoffmann-Dorr S et al (2005) Visible light (>395 nm) causes micronuclei formation in mammalian cells without generation of cyclobutane pyrimidine dimers. Mutat Res 572(1–2):142–149
29. Champion RH (1988) Urticaria: then and now. Br J Dermatol 119(4):427–436
30. Stratigos AJ et al (2003) Spectrum of idiopathic photodermatoses in a Mediterranean country. Int J Dermatol 42(6):449–454
31. Uetsu N et al (2000) The clinical and photobiological characteristics of solar urticaria in 40 patients. Br J Dermatol 142(1):32–38

32. Ryckaert S, Roelandts R (1998) Solar urticaria. A report of 25 cases and difficulties in phototesting. Arch Dermatol 134(1):71–74
33. Nitiyarom R, Wongpraparut C (2014) Hydroa vaccin iforme and solar urticaria. Dermatol Clin 32(3):345–353, viii
34. Hasei K, Ichihashi M (1982) Solar urticaria. Determinations of action and inhibition spectra. Arch Dermatol 118(5):346–350
35. Leenutaphong V et al (1987) Plasmapheresis in solar urticaria. Photodermatol 4(6):308–309
36. Dawe RS, Ferguson J (2003) Diagnosis and treatment of chronic actinic dermatitis. Dermatol Ther 16(1):45–51
37. Lim HW et al (1994) Chronic actinic dermatitis. An analysis of 51 patients evaluated in the United States and Japan. Arch Dermatol 130(10):1284–1289
38. Paek SY, Lim HW (2014) Chronic actinic dermatitis. Dermatol Clin 32(3):355–361, viii–ix
39. Schulenburg-Brand D et al (2014) The cutaneous porphyrias. Dermatol Clin 32(3):369–384, ix
40. Ennever JF (1990) Blue light, green light, white light, more light: treatment of neonatal jaundice. Clin Perinatol 17(2):467–481
41. American Academy of Pediatrics Subcommittee on Hyperbilirubinemia (2004) Management of hyperbilirubinemia in the newborn infant 35 or more weeks of gestation. Pediatrics 114(1): 297–316
42. Maisels MJ, Kring EA, DeRidder J (2007) Randomized controlled trial of light-emitting diode phototherapy. J Perinatol 27(9):565–567
43. Onishi S et al (1986) Metabolism of bilirubin and its photoisomers in newborn infants during phototherapy. J Biochem 100(3):789–795
44. Lightner DA, Linnane WP 3rd, Ahlfors CE (1984) Bilirubin photooxidation products in the urine of jaundiced neonates receiving phototherapy. Pediatr Res 18(8):696–700
45. Jori G, Rossi E, Rubaltelli FF (1980) Phototherapy-induced covalent binding of bilirubin to serum albumin. Pediatr Res 14(12):1363–1366
46. Papageorgiou P, Katsambas A, Chu A (2000) Phototherapy with blue (415 nm) and red (660 nm) light in the treatment of acne vulgaris. Br J Dermatol 142(5):973–978
47. Cunliffe WJ, Goulden V (2000) Phototherapy and acne vulgaris. Br J Dermatol 142(5): 855–856
48. Rkein AM, Ozog DM (2014) Photodynamic therapy. Dermatol Clin 32(3):415–425, x
49. Piazena H, Kelleher DK (2010) Effects of infrared-A irradiation on skin: discrepancies in published data highlight the need for an exact consideration of physical and photobiological laws and appropriate experimental settings. Photochem Photobiol 86(3):687–705
50. Pujol JA, Lecha M (1992) Photoprotection in the infrared radiation range. Photodermatol Photoimmunol Photomed 9(6):275–278
51. Lee HS et al (2006) Minimal heating dose: a novel biological unit to measure infrared irradiation. Photodermatol Photoimmunol Photomed 22(3):148–152
52. Kligman LH (1982) Intensification of ultraviolet-induced dermal damage by infrared radiation. Arch Dermatol Res 272(3–4):229–238
53. Schroeder P et al (2008) Infrared radiation-induced matrix metalloproteinase in human skin: implications for protection. J Invest Dermatol 128(10):2491–2497
54. Krutmann J, Schroeder P (2009) Role of mitochondria in photoaging of human skin: the defective powerhouse model. J Investig Dermatol Symp Proc 14(1):44–49
55. Krutmann J, Morita A, Chung JH (2012) Sun exposure: what molecular photodermatology tells us about its good and bad sides. J Invest Dermatol 132(3 Pt 2):976–984
56. Shin MH et al (2012) Chronic heat treatment causes skin wrinkle formation and oxidative damage in hairless mice. Mech Ageing Dev 133(2–3):92–98
57. Menezes S et al (1998) Non-coherent near infrared radiation protects normal human dermal fibroblasts from solar ultraviolet toxicity. J Invest Dermatol 111(4):629–633
58. Jantschitsch C et al (2009) Infrared radiation confers resistance to UV-induced apoptosis via reduction of DNA damage and upregulation of antiapoptotic proteins. J Invest Dermatol 129(5):1271–1279
59. Zastrow L et al (2009) The missing link – light-induced (280–1,600 nm) free radical formation in human skin. Skin Pharmacol Physiol 22(1):31–44

60. Jung T et al (2010) Effects of water-filtered infrared A irradiation on human fibroblasts. Free Radic Biol Med 48(1):153–160
61. Miller K et al (2011) Erythema ab igne. Dermatol Online J 17(10):28
62. Paithankar DY et al (2002) Acne treatment with a 1,450 nm wavelength laser and cryogen spray cooling. Lasers Surg Med 31(2):106–114
63. Lloyd JR, Mirkov M (2002) Selective photothermolysis of the sebaceous glands for acne treatment. Lasers Surg Med 31(2):115–120
64. Hruza GJ, Avram MM (2013) Lasers and lights: procedures in cosmetic dermatology, 3rd edn. Elsevier
65. Anderson RR, Parrish JA (1983) Selective photothermolysis: precise microsurgery by selective absorption of pulsed radiation. Science 220(4596):524–527
66. Levine VJ, Geronemus RG (1995) Adverse effects associated with the 577- and 585-nanometer pulsed dye laser in the treatment of cutaneous vascular lesions: a study of 500 patients. J Am Acad Dermatol 32(4):613–617
67. Weiss RA, Weiss MA (1999) Early clinical results with a multiple synchronized pulse 1064 NM laser for leg telangiectasias and reticular veins. Dermatol Surg 25(5):399–402
68. Margolis RJ et al (1989) Visible action spectrum for melanin-specific selective photothermolysis. Lasers Surg Med 9(4):389–397
69. Lask G et al (1997) Laser-assisted hair removal by selective photothermolysis. Preliminary results. Dermatol Surg 23(9):737–739
70. McDaniel DH et al (1999) Laser hair removal: a review and report on the use of the long-pulsed alexandrite laser for hair reduction of the upper lip, leg, back, and bikini region. Dermatol Surg 25(6):425–430
71. Alster TS, Williams CM (1995) Treatment of keloid sternotomy scars with 585 nm flashlamp-pumped pulsed-dye laser. Lancet 345(8959):1198–1200
72. Lupton JR, Alster TS (2002) Laser scar revision. Dermatol Clin 20(1):55–65
73. Manuskiatti W, Fitzpatrick RE (2002) Treatment response of keloidal and hypertrophic sternotomy scars: comparison among intralesional corticosteroid, 5-fluorouracil, and 585-nm flashlamp-pumped pulsed-dye laser treatments. Arch Dermatol 138(9):1149–1155
74. Sadick NS et al (2000) Long-term photoepilation using a broad-spectrum intense pulsed light source. Arch Dermatol 136(11):1336–1340
75. Lev-Tov H et al (2013) Inhibition of fibroblast proliferation in vitro using red light-emitting diodes. Dermatol Surg 39(8):1167–1170
76. Lan CC et al (2009) Low-energy helium-neon laser induces melanocyte proliferation via interaction with type IV collagen: visible light as a therapeutic option for vitiligo. Br J Dermatol 161(2):273–280
77. Yu HS et al (2003) Helium-neon laser irradiation stimulates migration and proliferation in melanocytes and induces repigmentation in segmental-type vitiligo. J Invest Dermatol 120(1):56–64
78. Demidova-Rice TN et al (2007) Low-level light stimulates excisional wound healing in mice. Lasers Surg Med 39(9):706–715
79. Dougal G, Lee SY (2013) Evaluation of the efficacy of low-level light therapy using 1072 nm infrared light for the treatment of herpes simplex labialis. Clin Exp Dermatol 38(7):713–718
80. Calzavara-Pinton P et al (2010) A critical reappraisal of off-label indications for topical photodynamic therapy with aminolevulinic acid and methylaminolevulinate. Rev Recent Clin Trials 5(2):112–116
81. Wan MT, Lin JY (2014) Current evidence and applications of photodynamic therapy in dermatology. Clin Cosmet Investig Dermatol 7:145–163
82. Dolmans DE, Fukumura D, Jain RK (2003) Photodynamic therapy for cancer. Nat Rev Cancer 3(5):380–387
83. Meinke MC et al (2013) Radical protection by differently composed creams in the UV/VIS and IR spectral ranges. Photochem Photobiol 89(5):1079–1084
84. Castanedo-Cazares JP et al (2014) Near-visible light and UV photoprotection in the treatment of melasma: a double-blind randomized trial. Photodermatol Photoimmunol Photomed 30(1):35–42

85. Rajadhyaksha M, Anderson RR, Webb RH (1999) Video-rate confocal scanning laser microscope for imaging human tissues in vivo. Appl Opt 38(10):2105–2115
86. Rajadhyaksha M et al (1999) In vivo confocal scanning laser microscopy of human skin II: advances in instrumentation and comparison with histology. J Invest Dermatol 113(3): 293–303
87. Selkin B et al (2001) In vivo confocal microscopy in dermatology. Dermatol Clin 19(2):369–377, ix–x
88. Welzel J (2001) Optical coherence tomography in dermatology: a review. Skin Res Technol 7(1):1–9
89. Welzel J et al (1997) Optical coherence tomography of the human skin. J Am Acad Dermatol 37(6):958–963
90. van der Vorst JR et al (2013) Dose optimization for near-infrared fluorescence sentinel lymph node mapping in patients with melanoma. Br J Dermatol 168(1):93–98
91. Padilla-Medina JA et al (2014) Assessment technique for acne treatments based on statistical parameters of skin thermal images. J Biomed Opt 19(4):046019

Chapter 2
Photoprotection and Skin Cancer Prevention

Brian P. Hibler, Stephen W. Dusza, and Steven Q. Wang

Key Points

- Ultraviolet radiation is a major risk factor for the development of skin cancer, the most common form of cancer in the United States.
- Ultraviolet radiation causes both direct and indirect damages to DNA, leading to mutations and malignant transformation if the damage is not repaired.
- Skin cancer can be prevented by reducing intentional exposure to ultraviolet radiation and using photoprotective strategies, including sunscreens.
- Daily sunscreen application protects against the development of actinic keratoses, squamous cell carcinoma, nevi formation, and melanoma.

2.1 Introduction

Environmental exposures to both natural and man-made substances are a major risk factor for the development of many types of cancers. Skin serves as the interface between the body and the environment and is frequently exposed to potentially hazardous environmental elements. Viral and bacterial infections, smoking, radiotherapy, immunosuppressant drugs, artificial ultraviolet sources for phototherapy and tanning, and chemical carcinogens have all been shown to predispose individuals to skin cancers [1].

B.P. Hibler, BS • S.W. Dusza, DrPH • S.Q. Wang, MD (✉)
Dermatology Division, Memorial Sloan-Kettering Cancer Center, Basking Ridge, NJ, USA
e-mail: wants@mskcc.org

S.Q. Wang, H.W. Lim (eds.), *Principles and Practice of Photoprotection*,
DOI 10.1007/978-3-319-29382-0_2

Ultraviolet radiation (UVR) from sunlight is a major risk factor for melanoma and non-melanoma skin cancer (NMSC) [2]. Epidermal cells accumulate UVR-induced DNA damage which can lead to DNA base mutations and malignant transformation. This chapter discusses the biologic impact of UVR on the skin and its role in the development of both NMSC and melanoma. In addition, the role of photoprotection to prevent cutaneous malignancies is reviewed.

2.2 UV Radiation

Solar radiation is divided into ultraviolet (200–400 nm), visible light (400–700 nm), and infrared radiation (>700 nm) [3]. UVR plays a major role in the development of photoaging and skin cancer [4]. Due to inherent differences in biologic effects, the UV spectrum is further subdivided into UVC (200–290 nm), UVB (290–320 nm), UVA2 (320–340 nm), and UVA1 (340–400 nm) [4, 5]. The subdivision of the UVA range is due to a change in the slope of the action spectrum for erythema occurring near 340 nm, with UVA2 having more erythemogenic activity than UVA1.

The different types of UVR vary in their intensity at the Earth's surface and their effects on human skin. Nearly all of the UVC radiation from the sun is absorbed by the ozone layer, effectively negating its effects on the human body [6]. Approximately 95 % of the solar radiation reaching the Earth's surface is UVA, with the remaining 5 % UVB [7]. The intensity of UVB has been shown to increase between 4 and 10 % with every 1000 ft of elevation and by approximately 3 % for every degree of latitude as approaching the equator [8]. UVB, being a shorter wavelength compared to UVA, is only capable of penetrating down to the basal layer of the epidermis and superficial dermis, while UVA can penetrate deeper into the reticular dermis [9]. Compared to UVA, the erythemogenic potential of UVB is 1000 times greater [10]. UVA is generally more closely associated with tanning and photoaging changes such as loss of skin elasticity and wrinkling, although UVB can also produce the same effects [4, 11]. Both UVB and UVA have been implicated in the development of skin cancers.

2.3 DNA Damage by UVR

2.3.1 UVB Effects

UVB directly damages the DNA of keratinocytes. UVB is absorbed by DNA molecules within the keratinocytes, leading to the formation of dimeric photoproducts between adjacent pyrimidine bases. The two most common photoproducts are the cyclobutane pyrimidine dimer (CPD) and the 6-4 photoproduct (6-4PP), formed at a ratio of about 3:1 [12, 13]. The presence of these molecules prevents the replicative DNA polymerases from passing through the template strand, thereby blocking DNA synthesis [14]. Failure to repair these defects can lead to a collapse in the replication fork at the damaged site, causing a DNA double-strand breaks and ultimately cell death. Furthermore, the presence of UV-induced photoproducts can interfere with base pairing during DNA replication, leading to mutations.

Although normal cells maintain a high repair fidelity, errors in repair can lead to cytosine (C) → thymine (T) base substitution at dipyrimidine sites and CC → TT tandem base substitutions [14, 15]. These are known as "UV signature mutations," indicating damages from past UVR exposure [15]. While these mutations were once known as "UVB signature mutations," further studies have demonstrated that a high proportion of C → T transitions also occur with UVA-induced damage, but at a lower frequency (65 % for UVA vs. 85 % for UVB) [16, 17]. The rates of repair for 6-4PP and CPD photoproducts are different. Nearly 90 % of the 6-4PP lesions are repaired at 3 h post-UV exposure [12, 18]. In contrast, only 10 % of CPD lesions are repaired at 3 h and 50 % at 24 h after exposure [18]. Repair capacity diminishes with age, and there is a cumulative loss of 25 % in repair ability between the ages of 20 and 60 years; this difference may account for the increased risk of skin cancer that begins in middle age [19]. Individuals with defective nuclear excision repair pathways, such as patients with xeroderma pigmentosum, are exceptionally vulnerable to UV-induced cutaneous malignancies.

2.3.2 *UVA Effects*

UVA indirectly damages DNA via a free radical-mediated pathway [12]. UVA reacts with chromophores and photosensitizers, such as porphyrins, cytochromes, heme, riboflavin, and tryptophan, which generate free radicals [20–24]. In addition, UVA reacts with oxygen species and induces the formation of reactive oxygen species (ROS) [20]. Within 20 min of UVA exposure, expression of NADPH oxidase in human keratinocytes increases by 2-fold [25]. NADPH oxidase converts oxygen molecules to superoxide anions, which are ultimately converted to ROS such as hydrogen peroxide, superoxide anion ($\bullet O_2^-$), peroxide ($\bullet O_2^{-2}$), hydroxyl radical ($\bullet OH$), hydroxyl ion (OH^-), and singlet oxygen ($^1O_2$) [26]. These short-lived free radicals damage DNA in a myriad of ways, including cross-linking DNA to proteins and forming single-strand and double-strand breaks [12, 27]. It is important to note that UVB can also trigger oxidative damage [20, 28, 29].

Aside from these forms of nonspecific DNA damage, UVA-induced oxidation leads to specific DNA base mutations. The molecule 8-hydroxyguanine (8OH-G) is a mutagenic base that results from ROS interaction with guanine [30]. 8OH-G is preferentially generated with UV wavelengths greater than 350 nm and hence is thought to be UVA signature mutation [28]. This particular lesion has been shown to create G:C → T:A transversions in DNA [31]. In addition, UVA generates CPD mutations at nearly five times that of 8OH-G mutations [32]. However, compared to CPD mutations from UVB, the overall number of UVA-generated DNA photoproducts is significantly lower [20].

2.4 DNA Base Mutations in Malignant Transformation

Upon DNA damage, cells can either repair the mutation or, if the damage is beyond repair, target the cell for apoptosis. The *p53* tumor suppressor gene plays a major role in regulation of cell cycle checkpoint activity, DNA repair, and apoptosis. However, if the *p53* gene becomes mutated, these protective cellular mechanisms may fail, leading to carcinogenesis. Clones of cells with UV signature mutations (e.g., C → T and CC → TT transitions) in the *p53* tumor suppressor gene have been found in sun-exposed skin, actinic keratoses, squamous cell carcinoma, basal cell carcinoma, and melanoma, supporting its role in photocarcinogenesis [33, 34].

Under normal circumstances, p53 responds to DNA damage by blocking the progression of the cell cycle. Immediately after UV irradiation, *p53* transcription is upregulated and DNA damage leads to the alteration of the p53 protein, allowing for phosphorylation by other protein kinases [35]. Elevated levels of p53 that occur after UV exposure lead to induction of *p21* (also known as WAF1 or CIP1), which is responsible for cell cycle arrest and inhibiting apoptosis [36]. The p21 protein is capable of competitively forming a complex with cyclin-dependent kinase (CDK), blocking its interaction with cyclin and effectively inhibiting cell entry to the S phase where DNA replication takes place [37, 38]. Cell cycle arrest may also occur at checkpoints during S phase or after G2 (before mitosis) to ensure DNA fidelity [39]. By inhibiting progression of the cell cycle, the cell is providing itself time to repair, to prevent passage of mutated DNA onto daughter cells.

Upon cell cycle arrest, DNA repair mechanisms are activated to correct the UV-induced lesions. Two major mechanisms for DNA repair include base excision repair (BER) and nucleotide excision repair (NER). BER is used to remove damaged bases, such as the oxidized form of guanine (8OH-G) [40]. In this pathway, DNA glycosylases remove specific damaged or inappropriate bases forming a single-strand break, which is then repaired with small fragments of 1–12 nucleotides [41]. NER is used to repair a variety of bulky DNA damages, including CPDs and 6-4PPs, that commonly result from UVB exposure [42]. NER involves single-strand incisions flanking the lesion, followed by DNA repair synthesis and ligation. As mentioned earlier, 6-4PPs are repaired much more quickly than CPDs. This is thought to be because 6-4PPs are more destabilizing and cause a greater degree of unwinding in the DNA helix than CPDs [4, 43, 44]. Repair of these UV-specific CPD and 6-4PP lesions significantly decreases the overall apoptotic response [45].

If the DNA damage is beyond repair, apoptotic pathways are activated to prevent passage of daughter cells carrying those mutations. The molecule p53 can induce apoptosis through two major pathways, either the intrinsic mitochondrial pathway or the extrinsic death receptor pathway [46]. In the mitochondrial pathway, p53 upregulates pro-apoptotic genes, such as *Bax* and *Bak*, or p53 represses transcription of antiapoptotic genes, such as *survivin*. Furthermore, p53 induces caspase activation and apoptosis [46, 47]. To a lesser extent, p53 activates the death receptor pathway by promoting *fas* transcription and its cell-surface expression [48, 49]. Additionally, p53 induces DDB2 (damaged-DNA binding protein 2) which promotes programmed cell death by facilitating degradation of p21, an inhibitor of apoptosis [50]. Mutations in p53 can effectively inhibit these protective apoptotic pathways. The unregulated passage of DNA-carrying mutations to daughter cells during cell division leads to tumorigenesis.

Aside from the *p53* gene, there are other important genes affected by UVR. UV signature mutations have also been identified in the patched homologue (*PTCH*), smoothened (*SMO*) tumor suppressor genes, as well as the *ras* oncogene [12, 51–53]. Mutations in PTCH or SMO, two conducting proteins involved in the Hedgehog pathway, have been identified in up to 90 % of all BCCs [54]. As a result, molecules involved in this pathway represent an enticing target for novel treatment modalities. Inhibitors of this pathway, such as vismodegib, are now being employed to systemically treat locally advanced or metastatic BCCs. Other targeted therapies are sure to follow as the biological mechanisms and pathways underlying malignant transformation are further elucidated.

While *p53* mutations are commonly implicated in NMSC, they are not thought to play a major role in the development of melanoma. UVR has been shown to stimulate the clonal expansion of melanocytes expressing *BRAF* mutations in melanocytic nevi [55, 56]. The oncogenic BRAF V600E substitution has been shown to be an early event in melanomagenesis and is the most common somatic mutation identified in melanomas. Approximately 80 % of acquired human nevi and primary melanomas carry *BRAF* mutations [57]. A recent study using BRAF V600E mutant mice showed that UVR induced larger and more abundant nevi compared to non-UVR-exposed skin [55]. Additionally, all mutant mice developed melanomas within 7 months after UVR, whereas UVR did not induce melanoma in non-BRAF mutant mice. Finally, the application of broad-spectrum SPF 50 sunscreen blocked p53 induction, apoptosis, epidermal hypertrophy, and dermal thickening and also delayed the onset of UVR-driven melanoma. It should be noted that all sunscreen-protected mice did eventually develop tumors representing a significant increase over non-UVR-exposed mice, highlighting the damaging effects of UVR and need for enhanced photoprotection and UVR avoidance. Nevertheless, sunscreen did produce a significant reduction in tumors in those that were exposed to UVR and significantly prolonged the latency before tumor development, accentuating the role of sunscreen protection in addition to UVR avoidance for those at risk of melanoma.

2.5 Epidemiology of UV-Induced Cutaneous Malignancies

Skin cancer is the most common form of cancer in the United States [58–60]. Nearly five million people in the United States are treated for skin cancer every year with an estimated annual cost over $8 billion [61–63]. Basal cell carcinoma (BCC) and squamous cell carcinoma (SCC) account for nearly 95 % of skin cancers, and melanoma makes up approximately 5 %. In the United States in 2014, it is estimated that there would be over 76,000 new cases of invasive melanoma and 9710 melanoma-related deaths [64]. The risk of skin cancers is governed by both genetic factors and exposure to UV radiation.

2.5.1 Genetic Factors

Incidence rates of BCC and SCC are 5–10 times greater in the Caucasians than in darker-skinned individuals [58]. Individuals with blue or green eyes, red or blond hair, and lighter skin type have higher risk for developing skin cancer [65, 66]. Those individuals tend to have MC1R mutation and generate more pheomelanin than eumelanin [67]. Pheomelanin is less effective in absorbing UV, and furthermore, upon UVA exposure, pheomelanin are pro-oxidative and generate free radicals that can damage DNA and nearby cellular organelles. Other phenotypic traits associated with increased risks for skin cancer include high nevus count, tendency to sunburn, inability to tan, and a history of sunburn at a young age [68–70]. Additionally, individuals with a personal or family history of skin cancer are at an increased risk, suggesting the presence of additional genetic factors increasing susceptibility that have not yet been phenotypically identified.

2.5.2 Relationship to Ambient UV Radiation

The incidence of NMSC increases with higher exposure to ambient solar radiation and is greater in individuals with higher mean daily UV radiation [71]. Ecologic studies have shown that the incidence of skin cancer is higher in regions of low latitude and high UV index [72, 73]. The Nurses' Health Study reported an increased risk of skin cancer in individuals who lived in areas with moderate or high UV index (greater than or equal to 6), with more pronounced effects seen for women who grew up in states with higher UV indices [74]. Further studies have demonstrated that early childhood exposure to high UV radiation increases the risk of skin cancer. A migration study from Western Australia demonstrated that immigrants from Great Britain who arrived before the age of 10 years had similar rates of melanoma compared with the native-born population, whereas the incidence was nearly a quarter of the native rate in those who arrived after the age of 15 years [75]. Similar findings in migrant populations have been documented in other countries, including the United States [76–78].

Although a strong relationship exists between ambient solar radiation and the incidence of skin cancer, patterns of sun exposure appear to have an impact on the type of skin cancers. Chronic UV exposure has been implicated in the development of both precancerous actinic keratoses (AK) and SCCs [79–81]. These lesions tend to occur on sun-exposed sites, such as the head, neck, and dorsal hands. The association between BCC and sun exposure is more complex, because a large percentage of BCCs are located on non-sun-exposed sites [82, 83]. As a result, it is postulated that BCC may result from intermittent UV exposure or exposure early in life rather than cumulative UV exposure.

Likewise, the overall risk of melanoma appears to also be associated with more intense and intermittent exposure to high levels of UVR, often stemming from recreational activities or exposures occurring during childhood [66, 84, 85]. Melanoma is not often found on chronically sun-exposed sites, but rather is more common on locations that are sporadically exposed, such as the trunk in males and the legs in females [86]. However, certain subtypes of melanoma, such as lentigo maligna melanoma or desmoplastic melanoma, are more commonly found on chronically sun-exposed sites with a predilection for the head, neck, and upper extremities [87–90]. These lesions are often found on sun-damaged skin in older individuals [88, 91, 92]. These observations suggest that different subtypes of melanoma may result from either cumulative or intermittent sunlight exposure.

2.5.3 High-Risk Occupation and Behaviors

Aside from genetic traits, individuals with certain occupations and those who carry out high-risk behaviors have an increased probability of developing skin cancer. Outdoor workers tend to have extensive amounts of UV radiation. A systematic review and meta-analysis of 18 studies (6 cohort and 12 case–control) reported that 16 of the 18 studies (89 %) showed an increased risk of SCC in individuals with occupational UV exposure compared against individuals without UV exposure (OR = 1.77; 95 % CI = 1.40–2.22) [93]. As for BCC, a meta-analysis including 23 epidemiologic studies found a weaker, but still significant, association between occupational sun exposure and risk of BCC (OR = 1.43; 95 % CI = 1.23–1.66) [94]. The data on melanomas is mixed. While some studies have suggested that outdoor workers may not be at an increased risk of melanoma [95, 96], others have shown an increased risk among workers in UV-intense areas and a strong association between melanoma incidence and both intermittent and total UVR exposures [4, 97, 98]. These observations further emphasize the need for adequate protection for individuals who are exposed to the damaging effects of UVR in the workplace.

Individuals, especially young women, seeking indoor tanning are at high risk for developing skin cancer. A recent systematic review and meta-analysis concluded that there are an estimated 400,000 NMSCs and 6000 cases of melanoma annually in the United States attributable to indoor tanning [99]. In a study of tanning bed users, any use of tanning devices was associated with an increased risk of SCC (OR = 2.5; 95 % CI = 1.7–3.8) and BCC (OR = 1.5; 95 % CI = 1.1–2.1) [100]. A separate meta-analysis concluded that individuals with any history of indoor tanning had an increased risk of melanoma (OR = 1.16, 95 % CI = 1.05–1.28) [101]. The risk of skin cancer has a strong dose–response relationship with tanning, thought to be due to the accumulation of UV exposure [102]. Indoor tanning exposes users to elevated amounts of UV radiation, and in 2009, the World Health Organization (WHO) classified indoor tanning devices as group I human carcinogens due to numerous studies showing the link between tanning and increased cancer risk [103]. Furthermore, the FDA recently upgraded sunlamps to moderate-risk (class II) devices, requiring enhanced product labeling detailing the potential health effects of use [104]. As such, use of these devices should be strongly discouraged due to the adverse effects they can have on the skin.

2.6 Photoprotection

Numerous studies have shown that skin cancers can be prevented by reducing intentional exposure to UV radiation and improving photoprotective strategies. Effective photoprotection involves seeking shade, wearing protective clothing, and applying sunscreen properly. Although sunscreen is less effective than other protective measures, it is by far the most widely used vehicle for sun protection. A large body of clinical research has demonstrated that sunscreens, when used appropriately, can prevent skin cancers and precursor lesions.

2.6.1 Actinic Keratoses (AK)

A number of studies have demonstrated the protective effects of sunscreens on the development of AK [105–107]. The largest randomized controlled trial was conducted in subtropical Nambour, Australia, where 1621 adults were randomly assigned to two groups: daily use sunscreen vs. discretionary use of sunscreen [107]. Individuals in the daily use group were provided with free sunscreen (SPF 16) and instructed to apply it to all sun-exposed sites of the head, neck, arms, and hands. No sunscreens were provided to individuals in the discretionary use (control) group, but they were permitted to use sunscreens if they chose. After the first 2.5 years of intervention, there was a 21 % reduction of AKs in the daily use group compared to the control group in sunscreen-treated locations. However, no significant reduction between the two groups was observed after a further 2 years of follow-up. The acquisition rate of new AKs in the control group markedly decreased in the second 2-year period of the trial, which the investigators suggest may have been caused by an increase in sunscreen use by the control group.

Similar results showing the protective effects of sunscreen on AK development were observed in two smaller randomized controlled trials. In the first, conducted in Victoria, Australia, investigators studied the protective effects of using daily broad-spectrum sunscreen (SPF 17) to prevent the formation of new AKs and induce remission [105]. A total of 431 white residents who had between 1 and 30 AKs at baseline were enrolled. Sunscreen was applied daily to sun-exposed sites and the number of new lesions was recorded over a 7 month period. Participants in the sunscreen group developed fewer new lesions (difference = 0.72, 95 % CI = 0.15–1.28) and had 25 % remission of their existing AKs, compared to 18 % remission in the control group (OR = 1.45: 95 % CI = 1.10–1.88). Overall, participants in the vehicle control group had an average increase of one AK, while participants in the sunscreen group actually saw a decrease in the mean number of AKs by 0.6.

The last study was a randomized controlled trial in the United States assessing AK prevention by sunscreen use in 37 high-risk patients with a history of precancerous lesions or NMSC over a 2-year period [106]. The subjects in the sunscreen group were instructed to apply sunscreen (SPF 29) every day, while the control group applied the vehicle cream without active ingredients. After controlling for differences in risk factors, a 36 % decrease in the annual rate of new AKs was seen in the sunscreen group compared with the placebo group. These three studies demonstrate that daily use of sunscreen has protective benefits for AKs.

2.6.2 Non-melanoma Skin Cancer

The same population of Australian adults from the Nambour Trial was also observed over the same period from 1992 to 1996 to determine the effect of sunscreen use on the development of NMSC [108]. At enrollment, participants completed a survey and underwent a complete skin exam by a dermatologist. Any prevalent skin cancers were removed. Those randomized to the treatment group were instructed to apply a layer of SPF-16 sunscreen to all exposed sites on the head, neck, arms, and hands every morning, with reapplication after heavy sweating, bathing, or long sun exposure. The control group was permitted to use sunscreen at their discretion, and no sunscreen was provided. Compliance for the sunscreen group was assessed by weighing sunscreen bottles every 3 months. At follow-up clinics in 1994 and 1996, dermatologists blinded to treatment allocation reexamined all participants, with histologic confirmation of all clinically diagnosed skin cancers.

After 4.5 years of follow-up, the investigators observed that sunscreen use had no effect on either the incidence of BCC or in the total number of BCC tumors. However, the overall incidence of SCC, in terms of persons affected, was 12 % lower in the sunscreen treatment group ($n=22$) compared with the control group ($n=25$), but this difference was not statistically significant. The study found a 39 % reduction in the total number of SCC tumors among participants assigned to the daily sunscreen group, with 28 SCCs occurring in the sunscreen group compared with 46 SCCs in the control group (95 % CI=0.46–0.81).

A follow-up study was published in 2006 to assess for potential latency of sunscreen use [109]. Participants were followed for an additional 8 years. There was a rate reduction of 35 % (95 % CI=0.43–0.98) in the incidence of SCC, and there was a rate reduction of 38 % (95 % CI=0.38–0.99) in the total number of SCCs diagnosed in the sunscreen group. When the analysis was limited to the late follow-up period (2001–2004), there was a rate reduction of 51 % for both the incidence SCC and total tumor number. In contrast, the prolonged follow-up failed to demonstrate a statistically significant reduction in the incidence of BCC (persons affected) or total number of BCCs occurring in the daily sunscreen group. However, there was a

25 % reduction in the total number of BCCs in the treatment group in the late follow-up period (2001–2004), although this difference is not statistically significant (rate ratio = 0.75, 95 % CI = 0.49–1.14).

2.6.3 Nevi

Having many nevi or having at least 1 atypical nevus is the strongest constitutional risk factors for melanoma. Studies have shown that UVR promotes the growth of nevi [110–112]. Currently, there is only one randomized controlled trial conducted in Vancouver, British Columbia, that demonstrated the protective effect of broad-spectrum sunscreen in reducing the development of nevi in children [113]. Schoolchildren, ages 6–10, were randomized to either a sunscreen group and provided with SPF 30 broad-spectrum sunscreen or control group which received no sunscreen and were given no advice about sunscreen use. Each child's nevi were counted at the beginning and end of the 3-year trial. Based on an initial questionnaire and dermatologic examination, the authors found that factors such as hair color, skin response to sun exposure, facial freckling, and sunburn score in the first 5 years of life were all associated with nevus counts. Analysis revealed regular use of sunscreen was associated with a significant reduction in new nevi (median counts 24 vs. 28; $p = 0.048$). Additionally, a greater effect was seen for sunscreen used in individuals with a higher degree of freckling, with models suggesting that freckled children using sunscreen would develop 30–40 % fewer new nevi than untreated freckled children. These data demonstrate the importance of regular sunscreen use on attenuating the development of new nevi which are a known risk factor for melanoma.

2.6.4 Melanoma

There have been controversies regarding the protective role of sunscreens against the development of melanoma. Some of the early case–control studies suggested an increased risk of melanoma with sunscreen use [114–116]. A meta-analysis of the literature published between 1966 and 1999 found no association between sunscreen use and increased risk of melanoma (relative risk = 1.01; 95 % CI = 0.46, 2.28) [117]. A second review also found a similar result (odds ratio 1.0; 95 % CI = 0.8–1.2) [118]. However, these early case–control studies failed to account for skin sensitivity. Specifically, individuals who are more susceptible to burning and developing melanoma were more likely to use sunscreen, and hence there could be uncontrolled confounding by indication. Other explanations are related to inappropriate application of sunscreen with low SPF and lack of UVA protection.

The controversy was largely put to rest with the results from Nambour Trial in Queensland, Australia [119]. The participants were observed after long-term follow-up to assess whether application of sunscreen during the first 4.5 years had an effect on their risk of primary cutaneous melanoma. At the end of 10-year follow-up (nearly 15 years from the start of the trial), there were a total of 11 primary melanomas (3 invasive) in participants randomized to the sunscreen group and 22 primary melanomas (11 invasive) in the discretionary use (control) group. The study showed a 50 % reduction in the risk of overall melanomas in the sunscreen group ($p=0.051$) and a 73 % reduction in the risk of invasive melanomas among the daily sunscreen group ($p=0.045$). These results demonstrated that daily sunscreen use over a 4.5-year period appears to reduce the long-term melanoma incidence over a 10-year period, with the most pronounced effect seen for invasive melanoma.

It is important to note that the control group in the Nambour Trial for the AK, SCC, BCC, and melanoma studies was not given a placebo or inactive sunscreen, but rather was allowed to continue discretionary use of sunscreen. The design of the trial underestimates the full protective benefits of sunscreen against melanoma. Furthermore, the sunscreen used in the trial was SPF 16 and not UVA stable. Modern-day sunscreens have higher SPF values and are photostable, and theoretically they should offer superior protection.

2.7 Conclusion

UV radiation plays a key role in the development of both non-melanoma skin cancers and melanoma. It is imperative that clinicians continue to educate the general public regarding the benefit of ongoing photoprotection. The public message of photoprotection should encompass seeking shade when outdoor; wearing sun-protective clothing, hats, and sunglasses; and applying broad-spectrum sunscreens. Current scientific evidence demonstrates that sunscreens are safe and that daily application of sunscreen can prevent the incidence of AK, SCC, nevi, and melanoma.

References

1. Maru GB et al (2014) The role of inflammation in skin cancer. Adv Exp Med Biol 816:437–469
2. Young C (2009) Solar ultraviolet radiation and skin cancer. Occup Med 59(2):82–88
3. Dupont E, Gomez J, Bilodeau D (2013) Beyond UV radiation: a skin under challenge. Int J Cosmet Sci 35(3):224–232
4. Kozma B, Eide MJ (2014) Photocarcinogenesis: an epidemiologic perspective on ultraviolet light and skin cancer. Dermatol Clin 32(3):301–313, viii
5. Diffey BL (2002) What is light? Photodermatol Photoimmunol Photomed 18(2):68–74
6. Lautenschlager S, Wulf HC, Pittelkow MR (2007) Photoprotection. Lancet 370(9586): 528–537
7. Miller SA et al (1998) An analysis of UVA emissions from sunlamps and the potential importance for melanoma. Photochem Photobiol 68(1):63–70

8. Rigel DS, Rigel EG, Rigel AC (1999) Effects of altitude and latitude on ambient UVB radiation. J Am Acad Dermatol 40(1):114–116
9. de Laat A et al (1996) Cell cycle kinetics following UVA irradiation in comparison to UVB and UVC irradiation. Photochem Photobiol 63(4):492–497
10. Parrish JA, Zaynoun S, Anderson RR (1981) Cumulative effects of repeated subthreshold doses of ultraviolet radiation. J Invest Dermatol 76(5):356–358
11. Narayanan DL, Saladi RN, Fox JL (2010) Ultraviolet radiation and skin cancer. Int J Dermatol 49(9):978–986
12. Ichihashi M et al (2003) UV-induced skin damage. Toxicology 189(1):21–39
13. Kobayashi N et al (2001) Quantitation and visualization of ultraviolet-induced DNA damage using specific antibodies: application to pigment cell biology. Pigment Cell Res 14(2): 94–102
14. Ikehata H, Ono T (2011) The mechanisms of UV mutagenesis. J Radiat Res 52(2):115–125
15. Brash DE et al (1991) A role for sunlight in skin cancer: UV-induced p53 mutations in squamous cell carcinoma. Proc Natl Acad Sci U S A 88(22):10124–10128
16. Ikehata H et al (2008) UVA1 genotoxicity is mediated not by oxidative damage but by cyclobutane pyrimidine dimers in normal mouse skin. J Invest Dermatol 128(9): 2289–2296
17. Runger TM (2008) C→T transition mutations are not solely UVB-signature mutations, because they are also generated by UVA. J Invest Dermatol 128(9):2138–2140
18. Nakagawa A et al (1998) Three-dimensional visualization of ultraviolet-induced DNA damage and its repair in human cell nuclei. J Invest Dermatol 110(2):143–148
19. Wei Q et al (1993) DNA repair and aging in basal cell carcinoma: a molecular epidemiology study. Proc Natl Acad Sci U S A 90(4):1614–1618
20. Runger TM, Kappes UP (2008) Mechanisms of mutation formation with long-wave ultraviolet light (UVA). Photodermatol Photoimmunol Photomed 24(1):2–10
21. Wondrak GT, Jacobson MK, Jacobson EL (2006) Endogenous UVA-photosensitizers: mediators of skin photodamage and novel targets for skin photoprotection. Photochem Photobiol Sci 5(2):215–237
22. Peak JG, Peak MJ, MacCoss M (1984) DNA breakage caused by 334-nm ultraviolet light is enhanced by naturally occurring nucleic acid components and nucleotide coenzymes. Photochem Photobiol 39(5):713–716
23. Walrant P, Santus R (1974) N-formyl-kynurenine, a tryptophan photooxidation product, as a photodynamic sensitizer. Photochem Photobiol 19(6):411–417
24. McCormick JP et al (1976) Characterization of a cell-lethal product from the photooxidation of tryptophan: hydrogen peroxide. Science 191(4226):468–469
25. Fisher GJ et al (2002) Mechanisms of photoaging and chronological skin aging. Arch Dermatol 138(11):1462–1470
26. Chen L, Hu JY, Wang SQ (2012) The role of antioxidants in photoprotection: A critical review. J Am Acad Dermatol 67(5):1013–1024
27. Tran TT, Schulman J, Fisher DE (2008) UV and pigmentation: molecular mechanisms and social controversies. Pigment Cell Melanoma Res 21(5):509–516
28. Kielbassa C, Roza L, Epe B (1997) Wavelength dependence of oxidative DNA damage induced by UV and visible light. Carcinogenesis 18(4):811–816
29. Heck DE et al (2003) UVB light stimulates production of reactive oxygen species: unexpected role for catalase. J Biol Chem 278(25):22432–22436
30. Epe B (1991) Genotoxicity of singlet oxygen. Chem Biol Interact 80(3):239–260
31. Cheng KC et al (1992) 8-Hydroxyguanine, an abundant form of oxidative DNA damage, causes G----T and A----C substitutions. J Biol Chem 267(1):166–172
32. Cadet J et al (2012) Photoinduced damage to cellular DNA: direct and photosensitized reactions. Photochem Photobiol 88(5):1048–1065
33. Daya-Grosjean L, Dumaz N, Sarasin A (1995) The specificity of p53 mutation spectra in sunlight induced human cancers. J Photochem Photobiol B 28(2):115–124
34. Hussein MR (2005) Ultraviolet radiation and skin cancer: molecular mechanisms. J Cutan Pathol 32(3):191–205

35. Prives C, Hall PA (1999) The p53 pathway. J Pathol 187(1):112–126
36. Wilson GD (2004) Radiation and the cell cycle, revisited. Cancer Metastasis Rev 23(3-4):209–225
37. Sherr CJ, Roberts JM (1999) CDK inhibitors: positive and negative regulators of G1-phase progression. Genes Dev 13(12):1501–1512
38. Matsumura Y, Ananthaswamy HN (2004) Toxic effects of ultraviolet radiation on the skin. Toxicol Appl Pharmacol 195(3):298–308
39. Houtgraaf JH, Versmissen J, van der Giessen WJ (2006) A concise review of DNA damage checkpoints and repair in mammalian cells. Cardiovasc Revasc Med 7(3):165–172
40. Aburatani H et al (1997) Cloning and characterization of mammalian 8-hydroxyguanine-specific DNA glycosylase/apurinic, apyrimidinic lyase, a functional mutM homologue. Cancer Res 57(11):2151–2156
41. Kim YJ, Wilson DM 3rd (2012) Overview of base excision repair biochemistry. Curr Mol Pharmacol 5(1):3–13
42. Reardon JT, Sancar A (2005) Nucleotide excision repair. Prog Nucleic Acid Res Mol Biol 79:183–235
43. Black H et al (1997) Photocarcinogenesis: an overview. J Photochem Photobiol B Biol 40(1):29–47
44. Jing Y, Kao JF, Taylor JS (1998) Thermodynamic and base-pairing studies of matched and mismatched DNA dodecamer duplexes containing cis-syn, (6-4) and Dewar photoproducts of TT. Nucleic Acids Res 26(16):3845–3853
45. Lo HL et al (2005) Differential biologic effects of CPD and 6-4PP UV-induced DNA damage on the induction of apoptosis and cell-cycle arrest. BMC Cancer 5:135
46. Amaral JD et al (2010) The role of p53 in apoptosis. Discov Med 9(45):145–152
47. Hoffman WH et al (2002) Transcriptional repression of the anti-apoptotic survivin gene by wild type p53. J Biol Chem 277(5):3247–3257
48. Muller M et al (1998) p53 activates the CD95 (APO-1/Fas) gene in response to DNA damage by anticancer drugs. J Exp Med 188(11):2033–2045
49. Bennett M et al (1998) Cell surface trafficking of Fas: a rapid mechanism of p53-mediated apoptosis. Science 282(5387):290–293
50. Li H, Zhang XP, Liu F (2013) Coordination between p21 and DDB2 in the cellular response to UV radiation. PLoS One 8(11), e80111
51. Gailani MR et al (1996) The role of the human homologue of Drosophila patched in sporadic basal cell carcinomas. Nat Genet 14(1):78–81
52. Nishigori C et al (1994) Mutations in ras genes in cells cultured from mouse skin tumors induced by ultraviolet irradiation. Proc Natl Acad Sci U S A 91(15):7189–7193
53. Daya-Grosjean L, Couve-Privat S (2005) Sonic hedgehog signaling in basal cell carcinomas. Cancer Lett 225(2):181–192
54. Dreier J et al (2013) Basal cell carcinoma: a paradigm for targeted therapies. Expert Opin Pharmacother 14(10):1307–1318
55. Viros A et al (2014) Ultraviolet radiation accelerates BRAF-driven melanomagenesis by targeting TP53. Nature 511(7510):478–482
56. Rudolph P et al (1998) Enhanced expression of Ki-67, topoisomerase IIalpha, PCNA, p53 and p21WAF1/Cip1 reflecting proliferation and repair activity in UV-irradiated melanocytic nevi. Hum Pathol 29(12):1480–1487
57. Pollock PM et al (2003) High frequency of BRAF mutations in nevi. Nat Genet 33(1):19–20
58. Armstrong BK, Kricker A (2001) The epidemiology of UV induced skin cancer. J Photochem Photobiol B 63(1-3):8–18
59. Rogers HW et al (2010) Incidence estimate of nonmelanoma skin cancer in the United States, 2006. Arch Dermatol 146(3):283–287
60. Wang SQ, Halpern AC (2008) Public education in photoprotection. In: Clinical guide to sunscreens and photoprotection. CRC Press, Boca Raton, pp 281–291
61. United States. Public Health Service. Office of the Surgeon General. Human (2014) Reports of the surgeon general. In: The surgeon general's call to action to prevent skin cancer. Office of the Surgeon General (US), Washington (DC)

62. Jemal A et al (2011) Recent trends in cutaneous melanoma incidence and death rates in the United States, 1992-2006. J Am Acad Dermatol 65(5 Suppl 1):S17–S25.e1–3
63. Lazovich D, Choi K, Vogel RI (2012) Time to get serious about skin cancer prevention. Cancer Epidemiol Biomarkers Prev 21(11):1893–1901
64. Siegel R et al (2014) Cancer statistics, 2014. CA Cancer J Clin 64(1):9–29
65. Mitra D et al (2012) An ultraviolet-radiation-independent pathway to melanoma carcinogenesis in the red hair/fair skin background. Nature 491(7424):449–453
66. Gandini S et al (2005) Meta-analysis of risk factors for cutaneous melanoma: II. Sun exposure. Eur J Cancer 41(1):45–60
67. Raimondi S et al (2008) MC1R variants, melanoma and red hair color phenotype: a meta-analysis. Int J Cancer 122(12):2753–2760
68. Zanetti R et al (1996) The multicentre south European study 'Helios'. I: skin characteristics and sunburns in basal cell and squamous cell carcinomas of the skin. Br J Cancer 73(11): 1440–1446
69. Gallagher RP et al (1995) Sunlight exposure, pigmentary factors, and risk of nonmelanocytic skin cancer. I. Basal cell carcinoma. Arch Dermatol 131(2):157–163
70. Kricker A et al (1995) Does intermittent sun exposure cause basal cell carcinoma? a case-control study in Western Australia. Int J Cancer 60(4):489–494
71. Xiang F et al (2014) Incidence of nonmelanoma skin cancer in relation to ambient UV radiation in white populations, 1978-2012: empirical relationships. JAMA Dermatol 150(10):1063–1071
72. Rivas M, Rojas E, Calaf GM (2012) Prediction of skin cancer occurrence by ultraviolet solar index. Oncol Lett 3(4):893–896
73. Eide MJ, Weinstock MA (2005) Association of UV index, latitude, and melanoma incidence in nonwhite populations--US Surveillance, Epidemiology, and End Results (SEER) Program, 1992 to 2001. Arch Dermatol 141(4):477–481
74. Qureshi AA et al (2008) Geographic variation and risk of skin cancer in US women. Differences between melanoma, squamous cell carcinoma, and basal cell carcinoma. Arch Intern Med 168(5):501–507
75. Holman CD, Armstrong BK (1984) Cutaneous malignant melanoma and indicators of total accumulated exposure to the sun: an analysis separating histogenetic types. J Natl Cancer Inst 73(1):75–82
76. Mack TM, Floderus B (1991) Malignant melanoma risk by nativity, place of residence at diagnosis, and age at migration. Cancer Causes Control 2(6):401–411
77. Levine H et al (2013) Country of origin, age at migration and risk of cutaneous melanoma: a migrant cohort study of 1,100,000 Israeli men. Int J Cancer 133(2):486–494
78. Autier P et al (1997) Melanoma risk and residence in sunny areas. EORTC Melanoma Co-operative Group. European Organization for Research and Treatment of Cancer. Br J Cancer 76(11):1521–1524
79. Kennedy C et al (2003) The influence of painful sunburns and lifetime sun exposure on the risk of actinic keratoses, seborrheic warts, melanocytic nevi, atypical nevi, and skin cancer. J Invest Dermatol 120(6):1087–1093
80. Strickland PT et al (1989) Quantitative carcinogenesis in man: solar ultraviolet B dose dependence of skin cancer in Maryland watermen. J Natl Cancer Inst 81(24):1910–1913
81. Woodhead AD, Setlow RB, Tanaka M (1999) Environmental factors in nonmelanoma and melanoma skin cancer. J Epidemiol 9(6 Suppl):S102–S114
82. Raasch B et al (1998) Body site specific incidence of basal and squamous cell carcinoma in an exposed population, Townsville, Australia. Mutat Res 422(1):101–106
83. Franceschi S et al (1996) Site distribution of different types of skin cancer: new aetiological clues. Int J Cancer 67(1):24–28
84. Jhappan C, Noonan FP, Merlino G (2003) Ultraviolet radiation and cutaneous malignant melanoma. Oncogene 22(20):3099–3112
85. Gallagher RP et al (2010) Ultraviolet radiation. Chronic Dis Can 29(Suppl 1):51–68
86. Bataille V (2013) Sun exposure, sunbeds and sunscreens and melanoma. What are the controversies? Curr Oncol Rep 15(6):526–532

87. Kraft S, Granter SR (2014) Molecular pathology of skin neoplasms of the head and neck. Arch Pathol Lab Med 138(6):759–787
88. Clark WH Jr, Mihm MC Jr (1969) Lentigo maligna and lentigo-maligna melanoma. Am J Pathol 55(1):39–67
89. Feng Z et al (2011) Incidence and survival of desmoplastic melanoma in the United States, 1992-2007. J Cutan Pathol 38(8):616–624
90. Wasif N, Gray RJ, Pockaj BA (2011) Desmoplastic melanoma - the step-child in the melanoma family? J Surg Oncol 103(2):158–162
91. Jain S, Allen PW (1989) Desmoplastic malignant melanoma and its variants. A study of 45 cases. Am J Surg Pathol 13(5):358–373
92. Chen LL et al (2013) Desmoplastic melanoma: a review. J Am Acad Dermatol 68(5): 825–833
93. Schmitt J et al (2011) Occupational ultraviolet light exposure increases the risk for the development of cutaneous squamous cell carcinoma: a systematic review and meta-analysis. Br J Dermatol 164(2):291–307
94. Bauer A, Diepgen TL, Schmitt J (2011) Is occupational solar ultraviolet irradiation a relevant risk factor for basal cell carcinoma? A systematic review and meta-analysis of the epidemiological literature. Br J Dermatol 165(3):612–625
95. Gallagher RP, Elwood JM, Yang CP (1989) Is chronic sunlight exposure important in accounting for increases in melanoma incidence? Int J Cancer 44(5):813–815
96. Garland FC et al (1990) Occupational sunlight exposure and melanoma in the U.S. Navy. Arch Environ Health 45(5):261–267
97. Whiteman DC et al (2006) Anatomic site, sun exposure, and risk of cutaneous melanoma. J Clin Oncol 24(19):3172–3177
98. Chang YM et al (2009) Sun exposure and melanoma risk at different latitudes: a pooled analysis of 5700 cases and 7216 controls. Int J Epidemiol 38(3):814–830
99. Wehner MR et al (2014) International prevalence of indoor tanning: a systematic review and meta-analysis. JAMA Dermatol 150(4):390–400
100. Karagas MR et al (2002) Use of tanning devices and risk of basal cell and squamous cell skin cancers. J Natl Cancer Inst 94(3):224–226
101. Colantonio S, Bracken MB, Beecker J (2014) The association of indoor tanning and melanoma in adults: systematic review and meta-analysis. J Am Acad Dermatol 70(5):847–857.e1–18
102. Lazovich D et al (2010) Indoor tanning and risk of melanoma: a case-control study in a highly exposed population. Cancer Epidemiol Biomarkers Prev 19(6):1557–1568
103. El Ghissassi F et al (2009) A review of human carcinogens Part D: radiation. Lancet Oncol 10(8):751–752
104. US Food and Drug Administration. FDA to require warnings on sunlamp products. FDA News Release 2014 May 29, 2014; Available from: http://www.fda.gov/NewsEvents/Newsroom/PressAnnouncements/ucm399222.htm
105. Thompson SC, Jolley D, Marks R (1993) Reduction of solar keratoses by regular sunscreen Use. N Engl J Med 329(16):1147–1151
106. Naylor MF et al (1995) High sun protection factor sunscreens in the suppression of actinic neoplasia. Arch Dermatol 131(2):170–175
107. Darlington S et al (2003) A randomized controlled trial to assess sunscreen application and beta carotene supplementation in the prevention of solar keratoses. Arch Dermatol 139(4):451–455
108. Green A et al (1999) Daily sunscreen application and betacarotene supplementation in prevention of basal-cell and squamous-cell carcinomas of the skin: a randomised controlled trial. Lancet 354(9180):723–729
109. van der Pols JC et al (2006) Prolonged prevention of squamous cell carcinoma of the skin by regular sunscreen use. Cancer Epidemiol Biomarkers Prev 15(12):2546–2548
110. Harrison SL, MacLennan R, Buettner PG (2008) Sun exposure and the incidence of melanocytic nevi in young Australian children. Cancer Epidemiol Biomarkers Prev 17(9): 2318–2324

111. Psaty EL et al (2010) Defining the patient at high risk for melanoma. Int J Dermatol 49(4):362–376
112. Bauer J et al (2005) Risk factors of incident melanocytic nevi: a longitudinal study in a cohort of 1,232 young German children. Int J Cancer 115(1):121–126
113. Gallagher RP et al (2000) Broad-spectrum sunscreen use and the development of new nevi in white children: a randomized controlled trial. JAMA 283(22):2955–2960
114. Westerdahl J et al (1995) Is the use of sunscreens a risk factor for malignant melanoma? Melanoma Res 5(1):59–65
115. Westerdahl J et al (2000) Sunscreen use and malignant melanoma. Int J Cancer 87(1): 145–150
116. Wolf P et al (1998) Phenotypic markers, sunlight-related factors and sunscreen use in patients with cutaneous melanoma: an Austrian case-control study. Melanoma Res 8(4):370–378
117. Huncharek M, Kupelnick B (2002) Use of topical sunscreens and the risk of malignant melanoma: a meta-analysis of 9067 patients from 11 case-control studies. Am J Public Health 92(7):1173–1177
118. Dennis LK, Beane Freeman LE, VanBeek MJ (2003) Sunscreen use and the risk for melanoma: a quantitative review. Ann Intern Med 139(12):966–978
119. Green AC et al (2011) Reduced melanoma after regular sunscreen use: randomized trial follow-up. J Clin Oncol 29(3):257–263

Chapter 3
Photoprotection for Photodermatoses

Daniel Gutierrez and Elma D. Baron

Key Points

- Photodermatoses represent a broad and extensive group of disorders caused by exposure to sunlight.
- Elucidation of action spectrum of a disease should be performed at the earliest convenience to assure most adequate management of the patient.
- The cornerstone of photoprotection in all photodermatoses involves the use of long-sleeve shirts, wide-brim hats, sunglasses, appropriate types and amounts of sunscreens, and sun avoidance during peak hours of sun intensity.
- If photosensitivity is due to administration of an exogenous agent or the result of an accumulation or deficiency of an endogenous entity, removal of the offending agent and correction of the deficiency are paramount to treatment.

3.1 Background

The spectrum of solar radiation is comprised of roughly 50 % visible light, 40 % infrared, and 9 % ultraviolet (UV) radiation (UVR) [1]. UVR is considered to be of greatest importance in healthcare due to its well-documented impact on

D. Gutierrez, BS
Department of Dermatology, University Hospitals Case Medical Center,
11100 Euclid, Ave. Lakeside 3500, Cleveland, OH 44106-5028, USA

E.D. Baron, MD (✉)
School of Medicine, Case Western Reserve University, Cleveland, OH, USA

Department of Dermatology, University Hospitals Case Medical Center,
11100 Euclid, Ave. Lakeside 3500, Cleveland, OH 44106-5028, USA

Louis Stokes Department of Veterans, Affairs Medical Center, Cleveland, OH, USA
e-mail: elma.baron@case.edu

S.Q. Wang, H.W. Lim (eds.), *Principles and Practice of Photoprotection*,
DOI 10.1007/978-3-319-29382-0_3

pathogenesis and clinical course of dermatologic diseases. In brief, UVR wavelengths range from 100 to 400 nm and are subdivided into the following groups: UVA, UVB, and UVC. Understanding these subdivisions within UVR is of great importance when evaluating and managing patients with photodermatoses, which are considered abnormal or adverse skin reactions to sunlight. The cutoffs of each subdivision vary slightly within the current literature; in this article, the most commonly accepted divisions will be used: UVA at 320–400 nm, UVB at 290–320 nm, and UVC at 200–290 [2]. Within the UVA continuum, UVA can be further subdivided into UVA1 at 340–400 nm and UVA2 at 320–340 nm. For phototherapeutic applications, UVB can be divided into broadband (BB) UVB at 290–320 nm and narrowband (NB) UVB at 311–313 nm.

Different UVR wavelengths penetrate human skin to varying degrees. The longer the wavelength, the deeper it penetrates human skin. UVA, having the longest wavelength of the UVR spectrum, will permeate deep into the dermis. UVB will extend through the epidermis as far as the dermal papillae. Finally, UVC light, due to its short wavelength, is completely absorbed by the Earth's ozone layer; rarely is UVC light implicated in human disease from sunlight exposure due to this. In addition to different depths of penetration, there exists variance among the biological effects each UVR subtype possesses on human tissues. Compounds ranging from porphyrins and nucleotides to exogenous photosensitizing agents deemed chromophores absorb light and produce a series of photochemical reactions. Exploiting the different wavelengths of light that excite different chromophores to produce desirable effects is the foundation of phototherapy. Though some of these effects can be desirable, others are not, and the reaction to light in these cases represents a pathologic mechanism.

The photodermatoses represent a heterogeneous group of disorders sharing the common trait of being precipitated by light. Each photodermatosis has a different action spectrum, or wavelength of light that will be absorbed by chromophores to elicit a cutaneous response. Even within the same photodermatosis, individuals can potentially have different action spectra. Knowledge of this is crucial for optimal management of each photodermatosis.

Photodermatoses can be divided into four distinct groups: (1) immunologically mediated photodermatoses (IMPs), (2) chemical- and drug-induced photosensitivity, (3) photoaggravated dermatoses, and (4) inherited disorders with defective DNA repair or with chromosomal instability [3]. In this review, we will discuss different strategies of photoprotection and management of the photodermatoses.

3.2 Immunologically Mediated Photodermatoses

The group of IMPs consists of five distinct conditions: actinic prurigo, chronic actinic dermatitis, hydroa vacciniforme, polymorphous light eruption (PMLE), and solar urticaria [3]. The pathophysiology underlying each of these photodermatoses has not been fully characterized. However, it is hypothesized that these disorders result from dysregulation of the immune system due to UVR in genetically susceptible individuals. Each of these conditions will be discussed separately.

3.2.1 Polymorphous Light Eruption

It is theorized that UVR-induced cutaneous photoantigens cause a delayed-type hypersensitivity reaction and result in the manifestation of polymorphous light eruption (PMLE) [4, 5]. Phototesting has consistently shown that UVA has been more effective than combined UVA/UVB or UVB alone in eliciting pathologic response [3]. Because the action spectrum of 90 % of those with PMLE is in the UVA range, sunscreen selection becomes of great importance to prevent disease exacerbations [6]. Many commercially available sunscreens focus on UVB light absorption and are not adequate for PMLE photoprotection. Therefore, broad-spectrum sunscreen with high UVA protection should be utilized for those with suspected PMLE.

An ideal sunscreen for patients with photodermatoses should have a sun protection factor (SPF) between 30 and 60 and should be applied adequately every 2 h when outdoor. The amount of sunscreen applied for SPF testing, as mandated by the Food and Drug Administration (FDA), is 2 mg/cm [2, 7]. In actual use, however, most apply only 0.5–1 mg/cm [2, 8, 9]. To test the efficacy of lower-than-recommended levels of sunscreen and UVA-specific protection in PMLE, Bissonnette and colleagues compared two SPF 45 sunscreens, one with a high-level UVA protection factor of 25 and another with a low UVA photoprotection factor of 5, when applied at both 2 mg/cm [2] and 1 mg/cm [2, 10]. Subjects were exposed to progressively increasing levels of combination UVA–UVB radiation for either 5 days or until an erythematous, vesicular, edematous, or popular response was noted. When comparing application levels at 2 mg/cm [2], 0 % of those in the high UVA protection sunscreen developed a PMLE exacerbation as compared to the 73 % of those in the low UVA sunscreen group. In contrast, 33 % of those in the high UVA protective sunscreen group developed an exacerbation compared to those 80 % when applied at 1 mg/cm [2]. This study showed that sunscreens with both high SPF and high UVA protective factor can successfully prevent exacerbations of PMLE even when applied at suboptimal levels [10]. This result strengthens the notion that both proper selection of sunscreen and proper application are crucial.

Prophylactic sun hardening, a form of desensitization to sunlight, can be administered to those with PMLE before prolonged sun exposure. Specific phototherapies used include BB-UVB, NB-UVB, and UVA alone or with psoralen (PUVA) [11]. Of note, NB-UVB treatments have increasingly begun to displace both PUVA and BB-UVB at some institutions because of the ability to avoid complications including psoralen-related gastrointestinal symptoms and lack of necessity to wear photoprotective glasses after treatment in addition to the theorized utility and safety in and pregnant [12]. Therefore, the most commonly used light source for hardening is currently NB-UVB. At a temperate climate, this is delivered in springtime with three times weekly treatment for 5 weeks. Patients are advised to continue with 20–30 min periods of sun exposure weekly between the peak hours UVB light from 10 AM to 2 PM without sunscreen to preserve newly gained hardening effects [12].

To manage patients with polymorphous light eruption, prednisolone has shown to be effective in suppressing exacerbation of symptoms [13]. Antihistamines to treat pruritic lesions can also be considered, but should be used only as adjunct to other therapies. *Polypodium leucotomos*, carotenoids, afamelanotide, and nicotinamide have been used as adjuncts to topical photoprotection. However, there lack of sufficient evidence assessing their to warrant recommendation at this time in lieu of other proven photoprotective. Above all, individuals should be counseled on the use of physical barriers for photoprotection: sunglasses, wide-brimmed hats, and long-sleeve shirts. Use of photoprotective clothing is a mainstay of preventing disease exacerbation.

3.2.2 Solar Urticaria

Solar urticaria is a very rare photodermatosis that results in wheal and flare development within minutes of light exposure with resolution within 24 h. The presumed pathophysiology is that of a type I hypersensitivity response in which chromophore absorption of a photon causes the formation of neoantigens capable of recognition by IgE antibodies [14]. These antibodies then bind to the Fc receptor on mast cells and upon re-exposure to light cause degranulation and release of inflammatory mediators. The action spectrum is vast among patients and extends over UV to the visible light spectrum [15] so much so that it has been reported that even infrared radiation causes exacerbation [16]. As the action spectrum is variable, phototesting should first be performed to determine a patient's action spectrum to best ensure adequate photoprotective strategies are used [6]. It should be emphasized that phototesting reading needs to be done immediately after exposure as the wheal and flare response will resolve.

General photoprotective strategies including sun avoidance, use of broad-spectrum sunscreen with high SPF, and use of tightly woven, thick, dark fabrics are initial precautions that can be taken to prevent acute flares. The visible light spectrum, in particular, is difficult to protect against. For topical visible photoprotection to be effective, the topical agent must be opaque. As such, there are no sunscreens currently available that provide coverage against the visible light spectrum. With respect to protection against visible light, it should be made known that the SPF of a sunscreen does not correlate to protection against the visible action spectrum [17]. Sunscreens with a higher concentration of iron oxides, which are pigmented, have been shown to be better at blocking visible light when compared to the sunscreens only containing micronized zinc oxide and titanium dioxide [17, 18]. No clinical trials have been performed evaluating the efficacy of such pigmented sunscreens in the idiopathic photodermatoses, there exists a likelihood of benefit given results from artificial sensitization against visible light [19].

Phototherapy, with UVA being the most commonly used light source, to facilitate hardening provides the next step of management for more severely affected patients. Recent evidence suggests that using wavelengths outside the action spectrum of a patient may induce tolerance [20, 21]. UVA rush-hardening protocols have reported, suggesting this as a viable option for treatment in the future [22]. An interesting agent for systemic photoprotection in solar urticaria involves the use of the α-melanocyte-stimulating hormone analogue, afamelanotide. In a cohort of 5 individuals receiving a single subcutaneous the urticarial dose necessary for eliciting wheal formation increased [23]. Dihydroxyacetone followed by an application of naphthoquinone over a period of 7 month yielded an SPF increase of 18 in 18 of the 30 patients tested [24]. Though quite promising, more trials are necessary in order to truly assess efficacy.

In the event of an exacerbation, topical corticosteroids and antihistamines can be used for symptomatic treatment. Although systemic corticosteroids are more effective at controlling flares, adverse side effects prevent their long-term use. In addition, IVIG [25, 26], plasmapheresis [27], and omalizumab [28, 29] have proven successful in select cases, supporting the proposed antibody-mediated pathophysiology. Most recently, a phase 3 multicenter study of omalizumab in 323 patients with chronic idiopathic or spontaneous urticaria, diseases similar to solar urticaria, had reported symptomatic relief in those where antihistamines had failed to alleviate symptoms of urticaria [30]. Based on these initial findings, it appears that immunomodulatory therapy should be more aggressively pursued as a treatment option for solar urticaria.

3.2.3 *Hydroa Vacciniforme*

Another rare photodermatosis, hydroa vacciniforme presents as one of two clinical phenotypes: classic hydroa vacciniforme and severe hydroa vacciniforme-like eruption. The classical variant most commonly affects children, declining in severity as adolescence is reached. Sun exposure triggers the formation of edematous, pruritic, or painful papules that progress to vesicles and eventually rupture. The ruptured vesicles heal, leaving a vacciniforme or varioliform pattern of scarring. The severe variant, in contrast, is most commonly described in adults and occurs concurrently with constitutional symptoms of fever, weight loss, and headache. It is frequently associated with T cell or natural killer cell lymphoma and has an aggressive course [31]. Histologically, epidermal necrosis with predominately neutrophilic and lymphocytic infiltrate is observed in both presentations [32]. As with the other photodermatoses, the pathogenesis is unclear. The action spectrum of those afflicted with the disease lies within the UVA spectra [33, 34]. However, it has been postulated that Epstein-Barr virus (EBV) infection is involved in the pathogenesis [31, 35, 36], especially because EBV DNA in blood and EBV-encoded small nuclear ribonucleic acid isolated from vesicles have been found in both the classic and severe hydroa vacciniforme-like variants.

Treatment of hydroa vacciniforme is difficult once visible lesions are present [37]. Photoprotective strategies geared toward preventing exacerbations are therefore critical. As with other photodermatoses, the most adequate method to avoid disease provocations involves the use of photoprotective clothing, sunscreens, and sun avoidance [37, 38]. Similarly, dark-tinted car windows and limiting heat exposure have been felt to ameliorate the severity of disease [37]. In addition to photoprotection, cases of associated with EBV should be managed by treatment of the viral infection. Successful treatment of EBV has resulted in increased ability to spend time in sunlight without the development of new skin lesions while also preventing any systemic manifestations associated with the infection [39].

3.2.4 Chronic Actinic Dermatitis

Chronic actinic dermatitis (CAD), also known as photosensitivity dermatitis, actinic reticuloid syndrome, photosensitive eczema, and persistent light reaction, is a photodermatosis of unknown, most likely immunologic, etiology that presents either as dermatitis with or without pseudolymphomatous lesions. In most severe cases, it may also present as erythroderma. Males, of any race above 50 years of age, are typically affected. Current literature, shows that CAD [40–42]. In addition, development of CAD in younger individuals is usually quite rare unless a history of atopic dermatitis [43] or HIV infection is noted [40]. Acute flares of the disease are characterized by scaly patches and papules mostly limited to sun-exposed areas. Later, eczematous plaques with lichenification become evident due to the chronicity of the disorder. Diagnosis of CAD includes fulfillment of the following criteria: dermatitis to a sun-exposed area without exposure to a photosensitizer; abnormal delayed erythema to UVA, UVB, or visible light; and histology suggesting photodermatitis (epidermal spongiosis, acanthosis, and a perivascular mononuclear cell infiltration in superficial and possibly deep dermis) [44].

Prophylactic photoprotective measures are the mainstay of management of the disease course. Choosing a broad-spectrum high SPF sunscreen is useful to prevent exacerbation of disease. A formulation with UV filters that are low in contact sensitization potential is advised so as to minimize the likelihood of development of dermatitis in patients [45, 46]. Like most photosensitive disorders, patients should seek shade during peak hours of sunlight and photoprotective clothing. Museum films that prevent transmission of UVR wavelengths can be used the aforementioned photoprotective strategies [47]. Given that the action spectra may lie within the visible light continuum, lifestyle changes to restrict exposure to both natural and artificial light sources may be necessary. Modifications of the home and work environment may also be necessary in particularly unrelenting disease. No reports of exacerbation of disease from neither televisions nor computer screens have been reported in the literature [45, 48].

If avoidance of the action spectrum is unfeasible, topical corticosteroids should be used for symptomatic relief. In particularly severe CAD, immunosuppressive therapy is indicated, of which azathioprine is the only clinically proven, efficacious treatment [49, 50]. Despite this, case reports have demonstrated that topical calcineurin inhibitors like tacrolimus [51–53] and pimecrolimus [54] can aid in the treatment of CAD. There exist anecdotal reports of benefit in severe CAD from other immunosuppressants typically used for unrelenting atopic dermatitis including mycophenolate mofetil [55] and cyclosporine [56, 57]. Hardening with artificial light sources is usually difficult to achieve as patients tend to be exquisitely photosensitive, making it difficult to increase the exposure dose. Because of the paucity of knowledge regarding immunosuppressive agents with potential for treatment, future clinical trials should focus on quantifying the effect of other immunosuppressants used in case reports compared to that of the azathioprine.

3.2.5 *Actinic Prurigo*

Actinic prurigo begins in childhood as a pruritic, papular, or nodular eruption on sun-exposed areas and appears hours to days after sun exposure. Sun exposure leads to an immediate edematous phase that transitions into an eczematous phase followed by a pruriginous phase [6]. Presentation of the disease varies, frequently having ocular manifestations as well as lower lip cheilitis. Unfortunately, the disease does not remit in adulthood. Indigenous populations of the Americas [58, 59]. Patients of Amerindian or mixed-Amerindian descent are often associated with human leukocyte antigen (HLA) DRB1*0407, an HLA-DR4 subtype [58, 60, 61]. HLA-DR4, of note, can be associated with a number of autoimmune disorders, most notably rheumatoid arthritis, and it has been proposed that certain HLA genes modify the response to UVR-induced neoantigens [62]. Though an important association, lack of associated HLA association does not preclude the development of the disease [63].

Both UVA and UVB have been shown to elicit a pathophysiological response [64]. Photoprotective strategies that should be utilized for actinic prurigo involve sun avoidance and use of photoprotective clothing, lip balm, and broad-spectrum sunscreens. Sunglasses blocking both UVA and UVB are strongly advocated to prevent any ocular symptoms that may arise. For optimal protection, sunglasses should wrap around and be fitted close to the face so as to prevent reflection of light from the interior portion of sunglasses back onto the face. As UVA could be part of an individual's action spectrum, environmental protective strategies to limit the amount of UVA light including UVA blocking films have been found helpful [47, 65]. It remains important to test for deterioration of photoprotective abilities of such films and replace them when necessary [65]. Topical corticosteroids are an effective treatment in some patients with acute exacerbations, though their side effects preclude chronic use. The role of phototherapy in these patients is limited. Thalidomide, through its immunomodulatory mechanism, is the most effective treatment for this condition; reports have shown its efficacy [66–68] and its potential for safe, long-term use [68].

3.3 Chemical- and Drug-Induced Photosensitivity

Chemical- or drug-induced sensitivity represents the most diverse group of photodermatoses and can be divided into exogenous and endogenous causes. Exogenous causes involve the ingestion, administration, or application of a medication, personal care product, or occupational agent causing adverse reactions to light. Meanwhile, photosensitivity due to endogenous agents is the result of accumulation of compounds in the body through either acquired or inherited mechanisms.

3.3.1 Exogenous Agents

Broadly, there are two categories of photosensitivity an individual may exhibit to exogenous agents: photoallergic and phototoxic. The pathogenic mechanism for each will be discussed.

3.3.2 Photoallergic Reactions

True photoallergic responses are much less common than phototoxic reactions. This type IV hypersensitivity response results from formation of a neoantigen due to any amount of UV exposure. Photoallergic reactions are usually not observed for 1–3 days; most common offending agents are topical agents, usually sunscreens. Following this period, the response manifests itself as an eczematous reaction spreading to areas unexposed to sunlight. Spongiosis is seen histologically. For classic photoallergic responses to develop, prior sensitization is necessary. Cross reactivity of many molecules, however, permit the development of photoallergic reactions from first exposure due to exposure of a structurally similar entity. The prototypical example of this phenomenon is photoallergy due to cross reactivity between thimerosal, a preservative used in skin antigen testing, and piroxicam. The thiosalicylic moiety in thiomersal is highly antigenic and causes allergic responses in some patients. Piroxicam, a nonsteroidal anti-inflammatory drug (NSAID), is photodecomposed when exposed to UVA into molecule that is structurally similar to the thiosalicylic moiety in thimerosal causing a photoallergic response upon the first exposure to the NSAID [69–71] Photoallergies can result from many topicals and systemic medications.

3.3.3 Phototoxic Reactions

Phototoxic reactions are significantly more common than photoallergic reaction and are observed within minutes to hours. These reactions occur on first exposure to an agent in the setting of sufficient amount of agent and UVA exposure. An exogenous agent will topically absorb photons causing it to reach an excited state. To reach the ground state, the agent becomes involved in a series of oxygen-dependent reactions eventually causing the formation of free radicals causing cellular damage. There are two types of phototoxic reactions. Type I phototoxic reactions involve a photosensitizer combining with cellular components or transferring hydrogen or electrons to other molecules, forming free radicals that cause cellular damage [72, 73]. Type II phototoxicity, on the other hand, involves the excited agent transferring electrons to oxygen directly, causing the formation of oxygen radicals [72, 73].

In contrast to photoallergic responses, phototoxic reactions are erythematous and sharply demarcated and only are present on sun-exposed portions of the body. There are, however, instances in which it may be hard to distinguish between photoallergic and phototoxic reactions simply based on morphology. Necrotic keratinocytes with a mild inflammatory response comprised of neutrophils and macrophages are seen histologically in phototoxic reactions.

3.3.4 Photoprotection for Exogenous Agents

The most effective way to prevent further photosensitivity is immediate removal of the offending substance. This is not feasible many times due to the importance of the medication in chronic disease management. In such cases, educating patients on proper photoprotective practices is necessary. Since UVA is the primary action spectrum implicated in these disorders, use of UVA blocking films in windows and use of UVA protective sunscreens are sometimes recommended. Avoidance of peak hours of sunlight should be emphasized as well.

3.3.5 Endogenous Agents

Photosensitivity from endogenous agents results from accumulation of different compounds likely secondary to enzymatic deficiency. Examples that will be discussed include cutaneous porphyrias, pellagra, and Smith-Lemli-Opitz syndrome.

3.3.6 Cutaneous Porphyrias

The porphyrias represent an inherited or acquired heterogeneous group of enzymatic defects in the heme biosynthesis pathway. Table 3.1 provides a summary of the heme biosynthetic pathway with enzymatic defects resulting in each porphyria. Each enzymatic defect beginning from uroporphyrinogen synthase onward produces a photosensitive phenotype. Porphyrinogens accumulate and then undergo spontaneous oxidation to the corresponding porphyrins. The resultant porphyrins are potent endogenous photosensitizing substances. The action spectrum of the porphyrias typically involves the Soret band, a peak in blue wavelength region of the visible light spectrum usually between 400 and 410 nm, with a less significant action spectrum in the visible red light spectrum at about 600–650 nm [74]. For this reason, UVA and UVB blocking sunscreens are typically ineffective in preventing exacerbation upon exposure to sunlight. Both zinc oxide and titanium dioxide sunscreens (non-nano-sized and opaque) may be helpful as well as use of opaque photoprotective clothing.

Table 3.1 Heme biosynthethic pathway with enzymatic defects in porphyria

Location	Heme biosynthesis		Enzyme	Pathology	Inheritance	Acute	Cutaneous manifestations	Treatment options
	Glycine + succinyl-CoA							
Mitochondria	↓	←	Aminolevulinic acid synthase 2	X-linked sideroblastic anemia	X-linked recessive	No	N/A	N/A
	Delta aminolevulinic acid							
	↓	←	Aminolevulinic acid dehydratase	ALA dehydratase porphyria	Autosomal recessive	Yes	N/A	Intravenous hematin
	Porphobilinogen							
	↓	←	Hydroxymethylbilane synthase	Acute intermittent porphyria	Autosomal dominant	Yes	N/A	Intravenous hematin
Cytosol	Hydroxymethylbilane							
	↓	←	Uroporphyrinogen synthase	Congenital erythropoietic porphyria (Günther disease)	Autosomal recessive	No	Bullae, vesicles, skin thickening, hypo- and hyperpigmentation, hypertrichosis, scarring, loss of nails, loss of digits	Hydroxyurea, red blood transfusion, activated charcoal, bone marrow transplant
	Uroporphyrinogen III							
	↓	←	Uroporphyrinogen dehydrogenase	Porphyria cutanea tarda (PCT)/ hepatoerythropoietic porphyria (HEP)	Type I/ III - sporadic type II: autosomal dominant	No	PCT: vesicles, bullae, erosions heal with hyperpigmentation or atrophy, periorbital hypertrichosis, milia HEP: similar to PCT	Hydroxychloroquine [111], Phlebotomy [111] HEP: same as PCT

	Coproporphyrinogen III							
	↓	←	Coproporphyrinogen oxidase	Hereditary coproporphyria	Autosomal dominant	Yes	Skin lesions similar to PCT	Intravenous hematin
	Protoporphyrinogen IX							
Mitochondria	↓	←	Protoporphyrinogen oxidase	Variegate porphyria	Autosomal dominant	Yes	Similar to PCT but with milder symptoms	Intravenous hematin, dihydroxyacetone [112]
	Protoporphyrin IX							
	↓	←	Ferrochelatase	Erythropoietic protoporphyria	Pseudo-dominant	No	Pruritus, wheals, painful edema, erythema, petechiae, purpura, lichenification, thick pseudovesicles	Afamelanotide [113], cholestyramine, chenodeoxycholic acid [74], cysteine [114], beta carotene, activated charcoal, blood transfusion, intravenous hematin
	Heme							

All information adapted from Sassa [115] unless otherwise stated
Not shown in the above, nonenzymatic conversion of hydroxymethylbilane to uroporphyrinogen I and then to coproporphyrinogen I accounts for the photosensitivity resulting from uroporphyrinogen synthase deficiency

3.3.7 Pellagra

Pellagra is a vitamin deficiency disease lack of niacin result in a classic presentation of diarrhea, dementia with hallucinations, and photosensitive dermatitis. The presentation of this photosensitivity is an erythematous, edematous eruption with eventual scaling and hyperpigmentation. Deemed the "Casal collar" after its discoverer, this eruption occurs in a C3 and C4 dermatomal distribution. The reason for photosensitivity remains unclear with multiple etiologies being proposed: urocanic acid deficiency, kynurenic acid accumulation, nicotinamide adenine dinucleotide and nicotinamide adenine dinucleotide phosphate deficiency, or porphyrin accumulation [75]. There have been no controlled phototesting studies to define the action spectrum of this disorder though photosensitivity varies within the UVA, UVB, and visible light spectra [75]. Avoidance of UVR along with immediate supplementation of niacin can prevent worsening and resolution of the disease process.

3.3.8 Smith-Lemli-Opitz Syndrome

Smith-Lemli-Opitz syndrome (SLOS) is a rare autosomal recessive disease with 7-dehydrocholesterol-reductase deficiency resulting in accumulation of 7-dehydrocholesterol with overall low serum cholesterol levels. The phenotypic presentation is diverse, usually presenting with craniofacial deformities (microcephaly, micrognathia, ptosis, cleft lip and palate), skeletal deformities (syndactyly of second and third toes), and CNS abnormalities (decreased frontal lobe size and cerebellar hypoplasia) in the setting of mental delay. Though the specific absorption wavelengths of 7-dehydrocholesteral are 274, 283, and 293 nm [76], the most severe cutaneous responses occur following UVA exposure at 350 nm [76–78]. Management involves a high cholesterol diet and bile acid replacement [79]. A lack of studies on potential photoprotective strategies for SLOS cases demonstrate that photoprotection with clothing was most effective [76]. Broad-spectrum sunscreens with high SPF and opaque films for house and car windows in preventing UVA transmission have been reported to be beneficial [76].

3.4 Photoaggravated Disorders

Photoaggravated disorders comprise the widest and least specific group of photodermatoses. The only unifying factor among the disorders involves exacerbation by UVR exposure. The list of photoaggravated disorders is extensive: acne vulgaris, atopic dermatitis, bullous pemphigoid, carcinoid syndrome, cutaneous T-cell lymphoma, Darier's disease, dermatomyositis, disseminated superficial actinic porokeratosis, erythema multiforme, Grover's disease, lichen planus, lupus erythematosus, pemphigus, pityriasis rubra pilaris, psoriasis, reticular erythematous mucinosis, rosacea, seborrheic dermatitis, and various viral infections [3]. We will be discussing photoprotective strategies primarily in regard to lupus erythematosus and dermatomyositis.

3.4.1 Lupus Erythematosus

Lupus erythematosus may be subdivided into the following categories: systemic lupus erythematosus, acute lupus erythematosus, subacute cutaneous lupus erythematosus, and chronic lupus erythematosus. Chronic lupus erythematosus can be further subdivided into lupus erythematosus tumidus, lupus erythematosus profundus, and discoid lupus erythematosus [80]. Photosensitivity is not limited solely to the development of cutaneous reactions but also to the development of malaise and arthralgia in patients [81].

Briefly, UVR has been established as a trigger for exacerbations of the disease through many now well-characterized mechanisms. In a genetically susceptible individual, ROS cause DNA to exhibit some antigenicity resulting in the formation of autoantibodies [82, 83]. In addition, these newly apoptotic cells generated by UV exposure in the upper epidermal layer are cleared more slowly [84], resulting in the persistence of the inflammatory response. Redistribution of intracellular Ro/SS-A and La/SS-B proteins to cell surfaces following UVR exposure [85, 86] results in cell death via antibody-dependent cellular cytotoxicity [87, 88]. UVA, on the other hand, is able to penetrate into the deep dermis and cause oxidation of DNA most frequently at the 8 position of guanine [89] with eventual cell apoptosis.

The photosensitivity of the subtypes of lupus varies: tumid lupus erythematosus being the most photosensitive followed by subacute cutaneous lupus erythematosus, systemic lupus erythematosus, and finally discoid lupus erythematosus [90]. The action spectrum varies as well. While some studies show that phototherapy with UVA can reduce disease severity [91, 92], both UVA and UVB have been shown to worsen disease manifestations as well [93, 94]. Nonsolar sources of both UVA [95] and UVB [96] have also been implicated in causing photoexacerbation of the disease.

Sunscreens play a significant role in the prevention of exacerbation of cutaneous lupus erythematosus. An intraindividual study regarding the efficacy of different sunscreen formulations protecting against cutaneous LE development subjected a cohort of 11 patients to photoprovocation using a combination of UVA and UVB radiation [97]. All using the formulation of sunscreen with UVA blocking Mexoryl SX and Mexoryl XL received complete protection against photoprovocation [97]. While other sunscreens without Mexoryl SX and Mexoryl XL protected some individuals against photoprovocation, the majority of individuals did not receive sufficient protection to prevent the development of UVR-induced skin lesions [97]. Similar findings from an intraindividual study of 25 patients comparing a vehicle control (esters, vitamin E, parabens, o-cymen-5-ol, phenoxyethanol) to a broad-spectrum SPF 60 test product containing ethylhexyl methoxycinnamate, titanium dioxide, zinc oxide, and methylene bis-benzotriazolyl tetramethylbutylphenol with vehicle products showed no cutaneous manifestations of lupus erythematosus in the sunscreen group. Notably, 14 of the 25 developed a positive result in vehicle-treated group [98]. Results from this study buttress those initial results of Stege and colleagues: a broad-spectrum sunscreen of sufficient strength and proper formulation with appropriate UV filters is capable of preventing the worsening of cutaneous lesions seen in lupus.

3.4.2 Dermatomyositis

Dermatomyositis, a disease related to polymyositis, presents with early proximal muscle weakness in the setting of pathognomonic erythematous to violaceous papules on metacarpophalangeal and interphalangeal edematous periorbital, heliotrope eruptions. Other commonly afflicted cutaneous areas include the anterior chest (V-neck sign) or upper back and shoulders (shawl sign). There remains a paucity of information regarding the mechanisms of photosensitivity in dermatomyositis. Cheong and colleagues utilized monochromatic irradiation to demonstrate that 5 out of 10 total patients were photosensitive and their action spectra included UVB and UVA light at 307.5, 340, and 360 nm, respectively [99]. Dourmishev and colleagues found that 8 out of their 19 patients with dermatomyositis undergoing photoprovocation with UBV light had comparable photosensitivity to those reported by Cheong [100]. There is a paucity of information in the current literature regarding photoprotective strategies in dermatomyositis. We can only advocate that broad-spectrum sunscreens should be used, along with general photoprotection practices.

3.5 Hereditary Photodermatoses

Hereditary photodermatoses are caused by enzymatic mutations leading to defects in DNA repair. Those afflicted with these disorders are not solely plagued by cutaneous complications, but have multisystem abnormalities and are at a high propensity for developing malignancies. The following disorders can typically be grouped under this category: ataxia–telangiectasia, Bloom syndrome, Cockayne syndrome, Hailey–Hailey disease, Hartnup disease, Kindler syndrome, Rothmund–Thomson syndrome, trichothiodystrophy, and xeroderma pigmentosum [3]. Though SLO is often considered hereditary photodermatosis, we choose to include it as a photosensitive disorder due to endogenous accumulation of precursors photosensitivity. Xeroderma pigmentosum will be discussed in depth as the model for which photoprotection for all other hereditary photodermatoses should be based upon.

3.5.1 Xeroderma Pigmentosum

Xeroderma pigmentosum is a rare autosomal recessive disorder of DNA repair resulting in cutaneous and ocular photosensitivity and increased propensity for development of skin cancers. UVA and UVB light are implicated in disease pathogenesis, the visible light spectrum is not a cause of disease manifestation. Patients have nucleotide excision repair and can therefore not repair bulky the cyclobutane pyrimidine dimers [89]. Inability to repair these products causes accumulation of DNA mutations and cell apoptosis. Mutations in any of the following genes may cause xeroderma pigmentosum: XP-A, XP-B (excision-repair cross-complementing group 3 [ERCC3]), XP-C, XP-D (ERCC4), XP-G (DNA damage-binding protein 2 [DDP2]), ERCC1, and XP-V (POLH gene [encoding DNA polymerase eta]) [101]. Blistering and extensive burning in response to only minimal sunlight is the hallmark of this photodermatosis. Typically presenting in early childhood, neonates cry when exposed to sunlight. Extreme freckling on sun-exposed areas before 2 years of age is invariably seen. In addition, poikiloderma, xerosis, and actinic keratosis are commonly seen. Ocular manifestations of the disorder are usually limited to the anterior eye, being the most sun-exposed portion, and consist of keratitis and corneal opacification with vascularization. In severe cases, the palpebrae may become atrophic or lost completely contributing to further ocular damage. Melanomas, squamous cell carcinomas, and basal cell carcinomas are common in this group of individuals.

Photoprotective strategies involve the utilization of adequate personal photoprotective precautions with alteration of the environment so as to reduce opportunities for potential UVR exposure. For example, outdoor activities should be limited before sunrise and after sunset.

Specific attention should be given to the lighting used in homes. It has been reported that compact fluorescent lamps [102–104], energy-efficient halogen lights [104], and mercury vapor tubes [105] can be major sources of UVA radiation. The use of double envelope lamps can help minimize the dosage of UVR in these scenarios [106]. Incandescent light bulbs [107] and LED lights [103] have been recommended in the household because of the negligible UVR emitted. In homes and in cars, film blocking UVA and UVB can be applied [108, 109].

An application of at least 30 SPF, broad-spectrum sunscreens to sun-exposed areas should be stressed and performed every day. The importance of reapplying every 2 h to potentially UVR-exposed areas cannot be understated. Dark, tightly woven clothing should be layered for optimal protection. In addition, gloves should be worn to shield the dorsum of the hands. Given the propensity for ocular manifestations, a UVR protective face shield paired with a hood that covers the entire head and neck should be worn when at risk for prolonged exposure to UVR. To supplement this, tight fitting, wraparound sunglasses covering UVA and UVB light should be worn simultaneously to assure sufficient photoprotection of the face and eyes.

There have been few trials addressing efficacy medical therapy after sun exposure to reduce skin cancer development for those with xeroderma pigmentosum. The most notable prospective trial evaluating topical application of T4 endonuclease V, encapsulated in liposomes, has been reported to decrease the incidence of actinic keratosis by 68 % and by 30 % in patients with xeroderma pigmentosum [110]. No adverse effects or development of antibodies against the molecule was seen in the study group [110]. Though no additional studies have been reported since, results from the trial suggest that targeted drug delivery of enzymes may be a safe, therapeutic option for treating those afflicted with such devastating disease, and more work regarding this treatment modality should be explored.

Photoprotection for hereditary photodermatoses can be cumbersome due to the extensive methods that must be utilized, and so special considerations must be made as to facilitate compliance with photoprotective strategies. The finances of patient care should be assessed with families. Affordable sunscreens are suggested so as to not economically burden families. Specialized photoprotective clothing also exists and may be purchased.

3.6 Conclusions

Photoprotection involves a set of actions individuals can take to minimize their exposure to the damaging effects of UVR. The use of photoprotective clothing, wide-brimmed hats, sunglasses, and sunscreens along with sun avoidance practices provides the cornerstone of photoprotection. Depending on the specific disorder and the action spectra of the photodermatosis, one or more aforementioned practices can be tailored for the prevention of disease in an individual. Follow-up with primary care physicians and dermatologists should occur regularly to assess for changes in disease manifestation and responses to treatment.

References

1. Brenner M, Hearing V (2008) The protective role of melanin against UV damage in human skin. Photochem Photobiol 84(3):539–549
2. Diffey B, Kochevar I (2007) Basic principles of photobiology. In: Lim H, Honigsmann H, Hawk JL (eds) Photodermatology. Informa Healthcare, New York, pp 15–27
3. Santoro FA, Lim HW (2011) Update on photodermatoses. Semin Cutan Med Surg 30(4):229–238
4. Hölzle E, Plewig G, von Kries R, Lehmann P (1987) Polymorphous light eruption. J Invest Dermatol 88(3 Suppl):32s–38s
5. Norris PG, Morris J, McGibbon DM, Chu AC, Hawk JL (1989) Polymorphic light eruption: an immunopathological study of evolving lesions. Br J Dermatol 120(2):173–183
6. Lehmann P, Schwarz T (2011) Photodermatoses: diagnosis and treatment. Dtsch Arztebl Int 108(9):135–141
7. Labeling and effectiveness testing; sunscreen drug products for over-the-counter human use. 21 CFR Parts 201 and 310. Sect. Vol. 76, No. 117 (17 June 2011)
8. Bech-Thomsen N, Wulf HC (1992) Sunbathers' application of sunscreen is probably inadequate to obtain the sun protection factor assigned to the preparation. Photodermatol Photoimmunol Photomed. 9(6):242–244
9. Azurdia RM, Pagliaro JA, Diffey BL, Rhodes LE (1999) Sunscreen application by photosensitive patients is inadequate for protection. Br J Dermatol 140(2):255–258
10. Bissonnette R, Nigen S, Bolduc C (2012) Influence of the quantity of sunscreen applied on the ability to protect against ultraviolet-induced polymorphous light eruption. Photodermatol Photoimmunol Photomed 28(5):240–243
11. Gruber-wackernagel A, Byrne SN, Wolf P (2008) Pathogenic mechanisms of polymorphic light eruption. J Natl Cancer Inst Monogr 1:341–354

12. Man I, Dawe RS, Ferguson J (1999) Artificial hardening for polymorphic light eruption: practical points from ten years' experience. Photodermatol Photoimmunol Photomed 15:96–99
13. Patel DC, Bellaney GJ, Seed PT, McGregor JM, Hawk JL (2000) Efficacy of short-course oral prednisolone in polymorphic light eruption: a randomized controlled trial. Br J Dermatol 143(4):828–831
14. Nitiyarom R, Wongpraparut C (2014) Hydroa vacciniforme and solar urticaria. Dermatol Clin 32(3):345–353, viii
15. Millard TP, Hawk JLM (2002) Photosensitivity disorders: cause, effect and management. Am J Clin Dermatol 3(4):239–246
16. Mekkes JR, de Vries HJ, Kammeyer A (2003) Solar urticaria induced by infrared radiation. Clin Exp Dermatol 28(2):222–3
17. Schalka S, Sant'Anna Addor FA, Agelune CM, de Melo C, Pereira V (2012) Sunscreen protection against visible light: a new proposal for evaluation. Surg Cosmet Dermatol 3(4):45–52
18. Sayre R, Kollias N, Roberts R (1990) Physical sunscreens. J Soc Cosmet Chem 41(2):103–109
19. Bissonnette R, Nigen S, Bolduc C, Méry S, Nocera T (2008) Protection afforded by sunscreens containing inorganic sunscreening agents against blue light sensitivity induced by aminolevulinic acid. Dermatol Surg 34(11):1469–1476
20. Wolf R, Herzinger T, Grahovac M, Prinz JC (2013) Solar urticaria: long-term rush hardening by inhibition spectrum narrow-band UVB 311 nm. Clin Exp Dermatol 38(4):446–447
21. Roelandts R (1985) Pre-PUVA UVA, desensitization for solar urticaria. Photodermatol 2(3):174–176
22. Masuoka E (2012) Fukunaga a, Kishigami K, et al. Successful and long-lasting treatment of solar urticaria with ultraviolet A rush hardening therapy. Br J Dermatol 167(1):198–201
23. Haylett AK, Nie Z, Brownrigg M, Taylor R, Rhodes LE (2011) Systemic photoprotection in solar urticaria with α-melanocyte-stimulating hormone analogue [Nle4-D-Phe7]-α-MSH. Br J Dermatol 164(2):407–414
24. Fusaro RM, Rice EG (2005) The maillard reaction for sunlight protection. Ann N Y Acad Sci 1043:174–183
25. Maksimovic L, Frémont G, Jeanmougin M, Dubertret L, Viguier M (2009) Solar urticaria successfully treated with intravenous immunoglobulins. Dermatology 218(3):252–254
26. Hughes R, Cusack C, Murphy GM, Kirby B (2009) Solar urticaria successfully treated with intravenous immunoglobulin. Clin Exp Dermatol 34(8):e660–e662
27. Collins P, Ahamat R, Green C, Ferguson J (1996) Plasma exchange therapy for solar urticaria. Br J Dermatol 134(6):1093–7
28. Güzelbey O, Ardelean E, Magerl M, Zuberbier T, Maurer M, Metz M (2008) Successful treatment of solar urticaria with anti-immunoglobulin E therapy. Allergy 63(11):1563–5
29. Waibel KH, Reese DA, Hamilton RG, Devillez RL (2010) Partial improvement of solar urticaria after omalizumab. J Allergy Clin Immunol 125(2):490–491
30. Maurer M, Rosén K, Hsieh HJ, Saini S, Grattan C, Gimenéz-Arnau A, Agarwal S, Doyle R, Canvin J, Kaplan A, Casale T (2013) Omalizumab for the treatment of chronic idiopathic or spontaneous urticaria. N Engl J Med 368(10):924–935
31. Iwatsuki K, Satoh M, Yamamoto T, Oono T, Morizane S, Ohtsuka M, Xu ZG, Suzuki D, Tsuji K (2006) Pathogenic link between hydroa vacciniforme and Epstein-Barr virus–associated hematologic disorders. Arch Dermatol 142(5):587–95
32. Jacyk WK, Moosa Y (2010) Crusts and vacciniforme scars on sun-exposed skin. Clin Exp Dermatol 35(1):97–98
33. Halasz CL, Leach EE, Walther RR, Poh-Fitzpatrick MB (1983) Hydroa vacciniforme: induction of lesions with ultraviolet A. J Am Acad Dermatol 8(2):171–176
34. Sunohara A, Mizuno N, Sakai M, Kawabe Y, Sakakibara S (1988) Action spectrum for UV erythema and reproduction of the skin lesions in hydroa vacciniforme. Photodermatol 5(3):139–145

35. Iwatsuki K, Ohtsuka M, Akiba H, Kaneko F (1999) Atypical hydroa vacciniforme in childhood: from a smoldering stage to Epstein-Barr virus-associated lymphoid malignancy. J Am Acad Dermatol 40(2 Pt 1):283–284
36. Yamamoto T, Tsuji K, Suzuki D, Morizane S, Iwatsuki K (2007) A novel, noninvasive diagnostic probe for hydroa vacciniforme and related disorders: detection of latency-associated Epstein-Barr virus transcripts in the crusts. J Microbiol Methods 68(2):403–407
37. Huggins RH, Leithauser LA, Eide MJ, Hexsel CL, Jacobsen G, Lim HW (2009) Quality of life assessment and disease experience of patient members of a web-based hydroa vacciniforme support group. Photodermatol Photoimmunol Photomed 25(4):209–215
38. Gupta G, Man I, Kemmett D (2000) Hydroa vacciniforme: a clinical and follow-up study of 17 cases. J Am Acad Dermatol 42(2 Pt 1):208–213
39. Almeida HL, Kopp J, Jorge VM, Sartori DS, Velloso CD (2013) Extensive hydroa vacciniforme. An Bras Dermatol 88(4):620–2
40. Meola T, Sanchez M, Lim HW, Buchness MR, Soter NA (1997) Chronic actinic dermatitis associated with human immunodeficiency virus infection. Br J Dermatol 137(3):431–436
41. Kerr HA, Lim HW (2007) Photodermatoses in African Americans: a retrospective analysis of 135 patients over a 7-year period. J Am Acad Dermatol 57(4):638–643
42. Lim HW, Buchness MR, Ashinoff R, Soter NA (1990) Chronic actinic dermatitis. Study of the spectrum of chronic photosensitivity in 12 patients. Arch Dermatol 126(3):317–323
43. Russell SC, Dawe RS, Collins P, Man I, Ferguson J (1998) The photosensitivity dermatitis and actinic reticuloid syndrome (chronic actinic dermatitis) occurring in seven young atopic dermatitis patients. Br J Dermatol 138(3):496–501
44. Yap LM, Foley P, Crouch R, Baker C (2003) Chronic actinic dermatitis: a retrospective analysis of 44 cases referred to an Australian photobiology clinic. Australas J Dermatol 44(4):256–262
45. Robert S, Dawe JF (2003) Diagnosis and treatment of chronic actinic dermatitis. Dermatol Ther 16(1):45–51
46. Moseley H, Cameron H, MacLeod T, Clark C, Dawe R, Ferguson J (2001) New sunscreens confer improved protection for photosensitive patients in the blue light region. Br J Dermatol 145(5):789–794
47. Dawe R, Russell SFJ (1996) Borrowing from museums and industry: two photoprotective devices. Br J Dermatol 135(6):1016–7
48. Paek SY, Lim HW (2014) Chronic actinic dermatitis. Dermatol Clin 32(3):355–361, viii–ix
49. Leigh IM, Hawk JL (1984) Treatment of chronic actinic dermatitis with azathioprine. Br J Dermatol 110(6):691–695
50. Murphy GM, Maurice PD, Norris PG, Morris RW, Hawk JL (1989) Azathioprine treatment in chronic actinic dermatitis: a double-blind controlled trial with monitoring of exposure to ultraviolet radiation. Br J Dermatol 121(5):639–646
51. Ma Y, Lu Z (2010) Treatment with topical tacrolimus favors chronic actinic dermatitis: a clinical and immunopathological study. J Dermatolog Treat 21(3):171–177
52. Evans AV, Palmer RA, Hawk JLM (2004) Erythrodermic chronic actinic dermatitis responding only to topical tacrolimus. Photodermatol Photoimmunol Photomed 20(1):59–61
53. Uetsu N, Okamoto H, Fujii K, Doi R, Horio T (2002) Treatment of chronic actinic dermatitis with tacrolimus ointment. J Am Acad Dermatol 47(6):881–884
54. Larangeira de Almeida H (2005) Successful treatment of chronic actinic dermatitis with topical pimecrolimus. Int J Dermatol 44(4):343–344
55. Thomson MA, Stewart DG, Lewis HM (2005) Chronic actinic dermatitis treated with mycophenolate mofetil. Br J Dermatol 152(4):784–786
56. Toonstra J, Henquet CJ, van Weelden H, van der Putte SC, van Vloten WA (1989) Actinic reticuloid. A clinical photobiologic, histopathologic, and follow-u study of 16 patients. J Am Acad Dermatol 21(2 Pt 1):205–214
57. Norris PG, Camp RD, Hawk JL (1989) Actinic reticuloid: response to cyclosporine. J Am Acad Dermatol 21(2 Pt 1):307–309

58. Wiseman MC, Orr PH, Macdonald SM, Schroeder ML, Toole JW (2001) Actinic prurigo: clinical features and HLA associations in a Canadian Inuit population. J Am Acad Dermatol 44(6):952–956
59. Birt AR, Davis RA (1971) Photodermatitis in North American Indians: familial actinic prurigo. Int J Dermatol 10(2):107–114
60. Suárez A, Valbuena MC, Rey M, de Porras Quintana L (2006) Association of HLA subtype DRB10407 in Colombian patients with actinic prurigo. Photodermatol Photoimmunol Photomed 22(2):55–58. doi:10.1111/j.1600-0781.2006.00205.x
61. Zuloaga-Salcedo S, Castillo-Vazquez M, Vega-Memije E et al (2007) Class I and class II major histocompatibility complex genes in Mexican patients with actinic prurigo. Br J Dermatol 156(5):1074–1075
62. Du P, Menage H, Vaughan RW, Baker CS et al (1996) HLA-DR4 May determine expression of actinic prurigo in British patients. J Invest Dermatol 106(2):362–364
63. Ferguson J, Ibbotson S (1999) The idiopathic photodermatoses. Semin Cutan Med Surg 18(4):257–273
64. Ker KJ, Chong WS, Theng CTS (2013) Clinical characteristics of adult-onset actinic prurigo in Asians: a case series. Indian J Dermatol Venereol Leprol 79(6):783–788
65. Kerr AC, Ferguson J (2007) Actinic prurigo deterioration due to degradation of DermaGard window film. Br J Dermatol 157(3):619–620
66. Crouch R, Foley P, Baker C (2002) Actinic prurigo: a retrospective analysis of 21 cases referred to an Australian photobiology clinic. Australas J Dermatol 43(2):128–132
67. Daldon PE, Pascini M, Correa M (2010) Case for diagnosis. Actinic prurigo. An Bras Dermatol 85(5):733–735
68. Yong-Gee SA, Muir JB (2001) Long-term thalidomide for actinic prurigo. Australas J Dermatol 42(4):281–283
69. Trujillo MJ, de Barrio M, Rodríguez A, Moreno-Zazo M, Sánchez I, Pelta R, Tornero P, Herrero T (2001) Piroxicam-induced photodermatitis. Cross-reactivity among oxicams. A case report. Allergol Immunopathol (Madr) 29(4):133–136
70. Ikezawa Z, Kitamura K, Osawa J, Hariya T (1992) Photosensitivity to piroxicam is induced by sensitization to thimerosal and thiosalicylate. J Invest Dermatol 98(6):918–922
71. Gonçalo M, Figueiredo A, Tavares P, Ribeiro CA, Teixeira F, Baptista AP (1992) Photosensitivity to piroxicam: absence of cross-reaction with tenoxicam. Contact Dermatitis 27(5):287–290
72. Kutlubay Z, Sevim A, Engin B, Tüzün Y (2014) Photodermatoses, including phototoxic and photoallergic reactions (internal and external). Clin Dermatol 32(1):73–79
73. Björn LO, Huovinen P (2002) Phototoxicity. In: Björn LO (ed) Photobiology – the science of light and life, vol 18. Kluwer Academic Publishers, Dordrecht, pp 219–238
74. Chantorn R, Lim HW, Shwayder TA (2012) J Am Acad Dermatol 67(6):1093.e1–e18; quiz 1111–1112
75. Wan P, Moat S, Anstey A (2011) Pellagra: a review with emphasis on photosensitivity. Br J Dermatol 164(6):1188–1200
76. Charman CR, Ryan A, Tyrrell RM, Pearse AD, Arlett CF, Kurwa HA (1998) Photosensitivity associated with the Smith–Lemli–Opitz syndrome. Br J Dermatol 138(5):885–888
77. Anstey AV (1999) Photosensitivity in the Smith-Lemli-Opitz syndrome. Photodermatol Photoimmunol Photomed 15(6):217–218
78. Anstey AV, Ryan A, Rhodes LE, Charman CR, Arlett CF, Tyrrell RM, Taylor CR, Pearse AD (1999) Characterization of photosensitivity in the Smith-Lemli-Opitz syndrome : a new congenital photosensitivity syndrome. Br J Dermatol 141(3):406–415
79. Nwokoro NA, Mulvihill JJ (1997) Cholesterol and bile acid replacement therapy in children and adults with Smith-Lemli-Opitz (SLO/RSH) syndrome. Am J Med Genet 68(3):315–321
80. O'Gorman SM, Murphy GM (2014) Photoaggravated disorders. Dermatol Clin 32(3):385–398, ix
81. Zandman-Goddard G, Solomon M, Rosman Z, Peeva E, Shoenfeld Y (2012) Environment and lupus-related diseases. Lupus 21(3):241–250

82. Ashok B, Ali R (1999) Antigen binding characteristics of experimentally-induced antibodies against hydroxyl radical modified native DNA. Autoimmunity 29(1):11–19
83. Davis P, Russell A, Percy J (1976) Antibodies to UV light denatured DNA in systemic lupus erythematosus: detection by filter radioimmunoassay and clinical correlations. J Rheumatol 3(4):375–379
84. Kuhn A, Herrmann M, Kleber S, Beckmann-Welle M, Fehsel K, Martin-Villalba A, Lehmann P, Ruzicka T, Krammer PH, Kolb-Bachofen V (2006) Accumulation of apoptotic cells in the epidermis of patients with cutaneous lupus erythematosus after ultraviolet irradiation. Arthritis Rheum 54(3):939–950
85. LeFeber WP, Norris DA, Ryan SR, Huff JC, Lee LA, Kubo M, Boyce ST, Kotzin BL, Weston WL (1984) Ultraviolet light induces binding of antibodies to selected nuclear antigens on cultured human keratinocytes. J Clin Invest 74:1545–1551
86. Golan TD, Elkon KB, Gharavi AE, Krueger JG (1992) Enhanced membrane binding of autoantibodies to cultured keratinocytes of systemic lupus erythematosus patients after ultraviolet B/ultraviolet A irradiation. J Clin Invest 90(3):1067–1076
87. Furukawa F, Kanauchi H, Imamura S (1994) Susceptibility to UVB light in cultured keratinocytes of cutaneous lupus erythematosus. Dermatology 189(Suppl 1):18–23
88. Furukawa F, Kashihara-Sawami M, Lyons M, Norris D (1990) Binding of antibodies to the extractable nuclear antigens SS-A/Ro and SS-B/La is induced on the surface of human keratinocytes by ultraviolet light (UVL): implications for the pathogenesis of photosensitive cutaneous lupus. J Invest Dermatol 94(1):77–85
89. Baron ED, Suggs AK (2014) Introduction to photobiology. Dermatol Clin 32(3):255–266, vii
90. Medeiros V, Lim H (2010) Sunscreens in the management of photodermatoses. Skin Therapy Lett 15(6):1–3
91. Polderman MC, Huizinga TW, Le Cessie S, Pavel S (2001) UVA-1 cold light treatment of SLE: a double blind, placebo controlled crossover trial. Ann Rheum Dis 60(2):112–115
92. McGrath H, Martínez-Osuna P, Lee FA (1996) Ultraviolet-A1 (340–400 nm) irradiation therapy in systemic lupus erythematosus. Lupus 5(4):269–274
93. Walchner M, Messer G, Kind P (1997) Phototesting and photoprotection in LE. Lupus 6(2):167–174
94. Kuhn A, Sonntag M, Richter-Hintz D et al (2001) Phototesting in lupus erythematosus: a 15-year experience. J Am Acad Dermatol 45(1):86–95
95. Klein LR, Elmets CA, Callen JP (1995) Photoexacerbation of cutaneous lupus erythematosus due to ultraviolet A emissions from a photocopier. Arthritis Rheum 38(8):1152–1156
96. Rihner M, McGrath H (1992) Fluorescent light photosensitivity in patients with systemic lupus erythematosus. Arthritis Rheum 35(8):949–952
97. Stege H, Budde M, Grether-Beck S, Krutmann J (2000) Evaluation of the capacity of sunscreens to photoprotect lupus erythematosus patients by employing the photoprovocation test. Photodermatol Photoimmunol Photomed 16(6):256–259
98. Kuhn A, Gensch K, Haust M, Meuth A, Boyer F (2010) Photoprotective effects of a broad-spectrum sunscreen in ultraviolet-induced cutaneous lupus erythematosus : a randomized, vehicle-controlled, double-blind study. J Am Acad Dermatol 64(1):37–48
99. Cheong W, Hughes RV, Norris PG, Hawk JLM (1994) Cutaneous photosensitivity in dermatomyositis. Br J Dermatol 131(2):205–209
100. Dourmishev L, Meffert H, Piazena H (2004) Dermatomyositis: comparative studies of cutaneous photosensitivity in lupus erythematosus and normal subjects. Photodermatol Photoimmunol Photomed 20(5):230–234
101. Karalis A, Tischkowitz M, Millington GWM (2011) Dermatological manifestations of inherited cancer syndromes in children. Br J Dermatol 164(2):245–256
102. Fenton L, Ferguson J, Ibbotson S, Moseley H (2013) Energy-saving lamps and their impact on photosensitive and normal individuals. Br J Dermatol 169(4):910–915
103. Fenton L, Moseley H (2013) UV emissions from low energy artificial light sources. Photodermatol Photoimmunol Photomed 30(2–3):153–159

104. Fenton L, Ferguson J, Moseley H (2012) Analysis of energy saving lamps for use by photosensitive individuals. Photochem Photobiol Sci 11(8):1346–1355
105. Procaccini EM, Riccio G, Casula L, Posteraro G, Monfrecola G (1997) Thirty hours' evaluation of UVB-induced erythema by chromometry and microflowmetry. Dermatology 195(4):317–320
106. Khazova M, O'Hagan JB (2008) Optical radiation emissions from compact fluorescent lamps. Radiat Prot Dosimetry 131(4):521–525
107. Tamura D, DiGiovanna JJ, Khan SG, Kraemer KH (2014) Living with xeroderma pigmentosum: comprehensive photoprotection for highly photosensitive patients. Photodermatol Photoimmunol Photomed 30(2–3):146–152
108. Milota M, Jones DL, Cleaver J, Jamall IS (2011) Xeroderma pigmentosum family support group: helping families and promoting clinical initiatives. DNA Repair (Amst) 10(7):792–797
109. Webb S (2008) Xeroderma pigmentosum. BMJ 336(7641):444–446
110. Yarosh D, Klein J, O'Connor A, Hawk J, Rafal E, Wolf P (2001) Effect of topically applied T4 endonuclease V in liposomes on skin cancer in xeroderma pigmentosum: a randomised study. Xeroderma Pigmentosum Study Group. Lancet 357(9260):926–929
111. Cainelli T, Di Padova C, Marchesi L, Gori G, Rovagnati P, Podenzani SA, Bessone E, Cantoni L (1983) Hydroxychloroquine versus phlebotomy in the treatment of porphyria cutanea tarda. Br J Dermatol 108(5):593–600
112. Asawanonda P, Oberlender S, Taylor C (1999) The use of dihydroxyacetone for photoprotection in variegate porphyria. Int J Dermatol 38(12):916–8
113. Harms J, Lautenschlager S, Minder CE, Minder EI (2009) An alpha-melanocyte-stimulating hormone analogue in erythropoietic protoporphyria. N Engl J Med 360(3):306–307
114. Mathews-Roth MM, Rosner B (2002) Long-term treatment of erythropoietic protoporphyria with cysteine. Photodermatol Photoimmunol Photomed 18(6):307–309
115. Sassa S (2006) Modern diagnosis and management of the porphyrias. Br J Haematol 135(3):281–292

Chapter 4
Photoprotection and Photoaging

Ben J. Friedman, Henry W. Lim, and Steven Q. Wang

Key Points

- Photoaging refers to the long-term effects of ultraviolet radiation on chronically exposed skin.
- Clinical manifestations of photoaging include wrinkling, pigmentary alterations, and telangiectasias.
- Characteristic histopathological abnormalities underlie these clinical manifestations.
- Despite advances in skin rejuvenation technologies, photoprotection remains the most cost efficient and effective means of minimizing the clinical effects of photoaging.

4.1 Introduction

Situated at the interface between the viscera and the physical world, the skin provides protection from numerous environmental insults in real time. Although skin possesses remarkable resiliency, it undergoes characteristic, often undesirable

B.J. Friedman
Department of Dermatology, Henry Ford Medical Center,
Detroit, MI, USA

H.W. Lim
Department of Dermatology, Henry Ford Medical Center – New Center O,
Detroit, MI, USA

S.Q. Wang (✉)
Division of Dermatology, Memorial Sloan-Kettering Cancer Center, Basking Ridge, NJ, USA
e-mail: wants@mskcc.org

S.Q. Wang, H.W. Lim (eds.), *Principles and Practice of Photoprotection*,
DOI 10.1007/978-3-319-29382-0_4

functional and esthetic changes with time. One common paradigm in the study of skin aging is to differentiate between "intrinsic" and "extrinsic" skin aging, of which the first is a genetically influenced chronological process, while the latter is driven primarily by environmental factors [1]. Ultimately, both forms of aging interact in contributing to both a decline in skin structure and other cutaneous immunological, endocrinological, and neural functions. Recent work suggests that both genetic and environmental factors in skin aging may actually share common pathways [2].

Of the various harmful environmental factors contributing to extrinsic aging, ultraviolet (UV) light is considered to be the most significant and has also been the most widely studied. Photoaging (or dermatoheliosis) refers to the effects of long-term UV exposure and sun damage superimposed on intrinsically aging skin. Previous work has suggested that up to 80 % of facial aging may be attributable to UV, although other factors, such as cigarette smoking, may also promote premature facial wrinkling [3]. Photoaging is a universal phenomenon as the majority of light-skinned individuals manifest some form of chronic sun damage before the age of 50 [4].

Some of the clinico-morphological manifestations of photoaging include fine and coarse wrinkling, dyspigmentation, dry texture, increased laxity, telangiectasia, and solar purpura. These adverse changes in skin appearance and integrity often occur in parallel to the development of cutaneous malignances, a process referred to as photocarcinogenesis. Persons of lighter skin tone, or low Fitzpatrick skin type, and those with greater degrees of sun exposure (e.g., living in sunnier climates or working outdoors) are preferentially affected by photoaging [5–7]. Within individuals, sun-exposed areas such as the face, neck, extensor forearms and arms, and dorsal hands are among the most susceptible to these changes.

Underlying the clinico-morphological features of photoaged skin are specific histopathological alterations in epidermal and dermal structure. Ongoing research advances in photobiology have helped illuminate various key molecular pathways targeted by UV that induce these alterations. As the mechanisms of photoaging continue to be better understood, newer therapeutic strategies for reversing these processes and masking the photoaged phenotype continue to be developed. At the current time, the most cost-effective therapy still remains primary prevention in the form of sun avoidance, sun protective clothing, and use of sunscreens [8].

4.2 Clinical Manifestations of Photoaged Skin

The appearance of photoaged skin is characteristic, although interindividual variation does exist. These differences may depend on factors such as skin type, ethnic background, setting of greatest sun exposure (e.g., occupational vs. leisured), dress and hair styling practices, damage repair capacity, and other genetic predispositions [9, 10]. Individual features of photoaged skin may derive from damage at various levels of the skin, with key roles played by keratinocytes, melanocytes, endothelial cells, and fibroblasts serving as the cellular mediators of the observed changes. Pigmentary alterations and both fine and coarse wrinkling are

Table 4.1 Glogau classification of photoaging

Skin type	Clinical manifestations
I	No wrinkles Early photoaging: Mild pigmentary changes No keratoses Minimal wrinkles Minimal or no makeup
II	Wrinkles in motion Early to moderate photoaging: Early solar lentigines visible Keratoses palpable but not visible Parallel smile lines beginning to appear lateral to mouth Usually wears some foundation
III	Wrinkles at rest Advanced photoaging: Obvious dyschromia Visible keratoses Static wrinkling Always wears heavy foundation
IV	Only wrinkles Severe photoaging: Yellow-gray skin tone Prior skin malignancies Wrinkling without appreciable intervening normal skin Cannot wear makeup—"cakes and cracks"

Adapted from Ref. [13]

among the most prominent features seen with chronic UV exposure and are major constituents of various photoaging scales aimed at quantifying a given individual's degree of photodamage (Table 4.1) [11–14]. Other clinical features of photoaging include a dry leathery appearance, sallowness, vascular telangiectasia, sagging appearance, and fragility (aka solar purpura). This is in contrast to sun-protected skin, which ages in a more subtle fashion with increased laxity, fine wrinkling, and the development of seborrheic keratosis. It notably lacks the pigmentary and vascular changes characteristic of photoaging [15].

4.2.1 *Pigmentary Alteration*

Individuals of Caucasian and Asian descent who sustain chronic UV exposure are prone to developing solar lentigines (SLs). These benign lesions tend to present as fixed tan to dark brown macules and patches on chronically sun-exposed skin and are most commonly seen after the age of 50 (Fig. 4.1a) [16, 17]. SLs can be contrasted from ephelides, which, despite also being induced by UV and having a similar distribution and appearance to SLs, tend to be restricted to phototypes I and II, are dynamic (i.e., become more pigmented during the summer months), develop

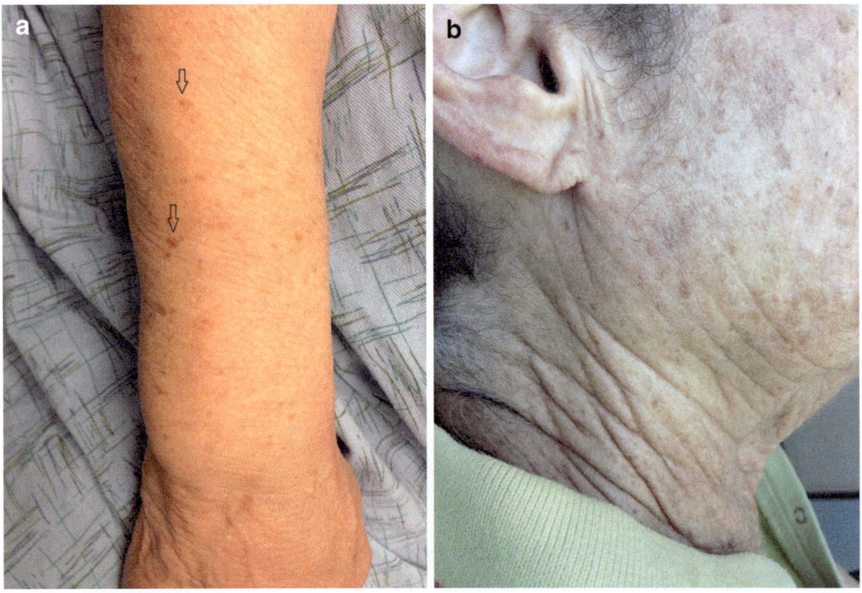

Fig. 4.1 *Clinical manifestations of photoaging*. (**a**) Multiple scattered solar lentigines are seen on this sun-damaged forearm (*indicated by black arrows*). (**b**) Coarse wrinkling is seen on the neck of this elderly Caucasian patient

early on in childhood and adolescence, and partially disappear with age [18]. SLs are actually seen more frequently in skin types III and IV, which has been thought to be a result of more active melanocytes in those skin types [19, 20].

There are multiple lines of evidence that support the relationship of SLs to sun exposure, beyond the observation that SLs have a predilection for sun-exposed skin. In one large epidemiological study ($n=962$), facial SLs were associated with cumulative lifetime sun exposure, while SLs on the back were associated with cumulative sun exposure and a sunburn history before the age of 20 [21]. Similar findings were captured by Ezzidine et al. who showed that SLs were associated with lifetime sun exposure in 523 French middle-age women [20]. A smaller case control study failed to demonstrate a link of SLs to cumulative or occupational sun exposure ($n=118$), but did find an association between SLs and both frequent sunburns and recreational sun exposure [19]. Additional indirect evidence supporting the link between photoaging and the development of SLs comes from the phenomenon of so-called PUVA lentigines. Patients treated with psoralens and ultraviolet A light (PUVA) for inflammatory skin conditions tend to develop lentigines in otherwise sun-protected areas [22, 23]. Although PUVA lentigines have definite histopathological differences as compared with SLs (including more active melanocytes with longer and more numerous dendrites and a higher frequency of basal keratinocytes containing large, single melanosomes), these may be explained by the higher potency and/or the pulse nature of PUVA treatment as compared with natural sunlight [24].

Hypermelanosis of the skin in the setting of chronic UV exposure may also manifest as mottled or heterogeneous pigmentation, diffuse hyperpigmentation, pigmented actinic keratoses, and/or pigmented seborrheic keratosis [25]. Malignant growths such as lentigo maligna and lentigo maligna melanoma represent less common causes of hypermelanosis in the skin, though they are almost exclusively seen in the context of sun damage. Idiopathic guttate hypomelanosis (IGH) is the most well-described yet poorly understood pattern of hypomelanosis seen in the context of skin aging. Seen in over 80 % of those over the age of 70, IGH occurs in all phototypes, though it is typically more apparent and striking in darker persons. IGH classically presents as well-circumscribed and sharply defined whitish macules with a predilection for the forearms and shins. Although chronic UV exposure has been postulated as a contributing factor to IGH, the cause may actually be multifactorial [26–28].

4.2.2 Wrinkling

One of the telltale signs of skin aging is wrinkling. These rippled changes in the skin surface presenting as variably sized creases and furrows may be most noticeable around the forehead, eyes, cheeks, and neck (Fig. 4.1b). In some patients, wrinkles may form interlacing patterns. Perhaps not surprisingly, studies have shown that there is a high correlation between perceived age and the degree of facial wrinkling in persons [29]. Various forms of wrinkling have been described. Dynamic wrinkles are those that temporarily result from contraction of underlying muscle fibers perpendicular to the direction of the visible skin lines. Over a period of time, these so-called facial expression lines may further deepen and develop a static component. Static wrinkles develop in thin stretched skin and are present even when underlying muscles are in a relaxed state.

The pathophysiology of wrinkling is complex, with likely contributions from intrinsic skin aging, constant gravitational forces, intermittent positional pressures, repetitive facial movements, pollution, and smoking [30]. Chronic UV exposure is thought to play a major role in accelerating and accentuating skin lines and wrinkles, though the precise histopathological correlate is still debated [31]. Furthermore, the presence of deep, coarser wrinkles are thought to be a more prominent feature of photoaged skin as compared with intrinsically aged skin [32]. In one recent cross-sectional study of a Mediterranean population ($n=574$), chronic sun exposure was found to be significantly associated with degree of wrinkling ($p<0.01$), as assessed by the Daniell skin-wrinkling grading system [33]. Multiple other studies have demonstrated similar associations [34–36].

4.2.3 Miscellaneous Phenotypes

There are a number of other phenotypic alterations that are seen with increasing age and have a predilection for sun-exposed skin and in which chronic UV exposure is thought to play a role. Sebaceous hyperplasia (SH) presents as small yellowish or skin-colored papules on the face or trunk, sometimes associated with a patulous follicle in which sebum can be extracted. UVA has been shown to be able to penetrate deep to the level of sebaceous glands, and experiments have shown that prolonged UV exposure in hairless mice induces prominent SH [37, 38] Colloid milia, a papular variant of solar elastosis (see Sect. 4.3), clinically manifests as closely spaced, dome-shaped translucent yellow papules with a predilection for the neck, face, and dorsal hands [39]. Poikiloderma of Civatte describes a pattern of reticulate hyperpigmentation, telangiectasia, and slight atrophy of the sides of the neck, lower anterior neck, and upper chest. The submental area, which is sun protected, is invariably spared in this condition [40]. Cutis rhomboidalis nuchae refers to deep furrowing, thickening, and a leathery appearance of the skin on the nape of the neck. Favre-Racouchot syndrome usually presents in older men as thickened yellow plaques with superimposed cysts and comedones in the periorbital and malar areas of the face [25].

4.3 Histopathology of Photoaged Skin

Multiple histopathological features characterize photoaged skin, which, in a given person, may differ both qualitatively and quantitatively in comparison to sun-protected skin. Of these features, the most recognizable and well described is solar elastosis (SE). SE is readily visualized in hematoxylin and eosin-stained sections as irregular deposits of basophilic material at the junction of the papillary and reticular dermis [1]. These deposits can extend to involve a variable thickness throughout the dermis (Fig. 4.2a). SE is thought to represent a degeneration of collagen, largely replaced by abnormally thickened, tangled, and subsequently granular-appearing amorphous elastin fibers [41–43]. Through various quantitative assays, it has been well documented that levels of type I and III collagen are significantly reduced in

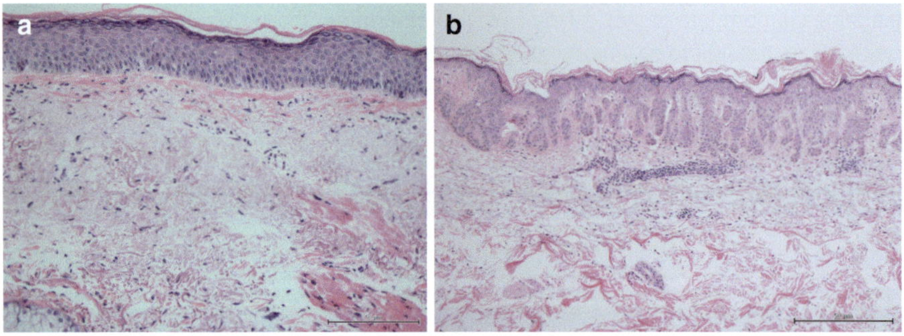

Fig. 4.2 *Histopathology of photoaging*. (**a**) Chronically sun-exposed skin demonstrating an effaced dermal-epidermal junction along with prominent solar elastosis filling the upper dermis. (**b**) Bulb-like elongation of the rete ridges with basilar hyperpigmentation, consistent with a solar lentigo

sun-exposed skin as compared with sun-protected skin [43, 44]. Additional dermal changes may include vasculature that is abnormally tortuous and dilated as well as postcapillary venules displaying concentric wall thickening with deposits of basement membrane-like material [45].

Epidermal thickness in photoaged skin can vary between individuals, demonstrating either atrophy with effacement of the dermal-epidermal junction, hypertrophy with acanthosis, or no appreciable change [43]. Basement membrane thickening can also be seen, which may signify chronic UV-mediated damage to the basal keratinocytes. Melanocytes are irregularly distributed along the basal layer and can vary widely in size, dendritic branching, and pigmentation [46, 47]. SL, when present, demonstrates bulb-like elongation of the rete ridges with increased pigmentation of the basal keratinocytes located at the rete tips (Fig. 4.2b). Not infrequently, biopsies of photoaged skin may display keratinocyte atypia, which presents as cellular crowding of large and hyperchromatic-appearing cells. The atypia may extend variably upward from the basal layer and is a marker of photo-carcinogenicity.

4.4 Molecular Mechanisms of Photoaging

Various cultural pressures combined with increased age expectancy have created a great demand for therapies which can restore a more youthful appearance. Crucial in the pursuit and ultimately the development of new antiaging therapies is achieving a more complete understanding of how chronic UV exposure initiates and propagates the clinical effects of photoaging. Perhaps not surprisingly, this area of photobiology has been and continues to be a subject of great interest and research. In recent years, there have been many new and exciting advancements in the field, which have begun to shed light on some of the key molecular pathways involved.

4.4.1 UV and Skin Biology

Both UVA (320–400 nm) and UVB (290–320) appear to contribute to photoaging, although UVA is thought to play a greater role among the two. This is largely due to the fact that UVA penetrates more deeply in the dermis and is at least 10 times more abundant than UVB when it reaches the earth's surface [48]. UVB is predominantly absorbed by DNA in the epidermis and in turn induces various forms of cellular damage through the formation of cyclobutane dimers. In this manner, UVB has been shown to be a key component in the pathogenesis of sunburn, cutaneous immunosuppression, and photocarcinogenicity [49]. In contrast, much of the damage inflicted by UVA is focused on dermal fibroblasts, extracellular matrix, and endothelial cells through the generation of reactive oxygen species (ROS). UVA-induced ROS have been shown to cause damage to various cellular compartments including lipid membranes, DNA, and mitochondria. This damage may take the form of lipid peroxidation, DNA strand breaks, and aberrant activation of transcription factors [50]. Epidermal melanin absorption of UV is perhaps the single most important endogenous protective factor against the deleterious effects of UVA and UVB and largely explains why darker individuals exhibit the clinical signs of photoaging much later in life as compared with fair-skinned individuals [51] (see 6.5.1).

4.4.2 UV and Extracellular Matrix

Induction of matrix metalloproteinases (MMPs) is thought to represent a key step in the development of the biochemical alterations seen in photoaged skin. MMPs represent a family of enzymes whose primary function is to degrade extracellular matrix (ECM). Moreover, each of the various MMPs serves to break down different components of the ECM. For example, MMP-1 (collagenase) has been shown to cleave collagen types 1, II, and III, while MMP-9 (92-kd gelatinase) is known to degrade collagen types IV, V, and gelatin [52]. The function and activity of these enzymes are regulated through complex processes, which intervene both at the level of MRNA transcription and posttranslational inhibition by tissue-specific inhibitors of MMPs (TIMPs) [53].

Multiple studies have confirmed the phenomenon that MMPs are induced by both UVA and UVB [54–56]. One paramount study demonstrated that in vivo exposure of human skin to low doses of UVB (0.1 minimal erythema dose), within hours, induced the expression of MMP-1, MMP-3 (stromelysin), and MMP-9 [57]. Also upregulated within minutes of UV exposure were NF-kB and AP-1, transcription factors known to stimulate the expression of MMPs [58, 59]. The implications of this work were that elevated MMPs, likely stimulated by the actions of AP-1 and NF-kB in the setting of chronic low intensity UV exposure, promote the gradual degradation of cutaneous collagen and elastin. Repetitive damage in this manner, if improperly repaired, has been proposed to contribute in the accumulation of solar elastosis and other features characteristic of premature, photoaged skin [60].

In addition to promoting collagen degradation, UV has also been implicated in reducing dermal collagen production [44]. In vivo, UV irradiation has been shown to reduce and ultimately deplete cutaneous procollagen levels within 24 h [61]. Collagen production is normally stimulated by TGF-B2. However, it has been shown that expression of TGF-B2 along with its receptor is markedly reduced in response to UV irradiation [62]. The upstream mediator of these changes may be c-Jun, which is the known inducible subunit of AP-1 [61]. In one in vitro model, overexpression of c-Jun in fibroblasts led to the decreased expression of type I collagen [61].

Subsequent investigations have begun to further fill in knowledge gaps regarding the specific mechanisms and mediators involved in UV-dependent collagen degradation and reduced collagen formation (Fig. 4.3) [63]. As mentioned above, UV radiation (especially UVA, but also UVB to some degree) promotes the formation of ROS. Accumulating evidence suggests that UV-induced ROS can actually mimic the effects of receptor ligands [7, 64, 65]. Support for this phenomenon comes from the fact that after only 15 min of exposure to UV, receptors for epidermal growth

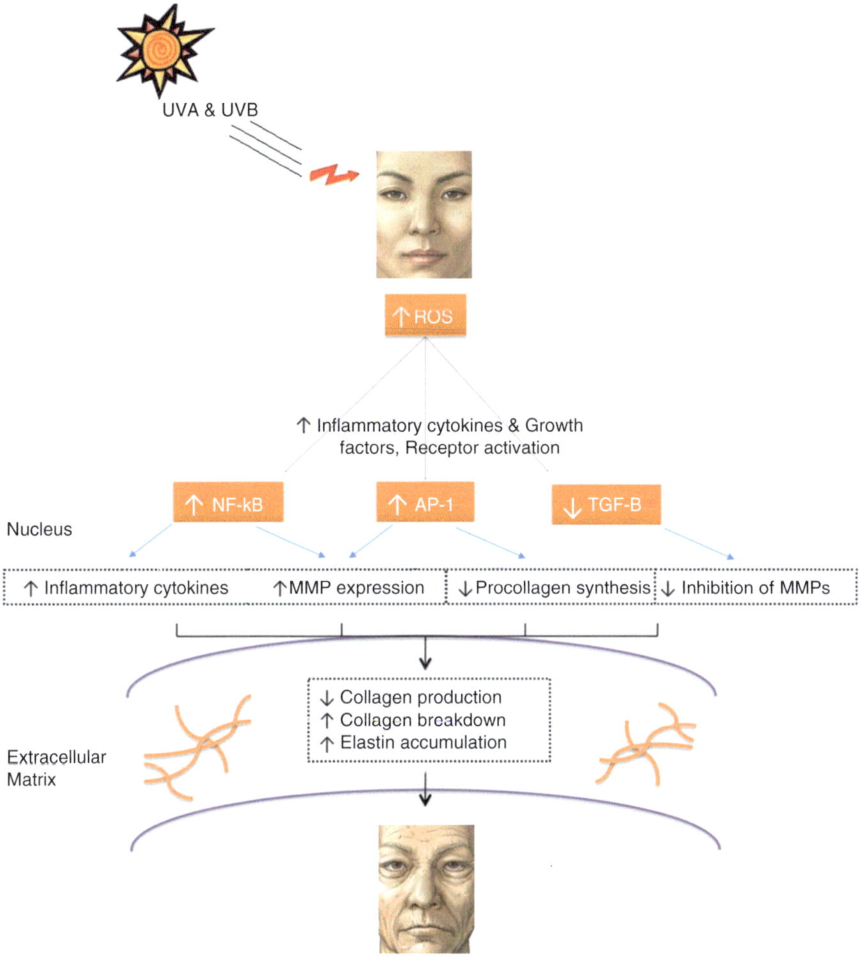

Fig. 4.3 Schematic demonstrating the various key molecular steps thought to be involved in photoaging (Adapted from Ref. [63])

factor (EGF), IL-1, and TNF-a are all activated in both keratinocytes and fibroblasts [7]. Activation of these key proinflammatory receptors has been proposed to result from ROS-induced oxidation and subsequent inhibition of protein-tyrosine phosphatases which normally function to downregulate these receptors [64, 66].

4.5 Photoprotection

Consistent use of a proper photoprotective regimen is likely as important in the management and prevention of photoaging as it is in the defense against the acute, harmful effects of UV [67]. The various forms of photoprotection which include endogenous factors, sun avoidance, shade, sun-protective clothing, and sunscreens are all likely to be important. Although there have been only a few controlled trials evaluating the long-term effects of photoprotection on photoaging (largely due to inherent difficulties in study design), various observational reports support its effectiveness in prevention [68, 69]. Despite the many new expensive technologies available for treating the clinical manifestations of photoaging, photoprotection remains the gold standard preventive strategy. It also continues to be the most cost-effective modality that can be offered to patients [70].

4.5.1 Natural Skin Protection

As mentioned above, darker skin types tend to display the clinical signs of photoaging much later in life as compared with lighter skin types [51]. This is largely attributable to the increase in melanin in darker skin, which absorbs and scatters detrimental UV rays [6]. An increase in melanin production occurs routinely in response to UV irradiation and is one natural defense mechanism against photocarcinogenesis and photoaging. This tanning response has previously been shown to be induced by oligonucleotides containing thymine dinucleotides (pTpT), which are formed as a result of UV damage [71]. Epidermal thickness is another inherent property of the skin influencing the penetration of UV. A reactive increase in skin thickness is a second intrinsic protective mechanism, with one study demonstrating increased epidermal and dermal mitotic activity 24–48 h after acute UV exposure [72].

The presence of antioxidants may also blunt the chronic effects of UV. The skin is equipped with a wide array of antioxidants, which normally serve to provide protection against oxidative stress developing in the context cellular respiration. A few notable ones include vitamin E, coenzymeQ10 (CoQ10), ascorbate, carotenoids, superoxide dismutase, catalase, and glutathione peroxidase [73]. There is indirect evidence to suggest that these antioxidants may also be important in the skin's defense against UV exposure, which, as previously discussed, is known to generate harmful ROS (see 6.4.1). UV irradiation has been shown to transiently deplete levels of cutaneous antioxidants [74]. It has been postulated that if such a depletion were to persist, increased tissue damage and subsequent premature photoaging might occur [75].

4.5.2 Sunscreen

There have been only two randomized control studies performed to date investigating the effects of sunscreen on photoaging. The first involved 53 patients with a history of skin cancer who were randomly assigned to apply either sunscreen or placebo at least twice a day. Skin biopsies were taken from preauricular skin at 0, 12, and 24 months, and epithelial thickness and dermal elastosis were assessed by blinded raters. Although 34 patients completed the study, complete data was only secured from 16. At 24 months, there was significantly less elastosis among the sunscreen group compared with the placebo group, but when repeated measurements were accounted for in the analysis, no differences were observed between the treatment groups [76].

The Nambour trial was a population-based intervention study conducted on a community of adult residents living in Queensland, Australia, in the early 1990s [77]. Subjects were categorized as daily sunscreen users versus discretionary sunscreen users, depending on whether they were randomized to apply study-provided sunscreen every day or to use their own discretion as to when/and if to apply sunscreen. 903 adults under the age of 55 (mean age 39 years) had silicone-based impressions taken on the dorsal left hand at baseline and then 4 years later. The presence and severity of photoaging was assessed by blinded raters using the Beagley and Gibson scale of microtopography grades, a previously validated method for predicting the extent of dermal elastosis [78]. At the conclusion of the follow-up period, the daily sunscreen group showed no detectable increase in skin aging. Moreover, as compared with discretionary sunscreen users, daily sunscreen users were 24 % less likely to show increased skin aging (relative odds = 0.76; 95 % CI = 0.50–0.98) [79].

4.6 Conclusion

Photoaging is a progressive process that results from cumulative sun exposure, superimposed on intrinsically aging skin. Some are more severely affected than others, though the phenomenon is largely universal. It represents a significant cost burden to many societies, given its aesthetic undesirability and the many existing cultural pressures to maintain a youthful appearance. The complicated mechanisms underlying photoaging continue to be better understood, though much still remains unknown. Although treatment options are increasing with time, prevention with photoprotection is the most cost-effective and safest approach to maintaining youthful-appearing skin over time.

References

1. Kligman AM (1969) Early destructive effect of sunlight on human skin. JAMA 210(13): 2377–2380
2. Goukassian DA, Gilchrest BA (2004) The interdependence of skin aging, skin cancer, and DNA repair capacity: a novel perspective with therapeutic implications. Rejuvenation Res 7(3):175–185
3. Uitto J (1997) Understanding premature skin aging. N Engl J Med 337(20):1463–1465
4. Drake LA et al (1996) Guidelines of care for photoaging/photodamage. American Academy of Dermatology. J Am Acad Dermatol 35(3 Pt 1):462–464

5. Fitzpatrick TB (1975) Soleil et peau. J Med Esthet 2:33–34
6. Kaidbey KH et al (1979) Photoprotection by melanin–a comparison of black and Caucasian skin. J Am Acad Dermatol 1(3):249–260
7. Fisher GJ et al (2002) Mechanisms of photoaging and chronological skin aging. Arch Dermatol 138(11):1462–1470
8. Seite S, Fourtanier AM (2008) The benefit of daily photoprotection. J Am Acad Dermatol 58(5 Suppl 2):S160–S166
9. Berneburg M, Plettenberg H, Krutmann J (2000) Photoaging of human skin. Photodermatol Photoimmunol Photomed 16(6):239–244
10. Goh SH (1990) The treatment of visible signs of senescence: the Asian experience. Br J Dermatol 122(Suppl 35):105–109
11. Glogau RG (1996) Aesthetic and anatomic analysis of the aging skin. Semin Cutan Med Surg 15(3):134–138
12. Larnier C et al (1994) Evaluation of cutaneous photodamage using a photographic scale. Br J Dermatol 130(2):167–173
13. Griffiths CE et al (1992) A photonumeric scale for the assessment of cutaneous photodamage. Arch Dermatol 128(3):347–351
14. Glogau RG (1994) Chemical peeling and aging skin. J Geriatr Dermatol 2:30–35
15. Gilchrest BA (1989) Skin aging and photoaging: an overview. J Am Acad Dermatol 21(3 Pt 2):610–613
16. Cario-Andre M et al (2004) Perilesional vs. lesional skin changes in senile lentigo. J Cutan Pathol 31(6):441–447
17. Hodgson C (1963) Senile lentigo. Arch Dermatol 87:197–207
18. Plensdorf S, Martinez J (2009) Common pigmentation disorders. Am Fam Physician 79(2):109–116
19. Monestier S et al (2006) Multiple senile lentigos of the face, a skin ageing pattern resulting from a life excess of intermittent sun exposure in dark-skinned caucasians: a case-control study. Br J Dermatol 154(3):438–444
20. Ezzedine K et al (2013) Freckles and solar lentigines have different risk factors in Caucasian women. J Eur Acad Dermatol Venereol 27(3):e345–e356
21. Bastiaens M et al (2004) Solar lentigines are strongly related to sun exposure in contrast to ephelides. Pigment Cell Res 17(3):225–229
22. Abel EA et al (1985) PUVA-induced melanocytic atypia: is it confined to PUVA lentigines? J Am Acad Dermatol 13(5 Pt 1):761–768
23. Rhodes AR, Stern RS, Melski JW (1983) The PUVA lentigo: an analysis of predisposing factors. J Invest Dermatol 81(5):459–463
24. Nakagawa H et al (1984) Morphologic alterations of epidermal melanocytes and melanosomes in PUVA lentigines: a comparative ultrastructural investigation of lentigines induced by PUVA and sunlight. J Invest Dermatol 82(1):101–107
25. Bilac C, Sahin MT, Ozturkcan S (2014) Chronic actinic damage of facial skin. Clin Dermatol 32(6):752–762
26. Loquai C et al (2005) Confetti-like lesions with hyperkeratosis: a novel ultraviolet-induced hypomelanotic disorder? Br J Dermatol 153(1):190–193
27. Whitehead WJ, Moyer DG, Vander Ploeg DE (1966) Idiopathic guttate hypomelanosis. Arch Dermatol 94(3):279–281
28. Kaya TI et al (2005) Idiopathic guttate hypomelanosis: idiopathic or ultraviolet induced? Photodermatol Photoimmunol Photomed 21(5):270–271
29. Warren R et al (1991) Age, sunlight, and facial skin: a histologic and quantitative study. J Am Acad Dermatol 25(5 Pt 1):751–760
30. Ernster VL et al (1995) Facial wrinkling in men and women, by smoking status. Am J Public Health 85(1):78–82
31. Kligman AM, Zheng P, Lavker RM (1985) The anatomy and pathogenesis of wrinkles. Br J Dermatol 113(1):37–42

32. Langton AK et al (2010) A new wrinkle on old skin: the role of elastic fibres in skin ageing. Int J Cosmet Sci 32(5):330–339
33. Ekiz O et al (2012) Factors influencing skin ageing in a Mediterranean population from Turkey. Clin Exp Dermatol 37(5):492–496
34. Chung JH et al (2001) Cutaneous photodamage in Koreans: influence of sex, sun exposure, smoking, and skin color. Arch Dermatol 137(8):1043–1051
35. Rexbye H et al (2006) Influence of environmental factors on facial ageing. Age Ageing 35(2):110–115
36. Raduan AP, Luiz RR, Manela-Azulay M (2008) Association between smoking and cutaneous ageing in a Brazilian population. J Eur Acad Dermatol Venereol 22(11):1312–1318
37. Lesnik RH, Kligman LH, Kligman AM (1992) Agents that cause enlargement of sebaceous glands in hairless mice. II. Ultraviolet radiation. Arch Dermatol Res 284(2):106–108
38. Zouboulis CC, Boschnakow A (2001) Chronological ageing and photoageing of the human sebaceous gland. Clin Exp Dermatol 26(7):600–607
39. Innocenzi D et al (1993) UV-induced colloid milium. Clin Exp Dermatol 18(4):347–350
40. Katoulis AC et al (2005) Poikiloderma of Civatte: a clinical and epidemiological study. J Eur Acad Dermatol Venereol 19(4):444–448
41. Mitchell RE (1967) A light and electron microscopical study of collagen degeneration. Aust N Z J Surg 36(4):310–318
42. Smith JG Jr et al (1962) Alterations in human dermal connective tissue with age and chronic sun damage. J Invest Dermatol 39:347–350
43. El-Domyati M et al (2002) Intrinsic aging vs. photoaging: a comparative histopathological, immunohistochemical, and ultrastructural study of skin. Exp Dermatol 11(5):398–405
44. Talwar HS et al (1995) Reduced type I and type III procollagens in photodamaged adult human skin. J Invest Dermatol 105(2):285–290
45. Lavker RM, Kligman AM (1988) Chronic heliodermatitis: a morphologic evaluation of chronic actinic dermal damage with emphasis on the role of mast cells. J Invest Dermatol 90(3):325–330
46. Gilchrest BA, Blog FB, Szabo G (1979) Effects of aging and chronic sun exposure on melanocytes in human skin. J Invest Dermatol 73(2):141–143
47. Breathnach AS, Wyllie LM (1964) Electron microscopy of melanocytes and melanosomes in freckled human epidermis. J Invest Dermatol 42:389–394
48. Yaar M, Gilchrest BA (2007) Photoageing: mechanism, prevention and therapy. Br J Dermatol 157(5):874–887
49. Benjamin CL et al (2008) p53 tumor suppressor gene: a critical molecular target for UV induction and prevention of skin cancer. Photochem Photobiol 84(1):55–62
50. Han A, Chien AL, Kang S (2014) Photoaging. Dermatol Clin 32(3):291–299, vii
51. Montagna W, Carlisle K (1991) The architecture of black and white facial skin. J Am Acad Dermatol 24(6 Pt 1):929–937
52. Sternlicht MD, Werb Z (2001) How matrix metalloproteinases regulate cell behavior. Annu Rev Cell Dev Biol 17:463–516
53. Scharffetter-Kochanek K (1997) Photoaging of the connective tissue of skin: its prevention and therapy. Adv Pharmacol 38:639–655
54. Fisher GJ et al (1997) Pathophysiology of premature skin aging induced by ultraviolet light. N Engl J Med 337(20):1419–1428
55. Scharffetter K et al (1991) UVA irradiation induces collagenase in human dermal fibroblasts in vitro and in vivo. Arch Dermatol Res 283(8):506–511
56. Koivukangas V et al (1994) UV irradiation induces the expression of gelatinases in human skin in vivo. Acta Derm Venereol 74(4):279–282
57. Fisher GJ et al (1996) Molecular basis of sun-induced premature skin ageing and retinoid antagonism. Nature 379(6563):335–339
58. Sato H, Seiki M (1993) Regulatory mechanism of 92 kDa type IV collagenase gene expression which is associated with invasiveness of tumor cells. Oncogene 8(2):395–405

59. Angel P et al (1987) Phorbol ester-inducible genes contain a common cis element recognized by a TPA-modulated trans-acting factor. Cell 49(6):729–739
60. Fisher GJ, Voorhees JJ (1998) Molecular mechanisms of photoaging and its prevention by retinoic acid: ultraviolet irradiation induces MAP kinase signal transduction cascades that induce Ap-1-regulated matrix metalloproteinases that degrade human skin in vivo. J Investig Dermatol Symp Proc 3(1):61–68
61. Fisher GJ et al (2000) c-Jun-dependent inhibition of cutaneous procollagen transcription following ultraviolet irradiation is reversed by all-trans retinoic acid. J Clin Invest 106(5): 663–670
62. Quan T et al (2002) Ultraviolet irradiation alters transforming growth factor beta/smad pathway in human skin in vivo. J Invest Dermatol 119(2):499–506
63. Chen L, Hu JY, Wang SQ (2012) The role of antioxidants in photoprotection: a critical review. J Am Acad Dermatol 67(5):1013–1024
64. Gross S et al (1999) Inactivation of protein-tyrosine phosphatases as mechanism of UV-induced signal transduction. J Biol Chem 274(37):26378–26386
65. Heck DE et al (2004) Solar ultraviolet radiation as a trigger of cell signal transduction. Toxicol Appl Pharmacol 195(3):288–297
66. Barford D, Jia Z, Tonks NK (1995) Protein tyrosinc phosphatases take off. Nat Struct Biol 2(12):1043–1053
67. Kimlin MG, Guo Y (2012) Assessing the impacts of lifetime sun exposure on skin damage and skin aging using a non-invasive method. Sci Total Environ 425:35–41
68. Ichihashi M et al (2003) UV-induced skin damage. Toxicology 189(1-2):21–39
69. Grob JJ et al (1993) Study of sunbathing habits in children and adolescents: application to the prevention of melanoma. Dermatology 186(2):94–98
70. Glaser DA (2003) Anti-aging products and cosmeceuticals. Facial Plast Surg Clin North Am 11(2):219–227
71. Gilchrest BA, Eller MS (1999) DNA photodamage stimulates melanogenesis and other photoprotective responses. J Investig Dermatol Symp Proc 4(1):35–40
72. Epstein JH, Fukuyama K, Fye K (1970) Effects of ultraviolet radiation on the mitotic cycle and DNA, RNA and protein synthesis in mammalian epidermis in vivo. Photochem Photobiol 12(1):57–65
73. Shindo Y et al (1994) Enzymic and non-enzymic antioxidants in epidermis and dermis of human skin. J Invest Dermatol 102(1):122–124
74. Fuchs J (1998) Potentials and limitations of the natural antioxidants RRR-alpha-tocopherol, L-ascorbic acid and beta-carotene in cutaneous photoprotection. Free Radic Biol Med 25(7):848–873
75. Shindo Y, Hashimoto T (1997) Time course of changes in antioxidant enzymes in human skin fibroblasts after UVA irradiation. J Dermatol Sci 14(3):225–232
76. Boyd AS et al (1995) The effects of chronic sunscreen use on the histologic changes of dermatoheliosis. J Am Acad Dermatol 33(6):941–946
77. Green A et al (1994) The Nambour skin cancer and actinic eye disease prevention trial: design and baseline characteristics of participants. Control Clin Trials 15(6):512–522
78. Hughes MC et al (2012) Validation of skin surface microtopography as a measure of skin photoaging in a subtropical population aged 40 and over. Photodermatol Photoimmunol Photomed 28(3):153–158
79. Hughes MC et al (2013) Sunscreen and prevention of skin aging: a randomized trial. Ann Intern Med 158(11):781–790

Chapter 5
Photoprotection, Photoimmunology and Autoimmune Diseases

Gillian M. Murphy and Nicola Ralph

Key Points

- There are several autoimmune diseases that are known to be aggravated by sun exposure, such as lupus erythematosus and dermatomyositis.
- Both UVB and UVA have been implicated in lupus erythematosus, and UVB has been implicated in dermatomyositis.
- Photoprotection is an important part of management in these patients.

5.1 Photoprotection

Photoprotection may be considered as innate mechanisms determined by genetic responses to minimize cellular damage to ultraviolet radiation (UVR) and visible light; but also measures adopted by the individual to reduce exposure to such radiation. Solar radiation has complex effects which include local effects on skin and eye but also systemic effects, mainly immunological. Local skin effects are determined by wavelength, the shortest wavelengths having mainly epidermal effects and longer wavelengths penetrating deeper into dermis and with visible light even through to fat and muscle. UVB has direct effects on cellular DNA; UVA though does have direct DNA effects and indirect effects mediated via oxidative stress. This chapter confines discussion to adopted measures for photoprotection which for the most

G.M. Murphy, MD, FRCI, FRCP Edin (✉)
National Photobiology Unit, Beaumont Hospital and Mater Misericordiae Hospital, Dublin, Ireland
e-mail: gillianmmurphy@gmail.com

N. Ralph, MRCP
National Photobiology Unit, Mater Misericordiae Hospital, Dublin, Ireland
e-mail: nicolaralph@hotmail.com

S.Q. Wang, H.W. Lim (eds.), *Principles and Practice of Photoprotection*,
DOI 10.1007/978-3-319-29382-0_5

part include behaviour to avoid undue exposure to UVR, the use of UV protective clothing and the use of sunscreens.

When UVR hits the skin, the photons are either absorbed, reflected back by the stratum corneum, or scattered within the skin and subsequently absorbed by chromophore(s). Keratin is very protective, so areas of the body with thick layers of keratin such as palms and heels are well protected. Melanin is more complex; dark-skinned people have mainly eumelanin as the protective pigment in skin, whereas fair-skinned people have pigment comprised of eumelanin and phaeomelanin, the latter being yellow/red in appearance. Eumelanin absorbs UVR and dissipates energy harmlessly. Phaeomelanin is more photochemically active and generates free radicals which lead to DNA damage. Over time direct DNA damage and indirect oxidative stress, unless repaired, can give rise to the adverse consequences of exposure to UV radiation which include photoaging, photodermatoses and photocarcinogenesis.

Photoprotection may be achieved by limiting ones' personal UVR exposure. The main ways to achieve this include sun avoidance at times of UVR increased intensity, i.e., midday ±3 h, awareness of the effects of latitude, altitude and prolonged exposure especially in summer months, seeking of shade, wearing of UVR protective clothing/broad-brimmed hat and the use of sun-protective products. The majority of our personal exposure to UVR comes from sun exposure. Other additional sources include artificial lighting, medical equipment, tanning booths, etc. The amount of sunlight we receive depends on ambient UV, our surrounding environment and our behaviour. Geographical location, cloud cover, terrain (snow, white sand, sparkling/rippling water) and surrounding environment (urban/open space) all affect our total exposure to UV radiation. Some of these considerations are beyond our control; however, our behaviour while outdoors can have a significant impact on our personal exposure to UV light. Our work environment; the time we spend outdoors, where we take part in physical activities; and overseas holidays all affect our total UV exposure.

Photoprotection can be achieved in four ways. The first three are essentially free and the last, the more expensive way of protecting oneself from UV radiation, is the most advertised method.

1. Sun avoidance – considerable protection from UV exposure can be achieved by avoiding the 3 h surrounding solar noon (for both temperate and tropical latitudes). During this time approximately 50 % of the day's total UV exposure during summer occurs.
2. Shade – this can be provided by natural objects such as trees and cliffs or by man-made buildings, umbrellas, etc. At noon, 50 % of the UV reaching our skin comes from direct sunlight and the other half is from scatter from the sky. Shade will remove all of the direct sunlight that reaches our skin. Shade can also remove part of the diffuse (scattered) sunlight.
3. Protective clothing/hats – the level of UV protection is primarily based on the tightness of the garment's weave; hence tightly woven cotton offers good protection. This has been extensively tested by the Australian Radiation

Protection and Nuclear Safety Agency (ARPANSA) [1] and other regulatory agencies. It has been shown that regular clothing provides good sun protection; hence specialized clothing is not necessary in order to be adequately protected from the sun.
4. Sunscreens – these are the most popular means of photoprotection. In order for them to provide good protection from UV exposure, they should have safe and effective ingredients, stability including photostability and a good physical structure which feels comfortable on the skin so that compliance rates are high and should be reliable (namely, realistic claims regarding their SPF/UVA protection/water resistance).

Ideally one should practice sun avoidance during peak times, first and foremost, followed by a combination of shade seeking, protective clothing/hat and the use of sunscreens.

5.2 Photoimmunology

This is the study of the effects of solar radiation on the immune system. Solar radiation is divided into different regions of the electromagnetic spectrum, UVC (<280 nm), UVB (280–315 nm) and UVA (315–400 nm), which is CIE (Commission Internationale l'Eclairage) [2] definition based on physiological effects by photons in those regions. The concept that UV, which is a part of the external environment, can affect the immune response, whose components are internal, arose from experiments in the 1970s by Kripke et al. [3] aimed at discovering a role for the immune response in rejecting UV radiation-induced skin cancer cells [4]. Their work demonstrated that UV radiation exerted suppressive effects on immune responses to UV-induced skin cancer cells and that the inhibition of tumour rejection could be adoptively transferred by T lymphocytes in an antigen-specific manner. Many laboratories have subsequently studied this topic and revealed details on how UV radiation induced the suppression of immune responses (also known as 'immune tolerance'). This suppression was observed not only for skin cancers but also infectious agents and chemical antigens. UVR affects the immune response by affecting the cells and other components of the immune system to alter the balance and functions of immune cells to infectious agents, chemicals and skin cancer. We know sunlight is immunosuppressive, as UVB depletes Langerhans cells and diminishes their function such that antigens are not presented efficiently to the immune system [5, 6]. Alterations in delayed hypersensitivity also occur such that if a universal allergen is applied to UV-irradiated skin, no response occurs; rather a population of antigen-specific T cells displaying tolerance to the antigen emerges. In mouse models, tolerance may be passively transferred to other mice conferring tolerance to the antigen. These observations also apply to UV-induced skin tumours, underwriting the importance of cell-based immunity in skin surveillance and the prevention of skin cancer. Chronically UV-exposed skin is immunosuppressed and

Table 5.1 Autoimmune photoaggravated dermatoses

Autoimmune diseases usually exacerbated by UVR:
1. Cutaneous lupus erythematosus
Subtypes:
SLE
Subacute cutaneous lupus erythematosus (SCLE)
Discoid lupus erythematosus (DLE)
Lupus tumidus
Rowell syndrome
Lupus profundus
2. Dermatomyositis
3. Sjogren's syndrome
4. MCTD
Diseases sometimes exacerbated by UVR:
1. Pemphigus
2. Psoriasis
3. Eczema
4. Rosacea
Diseases rarely exacerbated by UVR:
1. Bullous pemphigoid
2. Epidermolysis bullosa acquisita
3. Cutaneous T-cell lymphoma

more prone to develop viral warts. Acute exposure to UVR may also precipitate herpes simplex infections. Many viral diseases become more manifest in UV-damaged or the exposed skin. This has also been noted in many photoaggravated diseases.

5.3 Autoimmune Diseases

These are diseases in which impaired function and the destruction of tissue are caused by autoantibodies formation. Autoimmune diseases include a wide variety of disorders which can affect internal organs, muscles, joints and the skin. Some of these diseases may be exacerbated by UV radiation; hence photoprotection is imperative in the management of such diseases.

Photodermatoses may be classified into idiopathic photodermatoses, genodermatoses, photoaggravated dermatoses and photodermatoses which are secondary to exogenous agents including photoallergy/phototoxicity. In this chapter, we will discuss photoaggravated disorders of the autoimmune category (Table 5.1).

Immunologically mediated photodermatoses with no or minimal systemic manifestations other than in the skin include polymorphic light eruption (PLE), juvenile spring eruption, actinic prurigo, solar urticaria, chronic actinic dermatitis and hydroa vacciniforme; these are covered in another chapter.

5.3.1 *Lupus Erythematosus*

5.3.1.1 Introduction

Lupus erythematosus encompasses a number of related conditions, the common feature being underlying autoimmunity against nuclear constituents. Photosensitivity is a common feature for all subsets.

5.3.1.2 History

In the mid-nineteenth century, Cazenave first coined the term lupus erythematosus [7] and helped to differentiate it from lupus vulgaris, a cutaneous form of tuberculosis. In the mid-twentieth century, Dubois described the spectrum of disease seen with lupus ranging from cutaneous involvement to a multisystem disease [8].

5.3.1.3 Epidemiology

The epidemiology of lupus erythematosus varies depending on the subtype. Systemic lupus erythematosus (SLE) is more common in females (6F:1M) with a higher prevalence in African-American populations compared to white populations [9]. Subacute cutaneous lupus erythematosus (SCLE) and discoid lupus erythematosus (DLE) also occur more commonly in females but the ratio at 3F:1M is not as marked as for SLE [10]. The mean age at presentation for SCLE is in the sixth decade. DLE can be seen in any age group but it most commonly presents in the fifth decade [10]. The association between photosensitivity and lupus varies throughout the world with a higher prevalence of photosensitivity in lupus in Asia compared with Africa [11].

5.3.1.4 Pathogenesis

LE represents an autoimmune disease characterized by photosensitivity, apoptosis of keratinocytes and an inflammatory infiltrate in the superficial and/or deep compartments of the skin. The underlying pathogenesis, while not fully understood, reflects an interaction between host factors, such as susceptibility genes, sex hormones and environmental factors, including viruses, drugs and ultraviolet radiation.

UVR results in the aggravation of LE through a variety of mechanisms [12–14]. UV-generated reactive oxygen species render DNA antigenic. The resultant autoantibodies recognize both this altered DNA but also native DNA [15, 16]. UVB displaces the typically intracellular antigens Ro/SS-A and La/SS-B to the surface of the keratinocyte [17–19], resulting in antibody-mediated cytotoxic keratinocyte damage [20]. UV-induced destruction of keratinocytes through apoptosis occurs even in a normal setting; however in lupus slow clearance of apoptotic cells leads to prolonged exposure of DNA and extractable nuclear antigen to the immune system, generating anti-DNA and ENA antibodies [21, 22]. The mechanisms underlying this process have been reviewed recently [23, 24]. UV light also up-regulates adhesion molecules, such as ICAM-1 [25] in patients with LE. Nitric oxide synthase capable of inducing cytokines (iNOS) is released from keratinocytes following UV irradiation. In patients with LE this release is delayed but prolonged [26]. The promoter polymorphism 308A of TNF-α is seen with increased frequency in SCLE [27] and transcription is photoregulated [28].

The development of the skin lesions after UV injury may be delayed (days to 3 weeks) and the lesions may persist for months. This may make it difficult to elicit a history of photosensitivity from the patient, as the delay between UV exposure and exacerbation means patients may not make this association. UVA and UVB radiation are both implicated in the pathogenesis of LE in both in vitro [29] and in vivo [30] studies. One study documented that photosensitivity in cutaneous LE was UVB induced in 33 % of cases and UVA induced in 14 %, and in the majority of cases (53 %), it was mediated by a combination of UVB and UVA [14]. Nonsolar sources of UV, such as photocopiers [31], fluorescent and some energy-saving light sources [32], can aggravate LE. Interestingly, while UVB consistently aggravates LE, studies documented reduction in LE disease activity with UVA-1 (340–400 nm) irradiation [33–35]. Subtypes of LE appear to have varying degrees of photoaggravation, with lupus tumidus [36] and SCLE appearing to be the most photosensitive of the LE subtypes [37], although one study of phototesting with UVA, UVB and visible light in 100 patients (24 with SLE, 30 with SCLE and 46 with DLE) found no association between photosensitivity and LE subtype [38]. Phototesting is not routinely required in clinical practice to make a diagnosis of LE, as clinical history, examination, serologic studies and skin biopsy for histology and direct immunofluorescence suffice.

Polymorphous light eruption (PLE) is seen commonly in patients with LE (49 %), and the onset of PLE precedes the onset of LE by over 7 years in half of patients. This suggests that there may be features of pathogenesis common to both entities and that PLE may predispose to LE in a subset of patients [39].

5.3.1.5 Clinical Manifestations

The clinical presentation across the subtypes of LE is very diverse. The underlying disease process however is very similar. Patients with SLE can present acutely with internal organ damage secondary to circulating autoantibodies. No organ is protected from the immune-mediated destruction and SLE can present with arthralgia, central nervous system involvement, nephritis, pleuritis and vasculitis. At the other end of the spectrum, patients with other forms of LE may develop cutaneous lesions and never progress to systemic involvement.

Cutaneous manifestations of LE are varied and can be divided into LE-nonspecific and LE-specific lesions. LE-nonspecific mucocutaneous manifestations include oral ulcers, Raynaud's syndrome, scarring alopecia and vasculitis. The characteristic cutaneous manifestation of SLE is an erythematous, edematous, confluent eruption in a malar distribution; in the majority of cases, this malar rash is associated with underlying visceral involvement. SLE may present with erythema multiforme-like lesions, also known as Rowell syndrome. SCLE lesions include sharply demarcated psoriasiform plaques with fine scale and erosions and annular lesions with an erythematous border and a collarette of scale. DLE lesions are characteristically coin-shaped plaques on the face and neck, with fine scale and follicular plugging. There may be scarring and hypo/hyperpigmentation. Following a diagnosis of DLE, the probability of receiving a diagnosis of SLE is 9.8 % in the first year and 16.7 % after 3 years. The corresponding figures are higher for SCLE, at 22 % in the first year and 24.7 % after 3 years [9]. SLE classification criteria have been defined by the American College of Rheumatology [40, 41].

The cutaneous lesions of DLE heal with central atrophy associated with scarring. The cutaneous lesions of SCLE and SLE are non-scarring, although lesions of SCLE may result in hypo/hyperpigmentation. Lupus tumidus lesions include violaceous non-scaling papules and plaques on sun and non-sun-exposed sites.

There is a seasonal variation in manifestations of LE with skin and joint symptoms flaring during summer months but an apparent increase in renal involvement in winter months [42, 43].

5.3.1.6 Investigations

Histological features are central to the diagnosis of cutaneous LE. There is a periadnexal and perivascular lymphocytic infiltrate in the dermis. At the dermo-epidermal junction, the lymphocytic infiltrate is lichenoid with liquefactive degeneration of the basal keratinocytes and epidermal cytoid bodies are present. Typically in DLE follicular plugging and basement membrane thickening are marked, although occasionally epidermal changes are not prominent and dermal changes predominate. There are minimal epidermal features in SCLE and the findings are a lymphocytic infiltrate with dermal vacuolar change. Mucin is abundant in lupus tumidus and direct immunofluorescence is positive in addition to the above-described dermal features.

5.3.1.7 Serology

SLE is the LE subtype most strongly associated with positive antinuclear antibody (ANA) and double-stranded DNA (ds-DNA) [10]. Given the propensity of SLE to affect internal organs, a comprehensive systemic workup including complete blood count, complement levels and renal function tests including urinalysis should be undertaken. The presence of anti-Ro (SS-A) and anti-La (SS-B) is associated with an abnormal photoprovocation reaction [44]. Anti-Ro (SS-A) is found in 72 % of patients with SCLE, 47 % of patients with acute cutaneous LE and 22 % of patients with chronic cutaneous LE. Anti-La antibodies are found in 36 % of patients with

SCLE, 27 % of patients with acute cutaneous LE and 7 % of patients with chronic cutaneous LE [9]. These antibodies are also associated with Sjogren's syndrome which may overlap with SCLE. Sjogren's syndrome may also be photoaggravated [45]. Anti-histone antibodies are commonly but not exclusively associated with drug-induced lupus. SCLE may be drug-induced and rarely may be a paraneoplastic disease.

5.3.1.8 Treatment

Essential lifestyle changes for patients with cutaneous lupus erythematosus are photoprotection [46] and smoking cessation. Broad-spectrum sunscreen is required [47] due to the implication of both UVA and UVB in the action spectrum of LE. Vitamin D levels may be reduced in patients with cutaneous LE who practice rigorous photoprotection; hence supplementation is often required [5]. Topical corticosteroids and antimalarials [48] are first-line treatment options for cutaneous LE. Second-line treatment options include dapsone [49], thalidomide [50], oral retinoids [51] and immunosuppressant medications such as mycophenolate mofetil [52, 53], azathioprine and methotrexate. Every patient with cutaneous and systemic LE should be evaluated to ensure no causative drug is implicated.

5.3.2 *Dermatomyositis*

This is an autoimmune disease of the skin and striated muscle. It is associated with an increased risk of malignancy, the risk being highest in the first 3 years after diagnosis of myositis but increased for up to 5 years [54].

5.3.2.1 History

Bohan and Peter compiled generally accepted diagnostic criteria in 1975 [55, 56]. A more recent revision of the classification means that myositis is no longer required for diagnosis [57].

5.3.2.2 Epidemiology

The incidence of dermatomyositis (DM) is 9 per million. There is a female predominance (3:1) [58]. In Europe there is an increasing prevalence of DM relative to polymyositis seen with decreasing latitude [59], and additionally an association exists between surface UV radiation intensity and expression of anti-Mi2 autoantibodies [60]. Dermatomyositis may occur at any age; however two peaks are seen: between the ages of 5–10 years in children and the sixth decade in adults.

5.3.3 *Pathogenesis*

The pathogenic trigger for dermatomyositis is thought to be antigen mimicry. It is driven by CD8+ T cells and is associated with other autoimmune diseases and with viral infections. The main target appears to be capillaries with immunological attack resulting in the development of ischaemic myocyte necrosis.

Dermatomyositis is frequently photoaggravated [61, 62]. The pathogenesis of photosensitivity in DM and LE may overlap with polymorphisms of TNF-α [63] and increased keratinocyte apoptosis occurring in both conditions [64].

5.3.3.1 Clinical Presentation

The skin and striated muscle may be affected to varying degrees. Cutaneous findings accompany muscle involvement in 60 % of cases and precede it in 30 %. Dermatomyositis sine myositis where there is no muscle involvement is described in approximately 10 % of cases. Cutaneous findings include blue/violaceous or erythematous plaques and patches which may be edematous affecting the face and the V of the neck. The pathognomonic heliotrope rash refers to a lilac discoloration of the eyelids with periorbital oedema. The dorsum of the hands may demonstrate mauve linear plaques along the back of the fingers and dusky erythematous papules with atrophy, termed Gottron's papules, over the joints. They tend to spare the skin in between the joints. These Gottron's papules represent a hyperkeratotic response to inflammation. The nail folds may be hyperkeratotic with haemorrhage. Capillary microscopy of the nail fold vessels shows coiling and enlargement. Photosensitivity is seen with poikilodermatous change (atrophy, hyper/hypopigmentation, telangiectasia).

Proximal muscles are those most affected; the quadriceps and triceps are symmetrically involved with a slow onset of weakness and myalgia. Patients may report difficulty getting up from a seated position. Distal muscles are involved in the advanced disease state. Involvement of the pharyngeal muscles may occur and manifests as dyspnoea or dysphagia. Complications include myocarditis, pulmonary fibrosis and vasculitis.

Dermatomyositis may be chronic or can spontaneously remit in 2–3 years. If an underlying malignancy is present, removal can result in rapid resolution of the symptoms.

5.3.3.2 Investigations

A muscle biopsy demonstrates CD 8+ T cells infiltrating the muscle fibres with associated apoptosis, atrophy, regeneration and hypertrophy. Deposition of antibodies and complement in the microvasculature precede inflammation and the perifascicular atrophy of muscle fibres and inflammation supports a microvascular pathology. Histology findings may be difficult to differentiate from LE. Epidermal atrophy, a sparse lymphocytic infiltrate and a vacuolar interface change are seen. Examination of a Gottron's papule may demonstrate acanthosis and a dense lichenoid infiltrate.

5.3.3.3 Serology

A positive antinuclear antibody test is present in over 90 % of cases with specific antibodies against mRNP, PM-Scl, Mi2 and Jo1 found in approximately 30 % of cases. Elevation of creatinine kinase and aldolase indicates muscle involvement and these enzyme levels can be monitored to track response to treatment. The diagnosis can be confirmed by a muscle biopsy and electromyography.

5.3.3.4 Phototesting

Routine photobiologic evaluation is not usually undertaken. However, in studies, approximately 50 % of patients with dermatomyositis have a reduced minimal erythema dose to UVB [62].

5.3.3.5 Treatment

Drug-induced dermatomyositis should be excluded. Photoprotection with clothing and broad-spectrum sunscreen use is advisable. First-line therapies for cutaneous disease include topical corticosteroids and antimalarials, such as hydroxychloroquine [65] or chloroquine. If muscle involvement occurs, prednisolone 1 mg/kg per day with options for steroid-sparing agents including methotrexate or azathioprine is used. High-dose intravenous immunoglobulin [66] has been used if there is failure to respond to first/second-line therapies or if there is significant muscle involvement.

5.3.4 Sjogren's Syndrome

This is an autoimmune disease which is characterized by its two most common symptoms – keratoconjunctivitis sicca (dry eyes) and xerostomia (dry mouth). It is often accompanied by other disorders of the immune system such as rheumatoid arthritis and lupus erythematosus. Patients have high levels of serum ENA predisposing to photosensitivity. Patients exhibit photosensitivity to UVB when phototested similar to LE. The exact cause is unknown, but may be due to having a genetic predisposition with a triggering factor such as a viral or bacterial infection. The mucous membranes and moisture-secreting glands (lacrymal and salivary) are affected, resulting in reduced tear and saliva production leading to the symptoms described. The condition is much more common in females and the diagnosis is usually made in those older than 40 years of age. People with this condition may also experience joint pains, fatigue, salivary gland swelling and xerosis. This condition may also have systemic involvement affecting organs such as the thyroid, lung, liver and kidneys. Due to this the cutaneous manifestations are often minimized, albeit relatively common. Cutaneous manifestations associated with primary SS include photosensitive rashes in the context of positive anti-Ro antibodies, alopecia, annular erythema, B cell lymphoma, vasculitis and vitiligo [67].

5.3.5 Mixed Connective Tissue Disease (MCTD)

MCTD is often referred to as an overlap disorder as it is a disease with signs and symptoms of a combination of disorders, mainly lupus erythematosus, polymyositis and systemic sclerosis; however, it is a distinct clinical entity. It is considered an autoimmune disease to which individuals who express specific HLA antigens such as HLA-DR4 or HLA-DBQ1 are genetically predisposed [68]. Some hypotheses implicate modified self-antigens and/or infectious agents in the pathogenesis. U1 ribonucleoprotein is a specific marker for disease. The diagnosis can be complicated due to the fact that many of the symptoms occur chronically over years rather than all occurring acutely.

The earliest symptoms often involve the hands whereby the fingers swell (dactylitis) and Raynaud's phenomenon occurs. With time this may evolve to present with a LE-like photodistributed cutaneous eruption; however, its photobiologic features have not been well studied. It may affect any age group but is most commonly diagnosed in young females. The female to male ratio is 4:1. People may develop systemic involvement including pulmonary, cardiac and renal involvement. Treatment of the cutaneous manifestations of this disorder is as described previously for lupus erythematosus. Other agents include oral hygiene to prevent dental caries, artificial saliva (saliva substitutes, mucin based), and saliva stimulants (organic acids, chewing gum and parasympathomimetic drugs). Artificial tears are also used to treat decreased lacrymal gland function.

5.3.6 Pemphigus

Pemphigus erythematosus (PE), also known as Senear-Usher Syndrome, is one of the six subtypes of pemphigus foliaceus (PF). PE affects all races and both genders. It typically affects adults aged 50–60 years, but children may rarely be affected. PE is a rare condition in which pemphigus foliaceus occurs with a positive antinuclear antibody, and it may represent an overlap of pemphigus and LE due to epitope spread. Chronically sun-exposed skin such as the face and scalp develop blisters that tend to ooze, crust and scale which may result in scarring and infection. Blisters do not occur on mucous membranes, helping to differentiate it from other subtypes of PF. The pathogenesis is thought to result from antibodies that attack desmosomes, bridges that connect epidermal cells. Destruction of these connections results in the blister formation, which are superficial and therefore rupture easily. PF can be photoaggravated [69, 70], as can pemphigus vulgaris [71]. While the action spectrum for this is unknown, photoprotection is advised.

5.3.7 Psoriasis

In the majority of patients with psoriasis, UV therapies are used to control the disease; however there is a defined subset of patients, 5–20 %, whom have an exacerbation of their psoriasis with UV exposure [72–74]. They tend to be older females with a positive family history of psoriasis and early onset of disease; patients are more likely to have psoriasis affecting their hands [75, 76]. There is a strong association with HLA-Cw*0602 [74]. Approximately 50 % develop PLE following sun exposure with subsequent development of psoriasis in the lesions of PLE, while the other 50 % have photoaggravated psoriasis with no associated PLE [73]. In the former group, symptoms of PLE followed by psoriasis were more easily provoked by UVA, while in the second group, UVB was the more effective photoaggravating spectrum [76]. If there is a question regarding photoaggravated psoriasis, patients should undergo confirmatory phototesting. Photoprotection is advisable in these patients.

5.3.8 Atopic Eczema

This is a common inflammatory skin disease which most frequently begins in childhood. It consists of erythematous scaly patches associated with intense pruritus resulting in excoriations, secondary infection and a significant impact on one's quality of life. Current therapies focus mainly on symptom control; however in recent years significant advances have been made in translational research similar to that which occurred in psoriasis over the past decade. The research has focused on elucidating immune pathways in AD including Th2, Th22 and Th17 pathways. An IL-4R antagonist (Dupilumab) is already in clinical trials with great promise and continued research into this area may bring new medications to target this disease. AD may flare due to a variety of reasons including infection, irritants and allergens (ingested, inhaled, contact), or it may also flare with time, following exposure to UVR. This diagnosis may be delayed due to the fact that the person has atopic dermatitis long standing and it may be simply treated as a flare; however with time it is noted that the patient is not responding to the standard treatments and the location of the rash is occurring on photo-exposed sites (face/neck/hands/forearms). Patients often undergo phototesting at this stage whereby they are noted to have photoaggravated atopic dermatitis; if they are elderly, they may fall into another cohort of patients with chronic actinic dermatitis. The action spectrum is usually similar to the erythema action spectrum, in which case the patient may be labelled "chronic actinic dermatitis". If the patient has UVA photosensitivity, then photosensitivity caused by a drug should be suspected.

5.3.9 *Chronic Actinic Dermatitis (CAD)*

This is a rare disease which mainly affects elderly men (~10 % female). It is also rarely found in HIV. They may give a history of previous atopy or allergic contact dermatitis to composítate [77]. They have severely lichenified, xerotic skin affecting the face, neck and dorsal hands most commonly with sparing behind the ears and inferior chin. Hypopigmentation may also be seen in CAD, and this seems to be post-inflammatory hypopigmentation. Skin biopsy from the affected areas may show an eczematous eruption particularly if biopsied following monochromator testing, but if severe it may also resemble a cutaneous T-cell lymphoma/reticulosis; hence, the other name it is also known by – actinic reticuloid – is sometimes used. There is a dense dermal lymphocytic dermatitis with atypical cerebriform lymphocytic cells identical to those in cutaneous T-cell lymphoma.

The eruption can be provoked by very minimal UV exposure. It is usually worse in the summer months and may improve in some individuals in the winter months. It is therefore more easily diagnosed in those with severe, year-round photosensitivity and disabling effects. If left untreated it may progress to erythroderma. Phototesting (monochromator) is essential to make the diagnosis of CAD. In the absence or abnormal tests, the diagnosis cannot be made. The pattern of the action spectrum in 90 % of patients with CAD implicates DNA as the chromophore, as the action spectrum is identical to the erythema action spectrum, i.e., UVB, but occurring at a lower dose [78]. The minority of patients exhibit UVA photosensitivity, but this is more commonly the pattern of drug-induced photosensitivity; thus drugs should be excluded in such cases [79].

Treatment includes UV protection (clothing, hat, broad-spectrum sunscreens) and sun avoidance during peak hours, topical tacrolimus, and, in more severe cases, azathioprine, cyclosporine, or mycophenolate mofetil. For patients who are extremely photosensitive (UVB, UVA extending into visible light), this condition can be an extremely debilitating disease.

5.3.10 *Rosacea*

This is a common inflammatory skin condition mainly affecting the face of middle-aged adults. Four major clinical subtypes have been identified: erythematotelangi-ectatic, papulopustular, phymatous and ocular. Rosacea is characterized by facial flushing, erythema, chronic inflammation in the form of papules and pustules and fibrosis. Some aspects of the pathophysiology of rosacea has been characterized in more detail in recent years; however the interplay of these dysregulated systems is still poorly understood. UVR effects on rosacea have yet to be fully understood as many trials to date show conflicting reports. Does the UVR induce damage to the dermal connective tissue permitting vasodilatation and vascular pooling which leads to erythema? Is it also that in the majority of rosacea patients who describe photoaggravated rosacea, there is failure to downgrade the immune response to UVR? Or does UVR actually have a beneficial effect by decreasing inflammation resulting in skin clearance as seen in some patients undergoing phototherapy for coexisting conditions?

5.3.11 Epidermolysis Bullosa Acquisita

This is a rare, acquired, chronic subepidermal bullous disease of the skin and mucosa due to autoantibodies to type VII collagen structures which are a major component of anchoring fibrils which attach the dermis to the epidermis. The autoantibodies which are either bound or circulating attack type VII collagen resulting in a reduction or change of normally functioning anchoring fibrils. Patients present with skin fragility, blistering, erosions, scarring, milia formation and sometimes loss of nails. There is not one satisfactory treatment for this condition but some therapeutic success has been achieved with the use of colchicine, dapsone, infliximab, intravenous immunoglobulins and plasmapheresis [80]. There have been rare case reports of this condition with sensitivity to both UVA and UVB radiation [81].

5.3.12 Cutaneous T-Cell Lymphoma (CTCL)

This is a type of lymphoma which presents in the skin but may evolve, often over many years to have systemic involvement. Mycosis fungoides, first described by a French physician Jean Luis Marc Alibert in 1806, is the most common type of CTCL. Patients present most commonly from the 4th decade onward with patches or plaques which can sometimes be misdiagnosed as eczema initially. Children may be affected but it is much more common in adults and also in males more so than females. Patients may also present with erythroderma and some progress to tumour stage with lymphadenopathy. Pruritus is commonly associated with this condition. Unfortunately there is no cure for this disease and the treatment is about control of skin eruption and symptomatic relief. One of the first-line treatments is phototherapy, both NB-UVB and PUVA. There are case reports of "photosensitive mycosis fungoides" [82], whereby patients may present with "actinic reticuloid"-type pattern of facial features, also known as chronic actinic dermatitis; however biopsies of the skin combined with T-cell gene rearrangement studies confirm it to be CTCL. These patients are not photosensitive and usually respond very well to PUVA despite the eruption clinically mimicking CAD. This disease may progress over a very short period of time to tumour stage or may smoulder for many decades.

Some of the photoaggravated autoimmune diseases have a known action spectrum; however, as the exact action spectra are not fully defined for all of the photoaggravated autoimmune diseases, a key component of their management includes photoprotection with behavioural change, UV protective clothing and broad-spectrum sunscreen.

References

1. Australian Radiation Protection and Nuclear Safety Agency. http://www.arpansa.gov.au. Accessed 13 May 2015
2. Commission Internationale de l'Eclairage. www.cie.co.at. Accessed 13 May 2015
3. Kripke ML (1974) Antigenicity of murine skin tumors induced by ultraviolet light. J Natl Cancer Inst 53:1333–1336
4. Schwarz T (2008) 25 years of UV-induced immunosuppression mediated by T cells – from disregarded T suppressor cells to highly respected regulatory T cells. Photochem Photobiol 84:10–18
5. Murphy GM, Norris PG, Young AR, Corbett MF, Hawk JL (1993) Low dose ultraviolet-B irradiation depletes human epidermal Langerhans cells. Br J Dermatol 129:674–677
6. Powles AV, Murphy GM, Rutman AJ et al (1989) Effect of simulated sunlight on Langerhans' cells in malignant melanoma patients. Acta Derm Venereol 69:482–486
7. Cazenave PL (1851) Lupus erythemateux (erythema centrifuge). Ann Mal de la Peau 3:297–299
8. Dubois EL (1966) Lupus erythematosus: a review of the current status of discoid and systematic lupus erythematosus and their variants. McGraw-Hill, Blakiston Division, New York
9. Gronhagen CM, Fored CM, Granath F, Nyberg F (2011) Cutaneous lupus erythematosus and the association with systemic lupus erythematosus: a population-based cohort of 1088 patients in Sweden. Br J Dermatol 164(6):1335–1341
10. Biazar C, Sigges J, Patsinakidis N et al (2013) Cutaneous lupus erythematosus: first multicenter database analysis of 1002 patients from the European Society of Cutaneous Lupus Erythematosus (EUSCLE). Autoimmun Rev 12(3):444–454
11. Scheinfeld N, Deleo VA (2004) Photosensitivity in lupus erythematosus. Photodermatol Photoimmunol Photomed 20(5):272–279
12. Baer RL, Harber LC (1965) Photobiology of lupus erythematosus. Arch Dermatol 92: 124–128
13. Everett MA, Olson RL (1965) Response of cutaneous lupus erythematosus to ultraviolet light. J Invest Dermatol 44:133–138
14. Lehmann P, Holzle E, Kind P, Goerz G, Plewig G (1990) Experimental reproduction of skin lesions in lupus erythematosus by UVA and UVB radiation. J Am Acad Dermatol 22(2 Pt 1):181–187
15. Ashok BT, Ali R (1999) Antigen binding characteristics of experimentally-induced antibodies against hydroxyl radical modified native DNA. Autoimmunity 29(1):11–19
16. Davis P, Russell AS, Percy JS (1976) Antibodies to UV light denatured DNA in systemic lupus erythematosus: detection by filter radioimmunoassay and clinical correlations. J Rheumatol 3(4):375–379
17. Jones SK (1992) Ultraviolet radiation (UVR) induces cell-surface Ro/SSA antigen expression by human keratinocytes in vitro: a possible mechanism for the UVR induction of cutaneous lupus lesions. Br J Dermatol 126(6):546–553

18. Golan TD, Elkon KB, Gharavi AE, Krueger JG (1992) Enhanced membrane binding of autoantibodies to cultured keratinocytes of systemic lupus erythematosus patients after ultraviolet B/ultraviolet A irradiation. J Clin Invest 90(3):1067–1076
19. Furukawa F, Kashihara-Sawami M, Lyons MB, Norris DA (1990) Binding of antibodies to the extractable nuclear antigens SS-A/Ro and SS-B/La is induced on the surface of human keratinocytes by ultraviolet light (UVL): implications for the pathogenesis of photosensitive cutaneous lupus. J Invest Dermatol 94(1):77–85
20. Bennion SD, Ferris C, Lieu TS, Reimer CB, Lee LA (1990) IgG subclasses in the serum and skin in subacute cutaneous lupus erythematosus and neonatal lupus erythematosus. J Invest Dermatol 95(6):643–646
21. Caricchio R, McPhie L, Cohen PL (2003) Ultraviolet B radiation-induced cell death: critical role of ultraviolet dose in inflammation and lupus autoantigen redistribution. J Immunol 171(11):5778–5786
22. Majai G, Kiss E, Tarr T et al (2014) Decreased apopto-phagocytic gene expression in the macrophages of systemic lupus erythematosus patients. Lupus 23:133–145
23. Janko C, Schorn C, Grossmayer GE et al (2008) Inflammatory clearance of apoptotic remnants in systemic lupus erythematosus (SLE). Autoimmun Rev 8(1):9–12
24. Yu C, Chang C, Zhang J (2013) Immunologic and genetic considerations of cutaneous lupus erythematosus: a comprehensive review. J Autoimmun 41:34–45
25. Norris DA, Lyons MB, Middleton MH, Yohn JJ, Kashihara-Sawami M (1990) Ultraviolet radiation can either suppress or induce expression of intercellular adhesion molecule 1 (ICAM-1) on the surface of cultured human keratinocytes. J Invest Dermatol 95(2):132–138
26. Kuhn A, Fehsel K, Lehmann P, Krutmann J, Ruzicka T, Kolb-Bachofen V (1998) Aberrant timing in epidermal expression of inducible nitric oxide synthase after UV irradiation in cutaneous lupus erythematosus. J Invest Dermatol 111(1):149–153
27. Millard TP, Kondeatis E, Cox A et al (2001) A candidate gene analysis of three related photosensitivity disorders: cutaneous lupus erythematosus, polymorphic light eruption and actinic prurigo. Br J Dermatol 145(2):229–236
28. Werth VP, Zhang W, Dortzbach K, Sullivan K (2000) Association of a promoter polymorphism of tumor necrosis factor-alpha with subacute cutaneous lupus erythematosus and distinct photoregulation of transcription. J Invest Dermatol 115(4):726–730
29. Golan TD, Foltyn V, Roueff A (1991) Increased susceptibility to in vitro ultraviolet B radiation in fibroblasts and lymphocytes cultured from systemic lupus erythematosus patients. Clin Immunol Immunopathol 58(2):289–304
30. Nived O, Johansen PB, Sturfelt G (1993) Standardized ultraviolet-A exposure provokes skin reaction in systemic lupus erythematosus. Lupus 2(4):247–250
31. Klein LR, Elmets CA, Callen JP (1995) Photoexacerbation of cutaneous lupus erythematosus due to ultraviolet A emissions from a photocopier. Arthritis Rheum 38(8):1152–1156
32. Rihner M, McGrath H Jr (1992) Fluorescent light photosensitivity in patients with systemic lupus erythematosus. Arthritis Rheum 35(8):949–952
33. McGrath H Jr (1999) Ultraviolet A1 (340-400 nm) irradiation and systemic lupus erythematosus. J Investig Dermatol Symp Proc 4(1):79–84
34. Molina JF, McGrath H Jr (1997) Long term ultraviolet-A1 irradiation therapy in systemic lupus erythematosus. J Rheumatol 24(6):1072–1074
35. McGrath H, Martinez-Osuna P, Lee FA (1996) Ultraviolet-A1 (340-400 nm) irradiation therapy in systemic lupus erythematosus. Lupus 5(4):269–274
36. Kuhn A, Sonntag M, Richter-Hintz D et al (2001) Phototesting in lupus erythematosus tumidus–review of 60 patients. Photochem Photobiol 73(5):532–536
37. Chlebus E, Wolska H, Blaszczyk M, Jablonska S (1998) Subacute cutaneous lupus erythematosus versus systemic lupus erythematosus: diagnostic criteria and therapeutic implications. J Am Acad Dermatol 38(3):405–412
38. Sanders CJ, Van Weelden H, Kazzaz GA, Sigurdsson V, Toonstra J, Bruijnzeel-Koomen CA (2003) Photosensitivity in patients with lupus erythematosus: a clinical and photobiological study of 100 patients using a prolonged phototest protocol. Br J Dermatol 149(1):131–137

39. Nyberg F, Hasan T, Puska P et al (1997) Occurrence of polymorphous light eruption in lupus erythematosus. Br J Dermatol 136(2):217–221
40. Tan EM, Cohen AS, Fries JF et al (1982) The 1982 revised criteria for the classification of systemic lupus erythematosus. Arthritis Rheum 25(11):1271–1277
41. Hochberg MC (1997) Updating the American College of Rheumatology revised criteria for the classification of systemic lupus erythematosus. Arthritis Rheum 40(9):1725
42. Duarte-Garcia A, Fang H, To CH, Magder LS, Petri M (2012) Seasonal variation in the activity of systemic lupus erythematosus. J Rheumatol 39(7):1392–1398
43. Szeto CC, Mok HY, Chow KM et al (2008) Climatic influence on the prevalence of noncutaneous disease flare in systemic lupus erythematosus in Hong Kong. J Rheumatol 35(6):1031–1037
44. Hasan T, Nyberg F, Stephansson E et al (1997) Photosensitivity in lupus erythematosus, UV photoprovocation results compared with history of photosensitivity and clinical findings. Br J Dermatol 136(5):699–705
45. Tsukazaki N, Watanabe M, Shimizu K, Hamasaki Y, Katayama I (2002) Photoprovocation test and immunohistochemical analysis of inducible nitric oxide synthase expression in patients with Sjogren's syndrome associated with photosensitivity. Br J Dermatol 147(6): 1102–1108
46. Stege H, Budde MA, Grether-Beck S, Krutmann J (2000) Evaluation of the capacity of sunscreens to photoprotect lupus erythematosus patients by employing the photoprovocation test. Photodermatol Photoimmunol Photomed 16(6):256–259
47. Kuhn A, Gensch K, Haust M et al (2011) Photoprotective effects of a broad-spectrum sunscreen in ultraviolet-induced cutaneous lupus erythematosus: a randomized, vehicle-controlled, double-blind study. J Am Acad Dermatol 64(1):37–48
48. Seiger E, Roland S, Goldman S (1991) Cutaneous lupus treated with topical tretinoin: a case report. Cutis 47(5):351–355
49. Neri R, Mosca M, Bernacchi E, Bombardieri S (1999) A case of SLE with acute, subacute and chronic cutaneous lesions successfully treated with Dapsone. Lupus 8(3):240–243
50. Duong DJ, Spigel GT, Moxley RT 3rd, Gaspari AA (1999) American experience with low-dose thalidomide therapy for severe cutaneous lupus erythematosus. Arch Dermatol 135(9): 1079–1087
51. Newton RC, Jorizzo JL, Solomon AR Jr et al (1986) Mechanism-oriented assessment of isotretinoin in chronic or subacute cutaneous lupus erythematosus. Arch Dermatol 122(2): 170–176
52. Schanz S, Ulmer A, Rassner G, Fierlbeck G (2002) Successful treatment of subacute cutaneous lupus erythematosus with mycophenolate mofetil. Br J Dermatol 147(1):174–178
53. Kreuter A, Tomi NS, Weiner SM, Huger M, Altmeyer P, Gambichler T (2007) Mycophenolate sodium for subacute cutaneous lupus erythematosus resistant to standard therapy. Br J Dermatol 156(6):1321–1327
54. Buchbinder R, Forbes A, Hall S, Dennett X, Giles G (2001) Incidence of malignant disease in biopsy-proven inflammatory myopathy. A population-based cohort study. Ann Intern Med 134(12):1087–1095
55. Bohan A, Peter JB (1975) Polymyositis and dermatomyositis (first of two parts). N Engl J Med 292(7):344–347
56. Bohan A, Peter JB (1975) Polymyositis and dermatomyositis (second of two parts). N Engl J Med 292(8):403–407
57. Sontheimer RD (1999) Cutaneous features of classic dermatomyositis and amyopathic dermatomyositis. Curr Opin Rheumatol 11(6):475–482
58. Bendewald MJ, Wetter DA, Li X, Davis MD (2010) Incidence of dermatomyositis and clinically amyopathic dermatomyositis: a population-based study in Olmsted County. Minnesota Arch Dermatol 146(1):26–30
59. Hengstman GJ, van Venrooij WJ, Vencovsky J, Moutsopoulos HM, van Engelen BG (2000) The relative prevalence of dermatomyositis and polymyositis in Europe exhibits a latitudinal gradient. Ann Rheum Dis 59(2):141–142

60. Okada S, Weatherhead E, Targoff IN, Wesley R, Miller FW (2003) Global surface ultraviolet radiation intensity may modulate the clinical and immunologic expression of autoimmune muscle disease. Arthritis Rheum 48(8):2285–2293
61. Cheong WK, Hughes GR, Norris PG, Hawk JL (1994) Cutaneous photosensitivity in dermatomyositis. Br J Dermatol 131(2):205–208
62. Dourmishev L, Meffert H, Piazena H (2004) Dermatomyositis: comparative studies of cutaneous photosensitivity in lupus erythematosus and normal subjects. Photodermatol Photoimmunol Photomed 20(5):230–234
63. Werth VP, Callen JP, Ang G, Sullivan KE (2002) Associations of tumor necrosis factor alpha and HLA polymorphisms with adult dermatomyositis: implications for a unique pathogenesis. J Invest Dermatol 119(3):617–620
64. Pablos JL, Santiago B, Galindo M, Carreira PE, Ballestin C, Gomez-Reino JJ (1999) Keratinocyte apoptosis and p53 expression in cutaneous lupus and dermatomyositis. J Pathol 188(1):63–68
65. Woo TY, Callen JP, Voorhees JJ, Bickers DR, Hanno R, Hawkins C (1984) Cutaneous lesions of dermatomyositis are improved by hydroxychloroquine. J Am Acad Dermatol 10(4): 592–600
66. Dalakas MC, Illa I, Dambrosia JM et al (1993) A controlled trial of high-dose intravenous immune globulin infusions as treatment for dermatomyositis. N Engl J Med 329(27): 1993–2000
67. Nishiyama S, Maywaki S, Hashimoto T (1995) Cutaneous manifestations of primary Sjogren syndrome. Nihon Rinsho 53(10):2551–2556
68. Yoshida K, Inoue H, Komai K, Yamane T, Hashiramoto A, Shiozawa K et al (2013) Mixed connective tissue disease is distinct from systemic lupus erythematosus: study of major histocompatibility complex class I polypeptide-related sequence A and HLA gene polymorphisms. Tissue Antigens 81(1):44–45
69. Igawa K, Matsunaga T, Nishioka K (2004) Involvement of UV-irradiation in pemphigus foliaceus. J Eur Acad Dermatol Venereol 18(2):216–217
70. Kano Y, Shimosegawa M, Mizukawa Y, Shiohara T (2000) Pemphigus foliaceus induced by exposure to sunlight. Report of a case and analysis of photochallenge-induced lesions. Dermatology 201(2):132–138
71. Reis VM, Toledo RP, Lopez A, Diaz LA, Martins JE (2000) UVB-induced acantholysis in endemic Pemphigus foliaceus (Fogo selvagem) and Pemphigus vulgaris. J Am Acad Dermatol 42(4):571–576
72. Farber EM, Bright RD, Nall ML (1968) Psoriasis. A questionnaire survey of 2,144 patients. Arch Dermatol 98(3):248–259
73. Ros AM, Eklund G (1987) Photosensitive psoriasis. An epidemiologic study. J Am Acad Dermatol 17(5 Pt 1):752–758
74. Rutter KJ, Watson RE, Cotterell LF, Brenn T, Griffiths CE, Rhodes LE (2009) Severely photosensitive psoriasis: a phenotypically defined patient subset. J Invest Dermatol 129(12): 2861–2867
75. Nalluri R, Arun B, Rhodes LE (2010) Photoaggravated hand and foot psoriasis. Photodermatol Photoimmunol Photomed 26(5):261–262
76. Ros AM, Wennersten G (1986) Photosensitive psoriasis–clinical findings and phototest results. Photodermatol 3(6):317–326
77. Murphy GH, White IR, Hawk JL (1990) Allergic airborne contact dermatitis to compositae with photosensitivity – chronic actinic dermatitis in evolution. Photodermatol Photoimmunol Photomed 7:38–39
78. Hd M, Harrison GI, Potten CS, Young AR, Hawk JL (1995) The action spectrum for induction of chronic actinic dermatitis is similar to that for sunburn inflammation. Photochem Photobiol 62:976–997
79. O'Reilly FM, McKenna D, Murphy GM (1999) Is monochromatic irradiation testing useful in the differentiation of drug-induced photosensitivity from: chronic actinic dermatitis? Clin Exp Dermatol 24:118–121

80. Ishii N, Hamada T, Dainichi T, Karashima T, Nakama T, Yasumoto S, Zillikens D, Hashimoto T (2010) Epidermolysis bullosa acquisita: what's new? J Dermatol 37(3):220–230
81. Jappe U, Zillikens D, Bonnekoh B, Gollnick H (2000) Epidermolysis bullosa acquisita with ultraviolet radiation sensitivity. Br J Dermatol 142(3):517–520
82. De Silva BD, McLaren K, Kavanagh GM (2000) Photosensitive mycosis fungoides or actinic reticuloid? Br J Dermatol 142(6):1221–1227

Chapter 6
Photoprotection and Vitamin D

James L. Griffith, Mohammed Al-Jamal, and Henry W. Lim

Key Points

- Vitamin D is unquestionably important in the development and maintenance of skeletal health but may have broader implications beyond bone health.
- There are varying definitions of vitamin D deficiency and recommended daily requirements. Current recommendation on vitamin D screening is that it should be done only for at-risk populations.
- Real-world application of sunscreen does not impact vitamin D status, although rigorous photoprotection practice does.
- Given the low cost, broad availability, and safety profile of oral vitamin D supplementation, replenishing vitamin D by solar and artificial ultraviolet radiation is not advised.

J.L. Griffith, MD • H.W. Lim, MD, FAAD (✉)
Department of Dermatology, Henry Ford Hospital,
3031 W. Grand Blvd., Suite 800, Detroit, MI 48202, USA
e-mail: jgriff10@hfhs.org; hlim1@hfhs.org

M. Al-Jamal, MD
Department of Dermatology, Henry Ford Hospital,
3031 W. Grand Blvd., Suite 800, Detroit, MI 48202, USA

Department of Dermatology, Prince Sultan Military Medical City, P.O. Box 59606,
Riyadh 11525, Saudi Arabia
e-mail: dr.aljamal_derma@yahoo.com

S.Q. Wang, H.W. Lim (eds.), *Principles and Practice of Photoprotection*,
DOI 10.1007/978-3-319-29382-0_6

6.1 Introduction

Vitamin D is a fat-soluble hormone obtained from sun exposure, diet, and oral supplements with many biologic effects. It is primarily known for its crucial role in the optimization of bone mass via its effects on parathyroid hormone and calcium and phosphorous homeostasis. However, it also may have extra-skeletal associations, such as cardiovascular disease, immune susceptibility, and cancers [1]. Thus, concern has developed whether photoprotection would affect vitamin D status. This chapter will discuss how humans acquire vitamin D, vitamin D's physiologic effects, associations with disease, impact of photoprotection, and recommendations to patients. Terms and conversions used in the discussion of vitamin D can be viewed in Table 6.1.

6.2 Sources of Vitamin D

6.2.1 Sunlight and Artificial Radiation

In the skin, vitamin D can be synthesized from 7-dehydrocholesterol (7-DHC) following ultraviolet B (UVB) exposure (Fig. 6.1). 7-DHC, which is found in the plasma membranes of keratinocytes and fibroblasts, undergoes nonenzymatic, photodecomposition to previtamin D3 after exposure to 300±5 nm of radiation. Previtamin D3 can then isomerize into cholecalciferol (vitamin D3) or further degrade to inactive products, lumisterol and tachysterol, with additional UVB irradiation. This latter pathway prevents vitamin D intoxication from prolonged sun exposure. Cholecalciferol is then released from the keratinocyte and fibroblast

Table 6.1 Common nomenclature used in vitamin D

Abbreviations/common nomenclature	Proper nomenclature
7-DHC	7-Dehydrocholesterol
Vitamin D	Refers to any form of the vitamin, especially calcitriol
Vitamin D2	Ergocalciferol
Vitamin D3	Cholecalciferol
25(OH)D	Calcidiol or calcifediol (25-hydroxyvitamin D)
$1,25(OH)_2D3$	Calcitriol (1, 25-dihydroxyvitamin D3)
$24, 25\ (OH)_2D$	24, 25-Dihydroxyvitamin D
IU	International Unit (40 IU of vitamin D=1 ng)
Serum 25(OH)D level	Serum concentration is reported as nmol/L or ng/mL (2.5 nmol/L=1 ng/mL)
Vitamin D deficiency[a]	Serum 25(OH)D levels below 12 ng/mL or 30 nmol/L
Vitamin D insufficiency[a]	Serum 25(OH)D levels below 20 ng/mL or 50 nmol/L

[a]Based on Institute of Medicine definition for at-risk populations [2]

plasma membrane and transported to the liver by serum vitamin D binding protein for conversion to 25(OH)D by 25-hydroxylase. 25(OH)D undergoes further hydroxylation to 1,25$(OH)_2$D by primarily renal 1-alpha-hydroxylase. However, keratinocytes, macrophages, T-lymphocytes, dendritic cells, bone, prostate, and placental cells also can convert 25(OH)D to 1,25$(OH)_2$D.

As cutaneous vitamin D synthesis requires UVB radiation, factors that attenuate or absorb UVB and the duration of exposure influence vitamin D production. Atmospheric ozone absorbs UVB radiation. However, its absolute and relative thickness in relation to the sun varies. The intensity of UVB radiation is greatly reduced early/late in the day, at higher latitude, at lower altitudes, and in the winter when the tilt of the earth is at its greatest. Analysis of published serum 25(OH)D levels in the northern hemisphere indicates there is insufficient ambient UVB for adequate vitamin D production during the winter at latitudes above 33° [3]. Additionally, UVB is reduced further exogenously by high nitrogen dioxide and ozone levels in polluted urban environments, such as Los Angeles, California, and Mexico City, Mexico [4].

Endogenously, UVB's effects on 7-DHC vary by skin phototype, as melanin mitigates UVB's penetration. A 1991 study of skin pigmentation and serum vitamin

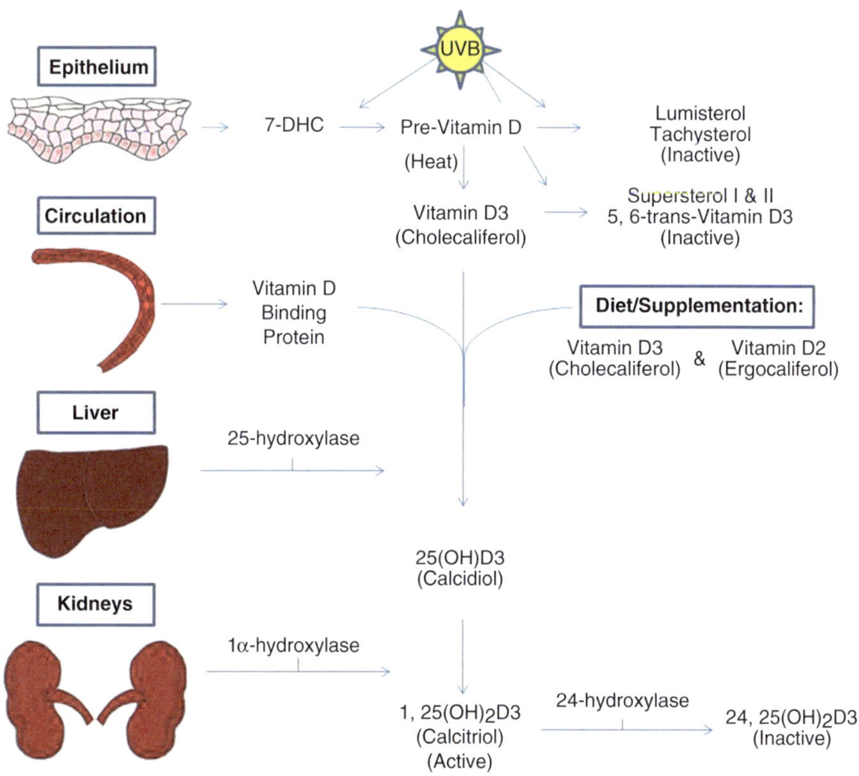

Fig. 6.1 Vitamin D production and metabolism. *Abbreviations*: *7-DHC* 7-dehydrocholesterol, *Active* active in calcium regulation, *Inactive* no activity in calcium regulation

D3 levels found significantly higher levels in Caucasian and Asian subjects compared to those of African American and East Indian descent [5]. Similar inverse relationships between skin pigmentation and serum vitamin D3 levels were also reported in subsequent 2004, 2010, and 2014 publications [6–8].

Artificial sources of UVB radiation can rapidly and effectively raise serum vitamin D levels at suberythemogenic levels via the same mechanisms as solar radiation without exogenous, atmospheric attenuators. However, it should be noted that ultraviolet exposure from artificial devices or natural sunlight can increase one's risk of skin cancers, and tanning booths are a poor source of artificial UVB for vitamin D as they primarily emit ultraviolet A (340–400 nm).

6.2.2 Diet and Supplementation

Exogenous vitamin D can be obtained through dietary intake, but only a few foods, such as cod liver, specific fish (mackerel, sockeye salmon, tuna), beef, egg yolks, shiitake mushrooms, and cheese, naturally contain high levels of vitamin D. Therefore, many countries, including the United States, fortify milk, orange juice, yogurt, cereal, and other foods to enhance the dietary sources of vitamin D. Additionally, vitamin D can be obtained through over-the-counter multivitamins and vitamin D supplements or prescription supplementation. Although fungal-/yeast-derived vitamin D2 (ergocalciferol) is available over the counter and by prescription, commercially synthesized vitamin D3 (cholecalciferol) is primarily utilized in fortification and supplementation. Following ingestion, both forms of exogenous vitamin D are metabolized by the liver to 25(OH)D. While the bioequivalence of D2 and D3 remains a controversial topic [9], a 2012 meta-analysis of randomized clinical trials found D3 superior in raising 25(OH)D levels [10].

6.3 Pathophysiologic Effects of Vitamin D

The active calcemic metabolite of vitamin D, 1, $25(OH)_2D3$, regulates transcription of up to 5 % of the human genome in at least 60 human cell types [11]. It does this by forming a heterodimeric complex with nuclear vitamin D receptor and retinoic acid X receptor. When deficient or insufficient, the genetic expression of at least 291 genes is altered over 150 % [4]. These changes have implications on bone, immunologic, cardiovascular, and cellular differentiation health.

Skeletally, vitamin D produces and maintains bone density through the hormonal regulation of calcium homeostasis. It does so directly by altering gastrointestinal absorption of calcium and phosphate while indirectly controlling parathyroid hormone's renal excretion and skeletal mobilization of calcium. Epidemiologic studies have shown 71 % of children with rachitic changes on radiographic studies were vitamin D deficient [4]. Additionally, a meta-analysis of 8 randomized controlled clinical trials (RCTs) reported 482–770 international units (IU) of vitamin D reduced hip fractures and non-vertebral fractures by 18 and 20 %, respectively, while no reduction was observed with less than 400 IU [12]. Interestingly, a meta-analysis of eight double-blind RCTs reported supplementation of greater than 700 IU of vitamin D reduced the fall risk of elderly patients by 19 % compared to those less than 700 IU [13]. These, as well as a myriad of other studies, conclusively demonstrated sufficient evidence for a dose-response relationship between vitamin D and bone health to merit a Dietary Reference Intake recommendation by the Institute of Medicine [2]. However, it should be noted that despite a 2 to 9 times higher prevalence of low vitamin D in the African American population compared to Caucasians, the fracture risk in the African Americans is half that of the Caucasian population [14]. The reported lower levels of vitamin D binding protein in African American, compared to Caucasian, hence resulting in similar levels of bioavailable vitamin D, may account for this finding [15].

Extra-skeletally, vitamin D appears to modulate the immune system, limit malignant potential, and mitigate vascular morbidity. Binding to T cells, B cells, natural killer, and monocyte vitamin D receptors, active vitamin D stimulates the innate immune system and repress of the adaptive system.

Clinically, this has implications in a variety of dermatologic and non-dermatologic conditions. Due to vitamin D's essential role in the containment and destruction of *Mycobacterium tubercul*osis, incorporation of vitamin D supplementation to the standard tuberculoid regimen in those with vitamin D deficiency induces accelerated clinical and radiographic improvement compared to the standard regimen alone [16]. Interestingly, this beneficial effect of vitamin D also has implications prior to clinical disease by reducing one's susceptibility and risk of progression from infection to disease [16]. Similarly, an inverse relationship between gastrointestinal cancer, breast cancer, all cancer mortality, and total life cancer incidence to vitamin D levels has been indicated [16]. Metabolites of 7-DHC and 1, 25 $(OH)_2D3$ also have pro-differentiation and apoptotic effects [17, 18]. Dermatologists take advantage of vitamin D's regulation of cell differentiation and T-cell activity through the topical management of psoriasis, atopic dermatitis, pityriasis alba, and other cutaneous conditions with vitamin D analogues [19]. However, the usefulness of oral vitamin D for these dermatologic conditions, excluding psoriasis, remains conflicted [19–23]. Lastly, vitamin D has receptors on vascular smooth muscle that appear to influence cardiovascular, cerebrovascular, and pregnancy-vasculature morbidity [24, 25].

Despite these and other published findings, the Institute of Medicine concluded that there were insufficient prospective trials to provide adequate evidence warranting any Dietary Reference Intake recommendations for extra-skeletal medical systems. [2] The United States Preventative Services Task Force (USPSTF) was also unable to find sufficient extra-skeletal evidence for recommendations [14]. Therefore, all daily vitamin D recommendations are based on date on skeletal health.

6.4 Photoprotection and Vitamin D

Individuals with limited sun exposure have an increased risk for vitamin D insufficiency and deficiency. A retrospective review of 165 patients with photosensitizing conditions found those practicing strict photoprotection (e.g., xeroderma pigmentosa) or developing symptoms within one hour of sun exposure (e.g., solar urticaria) reliably had vitamin D deficiency in the winter [4]. Additional investigations on erythropoietic protoporphyria and cutaneous lupus erythematosus reported approximately 2/3 of these cohorts were also at risk for vitamin D deficiency and inadequacy, respectively [26, 27]. In the later study, lower serum levels were associated with sun avoidance and daily sunscreen use [27]. However, approximately 50 % of healthy individuals not practicing photoprotection, but rather residing primarily indoors due to work, are at risk for vitamin D insufficiency [28, 29]. Interestingly, vitamin D supplementation provided near-normal serum levels in both healthy and photo-affected populations [29, 30].

While theoretically the use of sunscreens may cause similar vitamin D deficiency and insufficiency as sun avoidance, a 2009 review of published evidence failed to demonstrate the normal use of sunscreens and vitamin D insufficiency [31]. In laboratory setting, however, studies reported that daily application of SPF 8 can impair 90 % of cutaneous vitamin D production, and as little as 5 % of unprotected total body surface area is needed for a notable rise in serum levels following suberythemogenic UVB radiation in subjects with skin phototypes II–III [4, 32]. These findings seemed to be reflected in one of the first investigations on this topic, a randomized controlled trial on 40 fair-skinned patients with a history of skin cancer. However, while this study found subjects that applied para-aminobenzoic acid (PABA) sunscreen over their entire body had significantly lower serum 25(OH)D levels compared to controls with equivalent sun exposure, these levels remained within normal limits [4]. More recently, a randomized, double-blind, controlled trial on 113 Australian subjects divided evenly into daily application of SPF 17 sunscreen and placebo cream did not observe a decrease in vitamin D production with regular sunscreen use for individuals with adequate sun exposure [4]. Similar results were reported in two biannual, controlled studies evaluating daily SPF 15 use with serum and bone markers in one study and dual X-ray absorptiometry studies in the other [4]. A large cross-sectional survey in the United States with 5920 adults and a smaller Australian study found no association between frequent sunscreen use and vitamin D deficiency [4]. Both studies also discovered individuals frequently staying in the shade, or wearing long sleeve shirts, had significantly lower levels of vitamin D than those that did not. It has been speculated that these clinical results do not mirror strict laboratory findings; in laboratory settings, 2 mg/cm^2 of sunscreen was applied (the amount required by FDA for SPF testing), while in actual use, most individuals apply 0.5–1.0 mg/cm^2.

6.5 Recommendations

6.5.1 Vitamin D Levels

Recommendations for vitamin D screening in asymptomatic individuals and interpretation of the results remain a controversial topic between medical organizations. Currently, population-wide screening is not recommended by any national, primary care organization. However, screening is advised by the Endocrine

Society and American Geriatric Society for individuals at risk for vitamin D deficiency due to an underlying condition or behavior [33, 34]. Once tested, deciding the threshold for initiation of treatment varies based upon the organization focus: nutrition repletion, treatment of vitamin deficiencies in asymptomatic individuals, or prevention of a specific negative health outcome regardless of vitamin deficiency [14]. To add more confusion to this matter, serum levels of vitamin D can vary 10–20 % depending upon the assay method and laboratory performing the assessment [14]. Thus, while most practitioners follow the Institute of Medicine's published guidelines, which are discussed below, vitamin D level remains a heated debate.

In 2011, the Institute of Medicine published their evidence-based review and suggested recommendations on vitamin D deficiency and insufficiency for skeletal health. As serum 1,25(OH)D is under tight endocrine control, serum 25(OH)D is used for determining vitamin D status. Serum levels can be reported as either ng/mL or nmol/L (2.5 ng/mL = nmol/L). According to the IOM Committee, 25(OH)D levels of 16–20 ng/mL are sufficient for 97.5 % of the population. However, approximately 50 % of the population only requires 12–16 ng/mL of 25(OH)D to cover their requirements. Therefore, levels below 20 ng/mL suggest risk for insufficiency, and levels below 12 ng/mL indicate risk of deficiency. Levels above 20 ng/mL should not raise significant concern regarding potential adverse effects until levels exceed 50 ng/mL [2].

While these guidelines for vitamin D status are relevant for most conditions, special consideration should be noted for certain conditions, such as sarcoidosis. Patients with sarcoidosis may have falsely low 25(OH)D with sufficient 1, 25$(OH)_2$D due to macrophage conversion of 25(OH)D to 1, 25$(OH)_2$D. Thus, vitamin D supplementation in sarcoidosis may inadvertently cause hypervitaminosis D. Therefore, 1, 25$(OH)_2$D and parathyroid hormone should be evaluated in these patients. Low 1,25$(OH)_2$D with normal PTH merits 400–800 International Units (IU) per day of cholecalciferol, while normal vitamin D with elevated PTH levels warrants a consultation by endocrinology for concerns of hyperparathyroidism [35].

6.5.2 Vitamin D Supplementation

Based upon the IOM's recommended dietary allowances (RDAs) for adults and allowable intake (AI) for infants less than 1 year of age, the required daily nutrition to meet the skeletal requirements of vitamin D for 97.5 % of the population and ensure adequate nutrition (RDA and AI, respectively) is listed by age in Table 6.2. The upper daily intake limit unlikely to pose risk of hypervitaminosis D is 2500 IU/day for 1–3 years old, 3000 IU/day for 4–8 year olds, and 4000 IU/day for those greater than 9 years of age [36].

However, both adequate vitamin D levels and daily requirements of vitamin D are highly debated (Table 6.3).

Table 6.2 IOM recommended dietary allowances and allowable intake [36]

Age (years)	Dose (IU/day)
0–1	400
1–70[a]	600
>70	800

[a]Pregnancy and lactation do not require additional vitamin D supplementation above 600 IU/day

Table 6.3 Discrepancies in adequate vitamin D levels and daily requirements

Organization	25(OH)D level	Daily vitamin D intake
IOM	20 ng/mL (50 nmol/L)	400–800 IU
Endocrine Society	30 ng/mL (75 nmol/L)	400–2000 IU
American Geriatrics Society	30 ng/mL (75 nmol/L)	1000 IU (>65 years old)

Based on Institute of Medicine (IOM) [36], Endocrine Society [33], and American Geriatrics Society recommendations [34]

6.6 Conclusion

Vitamin D possesses a beneficial role in skeletal health and may have broader implications beyond calcemic health. While strict photoprotective measures can reduce serum vitamin D levels, frequent sunscreen use in the real world does not appear to impact vitamin D status. Instead, standard risk factors of low sun exposure, darker skin types, older age with history of falls and non-traumatic fractures, obesity, malabsorption syndromes, severe liver or renal disease, solely breastfed infants, granuloma-forming disorders, and specific medications (glucocorticoids, antiepileptic, antifungal, and autoimmune deficiency syndrome medications) may place individuals at increased risk for vitamin D deficiency or insufficiency [37]. While laboratory assessment and vitamin D supplementation should be considered in these at-risk groups, widespread testing of all individuals is not recommended. While there is much debate about vitamin D screening, definition of deficiency, and daily requirements, most medical bodies agree that replacing vitamin D by solar and artificial UV radiation or recommending against photoprotective practices is ill-advised, given the low cost, broad availability, and safety profile of oral vitamin D supplementation.

References

1. AlGhamdi K, Kumar A, Moussa N (2013) The role of vitamin D in melanogenesis with an emphasis on vitiligo. Indian J Dermatol Venereol Leprol 79(6):750–758
2. Institute of Medicine (US) Committee to Review Dietary Reference Intakes for Vitamin D and Calcium; Ross AC, Taylor CL, Yaktine AL et al (eds) (2011). Chapter 8: Implications and special concerns. In: Dietary reference intakes for calcium and vitamin D. National Academies Press (US), Washington (DC). Available from: http://www.ncbi.nlm.nih.gov/books/NBK56061/

3. Diffey BL (2010) Modelling the seasonal variation of vitamin D due to sun exposure. Br J Dermatol 162(6):1342–1348
4. Kannan S, Lim HW (2014) Photoprotection and vitamin D: a review. Photodermatol Photoimmunol Photomed 30(2-3):137–145
5. Matsuoka LY, Wortsman J, Haddad JG, Kolm P, Hollis BW (1991) Racial pigmentation and the cutaneous synthesis of vitamin D. Arch Dermatol 127(4):536–538
6. Bischoff-Ferrari HA, Dietrich T, Orav EJ, Dawson-Hughes B (2004) Positive association between 25-hydroxyvitamin D levels and bone mineral density: a population-based study of younger and older adults. Am J Med 116(9):634–639
7. Gozdzik A, Barta JL, Weir A, Cole DE, Vieth R, Whiting SJ, Parra EJ (2010) Serum 25-hydroxyvitamin D concentrations fluctuate seasonally in young adults of diverse ancestry living in Toronto. J Nutr 140(12):2213–2220
8. Au LE, Harris SS, Dwyer JT, Jacques PF, Sacheck JM (2014) Association of serum 25-hydroxyvitamin D with race/ethnicity and constitutive skin color in urban school children. J Pediatr Endocrinol Metab 27(11–12):1095–1100
9. Institute of Medicine (US) Committee to Review Dietary Reference Intakes for Vitamin D and Calcium; Ross AC, Taylor CL, Yaktine AL et al (eds) (2011) Chapter 3: Overview of vitamin D. In: Dietary reference intakes for calcium and vitamin D. National Academies Press (US), Washington (DC). Available from: http://www.ncbi.nlm.nih.gov/books/NBK56061/
10. Tripkovic L, Lambert H, Hart K, Smith CP, Bucca G, Penson S, Chope G, Hypponen E, Berry J, Vieth R, Lanham-New S (2012) Comparison of vitamin D2 and vitamin D3 supplementation in raising serum 25-hydroxyvitamin D status: a systematic review and meta-analysis. Am J Clin Nutr 95(6):1357–1364
11. Pike JW, Shevde NK, Hollis BW, Cooke NE, Zella LA (2008) Vitamin D-binding protein influences total circulating levels of 1,25-dihydroxyvitamin D-3 but does not directly modulate the bioactive levels of the hormone in vivo. Endocrinology 149(7):3656–3667
12. Bischoff-Ferrari HA, Willett WC, Wong JB, Stuck AE, Staehelin HB, Orav EJ, Thoma A, Kiel DP, Henschkowski J (2009) Prevention of nonvertebral fractures with oral vitamin D and dose dependency: a meta-analysis of randomized controlled trials. Arch Intern Med 169:551–561
13. Bischoff-Ferrari HA, Dawson-Hughes B, Staehelin HB, Oravek JE, Stuck AE, Theiler R, Wong JB, Egli A, Kiel DP, Henschkowski J (2009) Fall prevention with supplemental and alpha-hydroxylated vitamin D: a meta-analysis of randomized controlled trials. BMJ 339:3692–3703
14. LeFevre ML, on behalf of the U.S. Preventive Services Task Force (2015) Screening for vitamin D deficiency in adults: U.S. Preventive Services Task Force recommendation statement. Ann Intern Med 162:133–140
15. Powe CE, Evans MK, Wenger J, Zonderman AB, Berg AH, Nalls M, Tamez H, Zhang D, Bhan I, Karumanchi SA, Powe NR, Thadhani R (2013) Vitamin D-binding protein and vitamin D status of black Americans and white Americans. N Engl J Med 369(21):1991–2000
16. Salahuddin N, Ali F, Hasan Z, Rao N, Ageel M, Mahmood F (2013) Vitamin D accelerates clinical recovery from tuberculosis: results of the SUCCINCT Study [Supplementary Cholecalciferol in recovery from tuberculosis]. A randomized, placebo-controlled, clinical trial of vitamin D supplementation in patients with pulmonary tuberculosis'. BMC Infect Dis 13:22
17. Slominski AT, Kim TK, Janjetovic Z, Tuckey RC, Bieniek R, Yue J, Li W, Chen J, Nguyen MN, Tang EK, Miller D, Chen TC, Holick M (2011) 20-Hydroxyvitamin D2 is a noncalcemic analog of vitamin D with potent antiproliferative and prodifferentiation activities in normal and malignant cells. Am J Physiol Cell Physiol 300(3):C526–C541
18. Slominski AT, Janjetovic Z, Fuller B, Zmijewski MA, Tuckey RC, Nguyen MN, Sweatman T, Li W, Zjawiony J, Miller D, Chen TC, Lozanski G, Holick MF (2010) Products of vitamin D3 or 7-dehydrocholesterol metabolism by cytochrome P4850scc show anti-leukemia effects, having low or absent calcemic activity. PLoS One 5(3):e9907
19. Wat H, Dytoc M (2014) Off-label uses of topical vitamin D in dermatology: a systematic review. J Cutan Med Surg 18(2):91–108
20. Soleymani T, Hung T, Soung J (2015) The role of vitamin D in psoriasis: a review. Int J Dermatol 54(4):383–92

21. Kamangar F, Koo J, Heller M, Lee E, Bhutani T (2013) Oral vitamin D, still a viable treatment option for psoriasis. J Dermatolog Treat 24(4):261–267
22. Camargo CA, Ganmaa D, Sidbury R, Erdenedelger K, Radnaakhand N, Khandsuren B (2014) Randomized trial of vitamin D supplementation for winter-related atopic dermatitis in children. J Allergy Clin Immunol 134(4):831–835
23. Hata TR, Audish D, Kotol P, Coda A, Kabigting F, Miller J, Alexandrescu D, Boguniewicz M, Taylor P, Aertker L, Kesler K, Hanifin JM, Leung DY, Gallo RL (2014) A randomized controlled double-blind investigation of the effects of vitamin D dietary supplementation in subjects with atopic dermatitis. J Eur Acad Dermatol Venereol 28(6):781–789
24. LoPiccolo MC, Lim HW (2010) Vitamin D in health and disease. Photodermatol Photoimmunol Photomed 26:224–229
25. Sablok A, Batra A, Thariani K, Batra A, Bharti R, Aggarwal AR, Kabi BC, Chellani H (2015) Supplementation of Vitamin D in pregnancy and its correlation with feto-maternal outcome. Clin Endocrinol (Oxf) 83(4):536–541. [Epub ahead of print]
26. Holme SA, Ansley AV, Badminton MN, Elder GH (2008) Serum 25-hydroxyvitamin D in erythropoietic protoporphyria. Br J Dermatol 159:211–213
27. Cusack C, Danby C, Fallon JC (2008) Photoprotective behavior and sunscreen use: impact on vitamin D levels in cutaneous lupus erythematosus. Photodermatol Photoimmunol Photomed 24:260–267
28. Haney EM, Stadler D, Bliziotes MM (2005) Vitamin D insufficiency in internal medicine residents. Calcif Tissue Int 76:11–16
29. Vu LH, Whiteman DC, van der Pols JC, Kimlin MG, Neale RE (2011) Serum vitamin D levels in office workers in a subtropical climate. Photochem Photobiol 87:714–720
30. Reid SM, Robinson M, Kerr AC, Ibbotson SH (2012) Prevalence and predictors of low vitamin D status in patients referred to a tertiary photodiagnostic service: a retrospective study. Photodermatol Photoimmunol Photomed 28:91–96
31. Norval M, Wulf HC (2009) Does chronic sunscreen use reduce vitamin D production to insufficient levels? Br J Dermatol 161(4):732–736
32. Osmancevic A, Sandstrom K, Gillstedt M, Landin-Wilhelmsen K, Larko O, Wennberg Larko AM, F Holick M, Krogstad AL (2015) Vitamin D production after UVB exposure – a comparison of exposed skin regions. J Photochem Photobiol B 143:38–43
33. Holick MF, Binkley NC, Bischoff-Ferrari HA, Gordon CM, Hanley DA, Heaney RP et al; Endocrine Society (2011) Evaluation, treatment, and prevention of vitamin D deficiency: an Endocrine Society clinical practice guideline. J Clin Endocrinol Metab 96:1911–1930
34. American Geriatrics Society Workgroup on Vitamin D Supplementation for Older Adults (2014) Recommendations Abstracted from the American Geriatrics Society Consensus Statement on Vitamin D for Prevention of Falls and Their Consequences. J Am Geriatr Soc 62:147–152
35. Sage RJ, Rao DS, Burke RR, Lim HW (2011) Preventing vitamin D toxicity in patients with sarcoidosis. J Am Acad Dermatol 64(4):795–796
36. Ross AC, Manson JE, Abrams SA (2011) The 2011 report on dietary reference intakes for calcium and vitamin D from the Institute of Medicine: what clinicians need to know. J Clin Endocrinol Metab 96(1):53–58
37. Pramyothin P, Holick M (2012) Vitamin D supplementation: guidelines and evidence for subclinical deficiency. Curr Opin Gastroenterol 28(2):139–150

Chapter 7
Photoprotection and Skin of Color

Kesha J. Buster and Johnathan J. Ledet

Key Points

- UVR exposure is a risk factor for skin cancer in POC; however, melanin's photoprotective properties likely reduce this risk. Despite decreased skin cancer incidence, POC often have increased skin cancer morbidity and mortality.
- Darker constitutive pigmentation exhibits an inverse relationship with degree of photoaging; thus darker POC manifest photoaging much later in life.
- There is a lack of sufficient data regarding ideal photoprotection practices for POC.

7.1 Background: What Is Skin of Color?

Race is a poorly defined term that is a political and social construct more than a biologic phenomenon [12, 87]. Ethnicity is a somewhat broader term referring to ". . .large groups of people classed according to common racial, national, tribal, religious, linguistic, or cultural origin or background" [77]. Each of these terms is

K.J. Buster, MD (✉)
Private Practice, Buster Dermatology, PC, 3915 E. 51st Street, Tulsa, OK 74135, USA

Department of Dermatology, University of Alabama at Birmingham, 1530 3rd Avenue South EFH Suite 414,
Birmingham, AL 35294, USA
e-mail: kbuster07@yahoo.com

J.J. Ledet, MD
Department of Dermatology, NEA Baptist Clinic, 4802 E. Johnson Avenue,
Jonesboro, AR, USA

S.Q. Wang, H.W. Lim (eds.), *Principles and Practice of Photoprotection*,
DOI 10.1007/978-3-319-29382-0_7

multifaceted and self-defined. People of color (POC) is an encompassing phrase commonly used in the United States to refer to ethnic and racial minorities. The overall advantage of this phrase is ". . . its flexibility in accommodating various groups similarly disadvantaged, even if their disadvantages are based on different variables" [119]. Dermatologic health disparities have been identified in POC, particularly in regard to skin cancer [18]. Skin of color (SOC) consists of a wide spectrum of skin tones and racial/ethnic backgrounds. The construct SOC finds its utility in dermatology in a number of factors including that skin diseases sometimes present in drastically different fashion in people of darker skin color (e.g., sunburn/erythema in dark-skinned people can resemble hyperpigmentation). Thus the dermatologist is challenged to recognize a score of disease entities across the spectrum of skin tones. In addition, chief complaints of POC more commonly comprise various dyschromias, such as postinflammatory hyperpigmentation (PIH) [5, 50].

It is estimated that before the year 2050, more than half of those living in the United States will be POC and by 2060 "minorities" will comprise 57 % of the US population [17]. Data show that objective measures of pigmentation such as spectrometry, and colorimetry correlate poorly with self-identified race—a reflection of heterogeneous skin pigmentation found within racial groups [22]. Though racial categories can be useful (e.g., in health disparities research), the demographic ambiguity of a diverse and racially intermixed population may limit the utility of such groupings in dermatologic research. Mersha and Abebe [78] investigated the constraints of racial/ethnic categories in the "age of genomic research" and note that these categories may not be accurate predictors of treatment outcomes. However, the American Medical Association [6] recommends use of the terms of race/ethnicity that were used by the original investigator/author when writing about medical studies; thus such language will be used in this chapter except when using the unifying terms POC/SOC.

7.2 Skin Color Classification

Various systems have been developed to make the classification of skin color more phenotypically objective. Fitzpatrick skin-type scale, originally developed for Caucasian skin, is a frequently used and valid tool for categorizing skin according to ultraviolet radiation (UVR) sensitivity; however, it has been identified as less useful in POC including blacks, Asians, and likely other POC [31, 36, 92, 111, 127]. In an evaluation of various methods to measure skin color, Daniel et al. [27] found that a simple seven-point Likert scale for self-reported natural skin color (very fair/light to very dark) better correlated with spectrophotometry than did the Fitzpatrick skin-type scale. The study participants self-identified as Caucasian, Asian American/Pacific Islander, African American, Hispanic/Latino, or "other" ethnicity. Similarly, the Skin Color Chart is a tool developed by L'Oreal that has been validated in Caucasian, Asian, African American, and Indian skin ([30]; Del Bino S, 2015, personal communication). It allows for evaluation of skin color on any body surface based on a fan deck of 52 cards each with a three-centimeter hole through which skin color can be

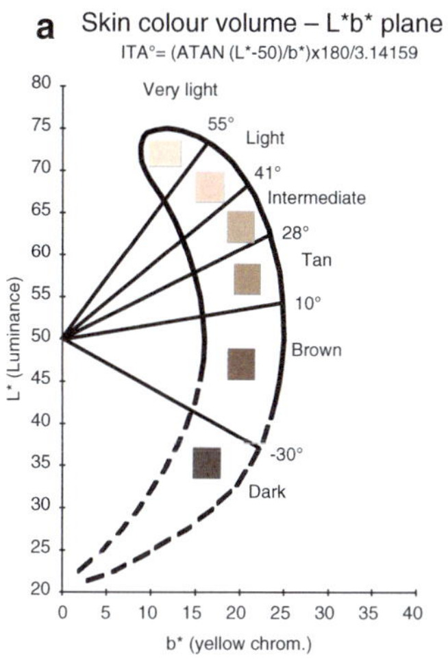

b

Individual Typology Angle ITA°	Skin classification
ITA° > 55°	Very light
41° < ITA°< 55°	Light
28° < ITA° < 41°	Intermediate
10° < ITA° < 28°	Tan
-30° < ITA° < 10°	Brown
ITA° < -30°	Dark

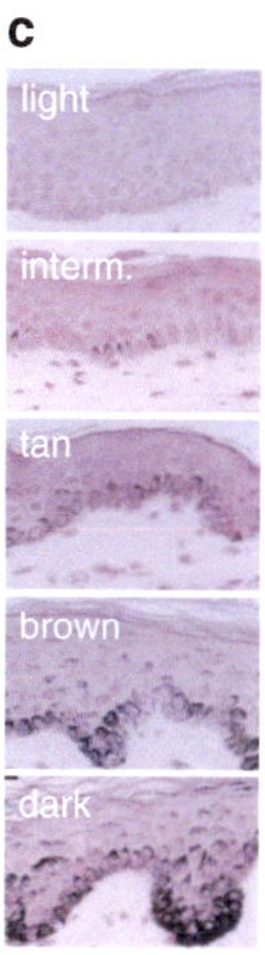

Fig. 7.1 (**a**) Skin colour volume on the L*b* plane (CIELAB 1976 system). The vertical axis L* is the luminance; the horizontal axis b* is the yellow–blue component. (**b**) The individual typology angle (ITA) allows skin colour classification into six groups, from very light to dark skin. (**c**) Fontana–Masson staining of melanin granules shows a good correlation between skin colour classification and melanin quantity and distribution (Reprinted with permission from Del Bino and Bernerd [31])

compared to the card [30]. In addition, colorimetric parameters have been used to create an individual typology angle (ITA)-based skin color classification system composed of 6 skin tones from very light to dark (Fig. 7.1) [23, 33]. ITA is both quantifiable and objective [33]. Visual phenotype/ethnically defined Caucasian skin had ITA values classifying it as light, intermediate, and tan [31]. Likewise defined Hispanic skin ITA values ranged from light to brown; and African skin ITA values ranged from intermediate to dark. Asian ITA scores showed a geographic split with northeast Asian skin ITA values of light, intermediate, and tan, and southeast Asian skin ITA values had a broad range from light to dark. Thus ITA-based skin color classification allows for precise evaluation of in vivo constitutive pigmentation. Furthermore, a correlation exists between ITA-determined skin color and DNA damage with greater levels of UVR-induced DNA damage correlating with lighter skin color [33]. These findings reveal that a spectrum of phenotypes exists in Caucasians and POC; thus objective measures of constitutive skin pigmentation could serve as concrete, consistent, and biophysiologically relevant criteria for defining skin color. Such phenotypically germane terminology is needed in dermatologic research as an alternative means of classification separate from race/ethnicity for greater clarity and consistency in medical literature. The authors and other researchers believe that such objective measurements could be used by dermatologists to make personalized photoprotection recommendations (e.g., maximum daily UVR exposure time, ideal sunscreens, skin cancer prevention strategies, etc.) ([31]; Del Bino S, 2015, personal communication).

Research has shown that epidermal melanin largely determines constitutive pigmentation [3, 4, 9, 110]. Though the beneficial effects of photoprotection in reduction of photoaging and cutaneous malignancy have been demonstrated for Caucasian individuals [42, 43, 89, 104, 117], it is less clear for POC. The role of sun protection in prevention and treatment of disorders of pigmentation such as melasma and postinflammatory hyperpigmentation (PIH) in skin tones across the spectrum is evident [14, 57, 63, 70]. However, there is a lack of sufficient data regarding ideal photoprotection practices for POC. In this chapter, the authors will review the effects of UVR on SOC and the role of photoprotection in POC, as well as controversies and recommendations.

7.3 Biological Effects of UVR on the Skin

7.3.1 Photocarcinogenesis

UVR exposure is a risk factor for skin cancer in POC including Hispanics, blacks, and Asians [25, 37, 48, 49, 52, 59, 61, 90]; however, due to the photoprotective effect of melanin, UVR may play a smaller role in skin cancer development in darkly pigmented skin [37]. Basal cell carcinoma (BCC) is most common on sun-exposed skin across the spectrum of skin types and ethnic backgrounds (Fig. 7.2a) [35, 37, 74, 82]. Though squamous cell carcinoma (SCC) is most common on non-sun-exposed skin in blacks [35, 48, 75, 106], several studies have shown increased nonmelanoma skin cancer (NMSC) in sun-exposed skin of blacks [83, 90]. Risk factors for malignant melanoma (MM) in darker POC are unclear and data are conflicting (see Fig. 7.2b for images). An evaluation of the Surveillance, Epidemiology, and End Results Program (SEER) data revealed no UVR index/lower latitude association with MM incidence in blacks or Hispanics [34]. However, several studies have identified an association between MM and UVR exposure in blacks (the United States), Hispanics (the United States), and Asians (India) [52, 61, 90, 98].

Despite decreased incidence, POC often have increased skin cancer morbidity and mortality [37, 49, 121, 124]. Groups with poorer skin cancer outcomes—including POC—more commonly have misperceptions regarding skin cancer (including expectation of symptoms, discounting importance of skin exams, and confusion on prevention strategies), and these may contribute to skin cancer disparities [19].

NMSC occurs with increased frequency in geographic areas with greater UVB exposure (SCC more than BCC) [101]. In the United States, this means areas of decreased latitude. During the 1980s and 1990s, the Earth experienced alarming loss of the ozone layer over midlatitudes of the Northern Hemisphere due to increased use of ozone-depleting substances over the previous decades [85]. With continued depletion, predictably, all humans, including POC, would have a progressively increased risk of NMSC due to increased UVB reaching the Earth's surface. A US National Cancer Institute study found that for each 1 % relative increase in UVB, there could be a 2 % increase in incidence of NMSC [101]. Similarly, a 2013 study found that NMSC incidence would increase by more than 1000 cases (26.9 %) yearly in Korea secondary to UVB from a constant 10 % decrease in ozone

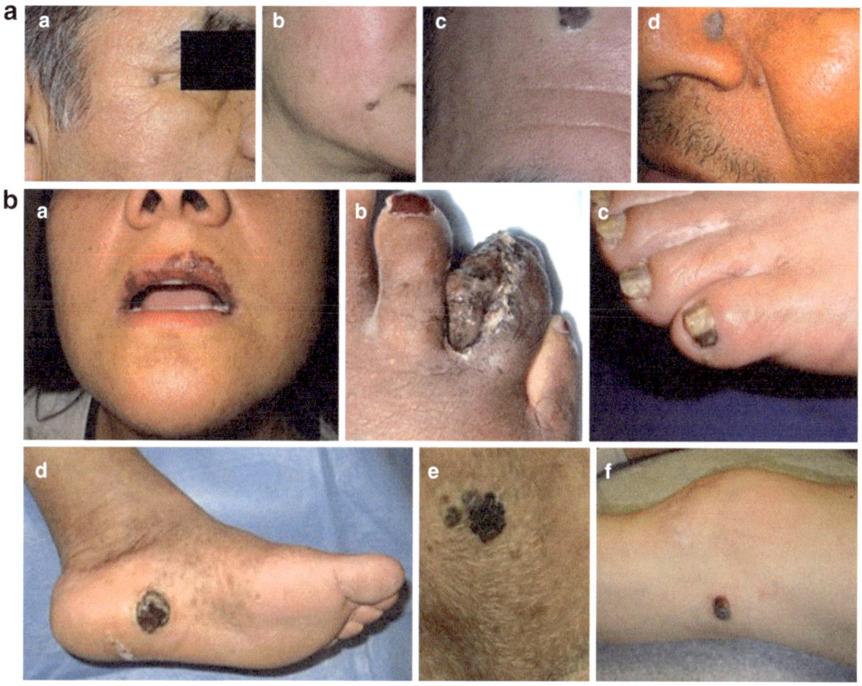

Fig. 7.2 (**a**) Nonmelanoma skin cancers in people of color. Pigmented basal cell carcinoma in elderly Hispanic man (right lateral orbital rim) (*a*); middle-aged Asian woman (right cheek) (*b*); middle-aged Hispanic man (right forehead) (*c*); middle-aged Hispanic man (left nasal ala) (*d*). (**b**) Melanomas in people of color. Lentigo maligna in middle-aged Hispanic woman (vermilion upper and lower lips) (*a*); melanoma in middle-aged black woman (right fourth toe) (*b*); Hispanic woman (left fifth toe) (*c*); middle-aged Hispanic man (left plantar foot) (*d*); elderly Hispanic man (right cheek) (*e*); and Asian woman (side of left leg) (*f*) (Reprinted with permission from Agbai et al. [1])

concentration [65]. Fortunately, international changes in production and use of ozone-depleting substances have led to a reversal of the damage that peaked in the late twentieth century and now the ozone layer is only approximately 3 % less than it was in the 1960s and 1970s [85].

The average UVB protective factor (ex vivo with solar simulator) of dark skin has been shown to be 13.4 vs. 3.4 in fair skin, translating to UVB transmission of 7.4 % vs. 29.4 %, respectively [54]. UVA protective factor is 5.7 in dark skin and 1.8 in fair skin indicating UVA transmission of 17.5 % vs. 55.5 %, respectively. Darker skin has greater melanin content [54, 126] which correlates with removal of UV-induced DNA damage [108] and decreased UVR sensitivity and likely accounts for the reduced skin cancer risk appreciated in POC. Despite the increased protection pigmentation provides against the effects of UVR, epidemiologic studies have shown that sunburn occurs even in darkly pigmented POC, though with decreased frequency compared with fair-skinned individuals [20, 21]. Similarly, UVR-induced skin damage has been documented in skin tones from very light to very dark. Light to tan skin develops cyclobutane pyrimidine dimers (CPD) in all epidermal layers, whereas brown and dark brown skin only form CPD in the suprabasal layers [31]. CPD develop secondary to UVR absorption and are subsequently found in skin cancers [112]. Immediately after UVR exposure, 79–100 % of melanocytes in light skin are CPD positive, whereas 17 % in brown skin and 15 % in dark skin are CPD positive [31]. Even at suberythemal doses, light, medium, and dark skin types incur DNA damage [105, 109], suggesting that photoprotection can be beneficial in all skin types. However, as noted above, the increased melanin content of darker skin does help protect it from photodamage [54]. Numerous studies have identified an inverse relationship between constitutive skin pigmentation and DNA damage [31–33, 97, 109]. Given this intrinsic photoprotection, the necessary level of external photoprotection for prevention of DNA damage and subsequent skin cancer in POC of different levels of skin pigmentation may vary.

7.3.1.1 Photocarcinogenesis and Photoprotection

Photoprotection is the backbone of prevention of acute and chronic effects of UVR, namely, sunburn and skin cancer. There is evidence that sunscreen use in whites is beneficial in the prevention and reduction of actinic keratoses, SCC, MM, and BCC [28, 42, 43, 89, 113, 117]. Further research is needed to determine if these benefits can be generalized to POC. As noted earlier in this chapter, numerous studies have shown that melanin protects the skin, but it does not prevent all DNA damage. Del Bino et al. [32] indicate that DNA of pigmented melanocytes from tan skin may serve as a UVR target and, thus, photoprotection should be recommended for not only light skin but also for moderately pigmented skin.

7.3.2 Photoaging

Photoaging has been defined as the combination of intrinsic aging and photodamage [116]. In contrast to intrinsic (chronological) aging, photoaging is associated with significant changes in skin composition including undesirable changes in texture, wrinkling, increased pigmentation, greater vascularity, laxity, and cutaneous malignancy [41, 103, 104, 116]. Compared to Caucasians, darker POC manifest photoaging much later in life, in approximately the 5th and 6th decade [50]. In one study comparing facial skin of black and white women from ages 20 to 50, blacks had no obvious wrinkles, while most white women 45–50 years old had wrinkles of the lateral canthi (crow's feet) and oral commissures [81]. Visual assessment has shown that African American skin exhibits photoaging changes of hyperpigmentation and uneven skin tone and white skin shows more severe fine lines, wrinkles, laxity, and overall photodamage [44].

Goh [38] observed photoaging as both hyperpigmentation and wrinkles in Asian (Singaporean, Malaysian, and Indonesian) skin. Similarly, Korean photoaging is exhibited as pigmentary changes (hyperpigmented macules and seborrheic keratoses) and wrinkles that gradually increase with age [26]. Mild hyperpigmentation is seen in the 50s, whereas fine wrinkles develop as early as the 40s. Koreans with sun exposure of more than 5 h/day had a 4.8-fold increase in wrinkling risk compared to those with 1–2 h of daily exposure. Dermatoheliosis typically appears in Thais by the age of 40 years, and by age 50 most exhibit extensive sun damage in the form of wrinkles, leathery texture, mottled pigmentation, and increased seborrheic keratoses [60]. Proximity to the equator and lack of efforts to use photoprotection are implicated in greater photodamage at younger age in Thai people.

There is little in the medical literature regarding photoaging in Hispanic populations. Sanchez [99] noted that photoaging was in the top 3 diagnoses recorded in 1000 Latino patients in a dermatology private practice. Photoaging in Hispanic patients of skin types III and IV was documented by Hernandez-Perez and Ibiett [51] in their small preliminary study evaluating the benefits of intense pulsed light in this population. Clinically, fine wrinkles were present and graded as moderate to severe.

Histologically, epidermal changes of photoaging include thickening and compaction of the stratum corneum, vacuolization and dysplasia of keratinocytes, irregular melanin deposition, and Langerhans cell loss [103]. Kotrajaras and Kligman [60] found many of these epidermal changes in photodamaged Thai skin (mostly skin type IV). Hispanic skin (El Salvador) exhibited epidermal disorder via loss of polarity and—in contrast to above—epidermal atrophy [51].

The histologic hallmark of photoaging is dermal solar elastosis [104]. Exposure of light skin (skin types II and III) to chronic (6 weeks) low levels of solar-simulated radiation (SSR) revealed early changes of solar elastosis including decreased procollagen I and deposition of alpha-1 antitrypsin and lysozyme on elastin fibers [104]. Progressive collagen loss and elastin increase are associated with increased sun exposure and age [120]. Photoaging biomarkers such as increase in matrix metalloproteinases and alteration/loss of dermal fibroblasts can primarily be attributed to UVA [9, 11, 71].

Dermal changes in photoaged Asian skin include solar elastosis, collagen loss, and increased glycosaminoglycans [60]. In older Thai people, the elastosis is extensive, only differing from “end-stage photodamaged Caucasoid skin” by not extending as deep in the dermis [60]. Histologic exam of Hispanic skin revealed a range of mild to severe solar elastosis [51]. In a study comparing black and white facial skin exposure to long-term UVR, Montagna and Carlisle [81] found no solar elastosis in the black skin regardless of age. Oxytalan fibers were still present in the skin of black subjects older than 50 years old, but these disappeared in white skin after the late 20s/early 30s. Interestingly, the amount and distribution of elastic fibers of a light-skinned black woman were similar to those in white skin. Only minor epidermal changes were present in black skin compared to extensive alterations in white skin. Similarly, Del Bino and Bernerd [31] found that UVR only caused damage in fibroblasts of light, intermediate, and tan-colored skin, not in brown or dark skin. These findings point to a correlation between constitutive pigmentation and photoaging and help explain the dermal changes of photoaging that are more appreciable in lighter skin.

In an analysis of ethnic variation in melanin content, Alaluf et al. [3] found that the quantity of epidermal melanin in heavily pigmented (i.e., African and Indian) skin is about double that is seen in relatively lightly pigmented (Mexican, Chinese, and European) skin. Prior to that, Yohn et al. [126] found that melanocytes of blacks have significantly more melanin than whites. The dispersion, size, and number of melanosomes are also on a spectrum with darker skin exhibiting greater dispersion, larger size, and increased numbers of melanosomes than lighter skin [3, 81, 114]. Melanosomes are largest in African skin and progressively decrease in size in Indian, Mexican, Chinese, and European skin [3]. Increased melanin correlates with higher constitutive pigmentation, which as aforementioned typically exhibits an inverse relationship with degree of photoaging.

7.3.2.1 Photoprotection and Photoaging

Avoidance of sun exposure and use of sunscreen are widely accepted photoprotective practices as they limit or eliminate UVR-induced DNA and collagen damage that lead to photoaging [10]. UVR also induces oxidative stress (which eventually leads to matrix metalloproteinase degradation of collagen), and antioxidants have been shown to inhibit the UVR cascade that leads to photoaging [56]. Some antioxidants (e.g., ferulic acid, vitamin C combined with vitamin E) also serve as photoprotectants [66, 67].

7.3.3 Pigmentary Disorders

A number of pigmentary disorders disproportionally affect POC and the importance of photoprotection in prevention and treatment of these conditions is often under-recognized as POC are less likely to practice sun-protective behaviors [14, 26, 60, 69, 91]. Two such disorders are highlighted below.

7.3.3.1 Melasma

Melasma is a common, acquired pigmentary disorder of the skin, which manifests as symmetric, irregularly shaped, hyperpigmented macules and patches on the sun-exposed surfaces of the body. The hyperpigmentation of melasma is caused by both melanocytosis and melanogenesis leading to an increase in epidermal and/or dermal pigment [47]. The pathogenesis of melasma is not fully understood as it is influenced by a variety of factors including genetic makeup, age, UVR exposure, hormonal status, and medications [45, 80, 95]. It is most commonly found in females with Fitzpatrick skin phenotypes III–V and is thought to affect over five million people in the United States making it a common reason to seek dermatologic care [45]. Visible light in addition to long-wavelength UVA and UVB has been found to increase pigmentation in melanocompetent skin [70]. A study by Kang et al. [55] showed skin affected by melasma to have upregulation of melanocyte markers TYR, MITF, SILV, and TYRP1. Numerous studies have also shown a significant vascular component in melasma verified through increased levels of vascular endothelial growth factor and stratum corneum hydration [58, 64].

Melasma can be very psychologically distressing to those affected [8]. Many POC are acutely aware of uneven pigmentation of their skin and having melasma heightens this issue. Melasma pigmentation is worse in environments with more intense UVR [96, 118].

Examination with a Wood's lamp was previously thought to differentiate epidermal from dermal pigment; however mixed patterns are commonly seen in melasma, and a histologic study by Sanchez et al. [100] confirmed dermal deposition of melanin in all cases examined. Grimes et al. [47] examined biopsy specimens from melasma-affected skin and perilesional normal-appearing skin in patients with Fitzpatrick phototypes IV through VI. All specimens had increased melanin in the dermis and epidermis compared to Wood's lamp examination predicting epidermal deposition in only some of the patients. Immunohistochemical staining with Mel-5 and electron microscopy showed that melanocytes increased in size, not number.

7.3.3.2 Postinflammatory Hyperpigmentation

Postinflammatory hyperpigmentation (PIH) is very common in POC and is a frequent reason POC present to the dermatologist [5, 50].

PIH is an acquired hypermelanosis that may result from the overproduction of melanin or irregular pigmentation after cutaneous inflammation or injury [46]. PIH may be caused by numerous skin disorders such as eczema, contact dermatitis, and acne but also can be seen after exogenous injury (e.g., burns, cuts, surgical scars, etc.). The exact mechanism of PIH is unknown; however, studies have shown that melanocyte activity is enhanced after stimulation with cytokines, prostanoids, chemokines, interleukins, prostaglandins, reactive oxygen species, and other inflammatory mediators [88, 115]. Epidermal melanin production increases and melanin is transferred to the surrounding keratinocytes. Damage to basal keratinocytes leads to melanin release into the dermis and macrophage (melanophage) phagocytosis takes place [29, 73]. Epidermal hyperpigmentation appears tan, brown, or dark brown, whereas dermal hyperpigmentation has a blue-gray appearance [62]. UVR may worsen PIH and reverse the progress made with therapy [50].

7.3.3.3 Photoprotection in Pigmentary Disorders

UV protection is a core element in the treatment of melasma, PIH, and other disorders of increased skin pigmentation. However, physicians are less likely to prescribe sunscreen for treatment of dyschromias in POC than whites. In an analysis of more than five million patient visits for the sole diagnosis of dyschromia, Kang et al. [57] found that sunscreen use was prescribed for 32 % of whites (3rd most common treatment prescribed for this population), 17 % of blacks (6th most common treatment), and 7 % for Asians (10th most common treatment). Though reasons for this discrepancy are unclear, authors speculate that it may be it is due to dermatologists' recognition of the photoprotective effect of melanin and decreased risk of sunburning in darker skin. However, they note that sunscreen is key in treating hyperpigmentation in all skin types.

Broad-spectrum sunscreen with good UVA protection plays a pivotal role in the treatment of melasma as it may help minimize melasma relapses. Lakhdar et al. [63] found that vigilant sunscreen use as the sole treatment in women (Fitzpatrick skin types II–V) during and after pregnancy led to fewer cases of melasma. With use of broad-spectrum (SPF 50, UVA protective factor 28) sunscreen every 2 h, nearly 80 % of women had lighter skin or the same skin tone at the end of the study. These results are encouraging, but outside a clinical study, compliance with sunscreen application every 2 h is likely to be poor. This is especially likely in POC since they, as noted earlier in this section, use sunscreen and other forms of sun protection less often.

Recently, the utility of *Polypodium leucotomos* extract (PLE) as a treatment for disorders of pigmentation has been evaluated. In a randomized double-blinded placebo-controlled trial (RCT) of 40 Hispanic women with moderate to severe facial melasma, Ahmed et al. [2] found that 240 mg of oral PLE three times daily plus once daily (morning) application of broad-spectrum sunscreen was not significantly better than sunscreen application alone. However, a smaller RCT ($n=21$) revealed significant improvement in women with epidermal melasma treated with twice daily PLE and broad-spectrum (SPF 45) sunscreen compared to sunscreen alone [72]. The skin types of the participants were not revealed in this study. Though, to date, there is no direct research implicating PLE as a useful agent in treatment of other common forms of hyperpigmentation in POC, this is an area worth exploring. A 2004 study in subjects of skin phototypes II and III revealed that PLE (7.5 mg/kg the night prior to exposure) decreased PUVA-induced acute phototoxicity as well as PUVA-induced hyperpigmentation [79]. A 2014 article on dermatologic applications for PLE reviewed research showing promising results for photodermatoses, pigmentary disorders, photoaging, and other dermatologic conditions [24]. Data from such studies indicate that PLE may have additional utility in prevention and treatment of pigmentary disorders in people of all skin types.

7.4 Conclusion

The most notable controversy regarding photoprotection in POC is the challenge of striking a balance between minimizing the risk of sunburn, skin cancer, and photoaging with the need for adequate vitamin D levels. POC are often at greater risk for vitamin D deficiency, which has been associated with a number of negative sequelae including cancer [86], diabetes mellitus [102], and death [107]. UVR is the major source of vitamin D in most countries [122, 125], but oral supplements can also increase vitamin D levels. The American Academy of Dermatology (AAD) recommends oral supplementation of vitamin D in those who are deficient/at risk for low vitamin D [1]. The Institute of Medicine notes that concerns regarding skin cancer preclude recommending vitamin D acquisition from sun exposure and currently lists 600 IU as the recommended daily allowance (RDA) of vitamin D for people from age one to 70 (800 IU for those over the age of 70) [76].

A recent study ($n = 29{,}518$) revealed concerns regarding rigorous sun protection. Swedish women who practiced sun avoidance had an increased risk of all-cause death and double mortality risk compared to women with highest sun exposure [68]. This inverse relationship was dose dependent, inferring a potential link to UVB and vitamin D. Similar results were found in a prior study [125]. Decreased cardiovascular disease and decreased overall mortality were associated with increased solar UV exposure, but increased cancer and overall mortality were associated with artificial UV (tanning bed) exposure. The fact that these studies were done in Sweden, a country of elevated latitude (and thus lower UVB irradiance) compared to the United States, is worth noting. Ecological studies in the United States have also identified an inverse association between UVB irradiance and at least 16 types of cancer including breast and prostate cancer [39, 40]. The association between low UVR dose and increased malignancy has been appreciated not only in Caucasians but also POC including African Americans, Asians, and other minorities [39]. Some advocate sun exposure based on skin type and UV index along with photoprotection against excess UVR as an answer to this problem [128]. However, some individuals have low vitamin D levels despite abundant sun exposure, suggesting varied response of the skin to UVB to create vitamin D [13]. A recent study of American blacks found low levels of vitamin D and vitamin D-binding protein, which appeared to result in 25-hydroxyvitamin D bioavailability equal to whites. Thus it may be that measurement of vitamin D-binding protein is needed to determine actual vitamin D status in diverse patient populations [94].

Some researchers note that if the negative associations with low UVR exposure and increased morbidity and mortality are predominantly the result of low vitamin D levels, then vitamin D supplementation and additional dietary fortification could be key solutions [53]. The question, however, remains whether orally supplemental vitamin D would eliminate the inverse relationship between UV exposure and mortality/malignancy. Although it is unclear if vitamin D obtained by oral supplementation is as effective in risk reduction as vitamin D created by the skin through exposure to UVB, a meta-analysis of 18 RCT revealed that daily vitamin D oral supplementation was associated with decreased overall mortality—though the study could make no conclusion on optimal dosing for the mortality reduction [7]. A more recent meta-analysis of 42 RCT found that oral vitamin D supplementation for greater than 3 years significantly reduced mortality [129]. These findings serve as strong evidence that oral supplementation is highly beneficial.

In response to the complex issues brought forth by the emerging research on vitamin D along with the need for photoprotection to reduce sunburn, skin cancer, and other solar effects, several organizations in the skin cancer capital of the world, Australia, along with New Zealand, convened in 2006 and developed a position

Table 7.1 Risks and benefits of sun exposure: position statement by Cancer Council Australia, the Australian and New Zealand Bone and Mineral Society, Osteoporosis Australia, and the Australasian College of Dermatologists [93]

1. For most people sun protection to prevent skin cancer is required when the UV index is moderate or above (i.e., UV index is 3 or higher). At such times sensible sun protection behavior is warranted and is unlikely to put people at risk of vitamin D deficiency
2. Most people probably achieve adequate vitamin D levels through the UVB exposure they receive during typical day to day outdoor activities. For example, it has been estimated that fair-skinned people can achieve adequate vitamin D levels (>50 nmol/L) in summer by exposing the face, arms, and hands or the equivalent area of skin to a few minutes of sunlight on either side of the peak UV periods on most days of the week. In winter, in the southern regions of Australia where UV radiation levels are less intense, maintenance of vitamin D levels may require 2–3 h of sunlight exposure to the face, arms, and hands or equivalent area of skin over a week
3. Some people are at high risk of skin cancer. They include people who have had skin cancer, have received an organ transplant, or are highly sun sensitive. These people need to have more sun protection and therefore should discuss their vitamin D requirements with their medical practitioner to determine whether dietary supplementation with vitamin D would be preferable to sun exposure
4. Some groups in the community are at increased risk of vitamin D deficiency. They include naturally dark-skinned people, those who cover their skin for religious or cultural reasons, the elderly, babies of vitamin D-deficient mothers, and people who are housebound or are in institutional care. Naturally dark-skinned people (Fitzpatrick skin types 5 and 6 – rarely or never burns) are relatively protected from skin cancer by the pigment in their skin; they could safely increase their sun exposure. Others on this list should discuss their vitamin D status with their medical practitioner as some might benefit from dietary supplementation with vitamin D

Table 7.2 AAD recommendations for photoprotection and early detection of skin cancer in people of color [1]

Seek shade whenever possible
Wear sun-protective clothing
Wear a wide-brimmed hat to shade the face and neck as well as shoes that cover the entire foot
Wear sunglasses with UV-absorbing lenses
Apply broad-spectrum sunscreen with an SPF 30 or greater. Sunscreens without inorganic filters (titanium dioxide and zinc oxide) are generally better accepted by people of color due to their better cosmesis on dark skin
Apply sunscreen to dry skin 15–30 min before going outdoors. When outdoors, reapply every 2 h to all exposed skin and after perspiring or swimming
Avoid exposure to indoor tanning beds/lamps
Take vitamin D supplement
Perform monthly self-skin examinations, paying close attention to subungual skin, palms, soles, mucous membranes, groin, and perianal area

statement with recommendations that attempt to strike a balance (See Table 7.1). In 2010 the British Association of Dermatologists (BAD) made a similar consensus statement with other national organizations advising minutes of regular midday sun exposure without sunscreen (avoiding burning) to promote vitamin D formation without unduly increasing skin cancer risk [15]. The AAD recommendations for photoprotection in POC are listed in Table 7.2.

Besides oral supplementation of vitamin D, personalized photoprotection is likely the key to the challenge of balancing the benefits of photoprotection with its potential risks (e.g., vitamin D deficiency and its associated sequelae). It has been suggested that modern humans take "prescriptions for sun exposure and diet that are appropriate to our ancestry, location and lifestyle" [53]. Seite et al. [103] note that effective UVR protection should be in the context of level of UVI (or similar measure of UVR exposure). Del Bino and Bernerd [31] note that objective phenotyping of skin color can lead to improved photoprotection strategies. Moyal [84] indicated that calculations on needed UVA protective factor have been made in Asia based on "meteorological daily dose according to season and weighted by different factors such as skin type, anatomical skin area, realistic conditions of sunscreen use and realistic duration of exposure to UVR" and that these should be adapted to consumer needs such as amount of time spent outdoors. To that effect, the BAD, in partnership with the UK's national weather service (the Met Office), developed a free phone app called World UV that utilizes UV index (UVI) of the user's location to provide recommendations on sun protection (either "no protection required" or "protection required") [16]. UVI serves as a measure of UVR at the surface of the Earth and was developed by the World Health Organization [123], in conjunction with other international groups, with the goal of serving as a daily tool for the general public to use as a guide for healthy sun protection behavior. The BAD World UV app also lists the UVI determined level of risk according to skin types 1–6 (from low risk to extremely high risk for skin damage). Though Fitzpatrick skin typing may not be ideal for SOC, this nevertheless is a practical educational tool for physicians and patients alike and allows for personalized photoprotection in a simple, modern, and informative format. As we continue to learn more about both the damaging and beneficial effects of UVR, the ability to make recommendations customizable to patients based on skin cancer risk factors, desired treatment outcomes, health needs, and aesthetic concerns is likely to become a reality.

Acknowledgments The authors thank Sandra Del Bino, MsD, and L'Oreal Research and Innovation for provision of Fig. 7.1.

References

1. Agbai ON, Buster K, Sanchez M, Hernandez C, Kundu RV, Chiu M, Roberts WE, Draelos ZD, Bhushan R, Taylor SC, Lim HW (2014) Skin cancer and photoprotection in people of color: a review and recommendations for physicians and the public. J Am Acad Dermatol 70(4):748–762. doi:10.1016/j.jaad.2013.11.038
2. Ahmed AM, Lopez I, Perese F, Vasquez R, Hynan LS, Chong B, Pandya AG (2013) A randomized, double-blinded, placebo-controlled trial of oral Polypodium leucotomos extract as an adjunct to sunscreen in the treatment of melasma. JAMA Dermatol 149(8):981–983. doi:10.1001/jamadermatol.2013.4294
3. Alaluf S, Atkins D, Barrett K, Blount M, Carter N, Heath A (2002) Ethnic variation in melanin content and composition in photoexposed and photoprotected human skin. Pigment Cell Res (Sponsored by the European Society for Pigment Cell Research and the International Pigment Cell Society) 15(2):112–118

4. Alaluf S, Atkins D, Barrett K, Blount M, Carter N, Heath A (2002) The impact of epidermal melanin on objective measurements of human skin colour. Pigment Cell Res (Sponsored by the European Society for Pigment Cell Research and the International Pigment Cell Society) 15(2):119–126
5. Alexis AF, Sergay AB, Taylor SC (2007) Common dermatologic disorders in skin of color: a comparative practice survey. Cutis 80(5):387–394
6. Association AM (2007) AMA manual of style: a guide for authors and editors, 10th edn. Oxford University Press, Oxford/New York
7. Autier P, Gandini S (2007) Vitamin D supplementation and total mortality: a meta-analysis of randomized controlled trials. Arch Intern Med 167(16):1730–1737. doi:10.1001/archinte.167.16.1730
8. Balkrishnan R, McMichael AJ, Camacho FT, Saltzberg F, Housman TS, Grummer S, Feldman SR, Chren MM (2003) Development and validation of a health-related quality of life instrument for women with melasma. Br J Dermatol 149(3):572–577
9. Battie C, Jitsukawa S, Bernerd F, Del Bino S, Marionnet C, Verschoore M (2014) New insights in photoaging. UVA induced damage and skin types. Exp Dermatol 23(Suppl 1): 7–12. doi:10.1111/exd.12388
10. Baumann L (2005) How to prevent photoaging? J Investig Dermatol 125(4):xii–xiii. doi:10.1111/j.0022-202X.2005.23810.x
11. Bernerd F, Asselineau D (1998) UVA exposure of human skin reconstructed in vitro induces apoptosis of dermal fibroblasts: subsequent connective tissue repair and implications in photoaging. Cell Death Differ 5(9):792–802. doi:10.1038/sj.cdd.4400413
12. Bigby M (2009) Epidemiology of cutaneous disease. In: Alexis AF, Taylor S (eds) Dermatology for skin of color, 1st edn. McGraw Hill Medical, New York
13. Binkley N, Novotny R, Krueger D, Kawahara T, Daida YG, Lensmeyer G, Hollis BW, Drezner MK (2007) Low vitamin D status despite abundant sun exposure. J Clin Endocrinol Metabol 92(6):2130–2135. doi:10.1210/jc.2006-2250
14. Briley JJ Jr, Lynfield YL, Chavda K (2007) Sunscreen use and usefulness in African-Americans. J Drugs Dermatol JDD 6(1):19–22
15. British Association of Dermatologists (2010) Vitamin D and the sun: consensus statement. http://www.bad.org.uk/for-the-public/skin-cancer/vitamin-d. Jan 2015
16. British Association of Dermatologists (2011) World UV App. v1.3.2 edn. 22 Design
17. Bureau USC (2012) U.S. Census Bureau Projections Show a Slower Growing, Older, More Diverse Nation a Half Century from Now. https://www.census.gov/newsroom/releases/archives/population/cb12-243.html. Accessed 10 Jan 2015
18. Buster KJ, Stevens EI, Elmets CA (2012a) Dermatologic health disparities. Dermatol Clin 30(1):53–59, viii. doi:10.1016/j.det.2011.08.002
19. Buster KJ, You Z, Fouad M, Elmets C (2012) Skin cancer risk perceptions: a comparison across ethnicity, age, education, gender, and income. J Am Acad Dermatol 66(5):771–779. doi:10.1016/j.jaad.2011.05.021
20. Centers for Disease Control and Prevention (2007) Sunburn prevalence among adults--United States, 1999, 2003, and 2004. MMWR Morb Mortal Wkly Rep 56(21):524–528
21. Centers for Disease Control and Prevention (2012) Sunburn and sun protective behaviors among adults aged 18–29 years--United States, 2000–2010. MMWR Morb Mortal Wkly Rep 61(18):317–322
22. Chan JL, Ehrlich A, Lawrence RC, Moshell AN, Turner ML, Kimball AB (2005) Assessing the role of race in quantitative measures of skin pigmentation and clinical assessments of photosensitivity. J Am Acad Dermatol 52(4):609–615. doi:10.1016/j.jaad.2004.03.051
23. Chardon A, Cretois I, Hourseau C (1991) Skin colour typology and suntanning pathways. Int J Cosmet Sci 13(4):191–208. doi:10.1111/j.1467-2494.1991.tb00561.x
24. Choudhry SZ, Bhatia N, Ccillcy R, Hougeir F, Lieberman R, Hamzavi I, Lim HW (2014) Role of oral *polypodium leucotomos* extract in dermatologic diseases: a review of the literature. J Drugs Dermatol 13(2):148–153

25. Chuang TY, Reizner GT, Elpern DJ, Stone JL, Farmer ER (1995) Nonmelanoma skin cancer in Japanese ethnic Hawaiians in Kauai, Hawaii: an incidence report. J Am Acad Dermatol 33(3):422–426
26. Chung JH, Lee SH, Youn CS, Park BJ, Kim KH, Park KC, Cho KH, Eun HC (2001) Cutaneous photodamage in Koreans: influence of sex, sun exposure, smoking, and skin color. Arch Dermatol 137(8):1043–1051
27. Daniel LC, Heckman CJ, Kloss JD, Manne SL (2009) Comparing alternative methods of measuring skin color and damage. Cancer Causes Control CCC 20(3):313–321. doi:10.1007/s10552-008-9245-3
28. Darlington S, Williams G, Neale R, Frost C, Green A (2003) A randomized controlled trial to assess sunscreen application and beta carotene supplementation in the prevention of solar keratoses. Arch Dermatol 139(4):451–455. doi:10.1001/archderm.139.4.451
29. Davis EC, Callender VD (2010) Postinflammatory hyperpigmentation: a review of the epidemiology, clinical features, and treatment options in skin of color. J Clin Aesthet Dermatol 3(7):20–31
30. de Rigal J, Abella ML, Giron F, Caisey L, Lefebvre MA (2007) Development and validation of a new Skin Color Chart. Skin Res Technol Off J Int Soc Bioeng Skin 13(1):101–109. doi:10.1111/j.1600-0846.2007.00223.x
31. Del Bino S, Bernerd F (2013) Variations in skin colour and the biological consequences of ultraviolet radiation exposure. Br J Dermatol 169(Suppl 3):33–40. doi:10.1111/bjd.12529
32. Del Bino S, Sok J, Bernerd F (2013) Assessment of ultraviolet-radiation-induced DNA damage within melanocytes in skin of different constitutive pigmentation. Br J Dermatol 168(5):1120–1123. doi:10.1111/bjd.12201
33. Del Bino S, Sok J, Bessac E, Bernerd F (2006) Relationship between skin response to ultraviolet exposure and skin color type. Pigment Cell Res (Sponsored by the European Society for Pigment Cell Research and the International Pigment Cell Society) 19(6):606–614. doi:10.1111/j.1600-0749.2006.00338.x
34. Eide MJ, Weinstock MA (2005) Association of UV index, latitude, and melanoma incidence in nonwhite populations–US Surveillance, Epidemiology, and End Results (SEER) Program, 1992 to 2001. Arch Dermatol 141(4):477–481. doi:10.1001/archderm.141.4.477
35. Fleming ID, Barnawell JR, Burlison PE, Rankin JS (1975) Skin cancer in black patients. Cancer 35(3):600–605
36. Galindo GR, Mayer JA, Slymen D, Almaguer DD, Clapp E, Pichon LC, Hoerster K, Elder JP (2007) Sun sensitivity in 5 US ethnoracial groups. Cutis 80(1):25–30
37. Gloster HM Jr, Neal K (2006) Skin cancer in skin of color. J Am Acad Dermatol 55(5):741–760, quiz 761–744. doi:10.1016/j.jaad.2005.08.063
38. Goh SH (1990) The treatment of visible signs of senescence: the Asian experience. Br J Dermatol 122(Suppl 35):105–109
39. Grant WB (2002) An estimate of premature cancer mortality in the U.S. due to inadequate doses of solar ultraviolet-B radiation. Cancer 94(6):1867–1875
40. Grant WB, Garland CF (2006) The association of solar ultraviolet B (UVB) with reducing risk of cancer: multifactorial ecologic analysis of geographic variation in age-adjusted cancer mortality rates. Anticancer Res 26(4A):2687–2699
41. Gray J, Hawk JLM (eds) (1998) The benefit of lifetime photoprotection. International Congress & Symposium Royal Society of Medicine Press, London
42. Green A, Williams G, Neale R, Hart V, Leslie D, Parsons P, Marks GC, Gaffney P, Battistutta D, Frost C, Lang C, Russell A (1999) Daily sunscreen application and beta carotene supplementation in prevention of basal-cell and squamous-cell carcinomas of the skin: a randomised controlled trial. Lancet 354(9180):723–729. doi:10.1016/S0140-6736(98)12168-2
43. Green AC, Williams GM, Logan V, Strutton GM (2011) Reduced melanoma after regular sunscreen use: randomized trial follow-up. J Clin Oncol Off J Am Soc Clin Oncol 29(3):257–263. doi:10.1200/JCO.2010.28.7078

44. Grimes P, Edison BL, Green BA, Wildnauer RH (2004) Evaluation of inherent differences between African American and white skin surface properties using subjective and objective measures. Cutis 73(6):392–396
45. Grimes PE (1995) Melasma. Etiologic and therapeutic considerations. Arch Dermatol 131(12):1453–1457
46. Grimes PE (2009) Management of hyperpigmentation in darker racial ethnic groups. Semin Cutan Med Surg 28(2):77–85. doi:10.1016/j.sder.2009.04.001
47. Grimes PE, Yamada N, Bhawan J (2005) Light microscopic, immunohistochemical, and ultrastructural alterations in patients with melasma. Am J Dermatopathol 27(2):96–101
48. Halder RM, Bang KM (1988) Skin cancer in blacks in the United States. Dermatol Clin 6(3):397–405
49. Halder RM, Bridgeman-Shah S (1995) Skin cancer in African Americans. Cancer 75(2 Suppl): 667–673
50. Halder RM, Nootheti PK (2003) Ethnic skin disorders overview. J Am Acad Dermatol 48(6 Suppl):S143–S148. doi:10.1067/mjd.2003.274
51. Hernandez-Perez E, Ibiett EV (2002) Gross and microscopic findings in patients submitted to nonablative full-face resurfacing using intense pulsed light: a preliminary study. Dermatol Surg Off Publ Am Soc Dermatol Surg [et al] 28(8):651–655
52. Hu S, Ma F, Collado-Mesa F, Kirsner RS (2004) UV radiation, latitude, and melanoma in US Hispanics and blacks. Arch Dermatol 140(7):819–824. doi:10.1001/archderm.140.7.819
53. Jablonski NG (2014) Is there a golden mean for sun exposure? J Intern Med 276(1):71–73. doi:10.1111/joim.12248
54. Kaidbey KH, Agin PP, Sayre RM, Kligman AM (1979) Photoprotection by melanin--a comparison of black and Caucasian skin. J Am Acad Dermatol 1(3):249–260
55. Kang HY, Suzuki I, Lee DJ, Ha J, Reiniche P, Aubert J, Deret S, Zugaj D, Voegel JJ, Ortonne JP (2011) Transcriptional profiling shows altered expression of wnt pathway- and lipid metabolism-related genes as well as melanogenesis-related genes in melasma. J Investig Dermatol 131(8):1692–1700. doi:10.1038/jid.2011.109
56. Kang S, Chung JH, Lee JH, Fisher GJ, Wan YS, Duell EA, Voorhees JJ (2003) Topical N-acetyl cysteine and genistein prevent ultraviolet-light-induced signaling that leads to photoaging in human skin in vivo. J Investig Dermatol 120(5):835–841. doi:10.1046/j.1523-1747.2003.12122.x
57. Kang SJ, Davis SA, Feldman SR, McMichael AJ (2014) Dyschromia in skin of color. J Drugs Dermatol JDD 13(4):401–406
58. Kim EH, Kim YC, Lee ES, Kang HY (2007) The vascular characteristics of melasma. J Dermatol Sci 46(2):111–116. doi:10.1016/j.jdermsci.2007.01.009
59. Koh D, Wang H, Lee J, Chia KS, Lee HP, Goh CL (2003) Basal cell carcinoma, squamous cell carcinoma and melanoma of the skin: analysis of the Singapore Cancer Registry data 1968–97. Br J Dermatol 148(6):1161–1166
60. Kotrajaras R, Kligman AM (1993) The effect of topical tretinoin on photodamaged facial skin: the Thai experience. Br J Dermatol 129(3):302–309
61. Krishnamurthy S (1992) The geography of non-ocular malignant melanoma in India: its association with latitude, ozone levels and UV light exposure. Int J Cancer 51(2):169–172
62. Lacz NL, Vafaie J, Kihiczak NI, Schwartz RA (2004) Postinflammatory hyperpigmentation: a common but troubling condition. Int J Dermatol 43(5):362–365. doi:10.1111/j.1365-4632.2004.02267.x
63. Lakhdar H, Zouhair K, Khadir K, Essari A, Richard A, Seite S, Rougier A (2007) Evaluation of the effectiveness of a broad-spectrum sunscreen in the prevention of chloasma in pregnant women. J Eur Acad Dermat Venereol JEADV 21(6):738–742. doi:10.1111/j.1468-3083.2007.02185.x
64. Lee DJ, Lee J, Ha J, Park KC, Ortonne JP, Kang HY (2012) Defective barrier function in melasma skin. J Eur Acad Dermat Venereol JEADV 26(12):1533–1537. doi:10.1111/j.1468-3083.2011.04337.x
65. Lee SG, Ko NY, Son SW, Bae HJ, Ha JS, Pak HY, Shin YS (2013) The impact of ozone depletion on skin cancer incidence in Korea. Br J Dermatol 169(5):1164–1165. doi:10.1111/bjd.12472

66. Lin FH, Lin JY, Gupta RD, Tournas JA, Burch JA, Selim MA, Monteiro-Riviere NA, Grichnik JM, Zielinski J, Pinnell SR (2005) Ferulic acid stabilizes a solution of vitamins C and E and doubles its photoprotection of skin. J Investig Dermatol 125(4):826–832. doi:10.1111/j.0022-202X.2005.23768.x
67. Lin JY, Selim MA, Shea CR, Grichnik JM, Omar MM, Monteiro-Riviere NA, Pinnell SR (2003) UV photoprotection by combination topical antioxidants vitamin C and vitamin E. J Am Acad Dermatol 48(6):866–874. doi:10.1067/mjd.2003.425
68. Lindqvist PG, Epstein E, Landin-Olsson M, Ingvar C, Nielsen K, Stenbeck M, Olsson H (2014) Avoidance of sun exposure is a risk factor for all-cause mortality: results from the Melanoma in Southern Sweden cohort. J Intern Med 276(1):77–86. doi:10.1111/joim.12251
69. Mahler HI (2014) Reasons for using and failing to use sunscreen: comparison among whites, Hispanics, and Asian/Pacific Islanders in Southern California. JAMA dermatology 150(1):90–91. doi:10.1001/jamadermatol.2013.4992
70. Mahmoud BH, Ruvolo E, Hexsel CL, Liu Y, Owen MR, Kollias N, Lim HW, Hamzavi IH (2010) Impact of long-wavelength UVA and visible light on melanocompetent skin. J Investig Dermatol 130(8):2092–2097. doi:10.1038/jid.2010.95
71. Marionnet C, Grether-Beck S, Seite S, Marini A, Jaenicke T, Lejeune F, Bastien P, Rougier A, Bernerd F, Krutmann J (2011) A broad-spectrum sunscreen prevents UVA radiation-induced gene expression in reconstructed skin in vitro and in human skin in vivo. Exp Dermatol 20(6):477–482. doi:10.1111/j.1600-0625.2011.01265.x
72. Martin L, Caperton C, Wollert-Lloyd H, Avashia N (2012) A randomized double-blind placebo controlled study evaluating the effectiveness and tolerability of oral Polypodium leucotomos in patients with melasma. J Am Acad Dermatol 66(4, Suppl 1):AB21
73. Masu S, Seiji M (1983) Pigmentary incontinence in fixed drug eruptions. Histologic and electron microscopic findings. J Am Acad Dermatol 8(4):525–532
74. Matsuoka LY, Schauer PK, Sordillo PP (1981) Basal cell carcinoma in black patients. J Am Acad Dermatol 4(6):670–672
75. McCall CO, Chen SC (2002) Squamous cell carcinoma of the legs in African Americans. J Am Acad Dermatol 47(4):524–529
76. Medicine Io (2011) Dietary reference intakes for adequacy: calcium and vitamin D; implications and special concerns. Dietary reference intakes for calcium and vitamin D. National Academies Press, Washington, DC
77. Merriam-Webster "Ethnicity". www.Merriam-Webster.com
78. Mersha TB, Abebe T (2015) Self-reported race/ethnicity in the age of genomic research: its potential impact on understanding health disparities. Hum Genomics 9(1):1. doi:10.1186/PREACCEPT-2695828013752627
79. Middelkamp-Hup MA, Pathak MA, Parrado C, Garcia-Caballero T, Rius-Diaz F, Fitzpatrick TB, Gonzalez S (2004) Orally administered Polypodium leucotomos extract decreases psoralen-UVA-induced phototoxicity, pigmentation, and damage of human skin. J Am Acad Dermatol 50(1):41–49. doi:10.1016/S0190
80. Moin A, Jabery Z, Fallah N (2006) Prevalence and awareness of melasma during pregnancy. Int J Dermatol 45(3):285–288. doi:10.1111/j.1365-4632.2004.02470.x
81. Montagna W, Carlisle K (1991) The architecture of black and white facial skin. J Am Acad Dermatol 24(6 Pt 1):929–937
82. Mora RG, Burris R (1981) Cancer of the skin in blacks: a review of 128 patients with basal-cell carcinoma. Cancer 47(6):1436–1438
83. Mora RG, Perniciaro C (1981) Cancer of the skin in blacks. I. A review of 163 black patients with cutaneous squamous cell carcinoma. J Am Acad Dermatol 5(5):535–543
84. Moyal D (2012) Need for a well-balanced sunscreen to protect human skin from both Ultraviolet A and Ultraviolet B damage. Indian J Dermatol Venereol Leprol 78(Suppl 1):S24–S30. doi:10.4103/0378-6323.97352
85. Newman P, Herman J (2009) Ozone and UV: Where are we now? Skin Cancer Found J 27:38–42

86. Obaidi J, Musallam E, Al-Ghzawi HM, Azzeghaiby SN, Alzoghaibi IN (2015) Vitamin d and its relationship with breast cancer: an evidence based practice paper. Glob J Health Sci 7(1):35687. doi:10.5539/gjhs.v7n1p261
87. Oppenheimer GM (2001) Paradigm lost: race, ethnicity, and the search for a new population taxonomy. Am J Public Health 91(7):1049–1055
88. Ortonne JP (1992) Retinoic acid and pigment cells: a review of in-vitro and in-vivo studies. Br J Dermatol 127(Suppl 41):43–47
89. Pandeya N, Purdie DM, Green A, Williams G (2005) Repeated occurrence of basal cell carcinoma of the skin and multifailure survival analysis: follow-up data from the Nambour Skin Cancer Prevention Trial. Am J Epidemiol 161(8):748–754. doi:10.1093/aje/kwi098
90. Pennello G, Devesa S, Gail M (2000) Association of surface ultraviolet B radiation levels with melanoma and nonmelanoma skin cancer in United States blacks. Cancer Epidemiol Biomarkers Prev Publ Am Assoc Cancer Res (Cosponsored by the American Society of Preventive Oncology) 9(3):291–297
91. Pichon LC, Corral I, Landrine H, Mayer JA, Norman GJ (2010) Sun-protection behaviors among African Americans. Am J Prev Med 38(3):288–295. doi:10.1016/j.amepre.2009.10.041
92. Pichon LC, Landrine H, Corral I, Hao Y, Mayer JA, Hoerster KD (2010) Measuring skin cancer risk in African Americans: is the Fitzpatrick Skin Type Classification Scale culturally sensitive? Ethn Dis 20(2):174–179
93. Position statement developed in 2006. http://www.dermcoll.edu.au/wp-content/uploads/2014/05/Risks_and_Benefits_of_Sun_Exposure03May07.pdf. Accessed Jan 2015
94. Powe CE, Evans MK, Wenger J, Zonderman AB, Berg AH, Nalls M, Tamez H, Zhang D, Bhan I, Karumanchi SA, Powe NR, Thadhani R (2013) Vitamin D-binding protein and vitamin D status of black Americans and white Americans. N Engl J Med 369(21):1991–2000
95. Resnik S (1967) Melasma induced by oral contraceptive drugs. JAMA 199(9):601–605
96. Rigopoulos D, Gregoriou S, Katsambas A (2007) Hyperpigmentation and melasma. J Cosmet Dermatol 6(3):195–202. doi:10.1111/j.1473-2165.2007.00321.x
97. Rijken F, Bruijnzeel PL, van Weelden H, Kiekens RC (2004) Responses of black and white skin to solar-simulating radiation: differences in DNA photodamage, infiltrating neutrophils, proteolytic enzymes induced, keratinocyte activation, and IL-10 expression. J Investig Dermatol 122(6):1448–1455. doi:10.1111/j.0022-202X.2004.22609.x
98. Rouhani P, Pinheiro PS, Sherman R, Arheart K, Fleming LE, Mackinnon J, Kirsner RS (2010) Increasing rates of melanoma among nonwhites in Florida compared with the United States. Arch Dermatol 146(7):741–746. doi:10.1001/archdermatol.2010.133
99. Sanchez MR (2003) Cutaneous diseases in Latinos. Dermatol Clin 21(4):689–697
100. Sanchez NP, Pathak MA, Sato S, Fitzpatrick TB, Sanchez JL, Mihm MC Jr (1981) Melasma: a clinical, light microscopic, ultrastructural, and immunofluorescence study. J Am Acad Dermatol 4(6):698–710
101. Scotto J, Fears T, Fraumeni JJ (1983) Incidence of non-melanoma skin cancer in the United States. http://www.ciesin.org/docs/001-526/001-526.html. Accessed Jan 2015
102. Scragg R, Sowers M, Bell C, Third National H, Nutrition Examination S (2004) Serum 25-hydroxyvitamin D, diabetes, and ethnicity in the Third National Health and Nutrition Examination Survey. Diabetes Care 27(12):2813–2818
103. Seite S, Fourtanier A, Moyal D, Young AR (2010) Photodamage to human skin by suberythemal exposure to solar ultraviolet radiation can be attenuated by sunscreens: a review. Br J Dermatol 163(5):903–914. doi:10.1111/j.1365-2133.2010.10018.x
104. Seite S, Fourtanier AM (2008) The benefit of daily photoprotection. J Am Acad Dermatol 58(5 Suppl 2):S160–S166. doi:10.1016/j.jaad.2007.04.036
105. Sheehan JM, Cragg N, Chadwick CA, Potten CS, Young AR (2002) Repeated ultraviolet exposure affords the same protection against DNA photodamage and erythema in human skin types II and IV but is associated with faster DNA repair in skin type IV. J Investig Dermatol 118(5):825–829. doi:10.1046/j.1523-1747.2002.01681.x

106. Singh B, Bhaya M, Shaha A, Har-El G, Lucente FE (1998) Presentation, course, and outcome of head and neck skin cancer in African Americans: a case-control study. Laryngoscope 108(8 Pt 1):1159–1163
107. Skaaby T (2015) The relationship of vitamin D status to risk of cardiovascular disease and mortality. Danish Med J 61(2)
108. Smit NP, Vink AA, Kolb RM, Steenwinkel MJ, van den Berg PT, van Nieuwpoort F, Roza L, Pavel S (2001) Melanin offers protection against induction of cyclobutane pyrimidine dimers and 6–4 photoproducts by UVB in cultured human melanocytes. Photochem Photobiol 74(3):424–430
109. Tadokoro T, Kobayashi N, Zmudzka BZ, Ito S, Wakamatsu K, Yamaguchi Y, Korossy KS, Miller SA, Beer JZ, Hearing VJ (2003) UV-induced DNA damage and melanin content in human skin differing in racial/ethnic origin. FASEB J Off Publ Fed Am Soc Exp Biol 17(9):1177–1179. doi:10.1096/fj.02-0865fje
110. Tadokoro T, Yamaguchi Y, Batzer J, Coelho SG, Zmudzka BZ, Miller SA, Wolber R, Beer JZ, Hearing VJ (2005) Mechanisms of skin tanning in different racial/ethnic groups in response to ultraviolet radiation. J Investig Dermatol 124(6):1326–1332. doi:10.1111/j.0022-202X.2005.23760.x
111. Taylor SC, Cook-Bolden F (2002) Defining skin of color. Cutis 69(6):435–437
112. Tewari A, Sarkany RP, Young AR (2012) UVA1 induces cyclobutane pyrimidine dimers but not 6–4 photoproducts in human skin in vivo. J Investig Dermatol 132(2):394–400. doi:10.1038/jid.2011.283
113. Thompson SC, Jolley D, Marks R (1993) Reduction of solar keratoses by regular sunscreen use. N Engl J Med 329(16):1147–1151. doi:10.1056/NEJM199310143291602
114. Toda K, Pathak MA, Parrish JA, Fitzpatrick TB, Quevedo WC Jr (1972) Alteration of racial differences in melanosome distribution in human epidermis after exposure to ultraviolet light. Nature New Biol 236(66):143–145
115. Tomita Y, Maeda K, Tagami H (1992) Melanocyte-stimulating properties of arachidonic acid metabolites: possible role in postinflammatory pigmentation. Pigment Cell Res (Sponsored by the European Society for Pigment Cell Research and the International Pigment Cell Society) 5(5 Pt 2):357–361
116. Tsoureli-Nikita E, Watson RE, Griffiths CE (2006) Photoageing: the darker side of the sun. Photochem Photobiol Sci Off J Eur Photochem Assoc Eur Soc Photobiol 5(2):160–164. doi:10.1039/b507492d
117. van der Pols JC, Williams GM, Pandeya N, Logan V, Green AC (2006) Prolonged prevention of squamous cell carcinoma of the skin by regular sunscreen use. Cancer Epidemiol Biomarkers Prev Publ Am Assoc Cancer Res (Cosponsored by the American Society of Preventive Oncology) 15(12):2546–2548. doi:10.1158/1055-9965.EPI-06-0352
118. Victor FC, Gelber J, Rao B (2004) Melasma: a review. J Cutan Med Surg 8(2):97–102. doi:10.1007/s10227-004-0158-9
119. Vidal-Ortiz S (2008) People of Color. In: Schaefer RT (ed) Encyclopedia of race, ethnicity, and society. SAGE Publications, Los Angeles, pp 1037–1039
120. Warren R, Gartstein V, Kligman AM, Montagna W, Allendorf RA, Ridder GM (1991) Age, sunlight, and facial skin: a histologic and quantitative study. J Am Acad Dermatol 25(5 Pt 1): 751–760
121. Weinstock MA (1993) Nonmelanoma skin cancer mortality in the United States, 1969 through 1988. Arch Dermatol 129(10):1286–1290
122. Weinstock MA, Moses AM (2009) Skin cancer meets vitamin D: the way forward for dermatology and public health. J Am Acad Dermatol 61(4):720–724. doi:10.1016/j.jaad.2009.04.016
123. World Health Organization (2002) Global solar UV index: a practical guide. http://www.who.int/uv/publications/en/UVIGuide.pdf. Accessed 21 Jan 2015
124. Wingo PA, Bolden S, Tong T, Parker SL, Martin LM, Heath CW Jr (1996) Cancer statistics for African Americans, 1996. CA Cancer J Clinicians 46(2):113–125

125. Yang L, Lof M, Veierod MB, Sandin S, Adami HO, Weiderpass E (2011) Ultraviolet exposure and mortality among women in Sweden. Cancer Epidemiol Biomarkers Prev Publ Am Assoc Cancer Res (Cosponsored by the American Society of Preventive Oncology) 20(4):683–690. doi:10.1158/1055-9965.EPI-10-0982
126. Yohn JJ, Lyons MB, Norris DA (1992) Cultured human melanocytes from black and white donors have different sunlight and ultraviolet A radiation sensitivities. J Investig Dermatol 99(4):454–459
127. Youn JI, Oh JK, Kim BK, Suh DH, Chung JH, Oh SJ, Kim JJ, Kang SH (1997) Relationship between skin phototype and MED in Korean, brown skin. Photodermatol Photoimmunol Photomed 13(5–6):208–211
128. Zeeb H, Greinert R (2010) The role of vitamin D in cancer prevention: does UV protection conflict with the need to raise low levels of vitamin D? Deutsches Arzteblatt Int 107(37): 638–643. doi:10.3238/arztebl.2010.0638
129. Zheng Y, Zhu J, Zhou M, Cui L, Yao W, Liu Y (2013) Meta-analysis of long-term vitamin D supplementation on overall mortality. PLoS One 8(12):e82109. doi:10.1371/journal.pone.0082109

Chapter 8
The Controversy of Sunscreen Product Exposure: Too Little, Too Much, or Just Right

J. Frank Nash and Paul R. Tanner

Key Points

- Sunscreen products have a controversial history. Fundamental to the controversies surrounding sunscreens is product use or exposure.
- It is alleged too little sunscreen product is applied reducing their effectiveness or, conversely, that too much product is used resulting in unfavorable health effects.
- The weight of evidence is supportive of daily use of sunscreens as part of a "safe sun strategy" including wearing protective clothing and seeking shade. Importantly, a consistent, simple public health message is required and supported broadly by all stakeholders.

8.1 Introduction

Exposure to sunlight, which is crucial for human survival, can have detrimental effects on our skin. The absence of hair covering our bodies makes human skin vulnerable to the effects of ultraviolet radiation (UVR) in sunlight. Acute overexposure to sunlight results in erythema, i.e., sunburn, and in more extreme cases edema, which are thought to be a manifestation of complex molecular events, including DNA damage and the release of cytokines [10, 22, 57]. Exposure to UVR also triggers melanogenesis or tanning, a protective mechanism but only to the extent that "damage" is the initiating biological event [32, 49].

J.F. Nash, PhD (✉) • P.R. Tanner
Central Product Safety, Global Product Stewardship,
The Procter & Gamble Company, Sharon Woods Innovation Center,
11530 Reed Hartman Highway, Cincinnati, OH 45241, USA
e-mail: nash.jf@pg.com

S.Q. Wang, H.W. Lim (eds.), *Principles and Practice of Photoprotection*,
DOI 10.1007/978-3-319-29382-0_8

Beyond the acute effects of sunlight overexposure, the prevailing view is that UVR-induced skin damage is cumulative [24, 26]. Such damage, over decades of life, may lead directly or significantly contribute to nonmelanoma and melanoma skin cancers [12, 68, 90] and photoaging, characterized by wrinkles, pigmentary unevenness, and telangiectasia [25, 67].

Public health education campaigns seem to be having the desired effect since there is general knowledge among teenagers and adults in the USA that exposure to UVR from sunlight can cause skin cancers and photoaging [21]. The use of sun-protective behaviors has held steady and actually increased from 2000 to 2010, although the percentage remains relatively low, i.e., less than 35 % for women and men [15]. Nevertheless, there still are many cases of skin cancers in the USA.[1] It is possible that there is a lag between widespread sun-protective activities and prevalence of skin cancers. However, it is equally likely that behaviors including indoor tanning and sunbathing contribute disproportionately to unfavorable long-term health effects. Thus, despite gains in awareness regarding the detrimental effects of sunlight, it would seem cosmetic/appearance benefits make it difficult for individuals to change behavior even when they know it is harmful [48, 78]. Further complicating the desire to intentional expose oneself to UVR is the evidence that such behavior may have some addictive components [27, 89].

Given the unequivocal cause-effect relationship between sunlight exposure and skin damage as well as the health-related messages advocating "active outdoor lifestyles," it would seem products whose singular purpose is to reduce the "dose" of solar UVR might be of unquestionable benefit. In the simplest of terms, sunscreens are such products. The ultraviolet (UV) filters are "active" ingredients applied to sun-exposed areas of the skin with the sole purpose of reducing the number of photons reaching areas where damage might occur. After absorbing energy, the UV filters dissipate it in the form of heat or phosphorescence [43, 72]. In some cases the photon energy is reflected or scattered, again reducing the energy reaching vital cells in the skin. Thus, when shade, clothing, or hats are not options in high-intensity exposure scenarios, sunscreens serve as the best alternative to protect against sunlight. As well, for daily incidental exposure, such products are, quite arguably, the most effective agents to reduce the signs of aging.

Despite this elementary proposition and decades of use, a host of controversies follow sunscreens. There are numerous issues, many of which have been reviewed elsewhere [14, 47, 50, 69, 86]. What these controversies share, to a large extent, is linked by "exposure," generally too little or too much. Thus, the purpose herein is not to repeat the arguments made by others but to consider the principle, underpinning the controversies regarding sunscreen use.

[1] www.skincancer.org.

8.2 Exposure: What Does It Mean?

For sunscreen products, there are many concerns related to efficacy and safety that might be classified as controversies. Importantly, in both cases these concerns have a shared origin, namely, exposure. For the purposes of this paper, exposure is a borrowed term from risk assessment where the magnitude, frequency, and duration of use are measured or estimated [45]. In toxicology, exposure is coupled with hazard, i.e., adverse effect, and dose-response data to determine risk. In the context of efficacy, magnitude, or dose, frequency or reapplication and duration of use will be discussed and how they are controversial relative to human health.

Exposure to sunlight is also part of the consideration. As stated, sunlight damages skin. Sunscreens or more accurately UV filters are without an endogenous biological target, i.e., lacking pharmacological activity. As such, application of such products to the skin has no effect in the absence of sunlight. Thus, for sunscreens, the product exposure is coupled inextricably to sunlight and serves as the basis for all the controversies.

8.3 Exposure: Efficacy Testing (Sun Protection Factor or SPF)

Arguably, the most contentious issue involving sunscreens is the widely held view, supported by numerous studies, that they are "under dosed," i.e., not enough is applied, under ad-lib conditions. This view is tied inseparably to the SPF test which has for decades been conducted using a dose of 2 mg/cm^2 [23, 29, 71]. The reason for using 2 mg/cm^2 in SPF test has little to do with consumer use. As with any procedure that may be used to support a product "claim," reproducibility is paramount to widespread acceptance. To have a universally applied laboratory result, the inter- and intralaboratory variability must be low; otherwise test results become untrustworthy. One of the primary sources of variability in the SPF test and known for many years is product application [71]. As the SPF test was being developed into a uniform, international method, largely led by the cosmetic trade association in Europe, Cosmetic Europe or CE, formerly COLIPA, it was agreed that 2 mg/cm^2 application dose was reproducible. There was never the intention of this efficacy test to "mirror" how a consumer used the product. It is, in fact, an unreasonable expectation given habits and practices differences and diverse product forms, e.g., water-resistant recreational products vs. moisturizers or lipsticks. As a result, the SPF test is conducted as a means for product comparison and not an absolute efficacy value. Unfortunately, too many professional/nonprofessionals interpret SPF as an in-use, absolute quantitative value of efficacy. As stated and generally speaking, it is not.

Finally, it is worth noting that there exists a standard method for determining in vivo SPF, ISO 24444, which has been adopted, worldwide, except for the USA, although in all methods, the application density is the same, i.e., 2 mg/cm^2.

8.3.1 What "Dose" Are Sunscreens Applied Under ad-lib Conditions and Why

It is a frequent comment that patients/consumers do not use enough sunscreen product, which, as presented above, is in reference and comparison to the amount of product used in SPF testing. However, there are two aspects that require some consideration. First, what are the data that ad-lib product dosage is below 2 mg/cm^2, and, second, what is the evidence that users of products under such "real-world" conditions are not protected?

There are a number of studies that support the view that people do not apply sunscreen product at 2 mg/cm^2. These data are summarized in Table 8.1. For 30 years, it has been reported that under "natural" or ad-lib conditions, e.g., beach or daily activities, of varying duration, product application is less than 2 mg/ cm^2. While the methods vary, the majority of the studies presented in Table 8.1 are single use, i.e., apply product and measure how much was used under "real-world" or laboratory conditions, with the exception of [60]. The point of all these studies is that 2 mg/cm^2 application is not what consumers use. What is underrepresented in this list of studies is the use of different forms, e.g., sprays, sticks, and nonrecreational sunscreen products, e.g., facial moisturizers with UV filters.

The reasons consumers may not apply 2 mg/cm^2 are complex and multifaceted. To begin with, the motives for selecting a sunscreen and the SPF have some effect on application amount. For example, a recreational product that is high SPF, e.g., 30–50+, applied to large body surface areas and water or sweat resistant may be used for high-intensity UVR exposure during mid-day sun with little/no shade, e.g., playing golf or going to the beach. In contrast, a daily facial moisturizer maybe selected for normal, everyday exposure, which may be intermittent and low intensity where limited skin is exposed to sunlight. Using these examples, a recreational product is likely applied at doses consistent with the results shown in Table 8.1 but perhaps reapplied following activities such as swimming or sweating. A daily moisturizer with SPF, on the other hand, may be applied once in the morning and not reapplied at all during the day. Finally, given the aesthetic differences between recreational and daily use products, the later may be applied at a dose approaching 2 mg/cm^2 (Nash and Tanner, unpublished data).

Importantly, variability in applied "dose" of sunscreen product is not unique to this category but is a question for any topically applied product, drug, or otherwise. In contrast to orally administered medicines, topically applied products do not dispense a fixed amount or dose with a "template" for surface area to be treated to best achieve the desired therapeutic or cosmetic effect. It is more common that product dose is left to the patient/consumer applying the product, e.g., apply generous amount. In this regard, aesthetics play a much greater role in topical product application.

Table 8.1 Summary of studies evaluating sunscreen application

Author (year)	Methods	Measurement technique	Product description	Measured "dose" (mg/cm^2)	
				Mean	Median
Stenberg and Larko (1985) [75]	50 individuals, one time full body use	Weight	5 creams in jars	0.9–1.3	–
Bech-Thomsen and Wulf (1992) [9]	42 individuals at beach, ad lib, one time full body use	Weight	Subject controlled	0.49	–
Azurdia et al. (1999) [6]	10 photosensitive patients, one time full body use	Fluorescence	Tube	–	0.5
Autier et al. (1999) [3]	124 students, ad-lib full body use over summer	Weight	2 sunscreens in tubes	–	0.39
Azurdia et al. (2000) [7]	6 photosensitive patients, single use on the head, neck, arms assessed before/after education	Fluorescence	Bottle	–	0.11 baseline 0.82–1.13 post education
Neale et al. (2002) [60]	595 individuals, ad-lib home use on the head, neck, hands, and arms for 4.5 years	Weight	Cream in bottle	0.99	0.79
Maier et al. (2003) [51]	28 individuals, lab study 18 individuals, ad-lib use skiing	Weight	2 lipsticks	–	0.86, 0.98 lab 1.58, 1.76 *ad-lib*
Lademann et al. (2004) [46]	60 individuals, ad-lib full body application 0.5-4 h prior to measurement	Tape strip, HPLC	Subject controlled	<0.2	–
Szepietowski et al. (2004) [77]	49 young adults, one time full body use	Weight	Emulsion Cream	0.92 0.96	–
Thieden et al. (2005) [79]	340 individuals, home use over 4 months UV tracked via dosimeter	–	Subject controlled	–	–
Reich et al. (2009) [70]	52 individuals – no instructions 53 individuals – instructions one time full body use	Weight	Cream in tube	0.68 0.86	–

(continued)

Table 8.1 (continued)

Author (year)	Methods	Measurement technique	Product description	Measured "dose" (mg/cm^2)	
				Mean	Median
Bauer et al. (2010) [8]	13 individuals, use on forearms	Swabs, spectrophotometer	–	1.4	–
De Villa et al. (2011) [16]	36 individuals, use on forearms	Tape strip, HPLC	Emulsion	–	0.43 (1 use) 0.95 (2 uses)
Diaz et al. (2012) [17]	87 children, 1 week full ad-lib use at home	Weight	Pump, bottle, and roll-on	–	0.75 (pump) 0.57 (bottle) 0.22 (roll-on)
Petersen et al. (2013) [66]	20 sun seekers on holiday, ad-lib full body use for 6 days	Weight	Subject controlled	0.79	–
Novick et al. (2015) [62]	52 individuals, lotion, stick use on the forearm, spray assessed by application on a paper towel	Weight	Lotion, spray, and stick	1.1 (lotion) 1.6 (spray) 0.35 (stick)	–

8.3.2 *What Factors Influence Topical Product Usability?*

Forgetting for the moment UV filters and film-forming characteristics which are critical for sunscreen product efficacy, attributes like the scent, feel, and optical appearance on the skin would be expected to impact how much and how often, i.e., frequency, it is used. If consumers do not like the feel, e.g., sticky and greasy, scent, e.g., chemical base odor, or on-skin appearance, e.g., shine and whiteness of the product, they will use less and perhaps avoid reapplication. Thus, formulating better sunscreen products is about much more than just performing well in SPF clinical tests or having "new" UV filters. What dose and reapplication translate into is compliance, which is rarely discussed when considering sunscreens.

Another characteristic that impacts sunscreen "dose" is film-forming properties and thickness. From a technical standpoint, the ability of a sunscreen product to form a uniform film on the skin is closely tied to efficacy [63, 74]. In fact, film formation/thickness is likely the key reason that product application is one of the primary sources of variability in SPF testing, as mentioned earlier. As well, the film formation/thickness has implications related to reapplication. To understand this, one needs to consider the topography of the skin (Fig. 8.1). Macroscopically, the surface of the skin is made up of hills and valleys. A thin layer applied over such topography may result in uneven coverage where "valleys" are filled/covered, but "peaks" are not. The analogy Diffey uses is that of painting a wall with an uneven surface [18]. The first coat/application doesn't provide adequate coverage, and therefore two coats (reapplication) are required. However, one goal of sunscreen

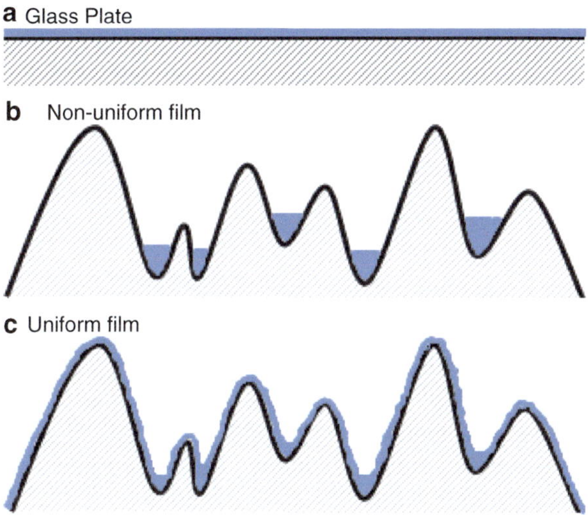

Fig. 8.1 Schematic representation of hypothetical sunscreen product applied at the same "dose" to (**a**) glass plate, (**b**) skin as a nonuniform film, and (**c**) skin as a uniform film

product development is to create products that have uniform film formation, high efficacy, under ad-lib conditions of use. In this regard, uniform coverage may be obtained at less than 2 mg/cm^2. Certainly, the more product applied, the more likely coverage will be achieved and in "lock-step" the more negative attributes such as greasiness and product remaining on the skin, i.e., not "absorbed,"[2] come into play. In general, the combination of product attributes, efficacy, and experience drives how much product is applied and/or reapplied.

8.3.3 What Is the Evidence That Sunscreens Do Not Work Under ad-lib Use?

Studies of acute sunscreen product failure under ad-lib use conditions are limited or a secondary objective. Some examples which have reported erythema/sunburn in people using sunscreen include McCarthy et al. [53] and Wright et al. [88]. Again, in these examples and other such studies, it is difficult to know if sunburn was due to inadequate "dose" or missed area on the body or overexposure to sunlight or combinations of these. For example, intentional misuse of sunscreen to prolong time spent in the sun for tanning purposes can result in sunburn suggestive of product failure [2–4]. What is not factored into "product failure" are the millions if not billions of product applications where sunburn has been prevented. Finally, the work of Green et al. in the Nambour Skin Cancer and Actinic Eye Disease Prevention

[2] "Absorption" in this context is a term used to describe whether a consumer "feels" product remaining on the skin after application. It is not used in the context of pharmacokinetics, i.e., absorption into the skin, but rather an aesthetic attribute.

Trial [34, 35, 41], Thompson et al. [80], Naylor et al. [59], and Gallagher et al. [28] are suggestive that repeated, regular application of sunscreen under ad-lib use prevent precursors as well as actual long-term skin damage supportive of the view that ad-lib sunscreen use is efficacious.

8.3.4 What Is the Frequency and Duration of Sunscreen Use?

The use of sunscreens is not limited to amount of product applied. The frequency of application or reapplication and duration of use are critical in understanding exposure and efficacy. In an experimental context, these have not received as much attention as the amount of product applied. As such, the number of prospective, stand-alone studies is less compared to those where amount of product applied has been investigated. Nonetheless, there are some studies that have investigated sunscreen product reapplication [13, 16, 64, 65, 82].

The duration of use has been studied in a limited number of prospective studies. The most important of such studies is that of Adele Green and colleagues [34, 35, 41]. Others, as mentioned above include the work of Thompson et al. [80], Naylor et al. [59], and Gallagher et al. [28].

Consumers do not apply enough sunscreen product to achieve the labeled SPF, but this does not mean the product failed or there is no efficacy. On the contrary, the preponderance of data supports the view that protection from harmful UVR is achieved under "normal" use conditions. There are numerous opportunities to reinforce behaviors including reapplication and daily use, which have been shown to have real benefits (see above) and, in theory, if started early in life would have the greatest impact [19, 76]. Unfortunately, the "controversies" related to amount/dose applied and lack of short-/long-term benefits obscure the benefits and public health message.

8.4 Exposure: Human Safety Assessment

The preceding discussion focused on "under dosing" or "too little" sunscreen product exposure. There is the other side of the coin that sunscreen use under ad-lib conditions represents a human health risk from "too much" exposure to such products. The focus of this "controversy" will be UV filters and their potential safety concerns including inhalation, endocrine, and systemic bioavailability. Like most sunscreen controversies, safety concerns have been addressed by others including but not limited to "nano" sunscreens and ingredients beyond UV filters, e.g., vitamin A analogs such as retinyl palmitate, and therefore the scope of the current discussion will be limited [14, 50].

For ingredients used in topically applied products, a common approach used to determine human safety is quantitative risk assessment (QRA). Such a method, modeled after National Research Council [54], is used frequently to assess many different chemicals used by humans and by design is a key part of toxicology/product safety [37]. Many authoritative, e.g., Scientific Committee Cosmetic Safety, and regulatory agencies, e.g., Environmental Protection Agency, around the world use QRA as part of their approach toward ensuring consumer safety.

In the USA, there are nine UV filters commonly used in sunscreen products [83]. It is beyond the scope of this paper to review the safety of each UV filter in any depth, and the interested reader may consider [30, 50, 58] for more information. However, among the human safety concerns related to these UV filters and sunscreen product exposure are: (1) spray products and inhalation, (2) endocrine disruption, and (3) systemic absorption from lifetime exposure, i.e., cradle to grave, including subpopulations, e.g., geriatric.

A complexity associated with safety controversies and sunscreens is "what drives the concern?" Is it the product, one of the UV filters, or a combination? The attempt here will be to outline the controversial concern and provide general comments with support by specific examples knowing that this will be limited by design.

Sunscreen spray products became more widely available in the decade of 2000 as a convenient means of product application particularly for children. Whereas pump sprays had been available for some time, the propellant-based continuous sprays represent a "new" form that has grown and by some estimates represents up to 50 % of recreational sunscreen product market in the USA [1, 20]. Spray products are thought to improve coverage, dosage, and drive compliance (see Novick et al. Table 8.1). The concern, however, is inhalation particularly among children. The toxicological profile of UV filters following the inhalation route of administration has not been systematically investigated. However, human exposure is intermittent, indirect, and restricted to nasal passages and to a lesser extent the upper respiratory tract based on the size of droplets [20]. Beyond the local effects in these tissues, i.e., nasal/upper part of the lung, systemic effects would be dependent on the exact UV filter and the availability of repeat exposure data perhaps generated from another route of administration, e.g., oral or diet. Whereas each marketed sunscreen spray product would need a safety evaluation based on specific properties and UV filters, in general, exposure to ingredients would be limited if not negligible.

UV filters have been shown to have endocrine effects in screening-type toxicological studies with benzophenone-3/oxybenzone [84], 4-methybenzylidene-camphor/4-MBC [56], and octyl methoxycinnamate/OMC [5], receiving the most attention [87]. Clearly, in vitro screening studies and findings in animals are suggestive of weak endocrine effects of select UV filters. The limited human studies have found internal concentrations of select UV filters in ng/ml range with no impact on measures of endocrine function, i.e., basal concentrations of hormones [42]. Greim, discussing endocrine disruption, made the following observation: "Overall, the science-based knowledge on the robustness of the endocrine system, the well-understood principles of substrate-receptor interactions, and the generally low exposure of humans to potentially endocrine-disrupting chemicals make it unlikely that the latter play a causative role in diseases and abnormalities observed in children and in the human population in general" [36]. That is not to dismiss the notion of subtle endocrine effects attributed to UV filters but in the context of systemic exposure following topical application, the risk is consider by many to be minimal if not negligible.

In the context of endocrine disruption, it is worth pointing out vitamin D might be considered as having endocrine properties and most notably is activated by sunlight in the skin. Hence, by definition, sunscreens "disrupt" vitamin D by reducing photochemical activation. So much has been written on this controversy, and still the debate continues. Suffice it to say that the argument persists with staunch supporters of sunscreens not affecting vitamin D under ad-lib use and equally dedicated opponents suggesting sunscreen use has an unfavorable effect on serum vitamin D and the risk outweighs any possible benefit [11, 31, 33, 39, 40, 44, 73]. Perhaps the only undisputable facts are that sunscreens, by design, have the potential to reduce photochemical conversation of vitamin D, while systemic endocrine effects mediated directly by UV filters is, at best, weak.

Systemic absorption and lifetime exposure to UV filters after topical application came to attention of the scientific community in the late 1990s following the Lancet publication by Hayden et al. [38]. Although studies preceding this exist, most had minimized the idea of systemic bioavailability of UV filters, perhaps in a dismissive manner. UV filters may penetrate into/through the skin [52, 55, 81, 85], to cite a few examples. Most studies have found limited penetration, but as analytical detection methods improve, it is quite likely to see more examples demonstrating systemic absorption from clinical investigations and in biomonitoring, e.g., NHANES.

The concern related to the potential topical bioavailability of UV filters is systemic toxicity. In years past, many risk assessments focused only on local effects, e.g., skin irritation, sensitization, phototoxicity, or photoallergy. With evidence of absorption following topical application, there are reasons to consider systemic toxicity. This, again, comes down to the data for individual UV filters supportive of repeat exposure. Importantly, the presence of a substance is not evidence of toxicity. This seems to be a common misconception.

The examples of human safety concerns, inhalation, endocrine effects, and systemic toxicity from topically applied sunscreens have been presented in a very superficial manner. The point of these examples is that there are fears of "too much" exposure to sunscreen/UV filters. This is largely independent of any benefits that use of such products might offer. The controversy regarding "too much" exposure to sunscreen products remains an active area of interest.

8.5 Conclusions

This everlasting controversy involving sunscreens is a variant of the story attributed to Robert Southey of "Goldilocks and the Three Bears." Goldilocks stubbles upon the home of the three bears while walking in the forest. Upon entering the house, she finds three bowls of porridge, three chairs, and three beds. She finds two of the porridge bowls, chairs, and beds unacceptable, i.e., too hot/cold, too big, and too hard/soft, respectively, but one "just right." When the bears return home, they eventually discover Goldilocks who in her fright flees never to be seen by the bears again. Sunscreens are considered to be used not enough or relied upon too frequently or by some "just right." Yet, in the end, the user is confused and possibly frightened away by all the controversy and divergent opinions.

Of course, this analogy isn't nearly as black and white for sunscreens. For years, the same "controversies" find their way into articles or on websites generally coinciding with the advent of summer. People don't apply enough, and the ingredients are unsafe, i.e., too much/toxic. The controversies will not go away, but that shouldn't be a cause to abandon efforts.

In the end, the responsibility to public health begs for a consistent message that can be applied for all to follow. A single message to limit sun exposure and follow the guidelines that have proven effective in Australia, namely, wear protective clothing, use a sunscreen product on skin exposure to sunlight and seek shade/shelter, may be the means of improving public health particularly as humans extend the life span and therefore cumulative exposure to sunlight. Rather than confuse people with messages of use an SPF 30 or SPF 15 daily, it should be agreed that a consistent message would benefit the public.

Beyond consistence in messaging, it would be of value to consider practical advice. For example, sunscreens in the USA and elsewhere are largely viewed as recreational products to be used as needed. So the idea of daily application hardly resonates with a typical user of such products. This is just common sense: Why apply a recreational product on days I will have little exposure to sunlight. Yet those days are thought to account for much of the cumulative damage [61]. Additionally, in a heterogeneous society like the USA, significant segments of the population including African-/Asian-Americans and Latinos may not use sunscreen products because they believe it is unnecessary, even though photodamage occurs in all skin types. Again, with regard to sunscreens, the idea of an SPF 30 applied daily in the context of recreational products, i.e., those applied to large surface areas, is unlikely and for the average person not affordable. Unfortunately, even well-meaning conscientious advocates may be missing an opportunity.

The controversy is around "just right." It is the responsible act to promote sun safety of which sunscreens are a key part. The single message might be: wear sunscreen, SPF 15 broad-spectrum or greater on exposed skin. Reapply as needed. If this encourages people to try sunscreen, it is quite possible that such trail will lead to retrial and rather than using high SPF, e.g., 30–50+, a new user can begin with a SPF 15.

References

1. Amber KT, Bloom R, Staropoli P, Dhiman S, Hu S (2014) Assessing the current market of sunscreen: a cross-sectional study of sunscreen availability in three metropolitan counties in the United States. J Skin Cancer 2014:285357
2. Autier P (2009) Sunscreen abuse for intentional sun exposure. Br J Dermatol 161(Suppl 3): 40–45

3. Autier P, Dore JF, Negrier S, Lienard D, Panizzon R, Lejeune FJ, Guggisberg D, Eggermont AM (1999) Sunscreen use and duration of sun exposure: a double-blind, randomized trial. J Natl Cancer Inst 91:1304–1309
4. Autier P, Dore JF, Reis AC, Grivegnee A, Ollivaud L, Truchetet F, Chamoun E, Rotmensz N, Severi G, Cesarini JP (2000) Sunscreen use and intentional exposure to ultraviolet A and B radiation: a double blind randomized trial using personal dosimeters. Br J Cancer 83:1243–1248
5. Axelstad M, Boberg J, Hougaard KS, Christiansen S, Jacobsen PR, Mandrup KR, Nellemann C, Lund SP, Hass U (2011) Effects of pre- and postnatal exposure to the UV-filter octyl methoxycinnamate (OMC) on the reproductive, auditory and neurological development of rat offspring. Toxicol Appl Pharmacol 250:278–290
6. Azurdia RM, Pagliaro JA, Diffey BL, Rhodes LE (1999) Sunscreen application by photosensitive patients is inadequate for protection. Br J Dermatol 140:255–258
7. Azurdia RM, Pagliaro JA, Rhodes LE (2000) Sunscreen application technique in photosensitive patients: a quantitative assessment of the effect of education. Photodermatol Photoimmunol Photomed 16:53–56
8. Bauer U, O'BRIEN DS, KIMLIN MG (2010) A new method to quantify the application thickness of sunscreen on skin. Photochem Photobiol 86:1397–1403
9. Bech-Thomsen N, Wulf HC (1992) Sunbathers' application of sunscreen is probably inadequate to obtain the sun protection factor assigned to the preparation. Photodermatol Photoimmunol Photomed 9:242–244
10. Bernard JJ, Cowing-Zitron C, Nakatsuji T, Muehleisen B, Muto J, Borkowski AW, Martinez L, Greidinger EL, Yu BD, Gallo RL (2012) Ultraviolet radiation damages self noncoding RNA and is detected by TLR3. Nat Med 18:1286–1290
11. Berwick M (2011) The good, the bad, and the ugly of sunscreens. Clin Pharmacol Ther 89:31–33
12. Brash DE (2015) UV signature mutations. Photochem Photobiol 91:15–26
13. Buller DB, Andersen PA, Walkosz BJ, Scott MD, Maloy JA, Dignan MB, Cutter GR (2012) Compliance with sunscreen advice in a survey of adults engaged in outdoor winter recreation at high-elevation ski areas. J Am Acad Dermatol 66:63–70
14. Burnett ME, Wang SQ (2011) Current sunscreen controversies: a critical review. Photodermatol Photoimmunol Photomed 27:58–67
15. CDC (2012) Sunburn and sun protective behaviors among adults aged 18–29 years – United States, 2000–2010. In: Moolenaar RL (ed). Office of Surveillance, Epidemiology, and Laboratory Services, Centers for Disease Control and Prevention (CDC), U.S. Department of Health and Human Service, Atlanta
16. De Villa D, Nagatomi AR, Paese K, Guterres S, Cestari TF (2011) Reapplication improves the amount of sunscreen, not its regularity, under real life conditions. Photochem Photobiol 87:457–460
17. Diaz A, Neale RE, Kimlin MG, Jones L, Janda M (2012) The children and sunscreen study: a crossover trial investigating children's sunscreen application thickness and the influence of age and dispenser type. Arch Dermatol 148:606–612
18. Diffey B (2001) Sunscreen isn't enough. J Photochem Photobiol B 64:105–108
19. Diffey BL (2011) The impact of topical photoprotectants intended for daily use on lifetime ultraviolet exposure. J Cosmet Dermatol 10:245–250
20. Durand L, Habran N, Denis C, Meulders L, Henschel V, Amighi K (2007) Influence of different parameters on droplet size and size distribution of sprayable sunscreen emulsions with high concentration of UV-filters. Int J Cosmet Sci 29:461–471
21. Eide MJ, Weinstock MA (2006) Public health challenges in sun protection. Dermatol Clin 24:119–124
22. Faustin B, Reed JC (2008) Sunburned skin activates inflammasomes. Trends Cell Biol 18:4–8
23. Ferguson J, Brown M, Alert D, Bielfeldt S, Brown J, Chardon A, Hourseau C, Mazilier C, Cuthbert J, D'Arcy-Burt K, Jolley J, Murdoch M, Finkel P, Masson P, Merot F, Maclennan A, Poret J, Siladgi S (1996) Collaborative development of a sun protection factor test method: a proposed European Standard. COLIPA Task Force 'Sun Protection Measurement', Europe. Int J Cosmet Sci 18:203–218

24. Fisher GJ, Kang S, Varani J, Bata-Csorgo Z, Wan Y, Datta S, Voorhees JJ (2002) Mechanisms of photoaging and chronological skin aging. Arch Dermatol 138:1462–1470
25. Fisher GJ, Talwar HS, Lin J, Voorhees JJ (1999) Molecular mechanisms of photoaging in human skin in vivo and their prevention by all-trans retinoic acid. Photochem Photobiol 69:154–157
26. Fisher GJ, Wang ZQ, Datta SC, Varani J, Kang S, Voorhees JJ (1997) Pathophysiology of premature skin aging induced by ultraviolet light. N Engl J Med 337:1419–1428
27. Flores KG, Erdei E, Luo L, White KA, Leng S, Berwick M, Lazovich D (2013) A pilot study of genetic variants in dopamine regulators with indoor tanning and melanoma. Exp Dermatol 22:576–581
28. Gallagher RP, Rivers JK, Lee TK, Bajdik CD, Mclean DI, Coldman AJ (2000) Broad-spectrum sunscreen use and the development of new nevi in white children: a randomized controlled trial. JAMA 283:2955–2960
29. Garzarella K, Caswell M (2013) Disparate SPF testing methodologies generate similar SPFs. J Cosmet Sci 64:297–307
30. Gasparro FP, Mitchnick M, Nash JF (1998) A review of sunscreen safety and efficacy. Photochem Photobiol 68:243–256
31. Gilchrest BA (2008) Sun exposure and vitamin D sufficiency. Am J Clin Nutr 88:570S–577S
32. Gilchrest BA, Park HY, Eller MS, Yaar M (1996) Mechanisms of ultraviolet light-induced pigmentation. Photochem Photobiol 63:1–10
33. Grant WB, Strange RC, Garland CF (2003) Sunshine is good medicine. The health benefits of ultraviolet-B induced vitamin D production. J Cosmet Dermatol 2:86–98
34. Green A, Williams G, Neale R, Hart V, Leslie D, Parsons P, Marks GC, Gaffney P, Battistutta D, Frost C, Lang C, Russell A (1999) Daily sunscreen application and betacarotene supplementation in prevention of basal-cell and squamous-cell carcinomas of the skin: a randomised controlled trial. Lancet 354:723–729
35. Green AC, Williams GM, Logan V, Strutton GM (2011) Reduced melanoma after regular sunscreen use: randomized trial follow-up. J Clin Oncol 29:257–263
36. Greim H (2005) Chemicals with endocrine-disrupting potential: a threat to human health? Angew Chem Int Ed Engl 44:5568–5574
37. Hartung T (2011) From alternative methods to a new toxicology. Eur J Pharm Biopharm 77:338–349
38. Hayden CG, Roberts MS, Benson HA (1997) Systemic absorption of sunscreen after topical application. Lancet 350:863–864
39. Holick M (2002) Does sunscreen block the skin's ability to make vitamin D? If so, how can I get enough of this vitamin without raising my risk of skin cancer? Health News 8:12
40. Holick MF, Matsuoka LY, Wortsman J (1995) Regular use of sunscreen on vitamin D levels. Arch Dermatol 131:1337–1339
41. Iannacone MR, Hughes MC, Green AC (2014) Effects of sunscreen on skin cancer and photoaging. Photodermatol Photoimmunol Photomed 30:55–61
42. Janjua NR, Kongshoj B, Andersson AM, Wulf HC (2008) Sunscreens in human plasma and urine after repeated whole-body topical application. J Eur Acad Dermatol Venereol 22:456–461
43. Jansen R, Osterwalder U, Wang SQ, Burnett M, Lim HW (2013) Photoprotection: part II. Sunscreen: development, efficacy, and controversies. J Am Acad Dermatol 69:867 e1–14; quiz 881–2
44. Kannan S, Lim HW (2014) Photoprotection and vitamin D: a review. Photodermatol Photoimmunol Photomed 30:137–145
45. Kleinjans JC (2003) Principles in toxicological risk analysis. Toxicol Lett 140–141:311–315
46. Lademann J, Schanzer S, Richter H, Pelchrzim RV, Zastrow L, Golz K, Sterry W (2004) Sunscreen application at the beach. J Cosmet Dermatol 3:62–68
47. Lautenschlager S, Wulf HC, Pittelkow MR (2007) Photoprotection. Lancet 370:528–537
48. Lazovich D, Forster J (2005) Indoor tanning by adolescents: prevalence, practices and policies. Eur J Cancer 41:20–27
49. Liu JJ, Fisher DE (2010) Lighting a path to pigmentation: mechanisms of MITF induction by UV. Pigment Cell Melanoma Res 23:741–745

50. Loden M, Beitner H, Gonzalez H, Edstrom DW, Akerstrom U, Austad J, Buraczewska-Norin I, Matsson M, Wulf HC (2011) Sunscreen use: controversies, challenges and regulatory aspects. Br J Dermatol 165:255–262
51. Maier H, Schauberger G, Brunnhofer K, Honigsmann H (2003) Assessment of thickness of photoprotective lipsticks and frequency of reapplication: results from a laboratory test and a field experiment. Br J Dermatol 148:763–769
52. Mavon A, Miquel C, Lejeune O, Payre B, Moretto P (2007) In vitro percutaneous absorption and in vivo stratum corneum distribution of an organic and a mineral sunscreen. Skin Pharmacol Physiol 20:10–20
53. Mccarthy EM, Ethridge KP, Wagner RF Jr (1999) Beach holiday sunburn: the sunscreen paradox and gender differences. Cutis 64:37–42
54. McClellan RO (1995) Risk assessment and biological mechanisms: lessons learned, future opportunities. Toxicology 102:239–258
55. Montenegro L, Puglisi G (2013) Evaluation of sunscreen safety by in vitro skin permeation studies: effects of vehicle composition. Pharmazie 68:34–40
56. Mueller SO, Kling M, Arifin Firzani P, Mecky A, Duranti E, Shields-Botella J, Delansorne R, Broschard T, Kramer PJ (2003) Activation of estrogen receptor alpha and ERbeta by 4-methylbenzylidene-camphor in human and rat cells: comparison with phyto- and xenoestrogens. Toxicol Lett 142:89–101
57. Murphy G, Young AR, Wulf HC, Kulms D, Schwarz T (2001) The molecular determinants of sunburn cell formation. Exp Dermatol 10:155–160
58. Nash JF (2006) Human safety and efficacy of ultraviolet filters and sunscreen products. Dermatol Clin 24:35–51
59. Naylor MF, Boyd A, Smith DW, Cameron GS, Hubbard D, Neldner KH (1995) High sun protection factor sunscreens in the suppression of actinic neoplasia. Arch Dermatol 131: 170–175
60. Neale R, Williams G, Green A (2002) Application patterns among participants randomized to daily sunscreen use in a skin cancer prevention trial. Arch Dermatol 138:1319–1325
61. Nole G, Johnson AW (2004) An analysis of cumulative lifetime solar ultraviolet radiation exposure and the benefits of daily sun protection. Dermatol Ther 17(Suppl 1):57–62
62. Novick R, Anderson G, Miller E, Allgeier D, Unice K (2015) Factors that influence sunscreen application thickness and potential preservative exposure. Photodermatol Photoimmunol Photomed 31(4):212–23
63. O'Neill JJ (1984) Effect of film irregularities on sunscreen efficacy. J Pharm Sci 73:888–891
64. O'Riordan DL, Lunde KB, Urschitz J, Glanz K (2005) A noninvasive objective measure of sunscreen use and reapplication. Cancer Epidemiol Biomarkers Prev 14:722–726
65. Odio MR, Veres DA, Goodman JJ, Irwin C, Robinson LR, Martinez J, Kraus AL (1994) Comparative efficacy of sunscreen reapplication regimens in children exposed to ambient sunlight. Photodermatol Photoimmunol Photomed 10:118–125
66. Petersen B, Datta P, Philipsen PA, Wulf HC (2013) Sunscreen use and failures – on site observations on a sun-holiday. Photochem Photobiol Sci 12:190–196
67. Poon F, Kang S, Chien AL (2015) Mechanisms and treatments of photoaging. Photodermatol Photoimmunol Photomed 31:65–74
68. Premi S, Wallisch S, Mano CM, Weiner AB, Bacchiocchi A, Wakamatsu K, Bechara EJ, Halaban R, Douki T, Brash DE (2015) Photochemistry. Chemiexcitation of melanin derivatives induces DNA photoproducts long after UV exposure. Science 347:842–847
69. Quatrano NA, Dinulos JG (2013) Current principles of sunscreen use in children. Curr Opin Pediatr 25:122–129
70. Reich A, Harupa M, Bury M, Chrzaszcz J, Starczewska A (2009) Application of sunscreen preparations: a need to change the regulations. Photodermatol Photoimmunol Photomed 25:242–244
71. Sayre RM, Powell J, Rheins LA (1991) Product application technique alters the sun protection factor. Photodermatol Photoimmunol Photomed 8:222–224

72. Shaath NA (1997) Evolution of modern sunscreen chemicals. Marcel Dekker, New York
73. Skolnick AA (1991) Sunscreen protection controversy heats up. JAMA 265:3218–3220
74. Sohn M, Heche A, Herzog B, Imanidis G (2014) Film thickness frequency distribution of different vehicles determines sunscreen efficacy. J Biomed Opt 19:115005
75. Stenberg C, Larko O (1985) Sunscreen application and its importance for the sun protection factor. Arch Dermatol 121:1400–1402
76. Stern RS, Weinstein MC, Baker SG (1986) Risk reduction for nonmelanoma skin cancer with childhood sunscreen use. Arch Dermatol 122:537–545
77. Szepietowski JC, Nowicka D, Reich A, Melon M (2004) Application of sunscreen preparations among young Polish people. J Cosmet Dermatol 3:69–72
78. Taylor MF, Westbrook D, Chang P (2015) Using UV photoaged photography to better understand Western Australian teenagers' attitudes towards adopting sun-protective behaviors. Int J Adolesc Med Health. ISSN (Online) 2191-0278, ISSN (Print) 0334-0139, DOI: 10.1515/ijamh-2014-0071, March 2015
79. Thieden E, Philipsen PA, Sandby-Moller J, Wulf HC (2005) Sunscreen use related to UV exposure, age, sex, and occupation based on personal dosimeter readings and sun-exposure behavior diaries. Arch Dermatol 141:967–973
80. Thompson SC, Jolley D, Marks R (1993) Reduction of solar keratoses by regular sunscreen use. N Engl J Med 329:1147–1151
81. Walters KA, Brain KR, Howes D, James VJ, Kraus AL, Teetsel NM, Toulon M, Watkinson AC, Gettings SD (1997) Percutaneous penetration of octyl salicylate from representative sunscreen formulations through human skin in vitro. Food Chem Toxicol 35:1219–1225
82. Wang SQ, Dusza SW (2009) Assessment of sunscreen knowledge: a pilot survey. Br J Dermatol 161(Suppl 3):28–32
83. Wang SQ, Tanner PR, Lim HW, Nash JF (2013) The evolution of sunscreen products in the United States – a 12-year cross sectional study. Photochem Photobiol Sci 12:197–202
84. Watanabe Y, Kojima H, Takeuchi S, Uramaru N, Sanoh S, Sugihara K, Kitamura S, Ohta S (2015) Metabolism of UV-filter benzophenone-3 by rat and human liver microsomes and its effect on endocrine-disrupting activity. Toxicol Appl Pharmacol 282:119–128
85. Watkinson AC, Brain KR, Walters KA, Hadgraft J (1992) Prediction of the percutaneous penetration of ultra-violet filters used in sunscreen formulations. Int J Cosmet Sci 14:265–275
86. Weinstock MA (1996) Controversies in the role of sunlight in the pathogenesis of cutaneous melanoma. Photochem Photobiol 63:406–410
87. Witorsch RJ, Thomas JA (2010) Personal care products an endocrine disruption: a critical review of the literature. Crit Rev Toxicol 40:1–30
88. Wright MW, Wright ST, Wagner RF (2001) Mechanisms of sunscreen failure. J Am Acad Dermatol 44:781–784
89. Zeller S, Lazovich D, Forster J, Widome R (2006) Do adolescent indoor tanners exhibit dependency? J Am Acad Dermatol 54:589–596
90. Ziegler A, Jonason AS, Leffell DJ, Simon JA, Sharma HW, Kimmelman J, Remington L, Jacks T, Brash DE (1994) Sunburn and p53 in the onset of skin cancer. Nature 372:773–776

Part II

Chapter 9
The Chemistry of Ultraviolet Filters

Nadim A. Shaath

Key Points

- This chapter describes the mechanism of action for both Inorganic particulates and organic ultraviolet filters. It classifies all ultraviolet filters in commerce today and lists their physical, chemical, and spectroscopic properties as well as their regulatory status.
- Synthetic approaches for the design of the current and future UV filters are discussed, and the photostability of ultraviolet filters is addressed.
- It concludes with an analysis of the future direction in designing new, safer, and more effective ultraviolet filters.

9.1 Introduction

The chemistry of ultraviolet filters is complex, and understanding the interaction between UV light and those compounds provides insights on how sunscreen works. Possessing the knowledge for a more intelligent design and development of novel UV filters can provide efficient and stable UV protection. Although much progress has been made in the advancement of ultraviolet filters in the past five decades, progress is slow and often hampered by regulatory restrictions [1, 2]. For example, little has changed in US regulations since 1978 when the Advanced Notice for Public Record (ANPR) was issued. At the time, 21 UV filters were considered Category I Ingredients (see Table 9.1), and their use in cosmetic formulations, at the percentages approved, allowed manufacturers to claim appropriate SPF (sun protection factor) on their labels.

N.A. Shaath, PhD
Alpha Research and Development, Ltd., White Plains, NY, USA
e-mail: alpharnd@aol.com

S.Q. Wang, H.W. Lim (eds.), *Principles and Practice of Photoprotection*,
DOI 10.1007/978-3-319-29382-0_9

Table 9.1 Twenty-one approved UV filters in 1978 in the USA

UVA absorbers/reflectors	%
Oxybenzone	2–6
Sulisobenzone	5–10
Dioxybenzone	3
Menthyl anthranilate	3.5–5
Red petrolatum	30–100
Titanium dioxide	2–25
UVB Absorbers	
Aminobenzoic acid	5–15
Amyl dimethyl PABA[a]	1–5
2-Ethoxyethyl p-methoxycinnamate	1–3
Diethanolamine p-methoxycinnamate[a]	8–10
Digalloyl trioleate[a]	2–5
Ethyl 4-bis(hydroxypropyl) aminobenzoate[a]	1–5
2-Ethylhexyl-2-cyano-3,3-diphenyl-acrylate	7–10
Ethylhexyl *p*-methoxycinnamate	2–7.5
2-Ethylhexyl salicylate	3–5
Glyceryl aminobenzoate[a]	2–3
Homomenthyl salicylate	4–15
Lawsone with Dihydroxyacetone[a]	0.25
Octyl dimethyl PABA	1.4–8
2-Phenylbenzimidazole-5-sulfonic acid	1–4
Triethanolamine salicylate	5–12

[a]These items have been deleted in the Final Monograph in 1999. Three additional items have been added since, namely, avobenzone (1–3 %), ecamsule (up to 10 %), and zinc oxide (2–25 %)

With the inclusion of any of those UV filters, protection from skin cancers was considered possible, and US companies could claim that "sunscreens reduce the risk of skin cancer and early skin aging when used as directed," if the final sunscreen product has SPF >15 and critical wavelength ≥370 nm. Despite the increased use of sun care products since then, incidences of skin cancer have quadrupled with no sign of abatement. Are people lulled into a false sense of security when they use sunscreens? All this sun damage begs the question: do sun care products provide enough protection? The search for the ultimate UV filter goes on, and protocols for superior protection are still underway with limited success.

In this chapter, I will review the approaches for designing the current UV filters that have been approved and are available for use worldwide. Understanding how filters work can help us to determine if they offer consumers adequate protection from the sun.

9.2 Mechanism of Sunscreen Action

Electromagnetic rays interact with UV filters by either absorbing or scattering of their energy. The dispersion of inorganic particulates scatters and reflects the harmful rays. Inorganic particulates, however, also have the ability to absorb the UV radiation.

When a molecule absorbs a UV photon, the electrons in its highest occupied molecular orbital (HOMO) are promoted to its lowest unoccupied molecular orbital (LUMO) as shown in Fig. 9.1.

This singlet excited state can be deactivated by a simple vibrational relaxation back to the ground state, through fluorescence of the molecule, or by undergoing photochemical reactions. On the other hand, under certain conditions, the singlet excited state can undergo an intersystem crossing that leads to a triplet excited state as shown in Fig. 9.2.

The energy in the triplet state may be dissipated in a number of ways, as shown in Fig. 9.2:

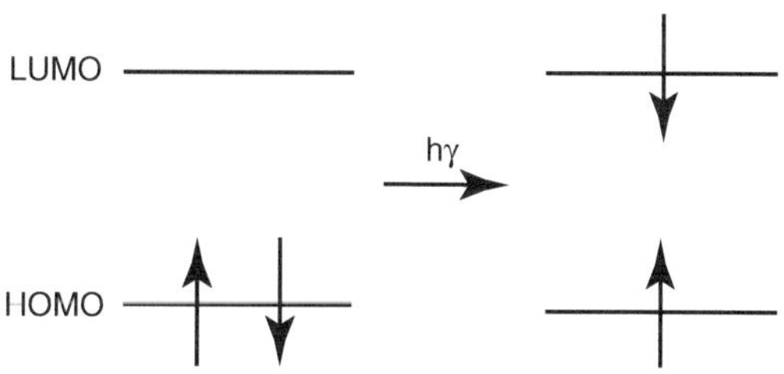

Fig. 9.1 Absorption of energy by an organic UV filter

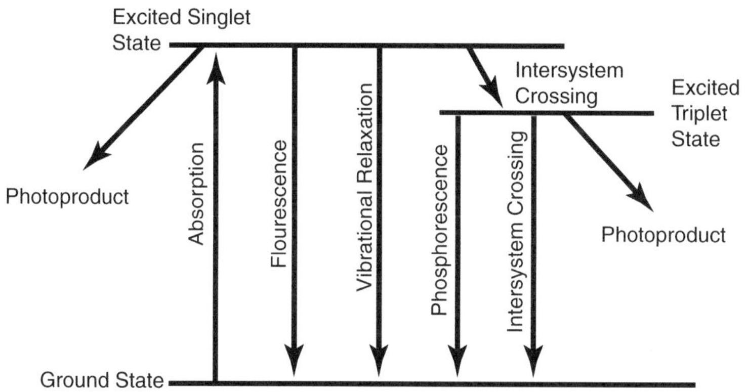

Fig. 9.2 Energy release pathways

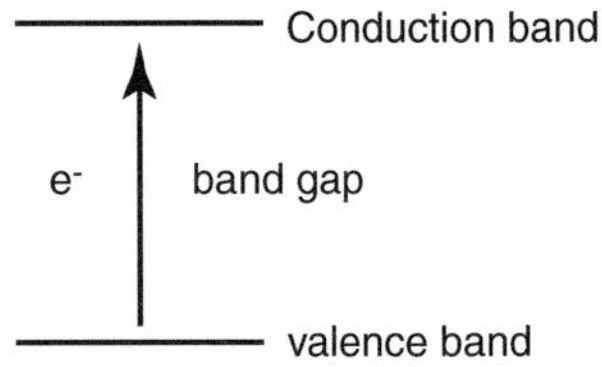

Fig. 9.3 The band gap energy in inorganic particulates between valence and conduction bands

1. Emission of a photon (phosphorescence)
2. Energy transfer to other receptor molecules (T-T transfer)
3. Photochemical reactions

The inorganic particulates, on the other hand, either scatter or absorb the UV radiation. These particulates are semiconductors with high bandgap energy between the valence and conduction band (between 380 and 420 nm) as shown in Fig. 9.3.

The wavelength of absorption varies with the particle size of the inorganic particulates. The smaller the primary particulate size is, the higher the bandgap energy.

9.3 Classification of Ultraviolet Filters

Ultraviolet filters can be broadly classified into two types: UV absorbers and inorganic particulates. There are only two inorganic particulates approved: zinc oxide and titanium dioxide. Both ingredients are considered broad spectrum since they absorb, scatter, and reflect UVB and UVA rays depending on their particle size. The remaining UV-absorbing molecules are classified as either UVB or UVA filters or both.

There are about 55 ultraviolet filters that are approved for use in sunscreen products globally, but only 10 of them are approved uniformly for international consumption [3, 4]. Table 9.2 lists their UV absorbance maxima (λmax) and their specific extinction E (1 %, 1 cm), namely, the nominal absorbance at the absorption maximum of a 1 % solution of the filter in a 1 cm optical pathway cuvette, the molar absorption coefficient ϵ (mol^{-1} cm^{-1}), along with the countries or regions where they are approved. Each filter is approved or rejected according to regional requirements. Note that currently there are only ten UV filters that are approved uniformly worldwide and are marked with an ^{XXX} in Table 9.2 under category country/region.

9.4 The Chemistry of Ultraviolet Filters

To illustrate the relationship between the chemical structures of all of these approved UV filters and their UV-absorbing characteristics, I will review one of the oldest UV filters in use, namely, PABA (para-aminobenzoic acid) and its derivatives. PABA has a λ max of 290 nm with an extinction coefficient E_1 (1 %, 1 cm)

Table 9.2 The properties of the 55 approved UV filters worldwide

INCI name	Country/region[a]	UV/region	$\lambda_{max, 1}$/nm	E_1(1 %, 1 cm)	ϵ_2/dm^3 mol^{-1} cm^{-1}	$\lambda_{max, 2}$/nm	E_2 (1 %, 1 cm)	ϵ_1/dm^3 mol^{-1} cm^{-1}
Benzophenone	AZ	UVA/B	284		10,300	340		8950
Benzophenone-1	JN, SA	UVA/B	291	630	12,265	328	420	10,265
Benzophenone-2	AZ, JN, SA	UVA/B	287	580	13,700	349	410	9400
Benzophenone-3 XXX	*ALL*	UVA/B	286	630	14,380	324	400	9180
Benzophenone-4	EU, US, AZ, CA, JN	UVA/B	286	440	13,400	324	360	8400
Benzophenone-5	EU, CA, JN, SA	UVA/B	286	430		323	345	
Benzophenone-6	JN, SA	UVA/B	284	490	13,500	323	390	12,950
Benzophenone-8	US, AZ, CA, SA	UVA/B	284	380	13,270	327	300	10,440
Benzophenone-9	JN, SA	UVA/B	284	260		331	175	
3-Benzylidene Camphor	EU, SA	UVB	289	890	21,360			
Benzylidene camphor sulfonic acid	EU, AZ, JN, SA	UVB	294	860	27,600			
Beta, 2-glucopyranoxy propyl hydroxy Benzophenone	JN, SA	UVA/B						
Bis-ethylhexyloxyphenol methoxyphenyl triazine	EU, AZ, SA	UVA/B	310	745	46,800	343	820	51,900
Butyl methoxydibenzoylmethane XXX	*ALL*	UVA	357	1110	34,140			
Camphor benzalkonium methosulfate	EU, AZ, SA	UVB	284	590	24,500			
Cinoxate	US, AZ, CA, JN, SA	UVB	308	825	20,650			
DEA methoxycinnamate	CA, SA	UVB	290	880	24,930			
Diethylamino hydroxybenzoyl hexyl benzoate	EU, AZ, JN, SA	UVA	354	925	35,900			
Diethylhexyl butamido triazone	EU, SA	UVB	311	1460	111,700			

(continued)

Table 9.2 (continued)

INCI name	Country/region[a]	UV/region	$\lambda_{max,1}$/nm	E_1(1 %, 1 cm)	ϵ_2/dm^3 mol^{-1} cm^{-1}	λ max,$_2$/nm	E_2 (1 %, 1 cm)	ϵ_1/dm^3 mol^{-1} cm^{-1}
Digalloyl trioleate	SA	UVB						
Diisopropyl methyl cinnamate	JN, SA	UVB						
Dimethoxyphenyl-[1-(3,4)]-4,4-dimethyl 1,3 Pentanedione	JN, SA	UVA						
Disodium phenyl dibenzimidazole tetrasulfonate	EU, AZ, SA	UVA	335	770	51,940			
Drometrizole	JN	UVA/B	300			340		
Drometrizole trisiloxane	EU, AZ, JN, SA	UVA/B	303	310	16,200	341	300	15,500
Ethyl Dihydroxypropyl PABA	CA,SA	UVB	312		27,000			
Ethylhexyl dimethoxy benzylidene dioxoimidazoline propionate	JN, SA	UVB						
Ethylhexyl dimethyl PABA XXX	*ALL*	UVB	311	990	27,300			
Ethylhexyl methoxycinnamate XXX	*ALL*	UVB	311	850	23,300			
Ethylhexyl salicylate XXX	*ALL*	UVB	305	165	4130			
Ethylhexyl triazone	EU, AZ, JN, SA	UVB	314	1550	119,500			
Ferulic acid	JN, SA	UVB						
Glyceryl ethylhexanoate dimethoxycinnamate	JN, SA	UVB						
Glyceryl PABA	CA, JN, SA	UVB	297	780	18,700			
Homosalate XXX	*ALL*	UVB	306	180	4300			
Isoamyl p-methoxycinnamate	EU, AZ, JN, SA	UVB	308	980	24,335			
Isopentyl trimethoxycinnamate trisiloxane	JN, SA	UVB						
Isopropyl benzyl salicylate	AZ, JN	UVB						
Isopropyl methoxycinnamate	JN, SA	UVB						
Lawsone + dihydoxyacetone	–	UVB						

Menthyl anthranilate	US, AZ, CA, JN, SA	UVA	336	190	5230			
4-Methylbenzylidene camphor	EU, AZ, CA, SA	UVB	300	930	23,655			
Methylene bis-benzotriazolyl tetramethylbutylphenol	EU, AZ, JN, SA	UVA/B	305	400	26,600	360	495	33,000
Octocrylene xxx	*ALL*	UVB	303	340	12,290			
PABA xxx	*ALL*	UVB	283	640	15,300			
PEG-25 PABA	EU, AZ, JN	UVB	309	180				
Pentyl dimethyl PABA	JN	UVB	310	310				
Phenyl benzimidazole sulfonic acid xxx	*ALL*	UVB	302	920	26,060			
Polyacrylamido methylbenzylidene camphor	EU, SA	UVB	297	610	19,700			
Polysilicone-15	EU, AZ, JN, SA	UVB	312	180	108,000			
Salicylic acid	AZ	UVB	300					
TEA salicylate	US, AZ, CA, SA	UVB	298	120	3000			
Terephthalylidene dicamphor sulfonic acid	EU, AZ, CA, JN, SA	UVA	345	750	47,100			
Titanium dioxide xxx	*ALL*	UVA/B						
Zinc oxide	EU, US, AZ, CA, JN, SA	UVA/B						

[a]*EU* EU, *US* USA, *AZ* AUS/NZ, *CA* Canada, *JN* Japan, *SA* S. Africa. For official regulations, consult specific country/region agencies

Note: *E* (1 %, 1 cm) is the "specific extinction," and ϵ ($dm^3 mol^{-1} cm^{-1}$) is the molar absorption coefficient

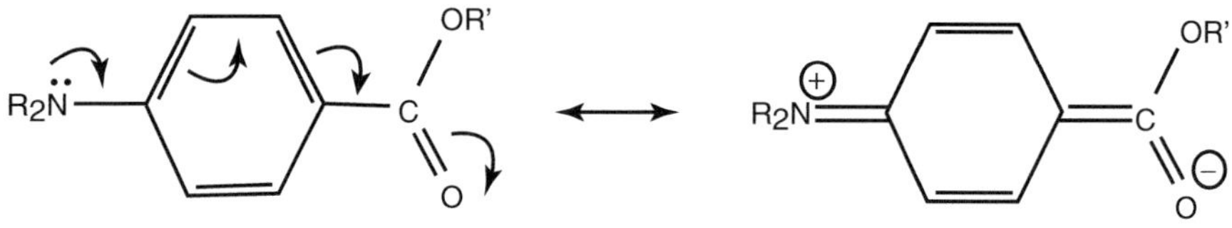

Fig 9.4 The electron delocalization in PABA molecule

of 640 or a ϵ_1(dm^3 mol^{-1} cm^{-1}) of 15,300. That characterizes this molecule as an efficient UVB filter which could yield SPF of over 8 by itself alone and in combinations can yield SPF well over 15 in cosmetic formulations. This molecule and its octyl (2-ethylhexyl) derivative, namely, padimate-O, were the workhorse molecules for producing efficient UVB protection in the USA in the past decades. These molecules have fallen out of favor recently as they tend to discolor and stain clothing and, most importantly, were implicated in a number of irritation cases by the consumer. Nevertheless, these molecules served as elegant examples of how sunscreen molecules exert their UV protection action. These molecules possess both an electron-releasing group (NR_2) and an electron-accepting group (–COOR), group that is situated in a para-position on the basic benzene (aromatic) molecule. This configuration allows for an efficient electron delocalization, with an energy requirement corresponding to an ultraviolet absorption of about 311 nm. Due to symmetry consideration and the ease of electron delocalization in the molecule, the absorption (as measured by its extinction coefficient) is quite high (990). Figure 9.4 illustrates that process.

If this PABA molecule was substituted differently on the benzene ring, say, an ortho-relationship instead of the para-relationship in PABA, the molecule would behave quite differently. In fact, menthyl anthranilate, another approved UV filter in the USA that has an ortho-relationship between its amine and ester grouping, is no longer a UVB filter. It is considered a UVA filter with a UV absorption of 336 nm but with a considerably weaker extinction coefficient E_1 (1 %, 1 cm) of 190. In examining the electron delocalization process in the ortho-disubstituted amine (menthyl anthranilate or meradimate), it is quite apparent that other processes are in play in this molecule, mostly through-space hydrogen bonding that eases the energy requirements of the electron delocalization. Since energy and wavelength are inversely proportional to one another, lower-energy requirements would produce a longer wavelength absorption. The through-space extra electron delocalization in the meradimate molecule produces a desired bathochromic (to higher wavelength) to UVA protection but, unfortunately, significantly lowers the ease of delocalization since the side chain hydrogen bonding electron transfer deviates from planarity, increases the energy requirements, and results in a lower extinction coefficient.

These two simple processes, namely, aromatic electron delocalization (contributing to the UV absorption) and the ortho-through-space hydrogen bonding (contributing to the ease of delocalization), are the basis of designing most of the ultraviolet

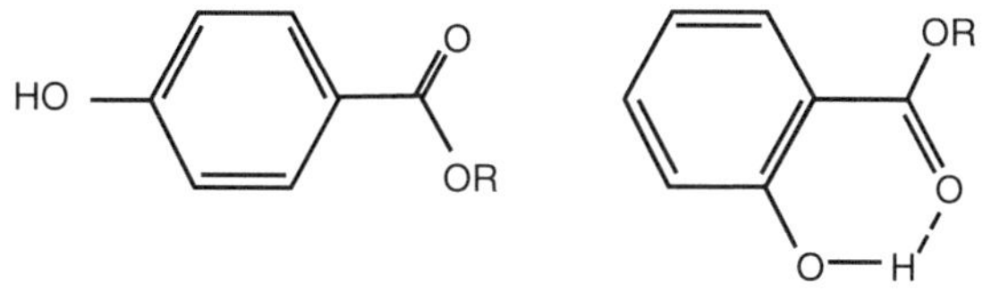

parabens (λ_{max}=260nm) salicylate (λ_{max}=300nm)

Fig 9.5 The para (parabens) with a lower λmax vs. the ortho (salicylates) with a higher λ max

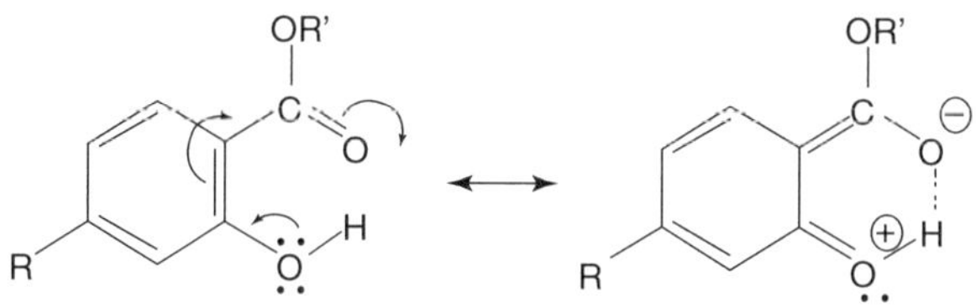

Fig 9.6 Resonance delocalizaton and through-space hydrogen bonding in salicylate

filters in the world today. Numerous similar examples to illustrate the forces at play in UV molecules are available. For instance, compare the parabens (para-disubstituted) to the salicylate (ortho-disubstituted molecules) in Fig 9.5.

Again, as predicted, the parabens would have a low UV absorbance of about 260 nm (that would not be considered a UVB filter) but with a considerable extinction coefficient, whereas the salicylates (homosalate or octisalate) have a higher UV absorbance of 306 nm (UVB filter) but with a lower extinction coefficient of 180 due to its ortho-through-space hydrogen bonding as shown in Fig. 9.6.

For a detailed review of the mechanism of all the other approved UV filters (cinnamates, benzopheones, dibenzoylmethanes, camphor, and triazone derivatives), consult other references [2].

9.5 New Molecules Appearing on the World Market

A series of molecules have recently been designed in Europe with high molecular weights (over 500 Da) to diminish their penetration into the skin. These molecules possess multiple chromophores that yield high extinction coefficients and also broad-spectrum protection [5]. They are, unfortunately, not yet approved in the USA. They are listed in Table 9.3.

In the USA, there are eight applications pending under the process termed TEA (Time and Extent Application) that, when approved, will undoubtedly enhance the UV protection of American consumers from the cancer-causing rays [6]. Two of the eight TEA ingredients, bemotrizinol and bisoctrizole, when approved for use in the USA, can be used to impart more photostable sunscreen formulations. See Table 9.4 below illustrating the properties of these two UVA ingredients.

Table 9.3 EU-approved UV filters for sunscreens designed with Dalton's of 500 or higher

Filter type	UV filter INCI name	COLIPA#	Trademark (supplier)	€/dm^3 mol^{-1} cm^{-1}	λ max (nm)	Mol. weight (Dalton)
UVB	Benzylidene malonate polysiloxane	S74 BMP	Parsol SLX (DSM)	108,000	314	~6000
	Dioctyl butamido triazone	S78 DBT	Uvasorb HEB (3V Sigma)	111,170	312	766
	Ethylhexyl triazone	S69 EHT	Uvinul T150 (BASF)	119,500	312	823
UVA	Disodium phenyl dibenzimidazole tetrasulfonate	S80 DPDT	Neo Heliopan AP (Symrise)	52,400	334	675
	Terephthalylidene dicamphor sulfonic acid	S71 TDSA	Mexoryl SX (L'Oreal)	47,100	345	607
UVA/UVB	Bis-ethylhexyloxyphenol methoxyphenyltriazine	S81 BEMT	Tinosorb S (BASF/Ashland)	42,800/47,500	310/343	629
	Drometrizole trisiloxane	S73 DTS	Mexoryl XL (L'Oreal)	15,900/15,500	303/341	501
	Methylene bis-benzotriazolyl tetramethylbutylphenol	S79 MBBT	Tinosorb M (BASF)	32,000/38,000	305/360	659

Table 9.4 Specifications of bemotrizinol and bisoctrizole [7]

Commercial name:	Tinosorb S, Eusolex S,	Tinosorb M
Structural formula:	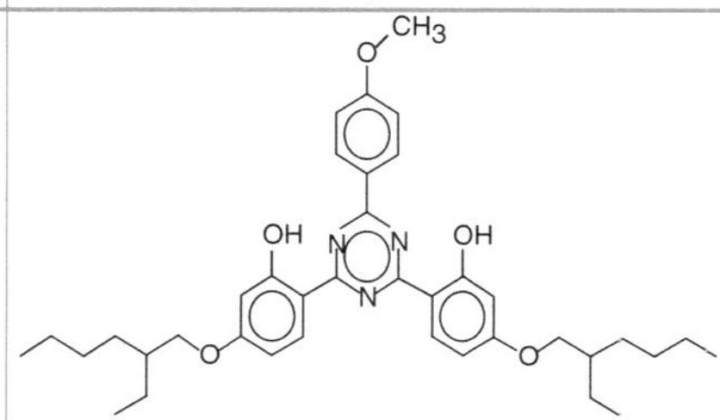	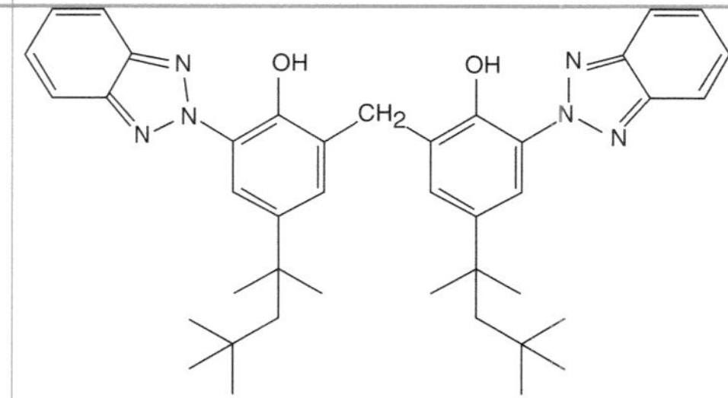
Molecular formula:	$C_{38}H_{49}N_3O_5$	$C_{41}H_{50}N_6O_2$
Molecular weight:	627.8 g/mol	658.86 g/mol
INCI name:	Bis-ethylhexyloxyphenol methoxyphenyl triazine (BEMT)	Methylene bis-benzotriazoyl tetramethylbutylphenol (and) aqua (and) decyl glucoside (and) propylene glycol (and) xanthan gum
USAN name:	Bemotrizinol	Bisoctrizole
CAS-no:	187393-00-6	103597-45-1
Physical Appearance:	Light yellow powder	Aqueous white dispersion (50 % active)
λmax:	310 and 340 nm	305 and 360 nm
E (1 %,1 cm):	819 (in ethanol, 340 nm)	480 (in water, 360 nm)
λc (critical wavelength)	373 nm	388 nm
UVA/UVB ratio:	0.73	1
Recommended level (%)	10 % in Australia and EU 3 % in Japan	20 % (10 % active) in Australia, EU, and Japan

9.6 Inorganic Particulates

These ingredients are chemicals that reflect, scatter, and absorb the UV radiation. They include titanium dioxide and zinc oxide. They are available in micronized and nanosized forms that enhance sun protection without imparting the traditional opaqueness that was aesthetically unappealing in cosmetic formulations. These metal oxides are reactive and insoluble in cosmetic formulations without chemical treatment. This treatment includes coating of the metal core and dispersion and suspension of the particles with oils, solubilizers, and emollients [8, 9]. Many users falsely believe that "natural" claims are admissible if only inorganic particulates are used in sunscreen products. Unfortunately, most of these chemical treatments render the inorganic particulates synthetic and unnatural.

There has been a shift to zinc oxide from titanium dioxide recently, mostly due to its broad-spectrum and higher UVA protection. It is also popular since it has a lower refractive index of 1.9–2.0 compared to titanium dioxide's 2.5–2.7, which leads to superior transparency. Recently, ZnO was also approved in Europe. In the USA, combinations of ZnO and TiO_2 with avobenzone are still not allowed.

Titanium is the ninth most common element on the Earth's crust. In nature, it exists only in combinations with other elements such as iron and oxygen. Three titanium ores are of commercial importance: ilmenite, rutile, and anatase. Ilmenite is a composite of oxides of iron and titanium. Rutile and anatase are also never pure and contain various amounts of metal including those that may pose health hazards to humans. Therefore, commercial TiO_2 is always synthetic [8]. Rutile and anatase have different crystalline structure and different physical and chemical properties. Of the three forms of TiO_2, rutile is the most thermally stable.

Zinc ranks 24th in abundance on the Earth's crust but never occurs free in nature. It is widespread around the world with important deposits located in North America and Australia. ZnO is produced by oxidizing vapors of Zn in burners. Pure ZnO is typically a white or yellow-white powder.

The optical behavior of ZnO and TiO_2 consists mainly of scattering or absorbing the light. The scattering from molecules and very tiny particles is predominantly Rayleigh scattering. When the particle size is at the same magnitude as the wavelength, Mie scattering predominates. The absorption, on the other hand, is a function of the number of atoms that interact with the light in its pathway. Light with a wavelength below 420 mm has enough energy to excite electrons in the valence band and can be absorbed by the inorganic particulate (see Fig. 9.3). Since the bandgap wavelength of ZnO is longer than that of TiO_2, ZnO absorbs a broader-spectrum range of UV light than TiO_2. TiO_2 is not considered an efficient UVA absorber; rather, it is an efficient UVB absorber. The attenuation of UVA by TiO_2, therefore, mainly takes place via scattering.

When using inorganic particulates, the following parameters need to be carefully evaluated:

(i) The type of metal
(ii) The particle size
(iii) The coating

(iv) The oil
(v) The dispersant
(vi) The loading
(vii) The absorption coefficient

Each of the above parameters may influence the behavior, the concentration, the solubility, the potential interactions, and, most importantly, the regulatory status of the particulate and the final cosmetic formulation.

9.7 The Photostability of UVA Absorbers

As described earlier, the exposure of UV-absorbing molecules to solar radiation may lead to photochemical reactions that can compromise both the physical attributes of the UV filters (color, appearance, etc.) and their chemical properties leading to undesirable reactions and by-products [10].

Avobenzone is one of the most important UVA filters in commerce today. Unfortunately, this molecule is photounstable. In its enol form, it exhibits an excellent UVA absorption at 357 nm, but in its diketo form, its absorption is in the UVC region and thereby is ineffective as a UVA or UVB filter. See Fig. 9.7.

Other studies have also shown that avobenzone (enol form) reacts with other molecules including ethylhexyl methoxycinnamate (USAN name, octinoxate) to yield photo-adducts [11]. It has also been reported that upon exposure to UV radiation, avobenzone tends to fragment into reactive species as shown in Fig. 9.8.

Approaches to improve the photostability of the UVA filters included the use of glass beads and microspheres and the use of ROS quenchers, triplet-triplet (T-T) and singlet-singlet (S-S) quenchers [10]. These quenchers, also termed excited-state quenchers (ESQ), have recently appeared on the US market to circumvent the photo-instability issues of avobenzone. The mechanism of T-T quenching has been extensively reviewed in the literature [12]. These UV-absorbing quenching

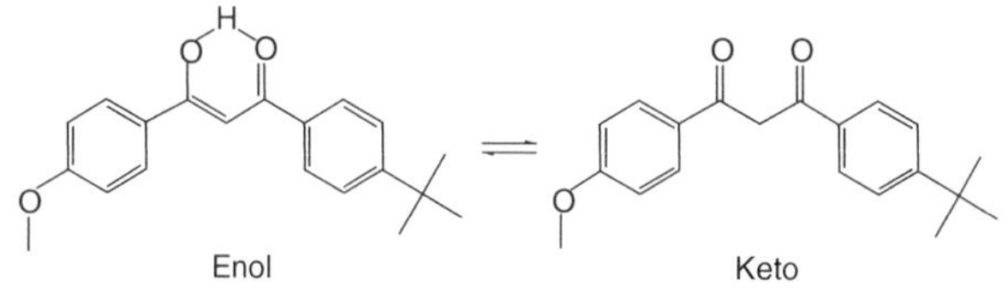

Fig 9.7 The keto-enol tautomerism of avobenzone

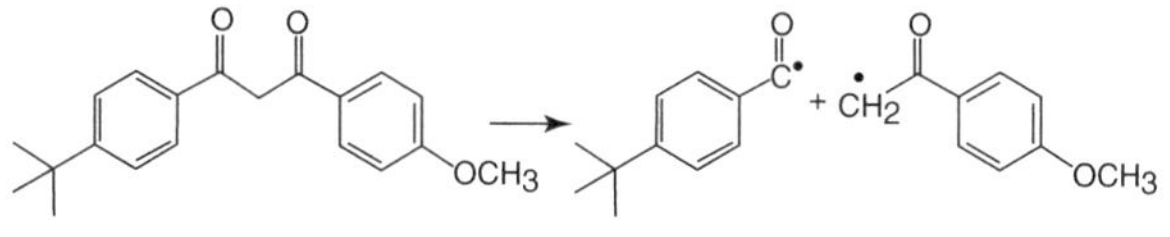

Fig. 9.8 The fragmentation of butyl methoxydibenzoylmethane (avobenzone)

molecules include octocrylene, 4 methyl benzylidene camphor, methoxycrylene, polyester 8, diethylhexyl naphthalate (DEHN), and diethylhexyl syringylidene malonate (DESM).

9.8 Future Direction

This illustration of the mechanism of UV action of the molecules we have today to combat the rising incidence of skin cancer reveals a deficiency in our arsenal for UV protection. The design of filters in the last century relied on small absorbing molecules that tend to penetrate the skin and potentially may interact with substrates in the body. In addition, the USA clearly has inadequate ingredients to protect consumers properly from the UVA radiation. The workhorse of the so-called UVA chemical absorbers, avobenzone, is photounstable and needs to be supported with quenchers and other ingredients to remain active as a UVA filter. In addition, protection from the infrared rays is not addressed. Whenever the subject of skin damage from the nonionizing infrared rays has come up in the past, it was summarily dismissed. IR rays were thought to be benign because of their relatively low energies and frequencies. They are the source of most of the "heat" produced from the sun. Recent evidence, however, has shown that the IR rays, particularly the IRA rays (750–1400 nm) penetrate much deeper into the skin, induce significant free radicals in the dermis and diminish the skin's antioxidant capacity [13]. IRA radiation has been reported to upregulate an enzyme that destroys the collagen fibers (the matrix metalloproteinase-1 (MMP-1) expression) [14]. Others recently reported that the ultraviolet filters used in today's sun care regimens prevent no more than 55 % of the damaging free radicals from the sun's UV radiation but none of the IRA-induced free radicals [15]. It is estimated that 65 % of the energy generated by the IRA radiation reaches the skin's dermal layers, the tissue responsible for the skin's structure with its fibers, elastin, and collagen. IRA biological effects cause the loss of elasticity and reduced firmness thus leading to the formation of wrinkles and the aging of the skin [16–19].

9.9 Conclusions

Protection from the burning (erythemal) UVB rays is a basic requirement. Protection from the UVA rays is paramount and so is protection from the damaging heat rays and the longer wavelength radiation of the infrared [20, 21]. In my opinion, our ingredients are woefully inadequate, especially the currently US-approved filters. We can no longer ignore the facts: sunscreen ingredients in cosmetics are not adequately preventing cancer incidence in the USA. We have lulled ourselves into a false sense of security. A cream or a lotion alone cannot, at this date, guard you entirely from the effects of the powerful sun. Heed all practical advice: wear protective clothing, seek shade, avoid noon sun exposure, and do use adequate and properly applied sunscreens. Until advanced ingredients are developed and approved, use all available measures to mitigate the effects of the total spectrum of the solar radiation.

References

1. Shaath NA (1986) The Chemistry of sunscreens. Cosmet Toilet 101(3):55
2. Shaath NA (2005) The Chemistry of ultraviolet filters. In: Shaath NA (ed) Sunscreens: regulations and commercial development, 3rd edn. Taylor & Francis, New York, pp 217–238
3. Shaath NA (2010) Ultraviolet filters. Photochem Photobiol Sci 9:407–418
4. Shaath NA (2007) The encyclopedia of UV filters. Allured Publications, Carol Stream
5. Herzog B, Hueglin D, Osterwalder U (2005) New sunscreen actives. In: Shaath NA (ed) Sunscreens: regulations and commercial development, 3rd edn. Taylor & Francis, New York, pp 291–320
6. Shaath NA (2013) The archaic TEA process revisited. The Sunscreen Filter. Happi, May 2013, pp 48–51
7. www.basf.com (Full report 2012) and www.ashland.com (Sunscreens with UVA protection 2014).
8. Schlossman D, Shao Y (2005) Inorganic ultraviolet filters. In: Shaath NA (ed) Sunscreens: regulations and commercial development, 3rd edn. Taylor & Francis, New York, pp 239–279
9. Shaath NA, Walele I (2005) Inorganic particulate ultraviolet filters. In: Shaath NA (ed) Sunscreens: regulations and commercial development, 3rd edn. Taylor & Francis, New York, pp 281–290
10. Shaath NA (2007) SPF boosters & photostability of ultraviolet filters. HAPPI, Oct 2007, pp 77–83
11. Sayre RM, Dowdy JC (2005) Unexpected photolysis of the sunscreen octinoxate in the presence of the sunscreen Avobenzone. Photochem Photobiol 81(2):452–456
12. Bonda C (2005) The photostability of organic sunscreen actives: a review. In: Shaath NA (ed) Sunscreens: regulations and commercial development, 3rd edn. Taylor & Francis, New York, pp 321–352
13. Holzer A, Athar M, Elmets C (2010) The other end of the rainbow: infrared and skin. J Invest Dermatol 130:1496–1498
14. Calles C et al (2010) Infrared A radiation influences the skin fibroblast transcriptome: mechanism and consequences. J Invest Dermatol 130:1424–1436
15. Haywood R et al (2003) Sunscreens inadequately protect against UVA induced free radicals in skin. J Invest Dermatol 121:862–868
16. Lademann J et al (2011) Interaction between carotenoids and free radicals in human skin. Skin Pharmacol Physiol 24:238–244
17. Darvin M et al (2010) Radical production by Infrared A irradiation in human tissue. Skin Pharmacol Physiol 23:40–46
18. Schiek S, Schroeder P, Krutmann J (2003) Cutaneous effects of Infrared radiation. Photodermol Photoimmunol Photomed 19:228–234
19. Cho S et al (2009) Effects of Infrared radiation and heat on human skin aging in vivo. J Invest Dermatol Symp Proc 14:15–19
20. Shaath NA (2012) Infrared radiation and skin protection. The Sunscreen Filter, HAPPI, March 2012, pp 50–53
21. Shaath NA (2012) Sun protection should protect from IRA damage. The Sunscreen Filter, HAPPI, May 2012, pp 53–56

Chapter 10
Chemistry of Sunscreens

Susan Daly, Hao Ouyang, and Prithwiraj Maitra

Key Points

- Sun filters can be classified as organic, organic particulates, polymeric, and inorganic particulates.
- The mechanism of action of all types of sun filters is primarily UV absorption.
- A global overview of sun filter approval levels, chemical structures, and absorbance properties is included in this chapter.
- Formulators must select the right combination of filters to deliver photostable, broad-spectrum protection, with high SPF, and optimal aesthetics to drive consumer compliance.
- Regulatory approvals, the breadth and height of a sun filter's UV absorbance, and the sun filter solubility or dispersibility are key parameters that formulators should consider during sunscreen design.

10.1 Introduction

Human skin is exposed daily to sunlight, which contains a significant amount of ultraviolet (UV) radiation. It is well known that UV radiation can be harmful and that UV exposure can play a significant role in development of skin damage [23, 27]. Various compounds have been used to protect skin from the harmful rays of the sun over the centuries. It is only over the last 100 years, however, that synthetic UV filters have been developed to protect individuals from sunburn and UV-induced skin cancer [35].

S. Daly • H. Ouyang • P. Maitra (✉)
JOHNSON & JOHNSON Consumer Companies, Inc,
199 Grandview Road, Skillman, NJ 08558, USA
e-mail: sdaly8@its.jnj.com; HOuyan4@its.jnj.com; pmaitra@its.jnj.com

S.Q. Wang, H.W. Lim (eds.), *Principles and Practice of Photoprotection*,
DOI 10.1007/978-3-319-29382-0_10

For practical and historical purposes, the UV spectrum has been divided into UVA1 (340–400 nm), UVA2 (320–340 nm), UVB (290–320 nm), and UVC (100–290 nm). UVC and some of the shorter UVB wavelengths emitted from the sun are filtered out by the ozone before they reach the Earth's surface. Both UVA and UVB rays can damage DNA, lipids, and proteins; produce inflammation; and ultimately result in burns, premature aging, and carcinogenesis [27, 30, 35]. An ideal sunscreen must protect the user from UV radiation across the light wavelength spectrum associated with harmful effects [24, 27].

10.2 Mechanism of Action of Sun Filters

Sunscreens protect skin from these harmful rays by forming a protective barrier on skin surface. Most sunscreen active ingredients are organic molecules with conjugated, aromatic chemical structures. The mode of action of these sunscreen active ingredients is primarily UV absorption [24]. By residing on skin surface as a film, these organic molecules effectively transform the harmful UV energy to harmless forms of energy and prevent the UV photons from entering into the skin [25, 30]. The electrons in these chemical structures are "active" because they are capable of energy transfer when hit by UV. Quantum mechanical calculations show that the energy of radiation quanta present in UVB and UVA lies in the same order of magnitude as the resonance energy of electron delocalization in aromatic compounds [35].

The electrons of sunscreen UV filters can accept the energy from UV photons and move to higher electronic energy states. This energy can then be quickly converted to heat by non-radiation energy dissipation or to other forms of light such as fluorescence, phosphorescence, or infrared rays [25]. The electrons will return back to the ground state during the energy transfer, ready to receive the next UV photon. The lifetime of excited states of these molecules is very short; therefore, as long as the chemical structure of the sunscreen is stable at excited states, the process of excitation and returning to ground states can occur continuously and repetitively without any loss of efficacy.

A few sunscreen active ingredients are not photostable. The chemical structures of these non-photostable molecules can change while the chemical is in the excited state (photochemical reactions). When that happens, the original molecules are broken down and not capable of repeating the excitation process and more importantly cannot absorb the next UV photons. With the degradation of the original active ingredients, free radicals (including singlet oxygen) may be generated that may then react with nearby molecules to form photobyproducts. Thus, the efficacy of the sunscreen decreases because less active ingredients remain to absorb more incoming photons.

Sun filters do not need to penetrate into the skin in order to be effective. As soon as the sunscreen film is present on skin surface, there will be at least some level of protection because of its inherent absorption properties. The final protection level may be enhanced as the product dries on the skin and the film structure is optimized [32].

10.3 Chemical Classification of Sun Filters

There are a number of different sun filters approved for the use in sunscreen products around the globe. Currently, 16 sun filters are approved for sunscreen products in the United States (Food and Drug Administration and Department of Health and Human Services [14, 15, 39]), 20 in Canada [18], 28 in the European Union [12, 22], 28 in the Association of Southeast Asian Nations [37], and 33 approved by MERCOSUR (Southern Common Market, consisting of Argentina, Brazil, Paraguay, Uruguay, and Venezuela) [37]. The complete listing of approved sun filters in these locations, along with the approved concentrations, is shown in Table 10.1.

Sun filter actives can be classified into the following categories: organic (traditional molecules or polymeric) or particulate (organic particulates or inorganic particulate), as described in subsequent sections 3.1 and 3.2, respectively.

10.3.1 Organic Filters

Organic filters are often referred to as "chemical" filters, but this can be misleading because it suggests that it is possible to have a sun filter that is "nonchemical." Strictly speaking, all active sun filter compounds, both organic and inorganic, are made up of chemical molecules originating from the periodic table, and all function primarily by absorbing light [26].

10.3.1.1 Organic Filters: Traditional Molecules

Traditional organic sun filters are aromatic, small molecules, with molecular weight values <900 g/mol. Today, the most widely used organic filters include avobenzone, oxybenzone, octocrylene, salicylate derivatives (homosalate and ethylhexyl salicylate), cinnamate derivatives (octyl-methoxycinnamate [OMC]), triazone derivatives (Uvinul T150 [ethylhexyl triazone]; UVASorb HEB [diethylhexyl butamido triazone]; Tinosorb S [bis-ethylhexyloxyphenol methoxyphenyl triazine]), benzoate derivatives (Uvinul A Plus [diethylamino hydroxybenzoyl hexyl benzoate]), benzotriazole derivatives (Mexoryl XL [drometrizole trisiloxane]), and camphor derivatives (Mexoryl SX [ecamsule]; terephthalylidene dicamphor sulfonic acid). Anthranilate derivatives (like meradimate) are less commonly used filters because of low efficacy.

Avobenzone (a dibenzoylmethane derivative) is one of the most efficient UVA-absorbing filters used around the globe, and it is the only UVA-absorbing organic sun filter approved in the USA. However, avobenzone is prone to photo instability because of an enol-to-keto tautomerization as shown in Fig. 10.1 [25]. The enol form of avobenzone absorbs in the UVA (315–400 nm), while the diketo form absorbs in the UVC (200–280 nm) and is prone to degradation [25]. Other photostabilizing ingredients must be used in combination with avobenzone to prevent light-induced degradation [7]. In order to achieve photostability of avobenzone, it must be combined with ingredients

Table 10.1 List of sun filters approved in the USA, Canada, European Union, ASEAN, and MERCOSUR; alternate names; and approved usage levels per region

Filter name	Other names	Coverage	US	Canada	EU	MERCOSUR	Australia	ASEAN
			Maximum allowed concentration (%)					
Benzophenone-3	*Oxybenzone* or 2-hydroxy-4-methoxybenzophenone	UVA/B	6	6	10	10	10	10
Benzophenone-4	*Sulisobenzone* or 2-hydroxy-4-methoxybenzophenone-5-sulfonic acid and its trihydrate	UVA/B	10	10	5**	10	10	5**
Benzophenone-5	2-Hydroxy-4-methoxybenzophenone-5--sulfonic acid (benzophenone-5) and its sodium salt Sulisobenzone sodium Sodium hydroxymethoxybenzophenone sulfonate	UVA/B	–	–	*	5	10	*
Benzophenone-8	Dioxybenzone or 2,2'-dihydroxy-4-methoxybenzophenone Dioxybenzone (2-hydroxy-4-methoxyphenyl)(2-hydroxyphenyl)methanone Methanone (2-hydroxy-4-methoxyphenyl)(2-hydroxyphenyl)	UVA/B	3	3	–	3	3	–
3-Benzylidene camphor	3-Benzylidene camphor	UVB	–	–	2	2	–	2
Bis-ethylhexyloxyphenol methoxyphenyl triazine	*Tinosorb S* or (1,3,5)-triazine-2,4-bis{[4-(2-ethyl-hexyloxy)-2-hydroxy]-phenyl}-6-(4-methoxyphenyl) or anisotriazine	UVA/B	–	–	10	10	10	10
Butyl methoxydibenzoyl methane	*Avobenzone* or 1-(4-tert-butylphenyl)-3-(4-methoxyphenyl) propane-1,3-dione	UVA	3	3	5	5	5	5

Camphor benzalkonium methosulfate	*Mexoryl SO* or N,N,N-trimethyl-4-(2-oxoborn-3-ylidene-methyl) anilinium methyl sulfate	UVB	–	–	6	6	6	6
Diethylamino hydroxybenzoyl hexyl benzoate	*Uvinul A plus* or benzoic acid, 2-[–4-(diethylamino)-2-hydroxybenzoyl]-, hexylester	UVA	–	–	10	10	10	10
Diethanolamine methoxycinnamate	DEA methoxycinnamate	UVA	–	10	–	–	–	–
Diethylhexyl butamido triazone	*UVASorb HEB* or benzoic acid, 4,4-((6-((4-(((1,1-dimethyleth yl) amino) carbonyl) phenyl) amino) 1,3,5-triazine-2,4-diyl) diimino) bis-(2-) ester) or dioctyl butamido triazone	UVB	–	–	10	10	–	10
Disodium phenyl dibenzimidazole tetrasulfonate	*Neo Heliopan AP* or monosodium salt of 2-2'-bis(1,4-phenylene)1H-benzimidazole-4,6-disulphonic acid) or bisimidazylate	UVA	–	–	10	10	10	10
Drometrizole trisiloxane	*Mexoryl XL* or phenol,2-(2H-benzotriazol-2-yl)-4-methyl-6-(2-methyl-3-(1,3,3,3-tetramethyl-I-(trimethylsilyl)oxy)-disiloxanyl)propyl)	UVA/B	–	15	15	15	15	15
Ethoxyethyl methoxycinnamate	Cinoxate	UVB	3	3	–	3	6	–
Ethylhexyl dimethylamino benzoate	Padimate O Octyl dimethyl *PABA* Ethylhexyl dimethyl PABA	UVB	8	8	8	8	8	8
Ethylhexyl methoxycinnamate	*OMC* or octinoxate Octyl methoxycinnamate	UVB	7.5	7.5	10	10	10	10

(continued)

Table 10.1 (continued)

Filter name	Other names	Coverage	US	Canada	EU	MERCOSUR	Australia	ASEAN
Ethylhexyl salicylate	*Octisalate* 2-Ethylhexyl salicylate Octyl salicylate	UVB	5	5	5	5	5	5
Ethylhexyl triazone	*Uvinul T150* 2,4,6-Trianilino-(p-carbo-2'-ethylhexyl-l'oxy)-1,3,5-triazine Octyl triazone	UVB	–	–	5	5	5	5
Homosalate	3,3,5-Trimethylcyclohexyl 2-hydroxybenzoate Salicilato de homomentila	UVB	15	15	10	15	15	10
Isoamyl p-methoxycinnamate	Amiloxate Isopentyl-4-methoxycinnamate	UVB	–	–	10	10	10	10
Methyl anthranilate	Meradimate	UVA	5	5	–	5	5	5
4-methylbenzylidene camphor	Enzacamene 3-(4'-methylbenxylidene)d-1 camphor 4 MBC	UVB	–	6	4	4	4	4
Methylene bis-benzotriazolyl tetramethylbutylphenol	*Tinosorb M* 2,2'-Methylene-bis-6-(2H-benzotriazol-2yl)-4-(tetramethyl-butyl)-1,1,3,3-phenol	UVA/B	–	–	10	10	10	10
Octocrylene	2-Cyano-3,3-diphenyl acrylic acid, 2-ethylhexyl ester	UVB	10	10	10	10	10	10
Para-aminobenzoic acid	*PABA* 4-Aminobenzoic acid	UVB	15	15	–	15	–	–
PEG-25 *PABA*	Ethoxylated ethyl-4-aminobenzoate	UVB	–	–	10	10	10	10

Phenylbenzimidazole sulfonic acid	*Neo Heliopan Hydro*, Ensulizole 2-Phenylbenzimidazole-5-sulfonic acid and its potassium, sodium, and triethanolamine salts Potassium, sodium, and TEA Phenylbenzimidazole sulfonate	UVB	4	4	8	8 (as acid)	4	8
Polyacrylamido methylbenzylidene camphor	*Mexoryl SW* Polymer of N-[(2 and 4)-[(2-oxoborn-3-ylidene)methyl]benzyl]acrylamide	UVB	–	–	6	6	–	6
Polysilicone-15	*Parsol SLX* Diethylbenzylidene malonate Dimethicone Diethylmalonylbenzylidene Oxypropene dimethicone Dimethicodiethylbenzalmalonate	UVB	–	–	10	10	10	10
Triethanolamine salicylate	*Neo Heliopan TES* Trolamine salicylate	UVB	12	12	–	12	12	–
Tris-biphenyl triazine (nano)	1,3,5 - Triazine, 2,4,6-tris [1,1-biphenyl]-4-1-; ETH-50	UVA/B	–	–	10	–	–	–
Terephthalylidene dicamphor sulfonic acid	*Mexoryl SX*	UVA	–	10	10	10	10	10
Benzylidene camphor sulfonic acid	Alpha-(2-oxoborn-3-ylidene)-toluene-4-sulfonic acid and its salts		–	–	6	6	6	6
Titanium dioxide		UVA/B	25	25	25	25	25	25
Zinc oxide		UVA/B	25	25	*	25	No limit	25

ASEAN Association of Southeast Asian Nations; *EU* European Union; *MBC* methylbenzylidene camphor; *MERCOSUR* Southern Common Market, consisting of Argentina, Brazil, Paraguay, Uruguay, and Venezuela; *OMC* octyl-methoxycinnamate; *PABA* para-aminobenzoic acid; *US* United States; *UVA* ultraviolet A; *UVB* ultraviolet B

* Inclusion in annex VI expected

** Sum of Benzophenone-4 and Benzophenone-5

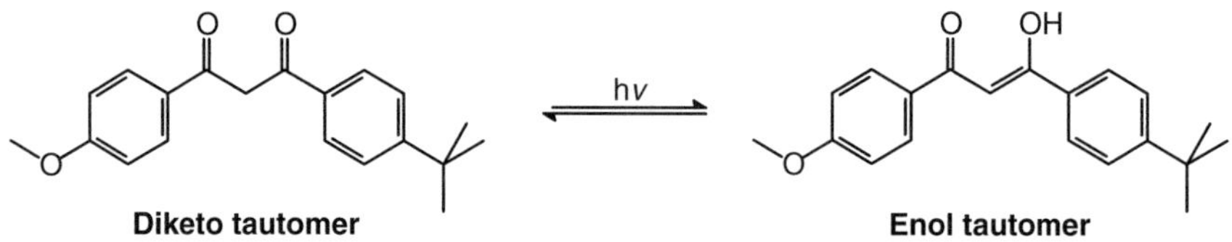

Fig. 10.1 The keto-to-enol tautomerization of avobenzone (Scheme 2 was reproduced with permission from Kockler et al. [25])

that are efficient in both triplet quenching and singlet quenching. Examples of triplet quenchers are the following UV filters: octocrylene, 4-methylbenzylidene camphor (ex-US), Tinosorb S (ex-US), or emollients such as diethylhexyl-2,6-naphthalate [7]. In addition, higher levels of oxybenzone are known to stabilize avobenzone by the singlet quenching mechanism [7]. A combination of singlet and triplet quenchers is most efficient in stabilizing avobenzone.

Cinnamates are very efficient UVB absorbers but also have issues with photostability. OMC is a member of the cinnamate class that is known to react with avobenzone to produce non-UV light-absorbing photoproducts. Hence, combinations of avobenzone and OMC are unfavorable and should be avoided because of enhanced photo instability [7, 33].

Salicylate derivatives are photostable, UVB-absorbing filters that have a long history of usage. They are excellent solubilizers for crystalline UV filters, including oxybenzone and avobenzone, however the absorption efficiency of these filters is quite low.

Oxybenzone (a benzophenone derivative) is used in many US sunscreen formulations with absorbance in the UVB (290–320 nm) and the UVA2 region (320–340 nm). Padimate O is a derivative of para-aminobenzoic acid that is a liquid and is oil soluble. It is a very effective UVB filter with one of the highest molar extinction coefficients of the approved filters. It is not widely used in products over concern that the parent molecule, para-aminobenzoic acid, has been associated with allergic reactions. Octocrylene is another oil-soluble UVB filter that has been widely used to provide increased sun protection factor (SPF) values and to also boost the photostability of avobenzone when used in combination. Ensulizole (phenylbenzimidazole sulfonic acid) is a water-soluble filter and is used in products formulated to feel lighter and less oily, such as daily use cosmetic moisturizers. Currently, it is not permitted to be combined with avobenzone in the USA and must be used in combination with on other UVA absorbers (such as zinc oxide) to provide broad-spectrum protection.

10.3.1.2 Organic Filters: Polymeric

Parsol SLX. Parsol SLX, or polysilicone-15, is made of organic chromophores attached to a polysiloxane chain and is approved for use outside North America. The average molecular weight is >6000 daltons [10], so it is envisioned that the molecule is large enough to reduce permeation through the skin [20], making it ideal for

Table 10.2 Relative lipophilicity of sunscreen chemicals based upon their calculated partition coefficients between octanol and water

CTFA name	Other names	Log *P* at 25 °C
Glyceryl PABA	1,2,3-Propanetriol,1-(4-aminobenzoate)	−0.02
Benzophenone-4	Sulisobenzone	−1.51
PABA	p-Aminobenzoic acid	0.74
Benzophenone-8	Dioxybenzone	2.15
Cinoxate	Ethoxyethyl methoxy cinnamate	2.55
Benzophenone-3	Oxybenzone	2.63
Ethyl dihydroxypropyl PABA	Ethyl-4-bis(2-hydroxypropyl-aminobenzoate)	2.84
Amyl dimethyl PABA	Amyl dimethyl PABA	4.53
Butylmethoxy dibenzoylmethane	Butylmethoxy dibenzoylmethane	4.86
Menthyl anthranilate	Methyl-O-aminobenzoate	5.05
Octyl salicylate	2-Ethylhexyl salicylate	5.30
Homosalate	Homomenthyl salicylate	5.61
Octyl methoxy cinnamate	Ethylhexyl-p-methoxycinnamate	5.65
Octocrylene	Octyl cyanodiphenylacrylate	5.69
Octyl dimethyl PABA	2-Ethylhexyl-p-dimethyl aminobenzoate	6.08

Modified with permission from Agrapidis-Paloympis et al. [1]
CTFA Cosmetic, Toiletry, and Fragrance Association; *PABA* para-aminobenzoic acid

mild applications. The polysiloxane backbone not only links the chromophores together, but it also provides a pleasant aesthetic to skin or hair [29]. Unfortunately, this polymeric filter only absorbs in the UVB ($\lambda_{max}=312$ nm) part of the spectrum and needs to be combined with UVA filters to achieve broad-spectrum protection.

10.3.1.3 Organic Filters: Solubility in Cosmetic Vehicles

In order for a UV-absorbing organic filter to be an effective sunscreen, it must be soluble in at least a portion of the sunscreen formulation. Today's organic sun filters are typically oil soluble or water soluble and occasionally alcohol soluble. The sun filter's partition coefficient (log *P*) between octanol and water gives an indication of the relative lipophilicity, where lower log *P* values indicate a higher degree of water solubility, as shown in Table 10.2 [1].

Oil-soluble filters are used in a wide variety of sunscreen products, including both recreational and daily use products. Recreational-use sunscreen products are typically formulated for enhanced water resistance through the addition of film-forming polymers. A high content of oily sun filter compounds can lead to a heavy and greasy aesthetic on the skin. For products that do not require a high level of water resistance, water-soluble sun filters may be used either alone or in combination with oil-soluble sun filters to create formulations with enhanced aesthetic properties and potentially improved user compliance. Ensulizole (2-phenylbenzimidazole-5-sulfonic acid), Neo Heliopan AP (disodium phenyl dibenzimidazole tetrasulfonate) and Mexoryl SX are examples of water-soluble sun filters.

Furthermore, filter solubility is important for maintaining formulation efficacy as some filters, including octyl triazone, benzophenone-3, butyl methylbenzylidene camphor, and methoxydibenzoylmethane, may crystallize out of solution if not properly solubilized [40], making the protective film less uniform on the skin. In addition, solvent polarity has been found to affect λ_{max} and critical wavelength in formulations [1].

10.3.2 *Particulate Filters*

While most organic filters must be dissolved into either the oil or water phases of a formulation to be effective, particulate sunscreens are not dissolved in either phase, and they exist in particle suspensions. Particulate filters are commonly used in mild and baby sunscreen products, and they have been demonstrated in several studies to stay on the surface of the skin [8, 16]. There are two types of particulate sunscreen filters: organic and inorganic.

10.3.2.1 Particulate Organic Filters

Methylene bis-benzotriazolyl tetramethylbutylphenol (i.e., MBBT or Tinosorb M) is considered to be an organic particulate filter. Pure MBBT is a solid powder with a particle size in the micron range, and the commercially available Tinosorb M is a MBBT suspension. The mechanism of action for Tinosorb M is mostly absorption with slight contributions from particulate scattering [19].

10.3.2.2 Inorganic Particulates

The inorganic particulate sunscreen class includes titanium dioxide (TiO_2) and zinc oxide (ZnO). It is important to point out that these particulate sunscreen active ingredients also absorb UV, with very little reflection and scattering in the UV portion of the spectrum [4], so it is not appropriate to call them "physical sunscreens." While the UV absorption action of Tinosorb M is not very different from other organic molecules, for TiO_2 and ZnO, the electrons in the crystals can freely move from the valence band to the conductance band when exposed to UV. This is because the energy band gap in TiO_2 or ZnO is lower than the energy conveyed by UV photons, allowing UV to excite the free electrons in these semiconductor-like materials.

Particulate inorganic sunscreen active ingredients also protect skin from harmful UV by absorbing, reflecting, and scattering; however, recent findings indicate that the primary means of protection is by absorption (roughly 95 %) and the remaining 5 % by scattering and reflecting. Incident light that is absorbed or backscattered by the particle sunscreens does not enter into the skin. Scattering of reflected photons increases the actual optical length of the UV photons as they pass through the absorbing sunscreen layer. The scattering by sunscreen particles depends on factors that include the volume concentration of the particles, the relative refractive index of the particle to the medium and/or coating, the particle size, and the scattering wavelength [11].

For the UV wavelength range, the absorption and scattering power of single TiO_2 or ZnO particles generally increases with the size of the particle, up to about 100 μm. We generally recognize, however, that absorption power increases monotonically when the particle size is smaller. This is because the number of particles has to increase with smaller and smaller particle size when evaluated for a fixed volume fraction (weight percentage). Therefore, the overall absorption power for the system becomes greater with smaller particle sizes. Based on both theoretical calculation and experimental measurement, the light scattering of particulate sunscreen ingredients (TiO_2, ZnO, and Tinosorb M) does not contribute significantly to the attenuation of UV (290–370 nm) when compared absorption. For long UVA and visible light wavelength range (370–760 nm), however, reflection contributes much more to the protective effects of TiO_2 and ZnO particles when applied on skin surface because of very limited absorption of these ingredients within the visible wavelength range. Since absorption and scattering of UV light depend on both the volume fraction of particles in the medium and also the uniformity of the particles, dispersion of particles in sunscreen formulation plays a critical role in the efficacy of UV attenuation. It is also critical to make sure the inorganic particles are photostable and do not lead to generation of free radicals. Effective surface treatment of inorganic particles ensures photostability of these inorganic sunscreens. Examples of surface treatments include alkoxy silane, dimethicone, methicone, polyhydroxystearic acid and aluminum stearate, silica, alumina, etc. Photostability also depends on the type of the inorganic crystal. For example, antase is known to be less stable than rutile grade TiO_2.

ZnO has gained popularity as a mild, safe, and effective sun filter in the past 10 years. It is the only other effective UVA1 filter besides avobenzone that is approved in the USA. TiO_2 has high UVB efficacy, but does not provide significant UVA protection. On the other hand, ZnO provides very uniform UVB and UVA protection across the whole spectrum, providing a flat spectral absorption curve [36]. Figure 10.2a shows a comparison between absorbance of TiO_2 and ZnO. It is desirable to maximize light attenuation while limiting the scattering in the visible region, as consumers do not like to see a white/blue haze on their skin. Formulators need to balance the particle size, dispersion, solvent, and volume fraction to achieve an aesthetically acceptable and effective inorganic sunscreen product.

10.4 Sun Filter Efficacy: Breadth and Height of UV Absorbance

A key performance metric for sun filters is absorbance intensity and breadth of coverage. Dilute solution UV spectroscopy is used to determine filter efficacy and is commonly reported as a specific extinction, E(1 %, 1 cm), value. E(1,1) corresponds to the absorbance at the peak wavelength (λ_{max}) for a 1 % solution in a cuvette with a 1 cm

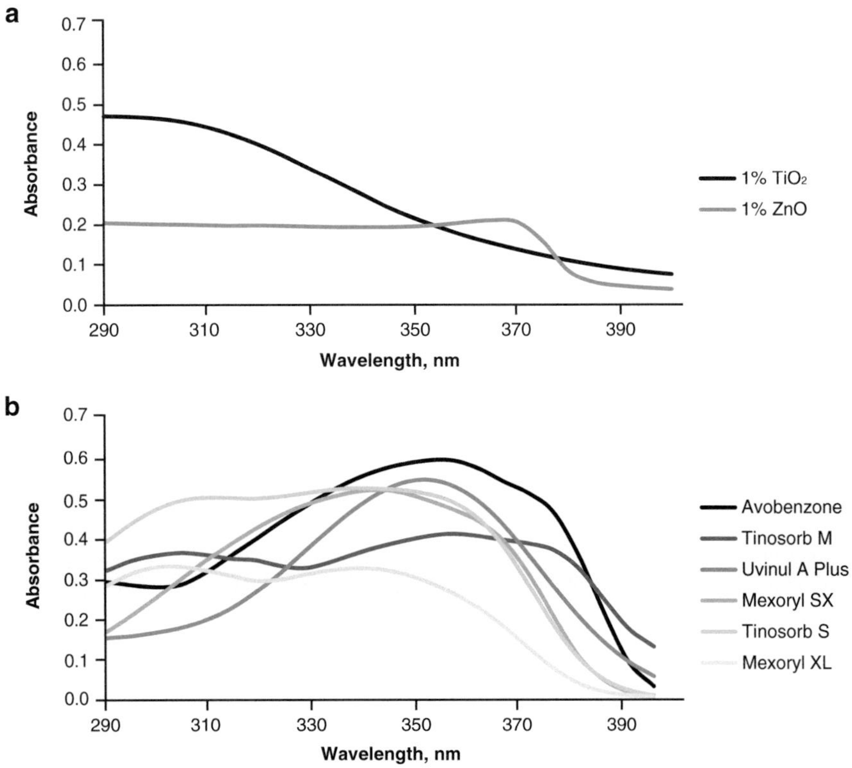

Fig. 10.2 The absorbance spectra for various sunscreen agents at 1 %; (**a**) TiO2 and ZnO, and (**b**) key global UVA-absorbing filters

path length [35]. Table 10.3 shows the wavelength of absorbance maximum and specific extinction value for common organic filters, along with the molecular structures and molecular weight values [35].

Avobenzone is the most efficient UVA-absorbing filter with an E(1,1) value of 1,110 (357 nm), followed by Uvinul A plus (E[1,1] is 925 [354 nm]), Mexoryl SX (E[1,1] is 750 [345 nm]), and Tinosorb S (E[1,1] is 750 and 820 [310 and 343 nm, respectively]). Figure 10.2b shows the absorbance spectral overlay for key UVA filters (each at 1 %).

Although UVA protection is getting quite a bit of attention in recent years, UVB protection is critical to appropriate protection from the sun, as the action spectra for erythema, basal cell carcinoma, and squamous cell carcinoma are all known to be driven by UVB [6, 9]. Uvinul T150 (ethylhexyl triazone) and Uvinul HEB (diethylhexyl butamido triazone) are the two most efficient UVB filters with E(1,1) values of 1550 (at 314 nm) and 1460 (at 311 nm), respectively. Ethylhexyl diaminobenzoate, phenylbenzimidazole sulfonic acid, and several cinnamate derivatives are also very strong UVB absorbers. Benzophenone derivatives are modest UVB absorbers, and salicylate derivatives are typically relatively weak UVB absorbers.

Table 10.3 List of sun filters, chemical structures, molecular weight, lambda max values, and specific extinction values E(1 %, 1 cm)

Filter name	Chemical structure	Molecular weight (g/mol)	Coverage	λ MAX 1	λ MAX 2	E1 (1 %, 1 cm)	E2 (1 %, 1 cm)
Benzophenone-3	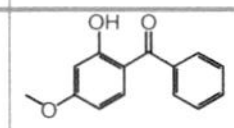	228	UVA/B	286	324	630	400
Benzophenone-4	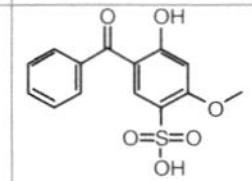	308	UVA/B	286	324	440	360
Benzophenone-5	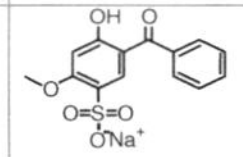	330	UVA/B	285	323	430	345
Benzophenone-8	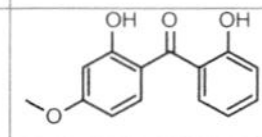	244	UVA/B	284	327	380	300
3-Benzylidene camphor	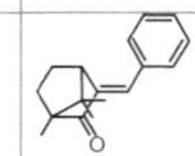	240	UVB	294		860	
Bis-ethylhexyloxyphenol methoxyphenyl triazine	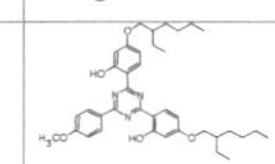	628	UVA/B	310	343	745	820
Butyl methoxydibenzoylmethane	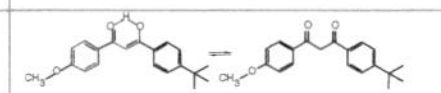	310	UVA	357		1,110	
Camphor benzalkonium methosulfate	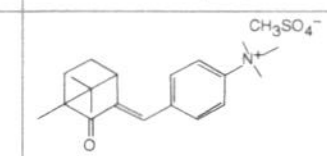	410	UVB	284		590	
Diethylamino hydroxybenzoyl hexyl benzoate	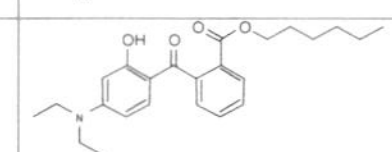	398	UVA	354		925	
Diethylhexyl butamido triazone	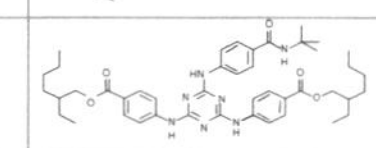	766	UVB	311		1,460	
Disodium phenyl dibenzimidazole tetrasulfonate	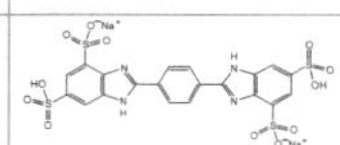	675	UVA	335		770	

(continued)

Table 10.3 (continued)

Filter name	Chemical structure	Molecular weight (g/mol)	Coverage	λ MAX 1	λ MAX 2	E1 (1 %, 1 cm)	E2 (1 %, 1 cm)
Drometrizole trisiloxane	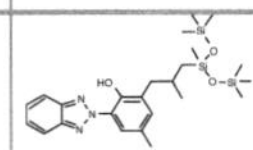	502	UVA/B	303	341	310	300
Ethoxyethyl methoxycinnamate	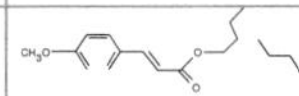	250	UVB				
Ethylhexyl dimethylamino benzoate	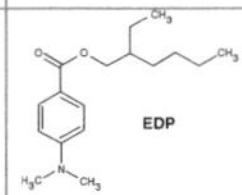	277	UVB	311		990	
Ethylhexyl methoxycinnamate	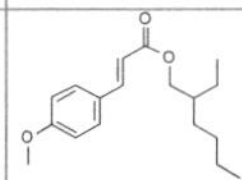	290	UVB	311		850	
Ethylhexyl salicylate	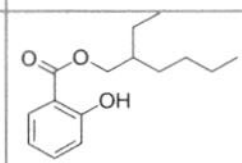	250	UVB	305		165	
Ethylhexyl triazone	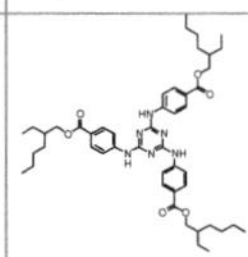	823	UVB	314		1,550	
Homosalate	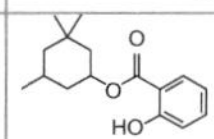	262	UVB	306		180	
Isoamyl p-methoxycinnamate	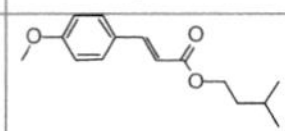	248	UVB	308		980	
Methyl anthranilate	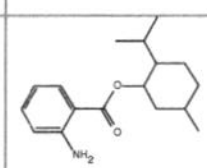	275	UVA	336		190	
4-Methylbenzylidene camphor	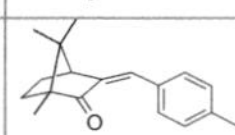	254	UVB	300		930	

Methylene bis-benzotriazolyl tetramethylbutylphenol	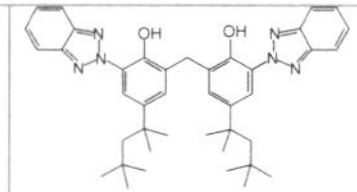	659	UVA/B	305	360	400	495
Octocrylene	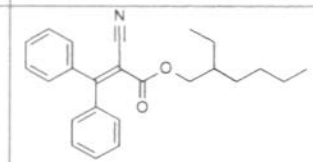	362	UVB	303		340	
Para-aminobenzoic acid	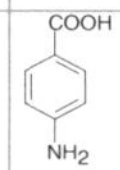	137	UVB	283		640	
PEG-25 para-aminobenzoic acid	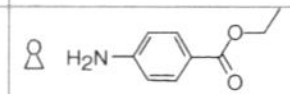	1,265	UVB	309		180	
Phenylbenzimidazole sulfonic acid	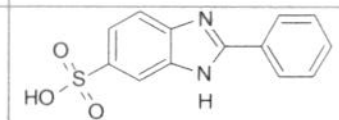	274	UVB	302		920	
Polyacrylamido methylbenzylidene camphor	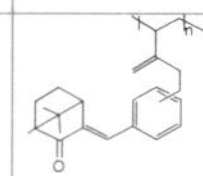	[323.44]n	UVB	297		610	
Polysilicone-15	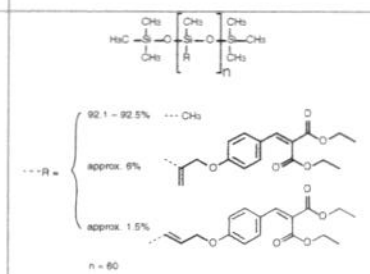	6,000	UVB	312		160–190	
Triethanolamine salicylate	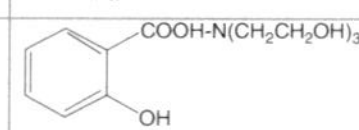	287	UVB	298		120	
Terephthalylidene dicamphor sulfonic acid	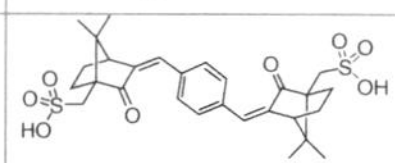	607	UVA	345		750	
Benzylidene camphor sulfonic acid	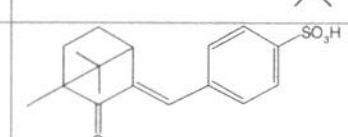	320		294		860	
Titanium dioxide	—	80	UVA/B	280–350			
Zinc oxide	—	81	UVA/B	280–390			

E specific extinction, *UVA* ultraviolet A, *UVB* ultraviolet B

In addition to absorbance intensity, it is also important to consider the breadth of protection. Avobenzone and Tinosorb M provide the widest long-range UVA1 protection, followed by Uvinul A plus, then Mexoryl SX, Tinosorb S, and Mexoryl XL. There are no approved sunscreens, however, that absorb significant amounts of light in the very longest part of the UVA spectrum and into the blue portion of the visible light spectrum. There is emerging research showing that light coming from these parts of the spectrum can contribute to skin pigmentation changes [3, 28].

Although extinction coefficients are widely used to provide quantitative comparison of sun filters, the relevancy of dilute solution spectroscopy measures to real-world sunscreen product application must be considered. As a sunscreen product dries to form a highly concentrated thin film, Beer's law does not apply, and so real-world sunscreen performance is most likely not dictated solely by the dilute solution absorbance values. The film structure and properties may be directly relevant to a sunscreen's final performance on skin as a thin film [32]. Thin-film transmission measurements on defined substrates are now used throughout the sunscreen industry to simulate real-world efficacy.

10.5 Combinations of Filters

There is no single sun filter available today that on its own can provide high-SPF and broad-spectrum protection without aesthetic drawbacks. With the current state of UV filter technology, sunscreen products today require the right combination of filters in the formulation to obtain both high efficacy in UV protection and optimal aesthetics to enhance compliance. Formulations containing oil-soluble filters may feel occlusive and or greasy [30]. Combinations of different filters may be used to improve the sensory profile, as well as provide broad-spectrum protection. In the USA, "broad spectrum" can be claimed if the in vitro determined critical wavelength value is ≥370 nm [15]. In Europe, products must achieve a 1:3 ratio of PFA (protection factor UVA):SPF [21]. Although many sunscreen products in the market claim broad spectrum, it is hard to differentiate between their UVA efficacies. Not all broad-spectrum sunscreens are created equal because they may have different degrees of UVA protection (amplitude of absorbance curve in UVA) with different filter combinations [5].

10.5.1 US-Approved Filter Combinations

A common combination of organic filters used in the US market to achieve high-SPF, broad-spectrum, and photostable protection is oxybenzone, octocrylene, homosalate, avobenzone, and 2-ethylhexyl salicylate (octisalate). This five-ingredient combination is found in many different product lines, and the proportions and concentrations are adjusted to provide the desired protection. Octocrylene, homosalate, and octisalate provide strong UVB protection, oxybenzone provides broad-spectrum UVB and UVA2 protection, and avobenzone provides the longer-wavelength UVA1 protection. In addition, both octocrylene and oxybenzone enhance the photostability of avobenzone by singlet and triplet quenching.

The inorganic filters TiO_2 and ZnO are often used together. ZnO is typically used to achieve breadth of protection, while TiO_2 brings higher SPF. The combination of avobenzone and ZnO is currently not permitted in the USA [14]. The agency did not approve the combination of ZnO with avobenzone in the latest monograph publications.

10.5.2 Ex-US Filter Combinations

In Europe and Latin America, many more filters are approved for combination use, such as Tinosorb S, Tinosorb M, Uvinul T150, Uvinul A Plus, Mexoryl SX, or Mexoryl XL. In Europe, it is common to omit oxybenzone. In Latin America, many formulations include a combination of traditional organic filters and a small amount of TiO_2. In Japan, very light and fluid textures are preferred, and mildness is very important; TiO_2, ZnO, OMC, and Tinosorb S are widely used ingredients.

10.5.3 SPF Boosting Through Formulation and Film Structure

Beyond the filter combinations selected for a sunscreen product formulation, formulation excipients, emulsion structure, and the sunscreen film structure are also important for determining the final sunscreen performance. The presence of film formers or emollients in the formulation [31, 34], the sunscreen rheological properties [2, 17], and the structures of the dried down sunscreen film [13, 38] have all been linked to sunscreen performance. Figure 10.3 illustrates how surface roughness plays a role in creating holes in a sunscreen film, and that the thickness of the sunscreen film above the skin peaks may be quite small [32]. It can be envisioned that the physical properties of the sunscreen film may act to increase the film thickness above the peaks and reduce settling into the valleys to create a more ideal film structure as in Fig. 10.3a [32].

10.6 Conclusion

A variety of organic sun filters are available for use with different properties, and it is important for formulators to understand their chemistry to maximize efficacy and create sunscreen products with an acceptable level of SPF and broad-spectrum protection. With the current state of sunscreen technology, it is necessary for formulators to select

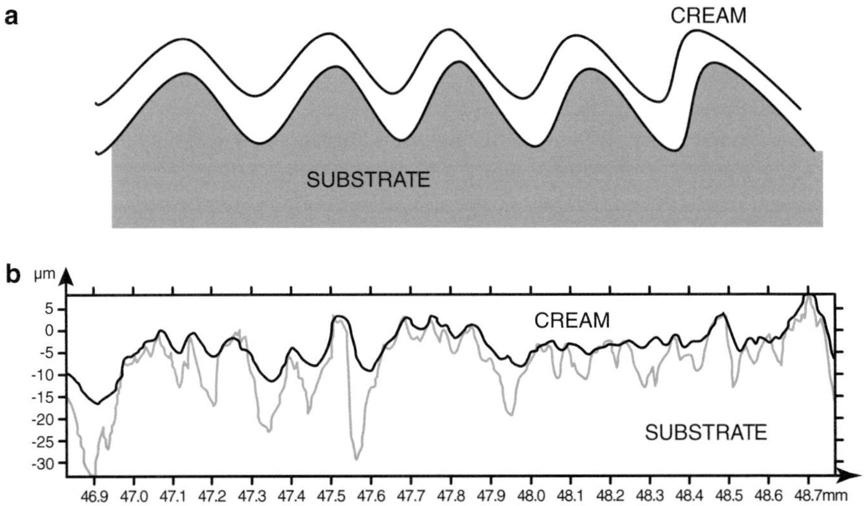

Fig. 10.3 Sunscreen distribution on a surface (**a**) ideal distribution (**b**) real distribution (Reproduced with permission from Osterwalder et al. [32])

a combination of sun filters to bring photostable, high-SPF, and broad-spectrum protection to consumers. There is a widespread misconception that inorganic sunscreens operate by a different mechanism than organic sun filters; the mechanism of action for both, however, involves UV absorbance. It is also critical for formulators to consider the aesthetic of filters and to design formulation vehicles to maximize the sunscreen product aesthetic, as sunscreen user compliance will continue to be the biggest challenge to protecting consumers from solar radiation.

Acknowledgment The authors would like to thank Alex Loeb, PhD, CMPP, of Evidence Scientific Solutions (Philadelphia, PA) for editorial support that was funded by JOHNSON & JOHNSON Consumer Companies, Inc. (Skillman, NJ).

References

1. Agrapidis-Paloympis L, Nash RA, Shaath NA (1987) The effect of solvents on the ultraviolet absorbance of sunscreens. J Soc Cosmet Chem 38:209–221
2. Anderson MW, Hewitt JP, Spruce SR (1997) Broad-spectrum physical sunscreens: titanium dioxide and zinc oxide. In: Lowe NJ, Shaath NA, Pathak MA (eds) Sunscreens: development, evaluation and regulatory aspects, vol 15, Cosmetic Science and Technology, vol 18. Marcel Dekker, Inc., New York, pp 353–398
3. Castanedo-Cazares JP, Hernandez-Blanco D, Carlos-Ortega B, Fuentes-Ahumada C, Torres-Álvarez B (2014) Near-visible light and UV photoprotection in the treatment of melasma: a double-blind randomized trial. Photodermatol Photoimmunol Photomed 30(1):35–42
4. Cole C, Shyr T, Ou-Yang H (2016) Metal oxide sunscreens protect skin by absorption not by reflection or scattering. Photodermatol Photoimmunol Photomed 32(1): 5–10

5. Cole CA (2014) Critical concepts about sunscreens. Pract Derm. (Suppl 2):1–4. http://practicaldermatology.com/pdfs/0414_insert2.pdf
6. Cole CA, Forbes PD, Davies RE (1986) An action spectrum for UV photocarcinogenesis. Photochem Photobiol 43(3):275–284
7. Cole CA, Vollhardt J, Mendrok C (2009) Formulation and stability of sunscreen products. In: Lim HW, Draelos ZD (eds) Clinical guide to sunscreens and photoprotection. Informa Healthcare, New York, pp 39–51
8. Cross SE, Innes B, Roberts MS, Tsuzuki T, Robertson TA, McCormick P (2007) Human skin penetration of sunscreen nanoparticles: in-vitro assessment of a novel micronized zinc oxide formulation. Skin Pharmacol Physiol 20(3):148–154
9. de Gruijl FR, van der Leun JC (1991) Development of skin tumors in hairless mice after discontinuation of ultraviolet irradiation. Cancer Res 51(3):979–984
10. DSM nutritional products AG (2013) PARSOL® SLX factsheet. http://www.respharma.com/Brochure/DSM/PARSOL%20SLX_Factsheet.pdf. Accessed 30 Oct, 2014
11. Egerton TA, Tooley IR (2012) UV absorption and scattering properties of inorganic-based sunscreens. Int J Cosmet Sci 34(2):117–122
12. European Union (2009) Regulation (EC) No 1223/2009 of the European Parliament and of the Council of 30 Nov 2009 on cosmetic products. Off J Eur Union L 342:59–209
13. Ferrero L, Pissavini M, Marguerie S, Zastrow L (2003) Efficiency of a continuous height distribution model of sunscreen film geometry to predict a realistic sun protection factor. J Cosmet Sci 54(5):463–481
14. Food and Drug Administration, Department of Health and Human Services (1999) Sunscreen drug products for over-the-counter human use; final monograph. Fed Regist 64(98): 27666–27693
15. Food and Drug Administration, HHS (2012) Over-the-counter sunscreen drug products; required labeling based on effectiveness testing. Fed Regist 76:95–107
16. Gamer AO, Leibold E, van Ravenzwaay B (2006) The in vitro absorption of microfine zinc oxide and titanium dioxide through porcine skin. Toxicol In Vitro 20(3):301–307
17. Gaspar LR, Maia Campos PM (2003) Rheological behavior and the SPF of sunscreens. Int J Pharm 250(1):35–44
18. Health Canada (2012) Draft: guidance document – Sunscreen monograph. http://www.hc-sc.gc.ca/dhp-mps/alt_formats/pdf/consultation/natur/sunscreen-ecransolaire-eng.pdf. Accessed 31 Oct 2014
19. Herzog B, Quass K, Schmidt E, Müller S, Luther H (2004) Physical properties of organic particulate UV absorbers used in sunscreens II. UV-attenuating efficiency as function of particle size. J Colloid Interface Sci 276(2):354–363
20. Household and Personal Products Industry (2010) DSM presents latest data on parsol SLX. http://www.happi.com/contents/view_breaking-news/2010-11-01/dsm-presents-latest-data-on-parsol-slx/. Accessed 30 Oct 2014
21. International Organization for Standardization (2012) ISO 24443:2012 determination of sunscreen UVA photoprotection in vitro. http://www.iso.org/iso/catalogue_detail?csnumber=46522. Accessed 11 Nov 2014
22. Janousek A (1983) The current status of sunscreens in the EEC. Cosmet Toiletries 98(3):79–80
23. Jansen R, Osterwalder U, Wang SQ, Burnett M, Lim HW (2013) Photoprotection: part II. Sunscreen: development, efficacy, and controversies. J Am Acad Dermatol 69(6):867.e861–814
24. Jansen R, Wang SQ, Burnett M, Osterwalder U, Lim HW (2013) Photoprotection: part I. Photoprotection by naturally occurring, physical, and systemic agents. J Am Acad Dermatol 69(6):853.e851–812
25. Kockler J, Oelgemöller M, Robertson S, Glass BD (2012) Photostability of sunscreens. J Photochem Photobiol C Photochem Rev 13(1):91–110
26. Kollias N (1999) The absorption properties of "physical" sunscreens. Arch Dermatol 135(2): 209–210

27. Krutmann J, Morita A, Chung JH (2012) Sun exposure: what molecular photodermatology tells us about its good and bad sides. J Invest Dermatol 132(3 Pt 2):976–984
28. Mahmoud BH, Ruvolo E, Hexsel CL, Liu Y, Owen MR, Kollias N, Lim HW, Hamzavi IH (2010) Impact of long-wavelength UVA and visible light on melanocompetent skin. J Invest Dermatol 130(8):2092–2097
29. Maillan P, Gripp A, Sit F, Jermann R, Westenfelder H (2005) Protecting against UV: induced degradation and enhancing shine. Cosmet Toiletries 120(3):65–71
30. Mancebo SE, Hu JY, Wang SQ (2014) Sunscreens: a review of health benefits, regulations, and controversies. Dermatol Clin 32(3):427–438
31. O'Lenick TO, Lott D (2011) The effects of solvents on sunscreens: a new ester to improve efficiency. Cosmet Toiletries 126(6):431–436
32. Osterwalder U, Sohn M, Herzog B (2014) Global state of sunscreens. Photodermatol Photoimmunol Photomed 30(2–3):62–80
33. Ou-Yang H, Stanfield JW, Cole C, Appa Y (2010) An evaluation of ultraviolet A protection and photo-stability of sunscreens marketed in Australia and New Zealand. Photodermatol Photoimmunol Photomed 26(6):336–337
34. Prettypaul D, Fares H (2012) Microscopic evaluation of polymeric film properties of anhydrous sunscreen compositions and their relation to absorption and water resistance. J Cosmet Sci 63(3):213–221
35. Saath NA (2007) The encyclopedia of ultraviolet filters. Allured Publishing Corp, Carol Stream
36. Smijs TG, Pavel S (2011) Titanium dioxide and zinc oxide nanoparticles in sunscreens: focus on their safety and effectiveness. Nanotechnol Sci Appl 4:95–112
37. Stiefel C, Schwack W (2015) Photoprotection in changing times – UV filter efficacy and safety, sensitization processes and regulatory aspects. Int J Cosmet Sci 37(1):2–30. http://onlinelibrary.wiley.com/doi/10.1111/ics.12165/abstract
38. Teichmann A, Pissavini M, Ferrero L, Dehais A, Zastrow L, Richter H, Lademann J (2006) Investigation of the homogeneity of the distribution of sunscreen formulations on the human skin: characterization and comparison of two different methods. J Biomed Opt 11(6):064005
39. U.S. Department of Health and Human Services, Food and Drug Administration, Center for Drug Evaluation and Research (2011) Guidance for industry – enforcement policy – OTC sunscreen drug products marketed without an approved application (Draft guidance). http://www.fda.gov/downloads/drugs/guidancecomplianceregulatoryinformation/guidances/ucm259001.pdf. Accessed 30 Oct 2012
40. Woodruff J (2001) Factors affecting the formulation of sunscreen products. http://www.creative-developments.co.uk/papers/Factors%20affecting%20sun%20care%20formulations.html. Accessed 30 Oct 2014

Chapter 11
Global UV Filters: Current Technologies and Future Innovations

Uli Osterwalder and Lars Hareng

Key Points

- Tremendous progress has been made in sunscreen technology over the last two decades.
- Unfortunately, in the USA, UV filter technology is lagging 15 years behind compared to the rest of the world.
- In Europe and the rest of the world, development goes on, but it is slower than 20 years ago.
- The major weakness of sunscreen and photoprotection remains the lack of compliance by the user.
- Innovation in photoprotection education, including behavior modification and sunscreen use, is required.

11.1 Introduction

Sunscreens are used worldwide, especially by people with fairer skin phototypes in geographic areas with high sun exposure but also by people with darker skin to keep a uniform complexion, mainly of the face. This chapter focuses on global sunscreens, i.e., sunscreens that contain UV filters that are available and in use worldwide. Sunscreen is part of sun protection strategies consisting of seeking

U. Osterwalder (✉)
Personal Care, BASF PCN GmbH, Monheim, Germany
e-mail: uli.osterwalder@basf.com

L. Hareng
Regulatory Toxicology, BASF SE, Ludwigshafen, Germany

S.Q. Wang, H.W. Lim (eds.), *Principles and Practice of Photoprotection*,
DOI 10.1007/978-3-319-29382-0_11

shade, covering up with clothing and hats, and wearing sunglasses. Use of sunscreens has now been demonstrated to slow down the photoaging process and to decrease the development of squamous cell carcinoma, basal cell carcinoma, and melanoma [1–3].

A recent study confirmed the preventative role of sunscreen for malignant melanoma in mice, but the control sites that were covered by cloth had less melanoma, indicating that protection by sunscreen alone could not completely prevent skin cancer [4]. This chapter reviews what still can be done to improve sunscreens to become a yet more effective means of photoprotection.

11.2 Current Technology and Future Innovations

The basic requirements for UV filters in sunscreens are (1) efficacy, (2) safety, (3) registration, and (4) freedom to operate with respect to the status of intellectual property [5]. Efficient UV absorber molecules are the basis of all sunscreens. Efficacy indicates good UV absorbance in the spectral range between 290 and 400 nm. Good UV filters must also have the property of being able to be incorporated in sufficient amounts into cosmetic formulations. They may be dissolved in the oil phase or the water phase of sunscreen formulations, and thus the respective solubility must be high enough. Alternately, filters can be used as dispersions of fine particles of the absorbing substances.

11.2.1 Organic UV Filters

At present, all organic UV absorbers used in sunscreens possess aromatic moieties. The substituents at the aromatic ring are of great importance for the UV spectroscopic properties. An increase in the number of resonance structures stabilizes the excited state, thus leading to stronger absorption at longer wavelengths [6, 7].

Figure 11.1 shows the efficacy of some of the organic UV filters. A quick assessment of the performance of a UV filter can be simply gained by the use of a calculation tool, generally known as the "sunscreen simulator" which is freely accessible on the internet [8–13]. The sunscreen simulator results are presented in Fig. 11.1 as integrated transmission through the irregular sunscreen film on the skin. The UVB filters PABA (8 %) and EHMC (7.5 %) cover efficiently UVB and UVA2 but transmit practically 100 % of the radiation in the UVA1 region. The first UVA1 filter BMBM (avobenzone at 3 %) transmits about 35 % in the UVB but less than 20 % in the UVA1 region. The modern broad-spectrum UV filters BEMT (5 %) and MBBT (5 %) cover efficiently both UVA1 and UVB/UVA2. In the final sunscreen product, it is always the combination of several UV filters that determines its range and efficacy of protection. This can all be calculated on the sunscreen simulator [8, 13].

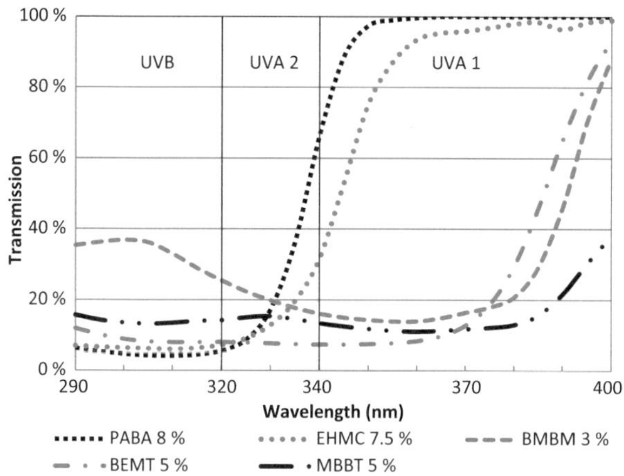

Fig. 11.1 Transmission of organic filters (Data obtained from the BASF sunscreen simulator, with the % applied as single UV filter in a sunscreen). *BEMT* bis-ethylhexyloxyphenol methoxyphenyl triazine, *BMBM* butyl methoxydibenzoylmethane, *EHMC* ethylhexyl methoxycinnamate, *MBBT* methylene bis-benzotriazolyl tetramethylbutylphenol (nano), *PABA* ethylhexyl dimethyl para-aminobenzoic acid

11.2.2 Particulate Organic UV Filters

Sunscreens, especially those with a high sun protection factor (SPF), contain a considerable amount of UV filters. Therefore, solubility of the active substance can be a significant problem [5]. For this reason, particulate organic UV filters were developed that allow high-SPF products to have relatively low concentrations of UV filters. Examples of these UV filters include bisoctrizole and tris-biphenyl triazine [14, 15]; the former is under consideration for approval through the time and extent application (TEA) process of the US Food and Drug Administration (FDA). These filters have extremely low solubility in oil and in water but can thus be micronized in an aqueous phase [16–18]. Particulate bisoctrizole shows a broad absorption up to 380 nm (Fig. 11.2). The UV absorbance spectrum of particulate bisoctrizole has a characteristic shape [19]. The spectrum of the particles extends toward longer UVA1 wavelengths with an additional shoulder around 320 and 380 nm caused by intermolecular interactions of the π-electrons inside the particles. Similar to small inorganic particle UV filters, the contribution to protection by scattering or reflectance is 5 % or less [20].

11.2.3 Inorganic UV Filters

Any inorganic material that absorbs in the UV range could potentially be used in sunscreens. Figure 11.3 shows transmission curves in the UV and also visible range of a few inorganic materials: titanium dioxide (TiO_2), zinc oxide (ZnO), cerium dioxide (CeO_2), CeO_2-doped ZnO, and various iron oxides [21–23]. "Doping" refers to the addition of

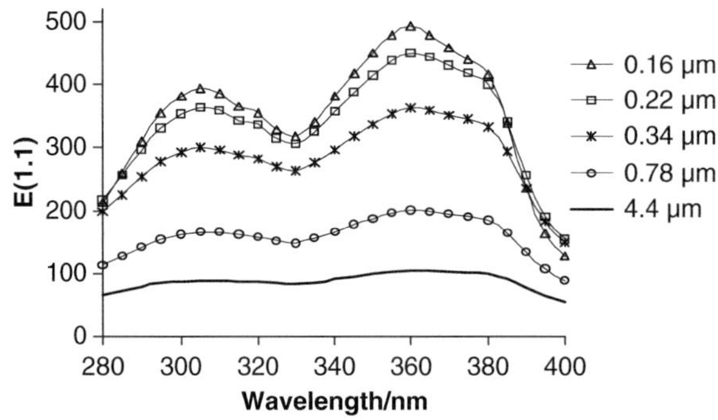

Fig. 11.2 Influence of particle size on efficacy of particulate UV filters (bisoctrizole, MBBT)

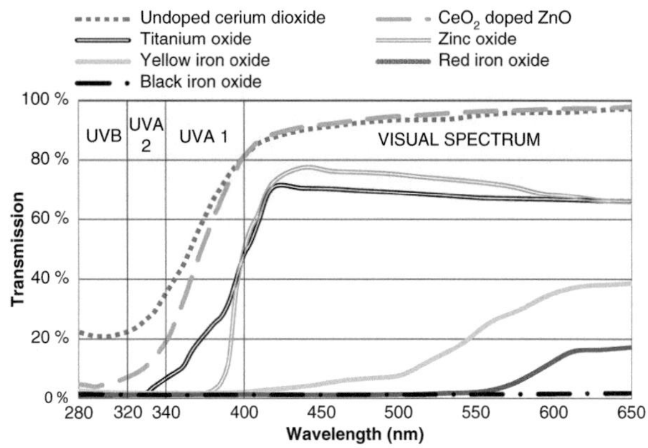

Fig. 11.3 Transmission of various inorganic UV filters in UV and VIS range (280–650 nm)

small amounts of foreign atoms altering the lattice properties. TiO_2, ZnO, and CeO_2 show good absorption in the UV range; the relatively low absorption in the visible range makes these materials colorless, hence qualifying them to be used in sunscreens. Cerium oxide is not listed in any country's positive list of sunscreen actives and is also slightly yellowish colored. The iron oxides are colored materials absorbing in the visible range in addition to the UV spectrum, which disqualifies them for use in sunscreens; however, they are used in other forms, such as BB creams (Blemish Balm all-in-one facial cosmetic product) or makeup and can contribute to photoprotection [24].

11.2.4 Future Innovations

Innovation differs from improvement in that innovation refers to the notion of doing something different rather than doing the same thing better. In the following paragraphs, three different approaches are outlined assessing future innovations in suncare.

Table 11.1 100 years of sunscreen – most important milestones

	Society/marketing	Technology	Standards/regulatory
1925	Nobel Prize for Light Therapy [25], Vit D [26]		
	Coco Channel makes tanned skin popular [27]	First Sunscreen [28]	
1950	Summer holidays in the sun become fashionable and affordable	UVB, PABA [30]	SPF Definition [33]
1975		More UVB (EHMC)	SPF FDA [29]
		First UVA filter (BMBM) [30, 32]	First UVA standards Boots, AUS, PPD [34]
2000	Suntan still in but protection becomes important "bronze and protect"	Photostability [32] EHT, TDSA, DTS	European recommendation on UVA, [35]
		Broad-spectrum UV filters MBBT, BEMT, DHHB [5, 31]	FDA final rule (labeling) [36]
2025	More awareness Sunbed bans Better compliance	Toward spectral homeostasis? Ideal sunscreen? New UV filters	Toward global harmonization of SPF and UVA methods/ standards Animal test ban

UVA ultraviolet A-rays, *UVB* ultraviolet B-rays, *AUS* Australian standards, *FDA* Food and Drug Administration, *PPD* persistent pigment darkening
Abbreviation of the INCI Name (International Nomenclature of Cosmetic Ingredients): *BEMT* bis-ethylhexyloxyphenol methoxyphenyl triazine, *BMBM* butyl methoxydibenzoylmethane, *DHHB* diethylamino hydroxybenzoyl hexyl benzoate, *DTS* drometrizole trisiloxane, *EHMC* ethylhexyl methoxycinnamate, *EHT* ethylhexyl triazone, *MBBT* methylene bis-benzotriazolyl tetramethylbutyl-phenol (nano), *PABA* ethylhexyl dimethyl PABA, *TDSA* terephthalylidene dicamphor sulfonic acid

11.2.5 1st Approach: The Best Predictor of Future Behavior Is Past Behavior

Innovations in sunscreens and UV filters over the last century were driven by changes in society, most importantly that tanned skin became fashionable (Table 11.1).

The development of UV filters started with the UVB filters salicylates and PABA [30]. The first UVA filter, avobenzone (BMBM) [30], was patented in 1973 and approved in Europe in 1978. Ten years later, it was available in the USA through the New Drug Application (NDA) route; another 10 years later, it was considered generally recognized as safe and effective (GRAS/E) and added to the FDA sunscreen monograph. The fact that avobenzone is not photostable triggered the search for alternatives. These were developed in the 1990s and brought into the market around 2000 [30]. They are all mentioned in Table 11.1 as UVA and broad-spectrum UV filters. In parallel to the development of new UV filters, there were successful attempts to improve the photostability of avobenzone. Indeed it is now common to stabilize avobenzone in sunscreen with other ingredients; the most effective ones are other UV filters such as octocrylene or bemotrizinol [32].

Extrapolation of technological progress of UV filters into the next 10–15 years shows that we can expect "more of the same," e.g., better coverage of the UV range where we still have a gap near the visible at the moment. This is illustrated by the following four examples.

Researchers in Japan found a novel UVB absorber to enhance the efficacy of UVA protection [37]. It is a new liquid UVB filter that could be used together with avobenzone in sunscreens as an alternative to octocrylene. No prediction can be made at this time when this UV filter would become available commercially.

A research group in Korea offers a solution to overcome perceived safety concerns about conventional sunscreens [38]. They synthesized silicon-based high-molecular-weight UV-absorbing polymers that are soluble in different solvents. Again, there is no concrete indication when this technology could become commercially available.

For the next two UV filters, a safety assessment by the European authorities has already been requested. The European Scientific Committee on Consumer Safety (SCCS) published an opinion on 2-(4-(2-(4-diethylamino-2-hydroxy-benzoyl)-benzoyl)-piperazine-1-carbonyl)-phenyl)-(4-diethylamino-2-hydroxyphenyl)-methanone (HAA299) in 2014 [39]. This new UV filter was developed by BASF SE (Germany), to cover the remaining gap in long UVA1 and in the visible light range up to ca. 450 nm. The final safety assessment in Europe is pending.

In early 2015 the European authorities published a request for a safety assessment for another particulate organic UV filter, phenylene bis-diphenyltriazine (INCI name), similar to the broad-spectrum UV filter bisoctrizole [40], i.e., covering the 290–400 nm range. However, it is difficult to predict when this filter will become commercially available.

11.2.6 Learnings from 1st Approach: Learning from the Past

In a foreseeable future, UV filter technology will bring UV coverage closer to ideal, i.e., covering the entire spectrum of UVB and UVA. But the use of sunscreen and the practice of photoprotection are still far from ideal [41]; this topic is covered in Chap. 11.3.

11.2.7 2nd Approach: General Morphological Analysis After Zwicky

Fritz Zwicky, a Swiss astrophysicist and aerospace scientist based at the California Institute of Technology (Caltech), called the morphological approach "totality research" which in an "unbiased way attempts to derive all the solutions of any

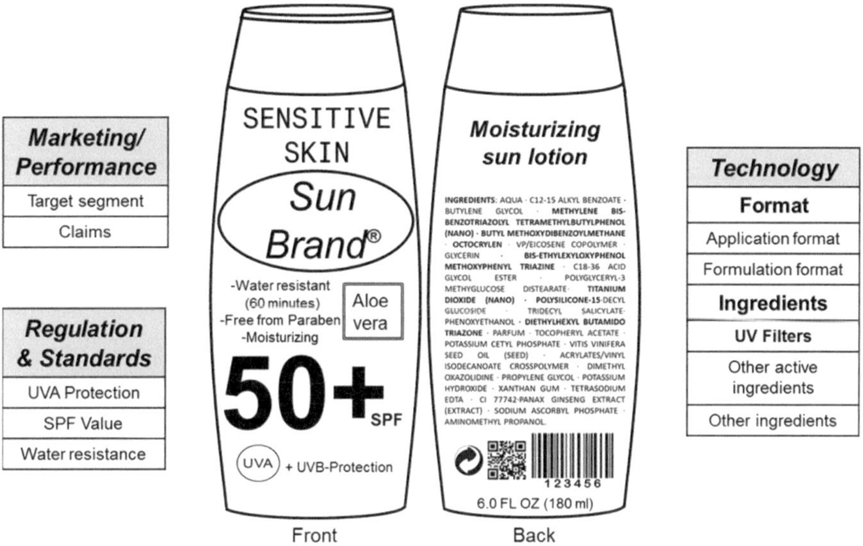

Fig. 11.4 Generic (hypothetical) sunscreen with three categories of parameters

given problem" [42]. Zwicky applied this method to such diverse fields as the classification of astrophysical objects, the development of jet and rocket propulsion systems, and the legal aspects of space travel and colonization. He founded the Society for Morphological Research and advanced the "morphological approach" for some 30 years, between the 1940s and his death in 1974.

"This approach may also help us discover new relationships or configurations, which are not so evident or which we might have overlooked by other – less systematic – methods. Importantly, it encourages the identification and investigation of boundary conditions, i.e., the limits and extremes of different contexts and factors."

The three steps of a systematic general morphological analysis (GMA) are, first, setting up the whole morphological box (x parameters with n values each); second, cross-consistency assessment in order to excluding impossible combinations and arriving at a manageable number of internally consistent configurations; and third, choosing single or multiple drivers, i.e., fixing one or more values of certain parameters in order to arrive at a "handful" of combinations.

The generic sunscreen in Fig. 11.4 shows the possible sunscreen variations. The core are always the UV filters, but not every type of UV filter is suitable for every kind of sunscreen, e.g., the particulate UV filters, inorganic or organic filters, are not suited for clear (transparent) formulations because a dispersion is always opaque, or certain UVA requirements can only be fulfilled with sufficient UVA or broad-spectrum UV filters.

The influencing parameters determining a sunscreen can be grouped into three categories: technology, marketing/society, and regulation/standards (Fig. 11.4).

Table 11.2 Morphological box with 3 parameters and 3 values (27 combinations)

		Selected parameters		
		UV filter	**Target segment**	**Product regulation**
Values	**1**	Organic	Toddler	Cosmetics
	2	Inorganic	Family	medicinal product
	3	Organic and inorganic	Sport	Natural product

Use of driver ("natural sunscreen") to narrow down the sunscreen product, e.g., from 27 (3 × 3 × 3) to 3 (1 × 3 × 1)

Since each parameter can assume many values, theoretically large numbers of combinations, representing new sunscreens, can be envisaged. To illustrate the morphological analysis, Table 11.2 shows an example of just one parameter of each category with three values. This gives already a theoretical total of 3 × 3 × 3 = 27 variations of sunscreens. This simplified example illustrates how these countless combinations can be reduced. If one was to choose only "natural sunscreen," e.g., as defined by European COSMOS (cosmetic organic standard) trade standards [43], then only inorganic UV filters (TiO_2 and ZnO) could be used and thus only 3 out of the 27 product variations are left to choose from. The fixed value of a parameter, in this case "natural sunscreen," is called a "driver" in the GMA nomenclature. Table 11.3 lists systematically parameters and values of sunscreens. Such a list is of course never exhaustive; there is always room for new ideas, but the systematic approach is also a checklist that helps in considering all aspects of the sunscreen product.

11.2.8 Learnings from 2nd Approach: General Morphological Analysis

Innovation has to be new but must also have an impact on the market place. From this morphological approach, it becomes apparent that the three categories, technology, marketing, and regulatory, all play an important role. Without UV filter technology, no progress in more efficient and broader UV coverage as well as yet higher safety could be achieved, but if the advantage is not perceived in public, the best technology cannot make an impact on the market [41].

Table 11.3 Lists systematically parameters and values of sunscreens

Technology (5 parameters)	Marketing/society (4 parameters)	Regulation/standards (3 parameters)
1. UV filter	6. Target segment	10. Product regulation
None	None	None
Organic	Baby, toddler, kids	Cosmetics
Inorganic	Family, men	Quasi drug
Organic and inorganic	Sport, winter, beach	Therapeutic good
2. Other ingredients	Tanned skin	Natural product
None	Sensitive skin	Medical device
Emulsifier	Dry skin	Medicinal product (drug)
Emollient	7. Performance claims	11. SPF (sunburn protection)
Polymer	None	None
3. Other actives	Water resistant	6, 10, 15
None	IRA, RSF	20, 30
Vitamin E	Prevents skin cancer	50, 50+
Bisabolol	Antiaging	99, 100, 100+
Retinol A	Bronze and protect	12. UVA protection
4. Formulation format	Visible spectrum	None
Emulsion O/W	Long UVA I	EU ratio 1:3), 1:2, 1:1)
Emulsion W/O	8. Free from claims	FDA (370 nm)
Gel, oil, alcohol	None	BOOTS (3, 4, 5 star)
Water	Paraben, preservative	JCIA PA+, to-PA++++
5. Application format	Fragrance, alcohol	
Lotion, cream	Mineral oil, silicone	
Spray (pump)	Nano, GMO	
Aerosol spray	Octocrylene	
Stick, mousse	No human testing	
Powder, ointment	Noncomedogenic	
	9. Special claims	
	None	
	Wet skin application	
	Refresh, cool	
	Natural	
	No skin penetration	

Such a list is of course never exhaustive; there is always room for new ideas, but the systematic approach is also a checklist that helps considering all aspects of the sunscreen product

11.2.9 3rd Approach: Delphi Survey Among Sunscreen and UV Filter Experts

A third approach to learn more about future innovations in suncare is asking the opinion of experts. The Delphi method has been developed by the RAND Corporation [44]. Delphi is based on the principle that forecasts (or decisions) from a structured group of individuals are more accurate than those from unstructured groups [45, 46], based on the assumption that a group of experts can more accurately predict the future.

The following question was asked to about 40 experts from all over the world where sunscreens play an important role in sun protection: *What Innovations in sunscreens do you see happening in the next: (a) 1–2, (b) 3–5, and (c) 10–15 years?*

11.2.10 Learnings from 3rd Approach: Delphi Survey Among Sunscreen and UV Filter Experts

Regarding technology innovations, the experts confirm the trend of better UVA protection toward spectral homeostasis. Furthermore, better sunscreen formulations are expected based on new UVB and broad-spectrum UV filters (liquid UV filters or polymers). Some also predict the trend away from nanoparticles to continue.

Regarding marketing and performance innovations, the extension of UV protection claims beyond just SPF, but into protection in visible light and infrared range is predicted. Antioxidant claims are also anticipated. Furthermore a trend toward natural sunscreens and more public education are predicted.

Regarding regulatory/standards innovation, the pending issues at the US FDA (TEA UV filters, spray, SPF cap at 50+, etc.) are predicted to be resolved in the next few years. A worldwide ban of animal testing in cosmetics is anticipated as well as a ban of SPF in vivo testing on humans.

This 3rd approach is especially valuable in the context of the two previous ones. It confirms the extrapolation of the past (1st approach), but it also brings up some new ideas that reach outside the morphological box (2nd approach), e.g., a ban of human testing.

11.3 Efficacy (Sunscreen Performance)

Sunscreen performance depends mainly on its UV filter composition. The most frequently used UV filters are summarized in Table 11.4. It contains globally registered UV filters plus the TEA filters awaiting approval in the USA (see regulatory Chap. 11.5 for TEA).

The focus in sunscreen development has long been on increasing the sun protection factor (SPF) [47]. However, there is now a consensus to cap at SPF 50+ among authorities of many countries, except for Brazil which allows SPF 99, and the US FDA has yet to make a final decision. At the same time sunscreens improved significantly in UVA protection over the last two decades [48, 49]. This progress can be demonstrated in a comparison between Europe and the USA. In the USA often the question comes up on how much better can a sunscreen become if it was able to incorporate the more recently developed UV filters. After all, currently available sunscreens in the US achieve already the world's highest SPF and fulfill the US UVA protection criterion of the critical wavelength CW >370 nm [50]. One way to answer this question is looking at the transmission curve of different sunscreens. The transmission spectrum tells us how much of the damaging UV radiation is passing through onto the skin at every

Table 11.4 UV filters, globally approved and pending in the USA (TEA)

UV range (nm)		USAN	Trademark	INCI Abbr.[a]	Type/ stateb	Max. concentration limit (%)	
						USA (year of TEA filing)	EU
290–340	Global	Oxybenzone	Uvinul® M40	BP3	o/p	6	10
		Sulisobenzone	Uvinul® MS40	BP4	o/p	10	5
		Octinoxate	Uvinul® MC 80	EHMC	o/l	7.5	10
		Octisalate	Neo Heliopan® OS	EHS	o/l	5	5
		Homosalate	Eusolex® HMS	HMS	o/l	15	10
		Octocrylene	Uvinul® N 539 T	OCR	o/l	10	10
		Ensulizole	Eusolex® 232	PBSA	o/p	4	8
		Titanium dioxide	Eusolex® T2000	TiO2	i/p, d	25	25
	TEA (USA)	Iscotrizinol	(Uvasorb HEB)	DBT	o/p	10 (2005)	10
		Octyltriazone	Uvinul® T150	EHT	o/p	5 (2005)	5
		Amiloxate	Neo Heliopan® E1000	IMC	o/l	10 (2003)	10
		Enzacamene	Eusolex 6300	MBC	o/p	4 (2002)	4
290–400	Global	Avobenzone	Parsol® 1789	BMBM	o/p	3	5
		Zinc oxide[c]	Z-Cote® HP1	ZnO	i/p, d	25	25
	TEA (USA)	Bemotrizinol	Tinosorb® S	BEMT	o/p	10 (2005)	10
		Bisoctrizole	Tinosorb® M (active)	MBBT	o/d	10 (2005)	10
		Ecamsule	Mexoryl® SX	TDSA	o/p	3^d (2009)	10
		Drometrizole	Mexoryl® XL	DTS	o/p	10 (2007)	15

[a]Abbreviation of the INCI (International Nomenclature of Cosmetic Ingredients) name: *BEMT* bis-ethylhexyloxyphenol methoxyphenyl triazine, *BMBM* butyl methoxydibenzoylmethane, *BP3* benzophenone-3, *BP4* benzophenone-4, *DHHB* diethylamino hydroxybenzoyl hexyl benzoate, *DPDT* disodium phenyl dibenzimidazole tetrasulfonate, *DTS* drometrizole trisiloxane, *EHMC* ethylhexyl methoxycinnamate, *EHS* ethylhexyl salicylate, *EHT* ethylhexyl triazone, *HMS* homomenthyl salicylate, *IMC* isoamyl p-methoxycinnamate, *MBBT* methylene bis-benzotriazolyl tetramethylbutylphenol (nano), *OCR* octocrylene, *TDSA* terephthalylidene dicamphor sulfonic acid, TiO_2 titanium dioxide (nano), *ZnO* zinc oxide (nano)

[b]*o* organic. *i* inorganic. *p* powder. *d* dispersion. *l* liquid

[c]Europe, annex VI listing as (nano) expected 2015

[d]Approved in certain formulations up to 3 % via New Drug Application (NDA) Route

Table 11.5 Comparison of available US State of the Art Sunscreen with sunscreens modified with TEA ingredients, and ideal sunscreen (cloth)

	Best US Sunscreen[a]	**Modified US sunscreen with TEA ingredients**[a]	**Ideal sunscreen: cloth** [4]
SPF$_{calculated}$	37 (labeled up to 100)	35 (labeled up to 50+)	>>100
UVA-protect.: CW (nm) UVA/UVB UVA-PF/SPF	372 0.67 0.29 (<0.33; fail)	381 0.81 0.47 (>0.33; pass)	389 1 1
Composition: UVB/UVA2 UVA1, Broad-Spectrum	6 % BP3, 5 % EHS, 15 % HMS, 10 % OCR 3 % BMBM	5 % EHS, 5 % HMS, 1 % EHT – 3 % BEMT, 5 % MBBT	Cloth (black)
Total UV filters	39 %	19 %	n.a.
NTUV dose at 1 MED (Calculated)	3.2 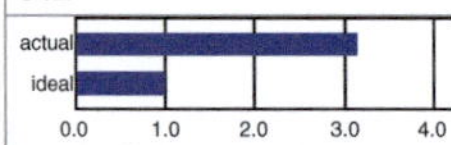	1.6 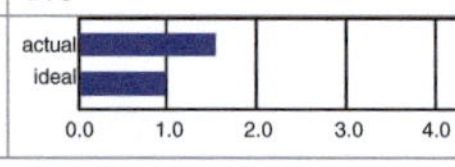	1.0 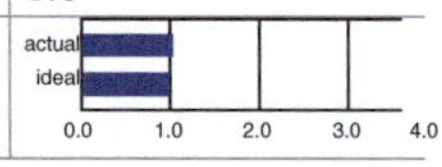

[a]Abbreviation of the INCI Name (International Nomenclature of Cosmetic Ingredients): *BEMT* bis-ethylhexyloxyphenol methoxyphenyl triazine, *BMBM* butyl methoxydibenzoylmethane, *BP3* benzophenone-3, *EHS* ethylhexyl salicylate, *EHT* ethylhexyl triazone, *HMS* homomenthyl salicylate, *MBBT* methylene bis-benzotriazolyl tetramethylbutylphenol (nano), *OCR* octocrylene *MED* 1 minimal erythema dose passes through sunscreen onto skin, *NTUV* normalized transmitted UV dose

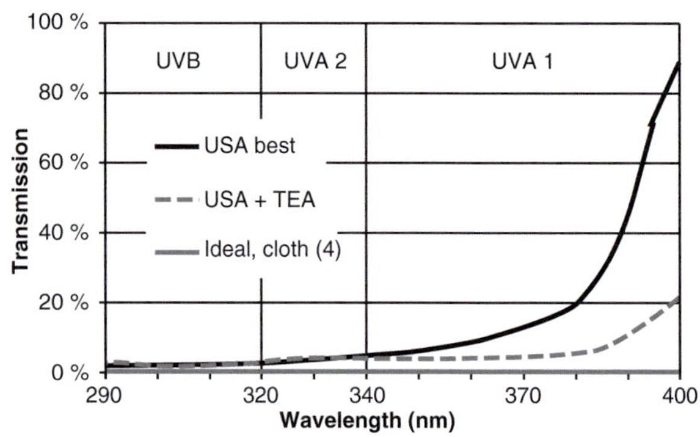

Fig. 11.5 Comparison of UV transmission curves. Sunscreen formulated with the highest allowable concentrations of UV filters available in the USA (USA-Best), incorporation of new filters into "USA-Best" sunscreen (USA + TEA), and ideal sunscreen (clothing) [4]

wavelength. The difference of sunscreens at equal SPF is mainly in the UVA1 region (340–400 nm). We know now that not only the erythemally weighted UV radiation is the cause of damage but also the extent of UVA1 radiation [51–54].

As shown in Table 11.5 and Fig. 11.5, much higher protection in the UVA1 spectrum can be achieved by the incorporation of TEA broad-spectrum filters; furthermore, a better protection can be achieved with lower total amounts of UV filter (19 % compared 39 %).

11.4 Safety

Sunscreen products are used widely, often daily across the whole population, which leads to high safety requirements irrespective of the regulatory environment. Therefore a UV filter-specific safety assessment is mandatory for its regulatory approval. In contrast to drugs, the deposition of UV filters on the skin is a prerequisite for their effectiveness and the uptake into the body is not intended. The protection against the known carcinogenic effect of UV light is to be emphasized as a health benefit of the UV filter besides its specific safety profile.

The safety assessment approach combines all relevant toxicological data to determine the UV filter intrinsic hazard profile that is to be compared to the exposure situation under conventional use of the sunscreen product. Such a hazard profile is initially determined by a basic set of studies addressing acute and topical toxicity of the UV filter such as skin/eye irritation, skin sensitization, and photo-induced toxicity. Furthermore, genotoxicity tests provide the basis for an adequate assessment of a potential mutagenic or cytogenetic effect of the UV filter and the absence of a genotoxic potential during the intended use in sunscreens is addressed by photogenotoxicity tests.

Repeated administration of the UV filter to animals in subacute, (sub-)chronic, or reproductive/developmental studies allows a thorough assessment of the systemic or reproductive toxicity potential. These studies help to identify target organs and are used for the determination of a UV filter-specific no observed adverse effect level (NOAEL). If no tissue changes indicate the onset of a tumor formation after repeated dosing, no genotoxic effects are observed, and no evident systemic uptake of the UV filter is found, a carcinogenic potential can be excluded in a weight of evidence without performing a definitive carcinogenicity test. However, if carcinogenic alerts exist, animal carcinogenicity studies are considered as a last resort to fully elucidate this endpoint [55].

Dermal penetration data [supported by studies on absorption, distribution, metabolization, and excretion if available] represent an important pillar to estimate the potential systemic human exposure with the UV filter during use. Based on standard exposure parameters for the use of sunscreen products [56] and UV filter-specific dermal penetration data, a systemic exposure dose of the UV filter for humans can be determined. This exposure dose takes into account the usual daily amount of sunscreen applied, the maximum concentration of the UV filter in sunscreens, and the dermal absorption of the UV filter as determined in the safety studies. In order to cover uncertainties due to variances in toxicological susceptibility between animals and humans and within the human population, the estimated human exposure dose needs to be at least 100-fold below the no observed adverse effect level identified in the relevant animal toxicity study in order to demonstrate the safe use of the UV filter in sunscreens [56].

11.5 Regulatory Approval Processes of UV Filters

Since safety is a prerequisite for the use of any consumer or medicinal product and since sunscreen products are used widely, often daily and on young children, high safety requirements apply. In Europe, UV filters must qualify for the positive list (Annex VI) of the European Cosmetics Regulation [57, 58], and in the USA, UV filters have to be listed in the FDA Over-the-Counter Sunscreen Monograph as active ingredients [29]. Similar requirements exist in most countries, e.g., Australia, Japan, China, and Brazil [59–61].

11.5.1 Time and Extent Application (TEA) Process in the USA

For UV filters, the FDA sunscreen monograph [29] dictates the use of UV active ingredients in sunscreens. All ingredients listed on the sunscreen monograph may be combined into different sunscreens, with some important restrictions, e.g., no avobenzone/TiO_2 or avobenzone/ZnO combination is allowed. These restrictions go back to concerns about chemical interactions leading to photoinstability. The issue is still awaiting a final decision by the FDA [62].

Over the last two decades, new UV filters have been developed that are photostable and cover a broad range of the UV spectrum [5, 48, 49]. The USA is the only country that has not benefited from these innovations, because the US FDA has not added any new UV filters to the sunscreen monograph since the addition of avobenzone in 1997 [63]. In 2002 the time and extent application (TEA) process was enacted to extend the approval process to UV filters from abroad [64]; however, none of the eight UV filters that have been filed through the TEA process has yet been approved (Table 11.5). There is only one UV filter (avobenzone) for efficient UVA1 protection currently available in the USA. ZnO is much less efficient and offers little protection beyond 370 nm and not permitted in combination with avobenzone. On the other hand, there are a number of "new" UVA1 and broad-spectrum UV filters in the TEA pipeline that have all been available in the rest of the world for 15 years or more (bemotrizinol, bisoctrizole, ecamsule, and drometrizole).

Due to the lack of progress of the approval process, the Sunscreen Innovation Act (SIA) was signed into law by the President of the USA on November 29, 2014, stating defined time limits for the different steps of the approval process [65]. The SIA had been initiated by the multi-stakeholder PASS coalition [66] and was rated among the top health initiatives by the TIME magazine in 2014 [67]. In response, the FDA held a meeting of its advisory committee on nonprescriptive drugs in September 2014 [68–72], where the industry had an opportunity to explain their safety assessment approach (see Sect. 11.5). Early 2014, the FDA had already started to send response letters to the TEA applicants requesting more data [73–79]. Early 2015 it became apparent that there will not be any new UV filters on the US market any time soon [80]. The FDA maintains that "there is currently not enough data to determine that any of the ingredients under review are generally recognized as safe and effective" [81].

11.5.2 UV Filter Use in Market in USA vs. Europe and the Rest of the World

An evaluation at the launched products over the last few years in the high and very high SPF category done by the market research company MINTEL [24] shows that only a limited number of UV filters is used in the USA and Canada (North America) compared with the rest of the world (Fig. 11.6). US sunscreens that provide the required UVA protection are mainly composed of the five UV filters: avobenzone, homosalate (HMS), octisalate (EHS), octocrylene (OCR), and oxybenzone (BP3). Only avobenzone provides UVA1 protection (beyond 360 nm). The globally most frequently used UVB filter octinoxate (EHMC) is practically not used in sunscreens in the USA because it destabilizes avobenzone. In the rest of the world, it is used together with other UVA/broad-spectrum UV filters. Its slight photoinstability, partly due to internal cis/trans conversion, does not significantly affect its efficacy. TiO_2 and ZnO are less frequently used because they are not allowed in combination with avobenzone due to FDA monograph restrictions. US manufacturers have thus to make the decision to use either avobenzone or ZnO as UVA protection platform. Figure 11.6 shows that in the rest of the world many more UV filters are used, besides the global filters, mainly the TEA filters for UVA, bemotrizinol (BEMT), bisoctrizole (MBBT), drometrizole (DBT), and ecamsule (TDSA) and the UVB filters octyl triazone (EHT) and iscotrizinol (DBT). It should be noted that a global filter oxybenzone (BP3) is virtually not been used anymore in Europe, having been replaced by the new UVA filters. One reason is the mandatory declaration "contains oxybenzone" because of its allergy potential. Such phasing out of oxybenzone is not yet being possible in the US market for lack of available alternatives.

11.6 Conclusion

Tremendous progress has been made in sunscreen technology over the last two decades, with the development of new photostable filters that covers a broad range of UV radiation, including UVA1. Unfortunately, in the USA, UV filter technology is lagging 15 years behind compared to the rest of the world. Until FDA provides approval of new UV filters that have been submitted through the TEA process, it is difficult for the sunscreen industry to introduce truly innovative new sunscreen products in the USA.

In Europe and the rest of the world, development goes on, but it is slower than 20 years ago. The animal test ban in the European Cosmetics regulation may further slow down technology innovations, but it could also trigger a regulatory shift away from cosmetics toward medical device.

The major weakness of sunscreen and photoprotection remains the lack of compliance by the user. To solve this problem, innovation in photoprotection education, including behavior modification and sunscreen use, is required.

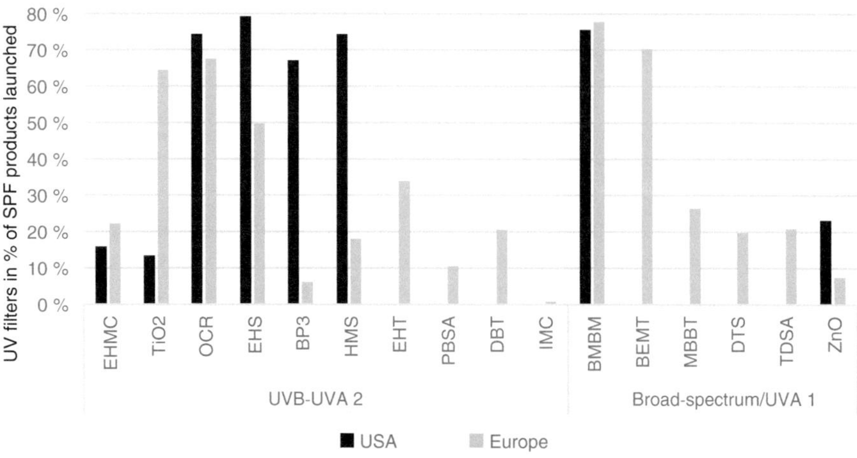

Fig. 11.6 UV filters used in sunscreens launched (After MINTEL [24]). Please see footnote in Table 11.4 for complete list of abbreviations

Acknowledgement Thanks go to those who have contributed to the Delphi survey, although they will remain anonymous to the reader; further to Prof. Brian Diffey for all his scientific contributions to the topic over the last three decades and the valuable discussions; furthermore to our BASF colleagues Drs. Bernd Herzog, Mechtild Petersen-Thiery, and Myriam Sohn for valuable discussions; and last but not the least to the intern Felix Presencio who helped compiling and designing tables and figures.

References

1. Hughes MCB, Williams GM, Baker P, Green AC (2013) Sunscreen and maximum penetration is only 0.6 % of the applied prevention of skin aging. A randomized trial. Ann Intern Med 158:781–790
2. Green A, Williams G, Neale R et al (1999) Daily sunscreen application and beta-carotene supplementation in prevention of basal cell and squamous-cell carcinomas of the skin: a randomised controlled trial. Lancet 354:723–729
3. Green AC, Williams GM, Logan V, Strutton GM (2011) Reduced melanoma after regular sunscreen use: randomized trial follow-up. J Clin Oncol 29:257–263
4. Viros A, Sanchez-Laorden B, Pedersen M, Furney SJ, Rae J, Hogan K, Ejiama S, Romina Girotti M, Cook M, Dhomen N, Marais R (2014) Ultraviolet radiation accelerates BRAF-driven melanomagenesis by targeting TP53. Nature 511:478–482
5. Herzog B, Hueglin D, Osterwalder U (2005) New sunscreen actives. In: Shaath NA (ed) Sunscreens – regulations and commercial development, cosmetic science and technology, vol 28, 3rd edn. Taylor & Francis, Boca Raton, pp 291–320
6. Meyers T, Agin P (2015) Chapter 11: Chemistry of sunscreens – understanding properties of organic and inorganic UV filters. In: Lim H, Wang S (eds) Principles and practices of photoprotection. Springer, Heidelberg
7. Herzog B (2012) Photoprotection of human skin. In: Albini A (ed) Photochemistry, vol 40. RSC Publishing/The Royal Society of Chemistry, Cambridge, UK, pp 250–259
8. Anonymous. BASF sunscreen simulator, BASF SE, Ludwigshafen. 2010. Available at http://www.basf.com/sunscreen-simulator. Accessed 18 Jan 2015.

9. Ferrero L, Pissavini M, Marguerie S, Zastrow L (2003) Efficiency of a continuous height distribution model of sunscreen film geometry to predict a realistic sun protection factor. J Cosmet Sci 54:463–481
10. Herzog B, Mongiat S, Quass K, Deshayes C (2004) Prediction of sun protection factors and UVA parameters by using a calibrated step film model. J Pharm Sci 93:1780–1795
11. Wloka M, Lange RFM, Flösser-Müller H. An in vitro SPF screening approach considering photostability of the UV filters. In: Proceedings of International Sun Protection Conference, London. 2005.
12. Stanfield J, Osterwalder U, Herzog B (2010) In vitro measurements of sunscreen protection. Photochem Photobiol Sci 9:489–494
13. Herzog B, Osterwalder U (2011) Silico determination of topical sun protection. Cosmetic Sci Technol 62:1–8
14. OJ European Union (2000) 24th Commission Directive of 29 Feb 2000, adapting to technical progress annexes II, III, VI and VII to council directive 76/768/EEC on the approximation of the laws of the member states relating to cosmetic products, L 56/42.
15. OJ European Union (2014) Commission Regulation (EU) No 866/2014 of 8 August 2014 amending annexes III, V and VI to regulation (EC) No 1223/2009 on cosmetic product, L 238/7.
16. Herzog B, Hüglin D, Borsos E, Stehlin A, Luther H (2004) New UV absorbers for cosmetic sunscreens – a breakthrough for the photoprotection of human skin. Chimia 58:554–559
17. Opinion of the EU Scientific Committee on Cosmetic Products and Non-Food Products intended for Consumers. 1999.
18. Herzog B, Katzenstein A, Quass K, Stehlin A, Luther H (2004) Physical properties of organic particulate UV-absorbers used in sunscreens. I. Determination of particle size with fiber-optic quasi-elastic light scattering (FOQELS), disc centrifugation, and laser diffractometry. J Colloid Interface Sci 271:136–144
19. Herzog B, Quass K, Schmidt E, Müller S, Luther H (2004) Physical properties of organic particulate UV absorbers used in sunscreens II. UV-attenuating efficiency as function of particle size. J Colloid Interface Sci 276:354–363
20. Mueller S, Herzog B, Giesinger J, Quass K, Osterwalder U (2005) Micronization as a tool in the development of innovative UV filters. SOFW J 131:32–39
21. Kollias N (1999) The absorption properties of 'physical' sunscreens. Arch Dermatol 135:209–210
22. Shinryo Yabea S, Tsugio Satob T (2003) Cerium oxide for sunscreen cosmetic. J Solid State Chem 171:7–11
23. Herrling T, Seifert M, Jung K (2013) Cerium dioxide: future UV-filter in sunscreen? SOFW J 139(5):10–14
24. Anonymous, Ingredients analysis, MINTEL search. http://www.gnpd.com. Accessed 2 Feb 2015.
25. Anonymous, Niels Ryberg Finsen, http://en.wikipedia.org/wiki/Niels Ryberg Finsen. Accessed 14 Feb 2015.
26. Anonymous, Describing a visit by the Prince of Wales to the pretty town of Sigmaringen the reporter says: 'the castle possesses many delightful terraces which could be adapted for sunbathing". The Times. 1913. p. 6.
27. Anonymous, Sun Tanning, http://en.wikipedia.org/wiki/Sun_tanning. Accessed 14 Feb 2015.
28. Anonymous, Sunscreen, http://en.wikipedia.org/wiki/Sunscreen. Accessed 14 Feb 2015.
29. Food and Drug Administration (1999) Sunscreen drug products for over-the-counter human use; final monograph. Fed Regist 64(98):27666–27693
30. Shaat N (2005) Sunscreen evolution. In: Shaath NA (ed) Sunscreens – regulations and commercial development, cosmetic science and technology, vol 28, 3rd edn. Taylor & Francis, Boca Raton, pp 3–17
31. OJ European Union. Commission Directive 2005/9/EC of 28 Jan 2005 amending Council Directive 76/768/EEC, concerning cosmetic products, for the purposes of adapting annex VII thereto to technical progress, L 27/46.
32. Chatelain E, Gabard B (2001) Photostabilization of Butyl methoxydibenzoylmethane (Avobenzone) and Ethylhexyl methoxycinnamate by Bis-ethylhexyloxyphenol methoxyphenyl triazine (Tinosorb S), a new UV broadband filter. Photochem Photobiol 74(3):401–406

33. Schulze R (1956) Parfüm. Kosmet 37:310, 365
34. Osterwalder U, Champ S, Flösser-Müller H, Herzog B. Evolution of UVA protection. Cosmet Sci Technol. 2010;7:1–10.
35. OJ European Union (2006) Commission Recommendation of 22 Sept 2006 on the efficacy of sunscreen products and the claims made relating thereto, L265/39
36. Food and Drug Administration. Labeling and effectiveness testing; sunscreen drug products for over-the-counter human use. Available at: http://www.gpo.gov/fdsys/pkg/FR-2011-06-17/pdf/2011-14766.pdf. Accessed 15 Feb 2015.
37. Oguchi-Fujiyama N, Miyazawa K, Kikuchi A, Yagi M. A novel UV-B absorber to enhance the efficacy of UV-A protection based on an energy transfer system: design and properties of dioctyl 4-ethoxy-benzylidenemalonate. Poster at IFSCC Congress, Paris. 2014.
38. Kim YB. Soluble UV absorbing silicone polymer. Poster at IFSCC Congress, Paris. 2014.
39. Scientific Committee on Consumer Safety, OPINION ON 2-(4-(2-(4-Diethylamino-2-hydroxy-benzoyl)-benzoyl)-piperazine-1-carbonyl)-phenyl)-(4-diethylamino-2-hydroxyphenyl)-methanone (HAA299), http://ec.europa.eu/health/scientific_committees/consumer_safety/docs/sccs_o_159.pdf. Accessed 28 Feb 2015.
40. Scientific committee on consumer safety, Request for a scientific opinion: Phenylene Bis-Diphenyltriazine , (CAS n. 55514-22-2), S86 http://ec.europa.eu/health/scientific_committees/consumer_safety/docs/sccs_q_075.pdf. Accessed 28 Feb 2015.
41. Osterwalder U, Herzog B (2010) The long way towards the ideal sunscreen – where we stand and what still needs to be done. Photochem Photobiol Sci 9:470–481
42. Ritchey T. Outline for a morphology of modeling methods: contribution to a general theory of modelling. Acta Morph Gen. 2012. Available at http://www.amg.swemorph.com/pdf/amg-1-1-2012.pdf)
43. Anonymous, Cosmetic raw materials certified by ecocert under ecocert & cosmos standards, http://www.ecocert.com/en/cosmos. Accessed 14 Feb 2015.
44. Dalkey N, Helmer O (1963) An experimental application of the Delphi method to the use of experts. Manage Sci 9(3):458–467
45. Rowe G, Wright G (1999) The Delphi technique as a forecasting tool: issues and analysis. Int J Forecast 15:353–375
46. Rowe G, Wright G (2001) Expert opinions in forecasting. Role of the Delphi technique. In: Armstrong JS (ed) Principles of forecasting: a handbook of researchers and practitioners. Kluwer Academic Publishers, Boston
47. Osterwalder U, Herzog B (2009) Sun protection factors: worldwide confusion. Br J Dermatol 161(Suppl 3):13–24
48. Osterwalder U, Herzog B, Wang SQ (2011) Advance in sunscreens to prevent skin cancer. Expert Rev Dermatol 6:479–491
49. Osterwalder U, Sohn M, Herzog B (2014) Global state of sunscreen. Photodermatol Photoimmunol Photomed 30:62–80
50. Wang SQ, Tanner PR, Lim HW, Nash JF (2013) The evolution of sunscreen products in the United States – a 12-year cross sectional study. Photochem Photobiol Sci 12(1):197–202. doi:10.1039/c2pp25112d
51. Cadet J, Douki T, Ravanat JL (2015) Oxidatively generated damage to cellular DNA by UVB and UVA radiation. Photochem Photobiol 91(1):140–155. doi:10.1111/php.12368. Epub 2014 Nov 27
52. Tewari A, Sarkany RP, Young AR (2012) UVA1 induces cyclobutane pyrimidine dimers but not 6–4 photoproducts in human skin in vivo. J Invest Dermatol 132(2):394–400. doi:10.1038/jid.2011.283. Epub 2011 Oct 6
53. Tewari A, Grage MM, Harrison GI, Sarkany R, Young AR (2013) UVA1 is skin deep: molecular and clinical implications. Photochem Photobiol Sci 12(1):95–103. doi:10.1039/c2pp25323b
54. World Health Organization. Artificial tanning sunbeds risks and guidance, http://www.who.int/uv/publications/en/sunbeds.pdf?ua=1. Accessed 2015-02-20. 2003.
55. R.8 ECHA guidance on information requirements and chemical safety assessment. Version: 2. 2012.
56. White I et al The SCCS'S notes of guidance for the testing of cosmetic substances and their safety evaluation. 8th revision. SCCS/1501/12. 2012.
57. Cosmetic Products. Regulation (EC) no. 1223/2009 of the European parliament and of the council of 30 November 2009 on cosmetic products. Annex VI. 2009. Available at http://eur-

lex.europa.eu/LexUriServ/LexUriServ.do?uri=COM:2008:0049:FIN:EN:PDF. Accessed 13 Feb 2015.

58. Rogiers V, Pauwels M (2008) Safety assessment of cosmetics in Europe, current problems in dermatology. S Karger AG, Basel
59. Therapeutic Goods Administration. Australian regulatory guidelines for sunscreens, Version 1.0. 2012. https://www.tga.gov.au/publication/australian-regulatory-guidelines-sunscreens-args, Accessed 31 Jan 2016.
60. Xia J. Review of cosmetics regulations in Asia. http://www.skin-care-forum.basf.com/en/author-articles/review-of-cosmetics-regulations-in-asia/2012/12/07?id=a016034e-663a-4159-bf20-2cdae216763e&mode=Detail. Accessed 5 Apr 2015.
61. ANVISA Brazil. http://portal.anvisa.gov.br/wps/content/Anvisa+Portal/Anvisa/Inicio/Cosmeticos. Accessed 5 Apr 2015.
62. Hubbard WK, Sunscreen drug products for over-the-counter human use; Amendment to the tentative final monograph; Enforcement Policy Federal Register 63(204)/Thursday, October 22, 1998/Proposed Rules, p. 56587.
63. Food and Drug Administration. Sunscreen drug products for over-the-counter human use; marketing status of products containing Avobenzone, enforcement policy. Fed Regist. 62(83):23350. Wednesday, Apr 30, 1997. Rules and regulations.
64. Food and Drug Administration. Additional criteria and procedures for classifying over-the-counter drugs as generally recognized as safe and effective and not misbranded, final rule. Fed Regist. 67(15):3060. Wednesday, Jan 23 2002.
65. Reed J. Sunscreen Innovation Act (SIA), Public Law No. 113–195, 26 Nov. 2014.
66. Anonymous, On the Brink of Year Anniversary of the Sunscreen Innovation Act Becoming Law, Nothing Has Changed Except Rising Melanoma Rates, http://www.passcoalition.com/. Accessed 14 Feb 2014.
67. Sifferlin A. 11 remarkable health advances from 2014. Time. http://time.com/3640238/11-remarkable-health-advances-from-2014/. Accessed 5 Apr 2015.
68. Michele TM. FDA briefing document for a meeting of the Nonprescription Drugs Advisory Committee Sunscreen Active Ingredients Topic: sunscreen active ingredient safety testing 4, 5 Sept, 2014, and 6 Aug 2014.
69. FDA briefing document for a meeting of the Nonprescription Drugs Advisory Committee (NDAC). Sunscreen actives, topic: sunscreen active ingredient safety testing, 4, 5 Sept 2014.
70. Hong C, Neill R. FDA, summary minutes of the Nonprescription Drugs Advisory Committee (NDAC) meeting 4, 5 Sept 2014.
71. Michele TM. FDA, slides of the Nonprescription Drugs Advisory Committee (NDAC) meeting 4, 5 Sept 2014.
72. Hong C. FDA, transcripts of the Nonprescription Drugs Advisory Committee (NDAC) Meeting 4, 5 Sept 2014.
73. Kweder SL. FDA, feedback letter on safety and effectiveness data of *Amiloxate* submitted by Symrise Inc. and Ego Pharmaceuticals Pty. Ltd. 2014.
74. Kweder SL. FDA, feedback letter on safety and effectiveness data of *Diethylhexyl Butamido Triazone* submitted by 3V Inc. 2014.
75. Kweder SL. FDA, feedback letter on safety and effectiveness data of *Octyl Triazone* submitted by BASF AG. 2014.
76. Kweder SL. FDA, feedback letter on safety and effectiveness data of *Drometrizole Trisiloxane* submitted by L'OREAL USA. 2014.
77. Kweder SL. FDA, feedback letter on safety and effectiveness data of *Bemotrizinol* submitted by Ciba Specialty Corp. 2014.
78. Ecamsule, FDA proposed order https://federalregister.gov/a/2015-03883
79. Enzacamene, FDA proposed order. https://federalregister.gov/a/2015-03884
80. Editorial, Washington's Skin Cancer Hostages – The FDA is defying Congress and Obama on better sunscreens, WSJ. 2015. http://www.wsj.com/articles/washingtons-skin-cancer-hostages-1426287044. Accessed 5 Apr 2015.
81. Michele TM. FDA is systematically screening for safe sunscreens, letters. WSJ. 2015. http://www.wsj.com/articles/fda-is-systematically-screening-for-safe-sunscreens-letters-to-the-editor-1427649129

Chapter 12
Organotypic Models for Evaluating Sunscreens

Claire Marionnet and Françoise Bernerd

Key Points

- The development of reconstructed skins has made possible in vitro assessment of the effects of different types of UV exposure (UVB, UVA, or solar simulation) in a three-dimensional context and in a cutaneous structure, including different types of skin cells.
- Reconstructed skin shows numerous biological endpoints which are predictive of in vivo response, hence allowing a better understanding of the precise biological processes involved.
- Reconstructed skin can be used to evaluate the photoprotection afforded by sunscreens in vitro, providing additional biological data on sunscreen efficacy to correlate with protection factors assessed in vivo.
- The combination of 3-D skin models and new biological approaches such as transcriptomic or proteomic will indisputably increase the added value of such systems for evaluating sunscreen performance.

12.1 UV Exposure and Clinical Consequences

Skin, the largest organ of the human body, represents the main barrier ensuring a key function of protection against external/environmental harm. Among this, solar and especially ultraviolet (UV) rays can be considered as one of the major contributors. The protective properties of the skin are supported by the whole skin structure in a

C. Marionnet • F. Bernerd (✉)
Department of Biological and Clinical Research,
L'Oréal Research and Innovation, 1 avenue Eugène Schueller,
Aulnay sous Bois 93600, France
e-mail: fbernerd@rd.loreal.com

S.Q. Wang, H.W. Lim (eds.), *Principles and Practice of Photoprotection*,
DOI 10.1007/978-3-319-29382-0_12

coordinate manner between the different compartments. The most superficial cutaneous layer, the epidermis, mainly composed of keratinocytes (approx. 90 %), undergoes a stratification process and a specific and fine-tuned program of keratinocyte differentiation that leads to the formation of a compact stratum corneum. The latter ultimately constitutes the first line of defense of the skin (for review, [67, 99]). The epidermis is also the place of residence for the following: (1) melanocytes, the pigmentary cells responsible for melanin synthesis [73], and (2) Langerhans cells, a member of the antigen-presenting cell family involved in immune function [27]. The underlying dermal compartment is mostly composed of extracellular matrix proteins (ECM) synthesized by dermal fibroblasts and provides a mechanical and thermal protective layer. It also hosts blood vessels as source of nutriments, nerve endings and various appendages such as hair follicles, sebaceous and sweat glands [56].

Beside some beneficial effects of sunlight, such as vitamin D production, acute or repetitive solar UV exposure can lead to harmful clinical consequences such as sunburn reaction associated with erythema and epidermal sunburn cells (SBC) formation but also middle- and long-term effects such as photoimmunosuppression, photoaging mostly characterized by dermal alterations and the development of solar elastosis and photocarcinogenesis, especially epidermal basal and squamous cell carcinomas [65]. It is also known that hyperpigmentation, including the physiological tanning response but also the appearance of hyperpigmented lesions such as actinic lentigines, is directly related to sun exposure. Considering all these phenomena, both compartments of the skin, dermis and epidermis, are affected. In addition, it is now proven that all UV rays that reach the Earth surface are involved. UVB rays (290–320 nm), the most energetic wavelengths, can directly induce DNA lesions such as cyclobutane pyrimidine dimers (CPDs) and 6,4-photoproducts. Most of the direct UVB effects are located within the epidermis due to low penetration of these wavelengths. Short (UVA2) or long (UVA1) UVA radiation (320–340 nm and 340–400 nm, respectively) are less energetic than UVB but show progressively higher penetration properties with increasing wavelength and can therefore reach the dermal compartment and its cells. Their major mode of action is the generation of reactive oxygen species (ROS) that, in turn, lead to activate various signaling pathways.

12.2 Organotypic Skin Models

For both designing and evaluating the most effective photoprotection strategies, it is crucial to understand and characterize the early biological events that occur following UV exposure. For practical and ethical reasons in vivo studies in human volunteers are often difficult to perform. In contrast, classical two-dimensional (2-D) skin cell cultures poorly reproduce physiological conditions and tissue organization, such as epidermal differentiation and cell-cell and cell-matrix interactions. Moreover, they cannot take into account the penetration of UV rays through the different skin compartments.

In vitro 3-D engineered skin models have been developed during the last 30 years on the basis of human skin cell culture and organotypic reconstruction techniques and

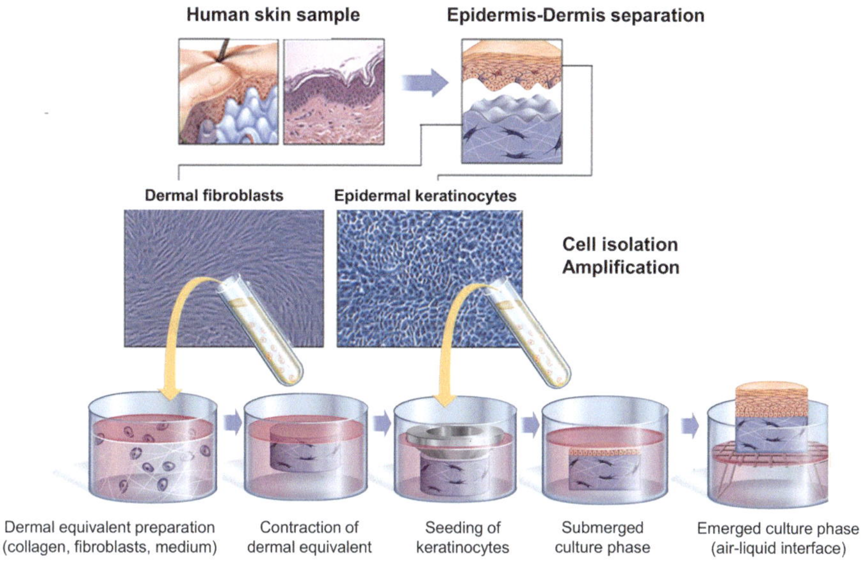

Fig. 12.1 Main steps of in vitro reconstruction of the full-thickness skin model. First, a human skin sample is trypsinized to separate dermis from epidermis. From both compartments, epidermal keratinocytes and dermal fibroblasts are isolated and amplified in their respective culture medium. The reconstruction starts with the production of the living dermal equivalent by mixing a collagen type I solution with medium and dermal fibroblasts. This gel is poured into a Petri dish and left in the incubator at 37 °C for 3–4 days to allow the contraction to proceed. Then the epidermis reconstruction starts by seeding epidermal keratinocytes on the top of the dermal equivalent. The ring allows for control of cell density. The culture is left for the immersion phase corresponding to the formation of a simple epithelium covering the dermal substrate. Afterward, the whole culture is raised to the air-liquid interface, fed by capillarity to promote the stratification and epidermal differentiation process. At the end of this phase (usually 7 days), a stratum corneum is formed (© L'Oréal Research and Innovation)

know-how. From the first reconstructed epidermis on a cell-free dermal substrate [100], the in vitro skin models have been perfected over the past decades by adding different cell types, improving the dermal equivalent and increasing the functionality of the models [5, 37, 42, 75]. Reconstruction of in vitro skin models usually follows similar key step process ([33, 40], and Fig. 12.1): (1) extraction of keratinocytes from the epidermis of skin biopsies and amplification and (2) seeding of keratinocytes on the top of a dermal equivalent which can be either a de-epidermized dermis (DED), an acellular collagen matrix, a polycarbonate membrane, or a living dermal equivalent composed of ECM and dermal fibroblasts. The keratinocytes are allowed to proliferate onto the surface of the support by being submerged by the culture medium. During this step, other epidermal cell types may be added – melanocytes or precursors for Langerhans cells (CD34+ cells) – depending on the model to be produced. In the last step, the whole culture system is placed in contact with air, corresponding to the air-liquid interface culture period. During that phase, the culture medium is added underneath the dermal support, and the system is fed by capillarity. This air-exposed phase period is mandatory for the stratification and full differentiation of the epidermal structure. Figure 12.2 illustrates different skin models.

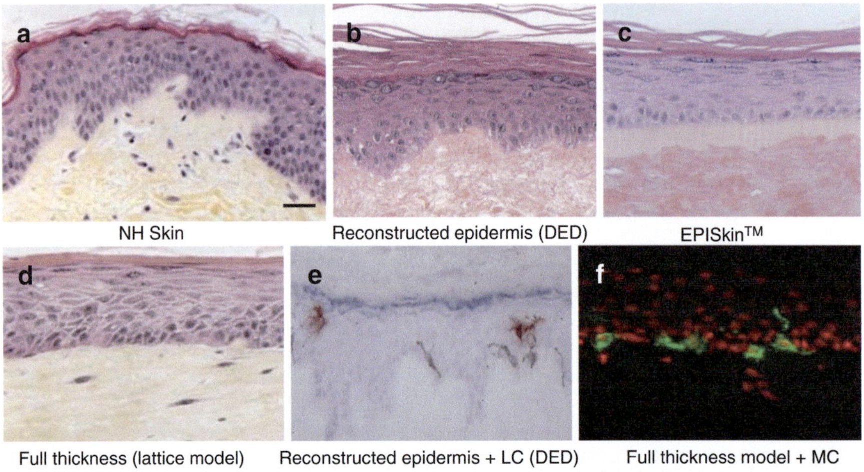

Fig. 12.2 Examples of organotypic skin models. (**a**) Normal human skin, bar = 50 μm. (**b**) Reconstructed epidermis on an acellular dead de-epidermized dermis (*DED*). (**c**) Reconstructed epidermis on an acellular collagen matrix Episkin™ model. (**d**) Full-thickness skin model composed of fibroblast-populated collagen matrix as dermal support and differentiated epidermis. (**a–d**) Hematoxylin-eosin staining. (**e**) Reconstructed epidermis on DED support; Langerhans cells (*brown*) stained with Langerin antibody. (**f**) Pigmented full-thickness skin model. Melanocytes (MD; *green*) are visualized using anti-tyrosinase-related protein (TRP)-1 antibody. Nuclei are counterstained with propidium iodide

12.3 Effects of UV on Organotypic Models

Reconstructed skin in vitro can be used to study damage induced by UVB or by UVA in order to determine the specific impact of each wavelengths range or that induced by the combination of UVB and UVA, to simulate solar exposure. Figure 12.3 illustrates the main biological effects induced by UVB, UVA or solar simulation that are further detailed.

12.3.1 Effects of UVB Exposure on Reconstructed Skin: A Major Impact on the Epidermis

Following UVB exposure of reconstructed human skin, major epidermal changes were observed, affecting keratinocyte homeostasis and increasing pigmentation process. The typical UVB-induced effects observed in human skin in vivo, such as DNA damage formation, p53 accumulation, SBC, and apoptotic features could be reproduced in skin reconstructed in vitro. These events represent the biological signature of a moderate sunburn reaction.

As found in vivo and due to the direct absorption of UVB photons by DNA, DNA damage such as pyrimidine dimers could be evidenced immediately following UVB

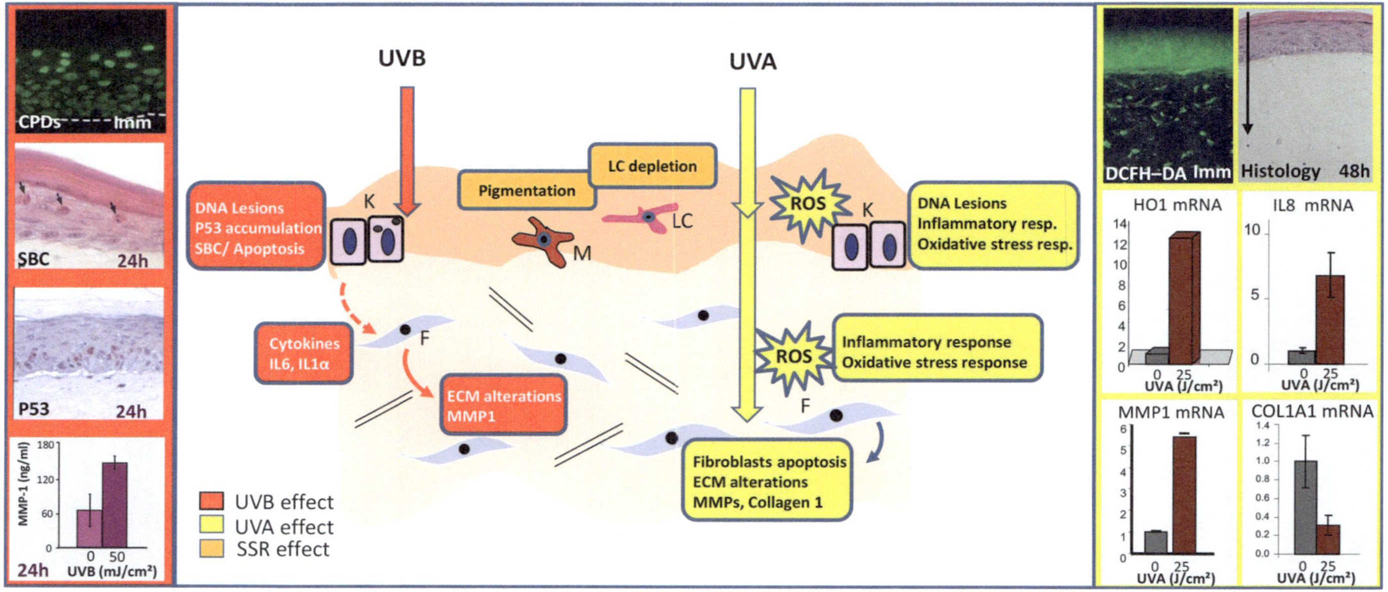

Fig. 12.3 Schematic representation of the main biological effects induced by UVB, UVA, or UV solar-stimulated radiation (*SSR*) exposure in a reconstructed skin model. *CPDs* cyclobutane pyrimidine dimers, *DCFH-DA* 2′, 7′ dichlorofluorescin diacetate, *ECM* extracellular matrix, *F* fibroblasts, *K* keratinocytes, *LC* Langerhans cells, *M* melanocytes, *MMP1* matrix metalloproteinase 1, *ROS* reactive oxygen species, *SBC* sunburn cell

exposure in epidermal keratinocytes of reconstructed skin, using immunostaining, LMPCR, and comet assay [12, 49, 115]. Using immunostaining, pyrimidine dimers were detected immediately after UVB exposure, in all nuclei of epidermal cells. Twenty-four hours later, the remaining positive nuclei persisted in upper suprabasal and granular layers of the epidermis [12]. Pyrimidine dimers were completely removed within the next few days by the nucleotide excision repair mechanism [15].

A direct consequence of such DNA lesions is the formation of SBC, the biological hallmark of a sunburn reaction. In reconstructed skin models, SBC displayed their typical histological features, i.e., a round shape, a loss of connection with the surrounding keratinocytes, a condensed pyknotic nucleus, and an eosinophilic cytoplasm together with a suprabasal localization 24 h post UVB exposure. Similarly to in vivo, these are progressively removed from the epidermis within a few days together with the formation of a parakeratotic horny layer and changes in expression of differentiation markers [12, 55]. Parallel to SBC formation, apoptosis was observed in viable epidermis of human reconstructed skin exposed to UVB, using TUNEL reaction. Apoptotic keratinocytes were especially detected in the deeper epidermal layers, with a density and a localization correlating with that of SBC [12, 55]. At the molecular level, UVB exposure altered the expression and posttranslational modifications of several actors of the apoptotic pathway. P53 accumulated in basal and suprabasal cells, while BCl2 expression decreased following UVB exposure [55, 118]. Moreover, other apoptotic-related biomarkers were induced such as galectin-7, a keratinocyte-specific protein or caspase 3 cleavage [17, 47]. Recently, the use of reconstructed skin model enabled to show that dermal fibroblasts can influence the impact of UVB exposure on epidermal keratinocytes by accelerating the removal of pyrimidine dimers and reducing keratinocyte apoptosis [47]. Apart from apoptotic SBC, structural UVB-induced alterations can be observed in the epidermis using electron microscopy, such as the formation of dense cytoplasmic bodies, as well as vacuolation and indentation of the nuclear envelope in basal cells [60]. These changes were similar to those observed in normal human skin following UV exposure [93, 94, 119]. UVB exposure also led to increased keratinocyte proliferative activity [12, 60] in agreement with hyperplasia observed in vivo [96].

The UVB photoproduction of vitamin D3 observed in human skin in vivo can be reproduced in models of human reconstructed skin, with the photoconversion of 7-dehydrocholesterol to previtamin D3 and its subsequent isomerization to vitamin D3 and ultimately calcitriol formation. The percentages of main photoproducts of 7-dehydrocholesterol were shown to be identical in reconstructed skin model and in human skin in vivo. Keratinocytes were absolutely required for calcitriol formation in reconstructed skin [70, 95].

In addition to the multiple direct effects of UVB on human epidermis, dermal compartment can also be impacted through the production of degrading enzymes, such as matrix metalloproteinases (MMPs) following UVB exposure. In human skin in vivo, increase in MMPs mRNA expression and MMP-1 activation after UVB exposure have been reported, and its involvement in premature aging has been pointed out [48]. Following UVB exposure of reconstructed human skin, MMP-1 protein expression was increased in fibroblasts, only in the presence of the epidermis.

This points out the indirect impact of UVB radiation on fibroblasts and ECM, *via* its direct action on epidermal keratinocytes and their release of diffusible IL1 and IL6 cytokines [45, 46]. UVB also increased the expression and activity of epidermal MMPs, such as MMP-2 and MMP-9 in a full-thickness skin model [2]. Reinforcing the involvement of UVB in photoaging process, Kurdykowski et al. showed the UVB modulation of hyaluronidases expression in reconstructed epidermis [66].

The use of reconstructed pigmented skin, including a mix of melanocytes and keratinocytes seeded onto a dermal equivalent or a de-epidermized dermis, enabled the impact of UVB exposure on pigmentation to be investigated. Sequences of repeated UVB exposures led to an increase in proliferation, dendricity, and activity of melanocytes and an increase in melanin production and in melanosome transfer from melanocytes to keratinocytes, resulting in a noticeable tanning of the reconstructed epidermis [20, 21, 38, 52, 69, 90, 116, 117].

12.3.2 Effects of UVA Exposure on Reconstructed Skin: A Major Impact in the Deeper Layers of the Skin

Studies of the impact of UVA in reconstructed human skin revealed that this 3-D skin model enabled to reproduce main features of UVA effects observed in human skin in vivo.

The immediate damage following UVA exposure in human skin in vivo is the generation of reactive oxygen species (ROS) leading to oxidative stress, as well as DNA damage, especially pyrimidine dimers and 8-oxo-7,8-dihydro-2′-deoxyguanosine (8-OHdG) accumulating in basal keratinocytes that may lead in the long term to DNA mutations [64, 114].

In reconstructed skin, UVA exposure also led to ROS formation, as visualized using DCFH-DA probe, in a UVA dose-dependent manner in both fibroblasts and keratinocytes. Increasing doses of UVA induced ROS deeply in the epidermal basal layer but also in the deepest dermal fibroblasts illustrating the high penetration properties of UVA wavelengths [80, 118]. Six hours after UVA exposure, cells of reconstructed skin responded to this oxidative stress with the upregulation of the expression of genes involved in oxidative stress management such as genes of the Nrf2 pathway. For example, a strong increase in HMOX1 and TXNRD1 mRNA could be observed in fibroblasts, together with a strong increase in TXNRD1, NQO1, and FTL mRNA in keratinocytes. A UVA induction of ferritin protein was detected in basal keratinocytes of reconstructed epidermis [109]. The expression of genes involved in the redox status of glutathione was also modulated [86]. ROS may lead to cell components alterations in reconstructed skin, such as lipid peroxidation and protein oxidation [54]. Lipid peroxidation can in turn lead to cell membrane damage and can also act as cell signal mediators since particular oxidized phospholipids could induce HMOX1 expression in reconstructed skin [54]. Protein oxidation phenomenon can be amplified by pheomelanin, acting as a photosensitizing agent, as shown by Maresca et al., in a reconstructed model including melanocytes [34, 77, 80].

As found in human skin in vivo, thymine dimers were also detected after UVA exposure, in basal keratinocytes of reconstructed skin using immunostaining, albeit in a much lower amount than post UVB exposure [13, 80, 114]. Immunostainings also revealed increased levels of 8-OHdG oxidative DNA lesion in epidermal and dermal cells nuclei following UVA exposure of living skin equivalents [36]. Furthermore, exposure to repeated low doses of UVA induced p53 mutations in basal keratinocytes of the epidermis [63].

Regarding histological alterations, in contrast to UVB, major features of UVA effects were located in the dermal compartment of reconstructed skin in vitro, in correlation with previous human in vivo studies showing that repetitive exposures to low UVA doses induced early morphological and biochemical alterations in the dermis [11, 68, 74].

Forty-eight hours after UVA exposure of reconstructed skin, the dermal fibroblasts localized in the superficial portion of the dermal equivalent disappeared, underlining the significant biological impact of UVA in deeper layers of skin and confirming that dermal fibroblasts were more sensitive to UVA-induced oxidative stress than keratinocytes [3, 88]. UVA cytotoxicity toward fibroblast was direct and mostly due to apoptosis, accompanied by an upregulation of the expression of genes related to cell death and apoptosis, such as DDIT3, IER3, BIRC3, and NR4A1, NR4A2, and NR4A3 [13, 43, 80]. This particular impact on dermis was emphasized by the upregulation of several MMP gene and protein expression (e.g., MMP-1, MMP-9, MMP-3) [78, 86]. It was shown that UVA exposure, in contrast to UVB exposure, induced the production of MMP1 by fibroblasts in a direct manner, since the removal of epidermis immediately after UVA exposure did not alter this effect [118]. The expression of COL1A1 gene was downregulated in fibroblasts of reconstructed skin exposed to UVA rays [79, 80, 86]. The epidermal structure and organization were to a lesser extent impacted by exposure to UVA, with a slight impact on the upper layers and parakeratosis [13]. Higher doses of UVA could lead to disorganization of the living epidermis together with a reduced skin barrier function, increase in phospholipid, and decrease of ceramide levels [103].

In vivo, UVA exposure also impacts skin immunity, with inflammatory effects and with immune suppression [28, 57, 58]. In line with these in vivo clinical features, UVA exposure of reconstructed skin leads to the upregulation of proinflammatory genes and/or proteins such as IL1, IL6, IL8, GM-CSF, COX-2, or PGE2 [32, 78, 80, 92]. In contrast, numerous genes encoding proteins involved in antiviral defense were strongly downregulated following UVA exposure in fibroblasts and keratinocytes of reconstructed skin, possibly related to photoimmune suppression observed in vivo [80].

Concerning pigmentation process, Duval et al., using a reconstructed epidermis including melanocytes, showed that UVA exposure led to the production and transfer of melanin to the neighboring keratinocytes and resulted in tanning of the reconstructed epidermis, like UVB exposure, and as observed in vivo [38, 97].

Altogether these results illustrated the penetration properties of UVA rays as attested by the direct UVA-induced biological damage in dermis and the particular vulnerability to UVA rays of the deepest epidermal layer, location of epidermal stem cells, proliferative keratinocytes, and melanocytes [59, 113]. The particular impact of UVA on the dermal compartment observed in vivo and in 3-D models in vitro may be involved in early events occurring during photoaging leading to drastic alterations of dermal structure and formation of the solar elastosis, classically observed in photoaged skin [25].

12.3.3 Effects of Solar Simulation Exposure on Reconstructed Skin

The effects of solar-simulated radiation (SSR), including UVA and UVB, have been studied in reconstructed human skin models. Today, two types of solar simulation can be distinguished: UV solar-simulated radiation (UV-SSR) and daily UV radiation (DUVR). Both include UVA and UVB rays, but in different proportion, the DUVR spectrum including a higher UVA proportion than the UV-SSR spectrum, in order to simulate two distinct types of sun exposure. UV-SSR spectrum mimics a condition of exposure under a summer zenithal sunlight (i.e., sunbathing on a beach in summer under a clear sky) and may rapidly lead to erythema in human skin in vivo therefore maximizing UVB impact. In turn, DUVR spectrum simulates a non-extreme condition of sun exposure corresponding to a western spring or autumn sunlight, with a solar elevation angle lower than 45°, which does not give rise to any visible immediate clinical damage [26, 53, 83, 106].

12.3.3.1 UV-SSR

It has been shown that UV-SSR induce DNA damage in keratinocytes of reconstructed skin, such as pyrimidine dimers, (6-4) photoproducts, photooxidative damage, and single-strand breaks [19, 22, 85, 98]. This was followed by an accumulation of p53 and an upregulation of genes controlled by p53 involved in DNA repair and in cell cycle regulation, such as p21, MDM2, and GADD45 genes. In addition, genes of the Nrf2 pathway were upregulated post UV-SSR exposure in keratinocytes [85]. The levels of HSP27, MnSOD, and PDX-2 proteins, also involved in oxidative stress response, were upregulated after UV-SSR exposure as revealed by proteomic profiling of reconstructed epidermis exposed to UV-SSR [62].

Histologically, changes induced by UV-SSR exposure of reconstructed skin closely resemble to those observed in vivo and those observed following pure UVB exposure. UV-SSR clearly impacted epidermis, with the induction of epidermal SBC formation 24 h after exposure, as well as an absence of laminin deposition at the basement membrane. Exposure to higher doses of UV-SSR led to an epidermal disorganization, a thickened stratum corneum and a reduction in the number of epidermal cell layers [19, 22, 46].

Repeated UV-SSR exposures also impacted the morphology of melanocytes in reconstructed skin: they became more dendritic, as observed in vivo. Exposure of pigmented reconstructed skin to UV-SSR induced an increase in melanin content and tanning of the 3-D model [4, 16, 39].

As immunosuppression is one of the main clinical consequences of UV exposure in vivo, 3-D models containing immune competent cells have been developed to study UV effects. In a reconstructed skin model including Langerhans cells, it was shown that UV-SSR exposure led to a significant decrease in the number of Langerhans cells and, for the remaining ones, a change in their morphology from a dendritic to a round cell shape [39]. These effects were reminiscent to those found in vivo associated with photoimmunosuppression [1, 7, 31, 91, 110]. Another model including Langerhans cells and dermal dendritic cells showed evidence of the migration of these cells into the dermal equivalent of the reconstructed skin exposed to UV-SSR, together with an increase in proinflammatory proteins such as TNF-α, IL1 β, IL6, IL8, and COX-2 [10, 76].

In addition to these epidermal direct effects, UV-SSR exposure of reconstructed human skin led to the increased production of MMP-1 by fibroblasts, *via* paracrine activation of epidermal keratinocytes, involving IL1 and IL6 cytokines, as it was observed after UVB exposure [46].

12.3.3.2 DUVR

While consequences of UV-SSR exposure on reconstructed skin closely resemble those observed after UVB exposure, DUVR induced features close to those found after UVA exposure. This may be related to the higher UVA/UVB ratio (23) in DUVR spectrum compared to that of UV-SSR (17).

DUVR exposure can immediately induce ROS formation in both deep keratinocytes and fibroblasts of the reconstructed skin, in a dose-dependent manner. In response to this oxidative stress, reconstructed skin cells exhibited a modulation of expression of numerous genes involved in antioxidant cell response, such as genes encoding metallothionein, Nfr2 target genes and proteins, sestrins, and methionine sulfoxide reductase A genes. The use of reconstructed skin model allowed to determine the specific responses of fibroblast and keratinocytes to oxidative stress induced by DUVR [81].

A histological analysis of reconstructed skin exposed to DUVR revealed that alterations were mostly located in the dermal compartment, with the disappearance of superficial fibroblasts, as observed after UVA exposure. In addition, several genes encoding ECM and dermal epidermal components and proteins of ECM maturation were affected by DUVR exposure. For instance, COL1A1 gene was downregulated, whereas MMP-1 and MMP-3 genes and proteins were upregulated in reconstructed skin exposed to DUVR [71, 79].

To a lesser extent than dermis, epidermis was impacted by DUVR exposure, with alterations of the granular layers also resembling those observed after UVA exposure, together with a thickened of the cornified layer. At molecular level, these changes were correlated with the modulation of expression of genes involved in the differentiation/proliferation balance, such as members of the epidermal differentiation complex, KI67, K6B, or ODC1. Altogether these epidermal changes could be linked to skin surface alterations (perturbation of hydration, skin microrelief, epidermal proliferation and thickening) observed in vivo following DUVR exposure [105, 111]. Few SBC and p53-positive keratinocytes could also be detected, as described in vivo [71, 81, 111].

The impact of DUVR on skin immunity was evidenced by the strong increase in the expression of genes encoding cytokines and inflammation markers such as IL1, IL6, IL8, CCL2, ICAM1, CSF2, TNF, and COX-2. Increase in IL6, IL8, TNF-α, and CSF2 expression was also shown at protein level. In contrast, TLR1, TLR3, and TNSF10 gene expression was downregulated [82].

12.4 Evaluation of Sunscreens in Organotypic Models

Reconstructed skins, including different types of skin cells, present a tissue organization close to that of in vivo human skin, with a correct epidermal differentiation, a dermal epidermal junction as well as cell-cell and cell-matrix interactions. Due to their 3-D architecture, they are useful tools to take into account the penetration of UV rays through the different skin compartments. Moreover major UV-induced damage observed in vivo can be reproduced in these 3-D skin models, with wavelength specific and common skin targets within epidermal and dermal compartments (Fig. 12.3).

Another great advantage of such 3-D skin models is the possibility to apply cosmetic/dermatologic formulations directly on the skin surface as it can be done in real-life situations. This aspect becomes paramount when dealing with sunscreen products that are only topically applied, forming a barrier between solar UV rays and skin cells.

By using classical endpoints and new ones such as gene expression profiling, reconstructed skins can be used to evaluate skin photoprotection incurred by chemical (organic) or physical (inorganic) sunscreens. Single absorbers or complex sunscreen formulations composed of a combination of filters, to provide the largest absorption profile comprising UVB+UVA wavelengths domains, have been tested. Table 12.1 summarizes the different studies found in the literature.

The first approach using reconstructed skin for the evaluation of photoprotective efficacy determined the global cellular viability, by performing the MTT (3-(4,5-dimethylthiazol-2-yl)-2,5-diphenyltetrazolium bromide) tetrazolium reduction assay [6, 92]. Augustin et al. tested photoprotection afforded by sunscreen ingredient, Eusolex™ 6300 (Merck, USA), a UVB blocking benzylidene camphor derivative (absorption peak at 300 nm), or Eusolex™ 8020 (Merck, USA), a UVA blocking dibenzoylmethane derivative (absorption peak at 350 nm), both diluted at 3 % and applied topically onto skin equivalents. After exposure to UVB or UVA, respectively, the residual cellular viability was found higher in photoprotected skin *versus* control, demonstrating the photoprotective effect of the filters [6]. Commercially available sunscreen products were also tested using the same protocol. A sunscreen product with a SPF (sunburn protection factor) 15 containing organic UVB or UVA filters and a sunscreen product, with ultra-high protection including mineral filters, showed both good efficacy regarding viability of skin equivalents following UVB or UVA exposure [6]. In an attempt to rank sunscreens

Table 12.1 Summary of studies using organotypic models for the evaluation of sunscreens

Sunscreen[a]	Protection factors[b]	Organotypic Model	Biological endpoints	UV source	Reference
Single absorbers (concentrations when available)					
Homosalate (8 %)	SPF 4.24	Full-thickness skin model (LSE ™)	MTT	UV-SSR	[92]
Photoplex™ (with PABA ester + BMDM)	PFA 1.8		MTT	UVA	
Padimate O (7 %)	PFA 1.31		MTT	UVA	
Benzophenone 3 (2 %, 5 %)	PFA 2.33, 3.97		MTT	UVA	
4-Methylbenzylidene camphor (3 %)	NA	Dermal equivalent	MTT	UVB	[6]
Isopropyl dibenzoylmethane (3 %)	NA	Full-thickness skin model	MTT IL1α	UVA	
2-EHMC (5 %)	SPF 5.8	Full-thickness skin model	SBC, CPDs	UVB	[18]
Terephthalylidene camphorsulfonic acid (5 %)	SPF 5.1		Dermal fibroblasts, histology, vimentin, MMP1	UVA	
Drometrizole trisiloxane	NA	Full-thickness skin model	SBC, CPDs Dermal fibroblasts, histology, vimentin	UVB UVA	[14]
Cinnamate	SPF 12	Reconstructed epidermis (DED model) +/– melanocytes	SBC, CPDs, protein oxidation, lipoperoxidation, vit E, SOD/Catalase ratio	UVB UVA UVA + UVB	[24]
TiO_2 (16 %)	SPF 28	Full-thickness skin model	6.4 PP, CPD, photooxidative damage	UV-SSR	[104]
Terephthalylidene camphorsulfonic acid (5 %)	SPF 5.1	Pigmented epidermis (DED model)	Pigmentation (visual, colorimetric L*)	UV-SSR	[39]
		Reconstructed epidermis (DED model) + Langerhans cells	Langerhans cells number and morphology (dendricity)	UV-SSR	

Terephthalylidene camphorsulfonic acid (1 % or 4 %)	NA	Reconstructed epidermis (Episkin™ model) + Langerhans cells	Langerhans cells number and morphology (dendricity), SBC	UV-SSR	[44]
Terephthalylidene camphorsulfonic acid (0.01 %)	NA	Reconstructed epidermis (Episkin™)	DNA lesions (comet assay)	UV-SSR	[49]
Complex formulations (concentrations of sunscreens when available)					
Chemical sunscreens[c]	SPF 4, 8, 12, 15	Full-thickness skin model (Skin[e]™)	IL1α release	UV-SSR	[102]
Physical sunscreen[c]	SPF 15				
4-Methylbenzylidene camphor (6 %), terephthalylidene camphorsulfonic acid (1 %), BMDM (2 %)	SPF 15	Full-thickness skin model	MTT, IL1 MTT	UVA UVB	[6]
TiO + TiO2	NA				
Terephthalylidene camphorsulfonic acid + TiO2	SPF 25 – PPD 5	Reconstructed epidermis (Episkin™)	MTT (phototoxicity induced by chlorpromazine)	UVA	[29]
Terephthalylidene camphorsulfonic acid, BMDM, 4-methylbbenzylidene camphor, TiO2	SPF 60 – PPD 12				
BMDM (3 %), benzophenone 3 (3 %), 2-ethylhexyl 2-hydroxybenzoate (5 %), 2-EHMC (7,5 %)	SPF 30	Full-thickness skin model	6,4PP, CPD, photooxidative damage	UV-SSR	[22]
Cinnamate, TiO2, ZnO	SPF 12	Reconstructed epidermis (DED) ± melanocytes	SBC, CPD, protein oxidation, lipoperoxidation, vit E, SOD/Catalase ratio	UVB UVA UVA + UVB	[24]
Cinnamate, TiO2, BMDM	SPF 12				
Octocrylene (7 %), BMDM (3 %)	SPF 7.4 – PPD 7.2	Full-thickness skin model	Histology, vimentin. SBC, CPD, histology, vimentin	UVA UV-SSR	[19]
2-EHMC (3,75 %), ZnO (7,5 %)	SPF 7.5 – PPD 2.8				

(continued)

Table 12.1 (continued)

Sunscreen[a]	Protection factors[b]	Organotypic Model	Biological endpoints	UV source	Reference
TiO_2 (11 %), ZnO (4 %)	NA	Reconstructed epidermis (SkinEthic™ RHE)	Histology, SBC, viability, p53 protein expression	UV-SSR	[51]
Octyl methoxycinnamate (4 %), methylene bis-benzothiazolyl tetramethylbutylphenol (4 %), TiO_2 (1 %), ZnO (0.5 %)	NA				
BMDM (1.5 %), ethylhexyl triazone (2 %), ethylbenzilidene camphor (5 %) in 15 % Miglyol®	SPF 25,2	Full-thickness skin model	Dermal fibroblasts, histology, vimentin, MMP1	UVA-UV-SSR	[84]
BMDM (1.5 %), ethylhexyl triazone (2 %), octyl methoxycinnamate (5 %) in 15 % vaseline oil	SPF 22,8				
BMDM (2 %), octocrylene (10 %), terephthalylidene camphorsulfonic acid (2 %)	SPF 15	Full-thickness skin model	Dermal fibroblasts, histology, vimentin, MMP1	DUVR	[71]
Octyl methoxycinnamate (6 %), ZnO (3 %)	SPF 15				
BMDM (3 %), terephthalylidene camphorsulfonic acid (3 %), octocrylene (5 %), drometrizole trisiloxane (1 %)	SPF 18				
Octocrylene (2.5 %), ethylhexyl methoxycinnamate (7.5 %), ethylhexyl salicylate (2.5 %), ZnO (6 %)	SPF 27				
2-EHMC, BEMT, methylene bis-benzotriazolyl, tetramethylbutylphenol	NA	Reconstructed epidermis (SkinEthic™ RHE)	Cell viability (LDH, ERK2 release), DNA damage (thymin dimers, DNA fragmentation), apoptosis (TUNEL, caspase 3 activation), SBC	UV-SSR	[8]

BMDM (3 %), homosalate (15 %), ethylhexyl salicylate (5 %), octocrylene (4.5 %), benzophenone 3 (6 %)	SPF 45	Full-thickness skin model (StrataTest™)	ROS (DCFH-DA), IL1α, IL1-RA, CPD	UV-SSR	[101]
BMDM (4 %), octocrylene (2.5 %), ethylhexyl salicylate (5 %), terephthalylidene dicamphor sulfonic acid (1 %), drometrizole trisiloxane (0.5 %), TiO_2 (4.5 %), ethylhexyl triazone (1 %), BEMT (3 %)	SPF 67.5- PPD 31.1	Full-thickness skin model	Gene expression/Protein expression	UVA	[78]
BMDM (3 %), octocrylene (5 %), ethylhexyl salicylate (5 %), terephthalylidene dicamphor sulfonic acid (3 %)	SPF 13- PPD 10.5	Full-thickness skin model	Gene expression/Protein expression	DUVR	[82]
Commercial sunscreens SPF >20+/UVA protection	SPF 20–50	Full-thickness skin model (EpiDerm™ Full Thickness)	DMPO protein-radical adduct	UV-SSR	[61]
BMDM (5 %), –2-EHMC (10 %)	SPF 15				
TiO_2 (7.5 %)	SPF 15				
UVA enhancer-TiO_2 (7.5 %)	SPF 15				
ZnO (4.12 %), octyl methoxycinnamate (5.5 %)	SPF 30	Full thickness skin model (EpiDerm™-FT)	CPDs, SBC	UV-SSR	[35]

[a]INCI names

[b]Protections factors determined in vivo. *NA* not available in the literature

[c]The composition is not available in the literature. *DED* dead de-epidermized dermis, *2-EHMC* 2ethylhexyl methoxycinnamate, *BMDM* butylmethoxy dibenzoylmethane, *MTT* 3-(4,5-dimethylthiazol-2-yl)-2,5-diphenyltetrazolium bromide, *BEMT* bis-ethylhexyloxyphenol methoxyphenyl triazine, *SPF* sunburn protection factor, *PPD* persistent pigment darkening [87], *PFA* protection factor UVA measured by delayed erythema or tanning 24 h after exposure to UVA [30], *DUVR* daily UV radiation, *CPD* pyrimidine dimers, *6,4PP* 6,4 photoproducts, *SBC* sunburn cells, *MMP1* matrix metalloproteinase 1

on their photoprotection efficacy, Nelson and Gay compared three UVA filters and one placebo having different UVA protection factors established in human skin by scoring delayed erythema or tanning 24 h after UVA exposure [30]. Placebo, 7 % padimate O, 2 % oxybenzones, and 5 % oxybenzones exhibited in vivo UVA protection factors of 1.15, 1.31, 2.33, and 3.97, respectively. Cytotoxicity measurements in Living Skin Equivalent (LSE™), a full-thickness skin model, exposed to UVA allowed the authors to calculate in vitro photoprotection values of sunscreens, by dividing the UVA_{50} in the sunscreen-applied skin equivalents by the UVA_{50} in the unprotected samples. All the tested filters exhibited a higher photoprotection efficacy compared to untreated skin. However, in vitro photoprotection values did not fully rank sunscreens as in vivo protection factors. The authors suggested that such discrepancy may be related to the different UVA light sources used in in vivo and in vitro studies, due to the use of different cut-off filters (2 mm WG-345 filter in vitro *vs* 3 mm WG-335 filter in vivo) [92].

Beyond cytotoxicity and because UVB and UVA induced specific damage in human skin, endpoints related to wavelength range have been used in photoprotection studies.

In vivo, one of the first approaches to evaluate protection of sunscreens is the determination of the SPF based on the prevention of cutaneous erythema, an endpoint mostly induced by UVB radiation. The clinical appearance of erythema has been correlated with the formation of epidermal SBC, whose apoptotic process is due to high levels of unrepaired DNA lesions. Moreover it has been shown in vivo that sunscreens with appropriate SPF values are efficient in preventing UV-induced DNA lesions [50, 72]. For these reasons, SBC and thymine dimer formation appeared to be relevant to evaluate photoprotection against UVB or UV-SSR-induced damage. Using these endpoints, the photoprotective efficiency of 2-ethylhexyl-p-methoxycinnamate (2-EHMC, Parsol™ MCX), a UVB absorber, with an in vivo SPF of 5.8, was tested in reconstructed skin exposed to UVB rays. By analyzing thymine dimers and SBC formation after application of 2-EHMC, the authors showed that the highest dose able to prevent SBC formation corresponded to five times the biological efficient dose previously determined in the in vitro model [18], in line with the in vivo SPF value (Fig. 12.4). Studying the protection afforded by the UVB filter cinnamate, or complex formulations including cinnamate, Cario-André et al. confirmed the relevance of using the prevention of SBC and CPD formation as endpoints after UVB or UVA+UVB exposure of reconstructed epidermis on dead de-epidermized dermis [24].

The quantification of UV-induced lesions, i.e., pyrimidine dimers, 6,4-photoproducts, and photooxidative damage, in the epidermis of reconstructed skin by alkaline gel electrophoresis and radioimmunoassay methods, was also used to evaluate chemical or physical sunscreens. This allowed the determination of a DNA protection factor (DNA-PF) defined as the frequency of lesions induced in unprotected reconstructed skin divided by the frequency of lesions induced in sunscreen-protected samples. Results suggested that, using this method, a 1-2 DNA-PF would correspond to an SPF 30 sunscreen [22, 104].

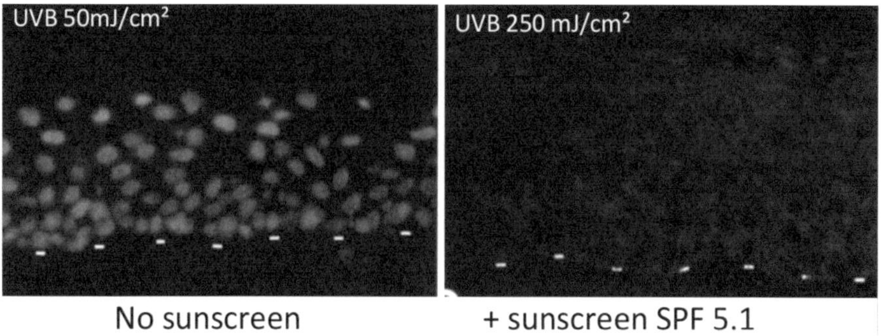

Fig. 12.4 Thymine dimers DNA lesions used for the evaluation of UVB photoprotection. Without prior sunscreen application, thymine dimers are immediately formed after exposure to pure UVB (50 mJ/cm^2) as revealed by the H3 antibody. When a sunscreen absorbing in the UVB range is applied prior to UVB exposure, the DNA lesions can be prevented. Note that the highest dose able to prevent thymine dimer formation is fivefold the biologically efficient dose, in line with the SPF value of 5.8 (Adapted from Bernerd et al. [18])

In addition to DNA damage and SBC formation, other UV-SSR-induced epidermal damages have been used in reconstructed epidermis for sunscreen evaluation after UV-SSR exposure, such as p53 protein expression and apoptosis [8, 51].

The contribution of UVA rays to photoaging and photocarcinogenesis are now well-established, therefore, evaluation of UVA photoprotection becomes crucial. Major alterations induced by UVA exposure are located in the deepest layers of the reconstructed skin, especially within the dermal compartment, with the apoptosis of dermal fibroblasts and MMP1 release in the culture medium. Using these endpoints, the photoprotection afforded by two UVA filters, terephthalylidene dicamphorsulfonic acid (Mexoryl™ SX) and drometrizole trisiloxane (Mexoryl™ XL), was assayed on a full-thickness reconstructed skin model. Each filter prevented the disappearance of fibroblasts and the MMP1 release in culture medium induced by UVA exposure. Since both products can also absorb UVB wavelengths, they were also shown to prevent UVB-induced SBC and thymine dimers. In contrast, 2-EHMC, a pure UVB absorber, was unable to prevent UVA-induced dermal alterations. These results demonstrated that using specific UVB and UVA endpoints, it became possible to discriminate the biological efficacy of single absorbers [14, 18]. These in vitro results fully correlate with in vivo data that showed the efficiency of Mexoryl™ SX in preventing dermal damage induced by repeated UVA exposures [107].

Such UVA- and UVB-specific endpoints were also useful to assess and compare the protection afforded by two sunscreen products with different absorption profiles. The tested products exhibited the same SPF values (7.4 and 7.3) but different UVA protection factors (7.2 and 2.8, respectively, as determined by the persistent pigment darkening, PPD, method). Following UVB exposure, the two products showed the same protection efficiency against SBC and pyrimidine dimers in agreement with their similar SPF values. In contrast, following UVA or UV-SSR exposure, dose-response experiments showed that the sunscreen with the highest UVA-PF provided a better protection with regard to dermal damage, as compared to the other one (Fig. 12.5) [19]. These results pointed out that the SPF value is, per se, not sufficient to reflect the efficiency of sunscreens over the entire solar UV spectrum and against the major biological damage induced by sun exposure. These in vitro results were also in agreement with an in vivo study using the same sunscreen products showing a higher efficacy of the product having a UVB-UVA balanced absorption profile [108].

Because of the major contribution of UVA rays in daily UV radiation exposure [79], the importance of UVA absorption by sunscreens was also demonstrated under a non-zenithal UV exposure condition. Two commercial sunscreens with similar SPF values (approx. 15) but with different absorption profiles in the UVA range were tested on reconstructed skins exposed to DUVR. The sunscreen formulation with the highest UVA-PF afforded a better protection of dermal damage such as fibroblast disappearance and MMP1 release than the other one. To test if a highest SPF could compensate a low UVA-PF, the protection against DUVR-induced damage of two other sunscreen products were compared: one product having an SPF of 27 and a low UVA absorption and the other having an SPF of 18 and a well-balanced UVB-UVA absorption profile. The study of prevention against dermal alterations indicated that a higher SPF value did not compensate for low UVA filtration, the SPF18 product with well-balanced UVA-UVB absorption being more effective than the SPF27 product [71].

Endpoints related to oxidative stress have been used to study UVA or UVB+UVA photoprotection, such as protein and lipid oxidation and antioxidant depletion. However, protective effects of sunscreens were not fully evidenced using these endpoints, partly due to the difficulty of spreading the cream onto reconstructed skin samples [24].

The importance of sunscreen photostability in photoprotection has also been addressed using a full-thickness model of reconstructed skin. A photostable sunscreen formulation was compared to a photounstable formulation after topical application on reconstructed skin further exposed to UVA or to UV-SSR. The results evidenced that only the photostable product ensured an efficient photoprotection against UVA or UV-SSR dermal damage and MMP1 production [84].

In order to assess some biological endpoints that could be related to other clinical consequences of UV exposure such as pigmentation or photoimmunosuppression, photoprotection against UV-induced pigmentation or UV-induced alterations of Langerhans cells can be tested in adapted 3-D models (Fig. 12.6). For example, the application of the broad-spectrum absorber Mexoryl™ SX on a model of reconstructed pigmented epidermis was able to prevent UV-induced pigmentation as visually assessed and by measuring the luminance L* factor [39]. In addition, in 3-D models comprising Langerhans cells, the same filter preserved the morphology and the number of Langerhans cells under UV-SSR exposure [39, 44].

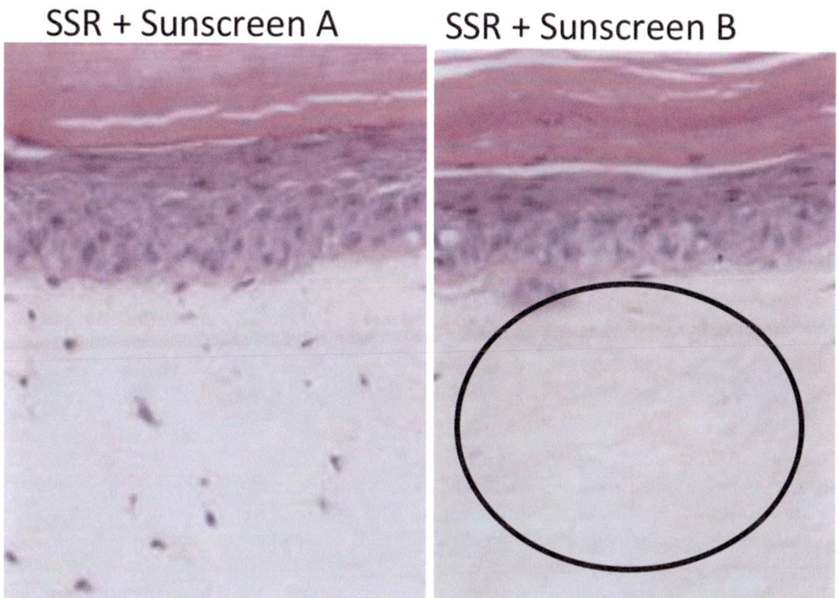

	SPF	UVA-PF (PPD)
A	7.4 ± 1.5	7.2 ± 1.8
B	7.5 ± 1.6	2.8 ± 0.8

Fig. 12.5 Dermal fibroblast alterations and disappearance used for evaluating UVA photoprotection. Sunscreen A or sunscreen B was applied onto full-thickness skins prior to exposure to the same dose of UV-SSR. Whereas sunscreen A, having the higher UVA protection factor (UVA-PF), is able to protect the skin against dermal damage, sunscreen B is not efficient in preventing the dermal fibroblasts disappearance (*oval*). No epidermal changes were observed in both cases under such a UV-SSR exposure due to the same SPF value of both sunscreens products (Adapted from Bernerd et al. [19])

More recent technologies such as transcriptomic and proteomic, which allow large-scale analyses of gene and protein expression to be performed, can also be useful in the field of photobiology. They evidenced that UV exposure induces numerous changes in gene and protein expression, revealing the diversity of biological functions that can be altered by UV radiation [9, 23, 41, 80, 89, 112]. Gene expression analysis was recently used to evaluate photoprotection efficacy of sunscreens. In a reconstructed skin model, the UVA protection incurred by a broad-spectrum sun care product was tested by studying the expression of more than 200 genes related to skin biology and stress, in dermal fibroblasts and in epidermal keratinocytes, respectively. The results showed that UVA exposure led to the

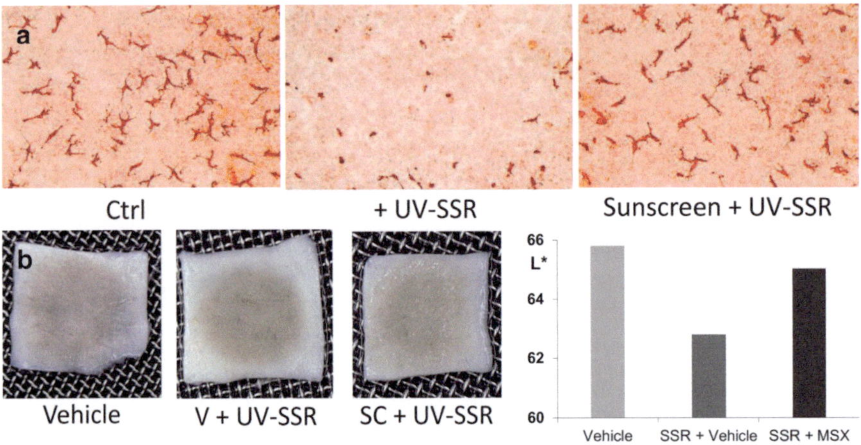

Fig. 12.6 Reconstructed epidermis containing Langerhans cells or melanocytes for the evaluation of photoprotection. (**a**) Epidermal sheets stained with anti-Langerin antibody. In control (*Ctrl*) sample, the Langerhans cells are randomly distributed throughout the epidermis while in the UV-SSR-exposed sample, Langerhans cells are sparse, and the remaining cells display a round and non-dendritic morphology. Application of the sunscreen before UV-SSR exposure prevented these alterations. (**b**) Reconstructed epidermis (DED model) containing melanocytes. The pigmentation is increased after exposure to UV-SSR, but this increase can be limited when the sunscreen is applied onto the sample prior to UV-SSR exposure. Pigmentation is assessed macroscopically and by measuring the luminance L*parameter (Adapted from Facy et al. [44] and Duval et al. [39]). *MSX* Mexoryl™ SX

modulation of gene expression in both cell types (32 modulated genes in fibroblasts and 44 in keratinocytes). The modulated genes were involved in ECM homeostasis, oxidative stress, heat shock response, cell growth, inflammation, and epidermal differentiation. Application of sunscreen on reconstructed skin before UV exposure mitigated these effects, with a reduction in the number of modulated genes (4 modulated genes in fibroblasts and 11 in keratinocytes) and in the intensity of modulation of the residual modulated genes (Fig. 12.7). The UVA-induced release of MMP1 protein and proinflammatory cytokines in the culture medium was also alleviated by using the sunscreen (Fig. 12.7). Prevention of gene expression modulation incurred by the sunscreen was confirmed in human skin in vivo by quantifying the expression of five genes involved in oxidative stress response and photoaging (HO-1, SOD2, GPX, CAT and MMP1), reinforcing the relevance of using the 3-D model to test photoprotection on such endpoints [78].

Gene expression analysis in fibroblasts and keratinocytes of reconstructed skin was also used to assess photoprotection efficiency of a broad-spectrum sunscreen (SPF 13, UVA-PF (PPD) 10.5) against DUVR. Again, this method demonstrated the protection afforded by the sunscreen, with very close gene expression profiles between unexposed samples and DUVR exposed but protected samples, as shown by hierarchical clustering, a decreased number of modulated genes, and a decrease in intensity of gene modulation for the residual modulated genes [82]. Thus, gene expression profiling constitutes a complementary approach to histological and biochemical studies for assessing of photoprotection in 3-D skin models.

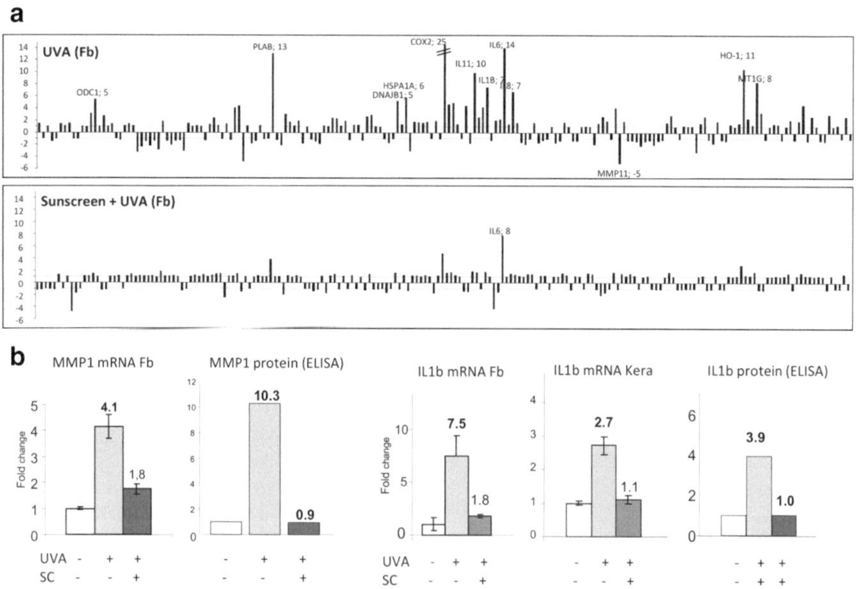

Fig. 12.7 The use of gene and protein expression for the evaluation of sunscreen efficacy. (**a**) Modulation levels of gene expression in fibroblasts of reconstructed skin exposed to UVA. *Bars* represent modulation ratios after UVA exposure for each studied transcript. Positive and negative values denote up- and downregulation of gene expression, respectively. Note the flatter aspect of the modulation profile when the broad-spectrum sunscreen was used (*lower panel*), as compared to unprotected samples (*upper panel*). (**b**) Examples of gene and soluble-protein expression after UVA exposure of reconstructed skin in the presence or absence of broad-spectrum sunscreen (Adapted from Marionnet et al. [78])

12.5 Conclusion

The development of organotypic skin models has made possible the in vitro assessment of the effects of different types of UV exposure (UVB, UVA, or solar simulation) in a three-dimensional context and in a cutaneous structure including different types of skin cells. Reconstructed skin appeared to be useful, showing predictive responses with numerous biological endpoints closely related to in vivo clinical data. It also allowed to increase the knowledge on the precise biological processes involved and can therefore be used to study the photoprotection afforded by sunscreens in vitro, providing additional biological data on sunscreen efficacy, complementing the in vivo protection factors (SPF or UVA-PF). Although these 3-D models did not follow a strict validation process for protection factor determination, they evidenced important concepts in photoprotection, such as the need of using a well-balanced photostable sunscreen absorbing over the entire UV spectrum of solar radiation for preserving essential biological functions. They also revealed from a biological point of view the limits of the SPF value for predicting the level of protection in the UVA range. The combination of 3-D skin models and new biological approaches such as transcriptomic or proteomic will indisputably increase the added value of such systems for evaluating sunscreen.

References

1. Aberer W, Schuler G, Stingl G et al (1981) Ultraviolet light depletes surface markers of Langerhans cells. J Invest Dermatol 76:202–210
2. Afaq F, Zaid MA, Khan N et al (2009) Protective effect of pomegranate-derived products on UVB-mediated damage in human reconstituted skin. Exp Dermatol 18:553–561
3. Applegate LA, Noel A, Vile G et al (1995) Two genes contribute to different extents to the heme oxygenase enzyme activity measured in cultured human skin fibroblasts and keratinocytes: implications for protection against oxidant stress. Photochem Photobiol 61:285–291
4. Archambault M, Yaar M, Gilchrest BA (1995) Keratinocytes and fibroblasts in a human skin equivalent model enhance melanocyte survival and melanin synthesis after ultraviolet irradiation. J Invest Dermatol 104:859–867
5. Asselineau D, Bernhard B, Bailly C et al (1985) Epidermal morphogenesis and induction of the 67 kD keratin polypeptide by culture of human keratinocytes at the liquid-air interface. Exp Cell Rės 159:536–539
6. Augustin C, Collombel C, Damour O (1997) Measurements of the protective effect of topically applied sunscreens using in vitro three-dimensional dermal and skin equivalents. Photochem Photobiol 66:853–859
7. Bacci S, Romagnoli P, Streilein JW (1998) Reduction in number and morphologic alterations of Langerhans cells after UVB radiation in vivo are accompanied by an influx of monocytoid cells into the epidermis. J Invest Dermatol 111:1134–1139
8. Bacqueville D, Mavon A (2009) Comparative analysis of solar radiation-induced cellular damage between ex vivo porcine skin organ culture and in vitro reconstructed human epidermis. Int J Cosmet Sci 31:293–302
9. Bart G, Hamalainen L, Rauhala L et al (2014) rClca2 is associated with epidermal differentiation and is strongly downregulated by ultraviolet radiation. Br J Dermatol 171:376–387
10. Bechetoille N, Dezutter-Dambuyant C, Damour O et al (2007) Effects of solar ultraviolet radiation on engineered human skin equivalent containing both Langerhans cells and dermal dendritic cells. Tissue Eng 13:2667–2679
11. Berneburg M, Kurten V, Grether-Beck S et al (1998) Induction of mitochondrial (MT) DNA mutations in human fibroblasts by in vitro ultraviolet A irradiation. J Invest Dermatol 110:489
12. Bernerd F, Asselineau D (1997) Successive alteration and recovery of epidermal differentiation and morphogenesis after specific UVB-damages in skin reconstructed in vitro. Dev Biol 183:123–138
13. Bernerd F, Asselineau D (1998) UVA exposure of human skin reconstructed in vitro induces apoptosis of dermal fibroblasts: subsequent connective tissue repair and implications in photoaging. Cell Death Differ 5:792–802
14. Bernerd F, Asselineau D (2001) Reconstructed human skin: effect of solar UV light and use to evaluate efficiency of sunscreens in vitro. Cosmet Dermatol 14:15–19
15. Bernerd F, Asselineau D, Vioux C et al (2001) Clues to epidermal cancer proneness revealed by reconstruction of DNA repair-deficient xeroderma pigmentosum skin in vitro. Proc Natl Acad Sci U S A 98:7817–7822
16. Bernerd F, Marionnet C, Duval C (2012) Solar ultraviolet radiation induces biological alterations in human skin in vitro: relevance of a well-balanced UVA/UVB protection. Indian J Dermatol Venereol Leprol 78(Suppl):S15–S23
17. Bernerd F, Sarasin A, Magnaldo T (1999) Galectin-7 overexpression is associated with the apoptotic process in UVB-induced sunburn keratinocytes. Proc Natl Acad Sci U S A 96:11329–11334
18. Bernerd F, Vioux C, Asselineau D (2000) Evaluation of the protective effect of sunscreens on in vitro reconstructed human skin exposed to UVB or UVA irradiation. Photochem Photobiol 71:314–320
19. Bernerd F, Vioux C, Lejeune F et al (2003) The sun protection factor (SPF) inadequately defines broad spectrum photoprotection: demonstration using skin reconstructed in vitro exposed to UVA, UVBor UV-solar simulated radiation. Eur J Dermatol 13:242–249

20. Bessou S, Surlève-Bazeille JE, Pain C et al (1996) Ex vivo study of skin phototypes. J Invest Dermatol 107:684–688
21. Bessou S, Surlève-Bazeille JE, Sorbier E et al (1995) Ex vivo reconstruction of the epidermis with melanocytes and the influence of UVB. Pigment Cell Res 8:241–249
22. Bissonauth V, Drouin R, Mitchell DL et al (2000) The efficacy of a broad-spectrum sunscreen to protect engineered human skin from tissue and DNA damage induced by solar ultraviolet exposure. Clin Cancer Res 6:4128–4135
23. Blumenberg M (2006) DNA microarrays in dermatology and skin biology. OMICS 10: 243–260
24. Cario-André M, Briganti S, Picardo M et al (2002) Epidermal reconstructs: a new tool to study topical and systemic photoprotective molecules. J Photochem Photobiol B 68:79–87
25. Chen VL, Fleischmajer R, Schwartz E et al (1986) Immunochemistry of elastotic material in sun-damaged skin. J Invest Dermatol 87:334–337
26. Christiaens FJ, Chardon A, Fourtanier A et al (2005) Standard ultraviolet daylight for nonextreme exposure conditions. Photochem Photobiol 81:874–878
27. Clausen BE, Kel JM (2010) Langerhans cells: critical regulators of skin immunity? Immunol Cell Biol 88:351–360
28. Clydesdale GJ, Dandie GW, Muller HK (2001) Ultraviolet light induced injury: immunological and inflammatory effects. Immunol Cell Biol 79:547–568
29. Cohen C, Roguet R, Cottin M (1998) The use of a reconstructed epidermis in the evaluation of protective effect of sunscreens against chemical phototoxicity by UVA. In: Rougier A, Schaefer H (eds) Protection of the skin against utraviolet radiations. John Libbey Eurotext, Paris, pp 195–199
30. Cole C, VanFossen R (1992) Measurement of sunscreen UVA protection: an unsensitized human model. J Am Acad Dermatol 26:178–184
31. Cooper KD, Oberhelman L, Hamilton TA et al (1992) UV exposure reduces immunization rates and promotes tolerance to epicutaneous antigens in humans: relationship to dose, CD1a-DR+ epidermal macrophage induction, and Langerhans cell depletion. Proc Natl Acad Sci U S A 89:8497–8501
32. Corsini E, Sangha N, Feldman SR (1997) Epidermal stratification reduces the effects of UVB (but not UVA) on keratinocyte cytokine production and cytotoxicity. Photodermatol Photoimmunol Photomed 13:147–152
33. Cotovio J, Pellevoisin C, Parsad D (2014) *In vitro* skin models. In: Srinivas CR, Verschoore M (eds) Basic science for modern cosmetic dermatology. Jaypee Brothers Medical Publishers, New Delhi, pp 25–46
34. Coulomb B, Lebreton C, Mathieu N et al (1996) UVA-induced oxidative damage in fibroblasts cultured in a 3-dimensional collagen matrix. Exp Dermatol 5:161–167
35. Dehaven C, Hayden PJ, Armento A, Oldach J (2014) DNA photoprotection conveyed by sunscreen. J Cosmet Dermatol 13:99–102
36. Dekker P, Parish WE, Green MR (2005) Protection by food-derived antioxidants from UV-A1-induced photodamage, measured using living skin equivalents. Photochem Photobiol 81:837–842
37. Duval C, Chagnoleau C, Pouradier F et al (2012) Human skin model containing melanocytes: essential role of keratinocyte growth factor for constitutive pigmentation-functional response to alpha-melanocyte stimulating hormone and forskolin. Tissue Eng Part C Methods 18: 947–957
38. Duval C, Regnier M, Schmidt R (2001) Distinct melanogenic response of human melanocytes in mono-culture, in co-culture with keratinocytes and in reconstructed epidermis, to UV exposure. Pigment Cell Res 14:348–355
39. Duval C, Schmidt R, Regnier M et al (2003) The use of reconstructed human skin to evaluate UV-induced modifications and sunscreen efficacy. Exp Dermatol 12 Suppl 2:64–70
40. Egles C, Garlick JA, Shamis Y (2010) Three-dimensional human tissue models of wounded skin. Methods Mol Biol 585:345–359

41. Enk CD, Shahar I, Amariglio N et al (2004) Gene expression profiling of in vivo UVB-irradiated human epidermis. Photodermatol Photoimmunol Photomed 20:129–137
42. Eungdamrong NJ, Higgins C, Guo Z et al (2014) Challenges and promises in modeling dermatologic disorders with bioengineered skin. Exp Biol Med (Maywood) 239:1215–1224
43. Evans-Johnson JA, Garlick JA, Johnson EJ et al (2013) A pilot study of the photoprotective effect of almond phytochemicals in a 3D human skin equivalent. J Photochem Photobiol B 126:17–25
44. Facy V, Flouret V, Régnier M et al (2005) Reactivity of Langerhans cells in human reconstructed epidermis to known allergens and UV radiation. Toxicol In Vitro 19:787–795
45. Fagot D, Asselineau D, Bernerd F (2002) Direct role of human dermal fibroblasts and indirect participation of epidermal keratinocytes in MMP-1 production after UV-B irradiation. Arch Dermatol Res 293:576–583
46. Fagot D, Asselineau D, Bernerd F (2004) Matrix metalloproteinase-1 production observed after solar-simulated radiation exposure is assumed by dermal fibroblasts but involves a paracrine activation through epidermal keratinocytes. Photochem Photobiol 79:499–505
47. Fernandez TL, Van Lonkhuyzen DR, Dawson RA et al (2014) Characterization of a human skin equivalent model to study the effects of ultraviolet B radiation on keratinocytes. Tissue Eng Part C Methods 20:588–598
48. Fisher GJ, Datta SC, Talwar HS et al (1996) Molecular basis of sun-induced premature skin ageing and retinoid antagonism. Nature 379:335–339
49. Flamand N, Marrot L, Belaidi JP et al (2006) Development of genotoxicity test procedures with Episkin, a reconstructed human skin model: towards new tools for in vitro risk assessment of dermally applied compounds? Mutat Res 606:39–51
50. Freeman SE, Ley RD, Ley KD (1988) Sunscreen protection against UV-induced pyrimidine dimers in DNA of human skin in situ. Photodermatol 5:243–247
51. Gelis C, Mavon A, Vicendo P (2003) Evaluation of biological effects of ultraviolet radiations and of photoprotection on human reconstructed epidermis. Nouvelles Dermatol 22:351
52. Gibbs S, Murli S, De Boer G et al (2000) Melanosome capping of keratinocytes in pigmented reconstructed epidermis–effect of ultraviolet radiation and 3-isobutyl-1-methyl-xanthine on melanogenesis. Pigment Cell Res 13:458–466
53. Grothmann K, Kaase H (1993) Testung von Lichtschutzmitteln: Vorschlag zur Definition einer Referenz-Spektralverteilung für UV-Sonnensimulatoren (Sun protection measurement: proposal for a definition of a UV solar simulator standard spectrum). Dermatol Monatsschr 179:108–111
54. Gruber F, Oskolkova O, Leitner A et al (2007) Photooxidation generates biologically active phospholipids that induce heme oxygenase-1 in skin cells. J Biol Chem 282:16934–16941
55. Haake AR, Polakowska RR (1995) UV-induced apoptosis in skin equivalents: inhibition by phorbol ester and Bcl-2 overexpression. Cell Death Differ 2:183–193
56. Haake A, Scott GA, Holbrook KA (2001) Structure and function of the skin: overview of the epidermis and dermis. In: Freinkel RK, Woodley DT (eds) The biology of the skin. Parthenon Publishing Group Limited, Lancs, pp 19–45
57. Halliday GM (2005) Inflammation, gene mutation and photoimmunosuppression in response to UVR-induced oxidative damage contributes to photocarcinogenesis. Mutat Res 571:107–120
58. Halliday GM, Byrne SN, Damian DL (2011) Ultraviolet A radiation: its role in immunosuppression and carcinogenesis. Semin Cutan Med Surg 30:214–221
59. Halliday GM, Cadet J (2012) It's all about position: the basal layer of human epidermis is particularly susceptible to different types of sunlight-induced DNA damage. J Invest Dermatol 132:265–267
60. Harriger MD, Hull BE (1994) Characterization of ultraviolet radiation-induced damage to keratinocytes in a skin equivalent in vitro. Arch Dermatol Res 286:319–324
61. Haywood R, Volkov A, Andrady C et al (2012) Measuring sunscreen protection against solar-simulated radiation-induced structural radical damage to skin using ESR/spin trapping: development of an ex vivo test method. Free Radic Res 46:265–275

62. Hensbergen PJ, Alewijnse AE, Kempenaar J et al (2005) Proteomic profiling identifies an UV-induced activation of cofilin-1 and destrin in human epidermis. J Invest Dermatol 124:818–824
63. Huang XX, Bernerd F, Halliday GM (2009) Ultraviolet A within sunlight induces mutations in the epidermal basal layer of engineered human skin. Am J Pathol 174:1534–1543
64. Javeri A, Huang XX, Bernerd F et al (2008) Human 8-oxoguanine-DNA glycosylase 1 protein and gene are expressed more abundantly in the superficial than basal layer of human epidermis. DNA Repair (Amst) 7:1542–1550
65. Kochevar I, Taylor R, Krutmann J (2008) Fundamentals of cutaneous photobiology and photoimmunology. In: Wolff K, Goldsmith LA, Katz SI (eds) Fitzpatrick's dermatology in general medicine, 7th edn. McGraw-Hill, New York, pp 797–808
66. Kurdykowski S, Mine S, Bardey V et al (2011) Ultraviolet-B irradiation induces differential regulations of hyaluronidase expression and activity in normal human keratinocytes. Photochem Photobiol 87:1105–1112
67. Kypriotou M, Huber M, Hohl D (2012) The human epidermal differentiation complex: cornified envelope precursors, S100 proteins and the 'fused genes' family. Exp Dermatol 21:643–649
68. Lavker RM, Veres DA, Irwin CJ et al (1995) Quantitative assessment of cumulative damage from repetitive exposures to suberythemogenic doses of UVA in human skin. Photochem Photobiol 62:348–352
69. Lee SJ, Jung TH, Kim H et al (2014) Inhibition of c-Kit signaling by diosmetin isolated from Chrysanthemum morifolium. Arch Pharm Res 37:175–185
70. Lehmann B, Genehr T, Knuschke P et al (2001) UVB-induced conversion of 7-dehydrocholesterol to 1α, 25- dihydroxyvitamin D3 in an in vitro human skin equivalent model. J Invest Dermatol 117:1179–1185
71. Lejeune F, Christiaens F, Bernerd F (2008) Evaluation of sunscreen products using a reconstructed skin model exposed to simulated daily ultraviolet radiation: relevance of filtration profile and SPF value for daily photoprotection. Photodermatol Photoimmunol Photomed 24:249–255
72. Ley RD, Fourtanier A (1997) Sunscreen protection against ultraviolet radiation-induced pyrimidine dimers in mouse epidermal DNA. Photochem Photobiol 65:1007–1011
73. Lin JY, Fisher DE (2007) Melanocyte biology and skin pigmentation. Nature 445:843–850
74. Lowe NJ, Meyers DP, Wieder JM et al (1995) Low doses of repetitive ultraviolet A induce morphologic changes in human skin. J Invest Dermatol 105:739–743
75. MacNeil S (2007) Progress and opportunities for tissue-engineered skin. Nature 445: 874–880
76. Mahns A, Wolber R, Stab F et al (2004) Contribution of UVB and UVA to UV-dependent stimulation of cyclooxygenase-2 expression in artificial epidermis. Photochem Photobiol Sci 3:257–262
77. Maresca V, Flori E, Briganti S et al (2006) UVA-induced modification of catalase charge properties in the epidermis is correlated with the skin phototype. J Invest Dermatol 126:182–190
78. Marionnet C, Grether-Beck S, Seite S et al (2011) A broad-spectrum sunscreen prevents UVA radiation-induced gene expression in reconstructed skin in vitro and in human skin in vivo. Exp Dermatol 20:477–482
79. Marionnet C, Lejeune F, Pierrard C et al (2012) Biological contribution of UVA wavelengths in non extreme daily UV exposure. J Dermatol Sci 66:238–240
80. Marionnet C, Pierrard C, Golebiewski C et al (2014) Diversity of biological effects induced by Longwave UVA rays (UVA1) in reconstructed skin. PLoS One 9:e105263
81. Marionnet C, Pierrard C, Lejeune F et al (2010) Different oxidative stress response in keratinocytes and fibroblasts of reconstructed skin exposed to non extreme daily-ultraviolet radiation. PLoS One 5:e12059
82. Marionnet C, Pierrard C, Lejeune F et al (2012) Modulations of gene expression induced by daily ultraviolet light can be prevented by a broad spectrum sunscreen. J Photochem Photobiol B 116:37–47

83. Marionnet C, Tricaud C, Bernerd F (2014) Exposure to non-extreme solar UV daylight: spectral characterization, effects on skin and photoprotection. Int J Mol Sci 16:68–90
84. Marrot L, Belaïdi JP, Lejeune F et al (2004) Photostability of sunscreen products influences the efficiency of protection with regard to UV-induced genotoxic or photoageing-related endpoints. Br J Dermatol 151:1234–1244
85. Marrot L, Planel E, Ginestet AC et al (2010) In vitro tools for photobiological testing: molecular responses to simulated solar UV of keratinocytes growing as monolayers or as part of reconstructed skin. Photochem Photobiol Sci 9:448–458
86. Meloni M, Farina A, de Servi B (2010) Molecular modifications of dermal and epidermal biomarkers following UVA exposures on reconstructed full-thickness human skin. Photochem Photobiol Sci 9:439–447
87. Moyal D, Chardon A, Kollias N (2000) Determination of UVA protection factors using the persistent pigment darkening (PPD) as the end point. (Part 1). Calibration of the method. Photodermatol Photoimmunol Photomed 16:245–249
88. Moysan A, Clement-Lacroix P, Michel L et al (1996) Effects of ultraviolet A and antioxidant defense in cultured fibroblasts and keratinocytes. Photodermatol Photoimmunol Photomed 11:192–197
89. Muller HK, Woods GM (2013) Ultraviolet radiation effects on the proteome of skin cells. Adv Exp Med Biol 990:111–119
90. Nakazawa K, Nakazawa H, Sahuc F et al (1997) Pigmented human skin equivalent: new method of reconstitution by grafting an epithelial sheet onto a non-contractile dermal equivalent. Pigment Cell Res 10:382–390
91. Neale R, Russell A, Muller HK et al (1997) Sun exposure, sunscreen and their effects on epidermal Langerhans cells. Photochem Photobiol 66:260–264
92. Nelson D, Gay RJ (1993) Effects of UV irradiation on a living skin equivalent. Photochem Photobiol 57:830–837
93. Nix TE Jr (1967) Ultraviolet-induced changes in epidermis. In: Zelickson AS (ed) Ultrastructure of normal and abnormal skin. Lea & Febiger, Philadelphia, pp 304–319
94. Nix TE Jr, Nordquist RE, Scott JR et al (1965) Ultrastructural changes induced by ultraviolet light in human epidermis: basal and spinous layers. J Invest Dermatol 45:52–64
95. Obi-Tabot ET, Tian XQ, Chen TC et al (2000) A human skin equivalent model that mimics the photoproduction of vitamin D3 in human skin. In Vitro Cell Dev Biol 36:201–204
96. Olsen WM (1988) Early cell kinetic effects of a single dose of monochromatic ultraviolet B irradiation on hairless mouse epidermis. J Invest Dermatol 91:585–589
97. Pathak MA, Fanselow DL (1983) Photobiology of melanin pigmentation: dose/response of skin to sunlight and its contents. J Am Acad Dermatol 9:724–733
98. Podda M, Traber MG, Weber C et al (1998) UV-irradiation depletes antioxidants and causes oxidative damage in a model of human skin. Free Radic Biol Med 24:55–65
99. Proksch E, Brandner JM, Jensen JM (2008) The skin: an indispensable barrier. Exp Dermatol 17:1063–1072
100. Prunieras M (1979) Epidermal cell cultures as models for living epidermis. J Invest Dermatol 73:135–137
101. Rasmussen C, Gratz K, Liebel F et al (2010) The StrataTest(R) human skin model, a consistent in vitro alternative for toxicological testing. Toxicol In Vitro 24:2021–2029
102. Reece BT, Deeds D, Rozen M (1992) As an in vitro method for screening sunscreen formulations for sun protection factor using a full-thickness skin model. J Soc Cosmet Chem 43:307–312
103. Robert M, Bissonauth V, Ross G et al (1999) Harmful effects of UVA on the structure and barrier function of engineered human cutaneous tissues. Int J Radiat Biol 75:317–326
104. Rouabhia M, Mitchell DL, Rhainds M et al (2002) A physical sunscreen protects engineered human skin against artificial solar ultraviolet radiation-induced tissue and DNA damage. Photochem Photobiol Sci 1:471–477

105. Seite S, Christiaens F, Bredoux C et al (2010) A broad-spectrum sunscreen prevents cumulative damage from repeated exposure to sub-erythemal solar ultraviolet radiation representative of temperate latitudes. J Eur Acad Dermatol Venereol 24:219–222
106. Seite S, Fourtanier A, Moyal D et al (2010) Photodamage to human skin by suberythemal exposure to solar ultraviolet radiation can be attenuated by sunscreens: a review. Br J Dermatol 163:903–914
107. Seite S, Moyal D, Richard S et al (1998) Mexoryl SX: a broad absorption UVA filter protects human skin from the effects of repeated suberythemal doses of UVA. J Photochem Photobiol B 44:69–76
108. Seite S, Moyal D, Verdier MP et al (2000) Accumulated p53 protein and UVA protection level of sunscreens. Photodermatol Photoimmunol Photomed 16:3–9
109. Seite S, Popovic E, Verdier MP et al (2004) Iron chelation can modulate UVA-induced lipid peroxidation and ferritin expression in human reconstructed epidermis. Photodermatol Photoimmunol Photomed 20:47–52
110. Seite S, Zucchi H, Moyal D et al (2003) Alterations in human epidermal Langerhans cells by ultraviolet radiation: quantitative and morphological study. Br J Dermatol 148:291–299
111. Seite S, Zucchi H, Septier D et al (2006) Elastin changes during chronological and photo-ageing: the important role of lysozyme. J Eur Acad Dermatol Venereol 20:980–987
112. Sesto A, Navarro M, Burslem F et al (2002) Analysis of the ultraviolet B response in primary human keratinocytes using oligonucleotide microarrays. Proc Natl Acad Sci U S A 99: 2965–2970
113. Tewari A, Grage MM, Harrison GI et al (2013) UVA1 is skin deep: molecular and clinical implications. Photochem Photobiol Sci 12:95–103
114. Tewari A, Sarkany RP, Young AR (2012) UVA1 induces cyclobutane pyrimidine dimers but not 6–4 photoproducts in human skin in vivo. J Invest Dermatol 132:394–400
115. Therrien JP, Rouabhia M, Drobetsky EA et al (1999) The multilayered organization of engineered human skin does not influence the formation of sunlight-induced cyclobutane pyrimidine dimers in cellular DNA. Cancer Res 59:285–289
116. Todd C, Hewitt SD, Kempenaar J et al (1993) Co-culture of human melanocytes and keratinocytes in a skin equivalent model: effect of ultraviolet radiation. Arch Dermatol Res 285:455–459
117. Topol BM, Haimes HB, Dubertret L et al (1986) Transfer of melanosomes in a skin equivalent model in vitro. J Invest Dermatol 87:642–647
118. Vioux-Chagnoleau C, Lejeune F, Sok J et al (2006) Reconstructed human skin: from photodamage to sunscreen photoprotection and anti-aging molecules. J Dermatol Sci Suppl 2:S1–S12
119. Wier KA, Fukuyama K, Epstein WL (1971) Nuclear changes during ultraviolet light-induced depression of ribonucleic acid and protein synthesis in human epidermis. Lab Invest 25:451–456

Chapter 13
UV Booster and Photoprotection

M. Sohn

Key Points

- The paradox of achieving great SPF values while using small amounts of UV filters explains the high interest in boosting the performance of the UV filter combination. As a prerequisite for performance, the UV filters must be uniformly dispersed and/or solved at first in the emulsion and then in the applied sunscreen film on the skin.
- Boosting the photoprotection is possible either by optimizing the efficacy of the UV-absorbing system or by improving the film-forming properties of the product during spreading.
- The optimization of the performance of the UV filtering system includes the combination of UVB- and UVA-absorbing molecules, the consideration of the photostability of the UV filters individually and in combination, as well as the synergy of water- and oil-dispersed UV filters. The addition of scattering particles was also shown to increase the efficiency of the UV filter system by increasing the optical path length.
- The improvement of film-forming properties and distribution of the UV molecules on the skin can be achieved by the addition of film formers, the choice of the sunscreen vehicle, and its viscosity.

M. Sohn
Global Technical Center Sun Care, BASF Grenzach GmbH,
Grenzach-Whylen, Germany

School of Life Sciences, Institute of Pharmaceutical Technology, University of Applied Sciences and Arts Northwestern Switzerland, Muttenz/Basel, Switzerland
e-mail: myriam.sohn@basf.com

S.Q. Wang, H.W. Lim (eds.), *Principles and Practice of Photoprotection*,
DOI 10.1007/978-3-319-29382-0_13

13.1 Introduction

The performance of a sunscreen in terms of SPF, UVA protection, and photostability primarily depends on the intrinsic absorbance and photostability properties of the UV filters contained in the product along with their used concentration. Over the last decade, we observed a growing appetite for increasing sunscreen performance with the development of products showing protection index as high as 50+. This phenomenon was supported by the placement in the market of new UV filters from early 2000s, exhibiting higher UV performance than the existing UV filters [1]. In most countries, the highest permitted SPF claim is 50+. However, in South America the maximum authorized SPF claim even attains a value up to 99. This race for higher and higher SPF values is a general trend observed in most countries across the globe. The tendency toward the development of sunscreen formulations with continuously larger SPF numbers resulted in using increased amount of UV filters challenging both the esthetics and the stability of the product. Paradoxically, there is a wish in reducing the concentration of UV filters in new sunscreen developments due to economical, ecological-, sensorial, or health-related reasons. Indeed, some UV filters are accused to show poor ecotoxicological profile, to have potential endocrine disruptor properties, or to induce photoallergy [2–5]. Further, the registered UV filters differ with respect to the regions. In the USA, for example, only 16 UV filters are registered compared to 27 in Europe.

Taken together, the requirements for achieving higher SPF values while using smaller amounts of UV filters explain the high interest in boosting the performance of the UV filtering system. A booster can be defined as a device or a thing that increases power or effectiveness. For sunscreens, boosting the UV filter system relates to the achievement of an improved ratio of "UV performance to UV filter concentration," literally attaining better UV performance with less UV filters. To this end, two routes are often pointed out, either by enhancing the efficacy of the UV-absorbing system or by improving the film-forming properties of the product during spreading. These two different aspects and strategies are discussed thereafter.

13.2 Optimizing the Efficacy of the UV-Absorbing System

13.2.1 Importance of UVA Protection

The erythema effectiveness spectrum displays human sensitivity to erythema, an immediate response to solar exposure. It results from the multiplication of the erythemal action spectrum [6] and the spectrum of the irradiation source [7] as shown in Fig. 13.1. In this graph, it is evident that human erythema originates mostly from UVB radiation that is responsible for about 85 % of this biological endpoint damage. However, a non-negligible part of the erythema effectiveness spectrum also extends over the UVA meaning that UVA markedly contributes to the erythema formation as well.

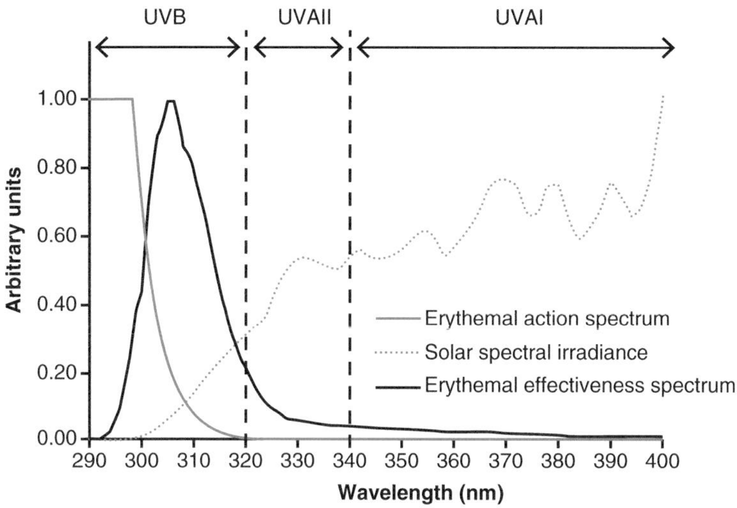

Fig. 13.1 Erythemal action spectrum [6], solar spectral irradiance [7], and erythema effectiveness spectrum, in arbitrary units. Approximately 85 % of erythema originates from UVB radiation, a non-negligible part also from UVA radiation

Fig. 13.2 SPF in silico of a combination containing 2 % UVB filter octyl triazone without and with the UVA filter diethylamino hydroxybenzoyl hexyl benzoate (*DHHB*) calculated using the BASF sunscreen simulator [10, 11]

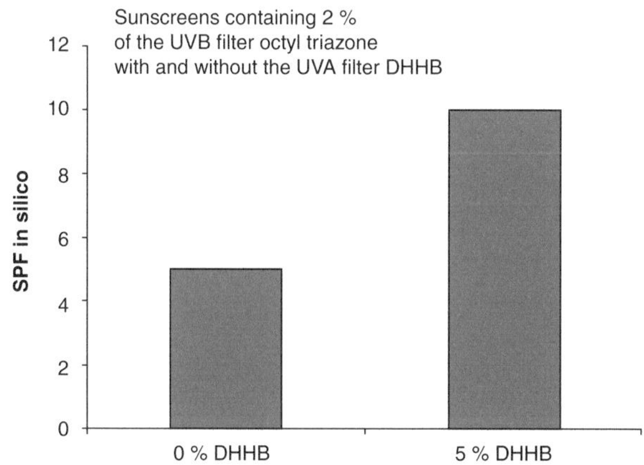

The addition of UVA filters are, therefore, a prerequisite to increase SPF values [8]. Indeed, a mere "UVB sunscreen" that would solely block radiations from 290 to 320 nm and transmit UVA radiation would reach in principle a maximum SPF of 11 only [9], because continuous level of erythemally active UVA2 radiation is transmitted. As a consequence, the addition of UVA filters is a requisite to obtain a substantial rise of the SPF value.

Figure 13.2 gives the SPF in silico value of an oil-in-water (O/W) sunscreen combination containing 2 % of the UVB filter octyl triazone without and with the UVA filter having the INCI diethylamino hydroxybenzoyl hexyl benzoate (DHHB).

Accordingly, the basic for sunscreen development and achievement of higher SPFs is the judicious combination of UVB and UVA filters. The presence of UVA filters is nowadays generally the case since UVA filters are incorporated to reach the minimal UVA protection that is required in most regions [7]. Therefore, an appropriate UV filter system should combine UVB and UVA filters to achieve optimized UV shield [12].

13.2.2 Photocompatibility of UV Filters

Besides their individual absorbance profile and extinction properties, UV filters are characterized also by their intrinsic photostability and photocompatibility with other UV filters. The two worldwide accepted UVA filter avobenzone and UVB filter octinoxate are known to be very photounstable under UV exposure [13], resulting in a loss of approximately 70 % and 40 % after ten Minimal Erythemal Dose (MED) for avobenzone and octinoxate, respectively [14]. Moreover, their combination leads to an increased photochemical instability due to a 2+2-hetero-photocycloaddition [15] producing non-UV-absorbing cyclobutylketone photoproducts. This issue often obliged sunscreen manufacturers to use either the one or the other filter in their sunscreen development.

Regarding octinoxate, it undergoes at first a trans-cis photoisomerization that equilibrates rapidly after UV irradiation [16]. Upon further UV irradiation, the molecule undergoes a irreversible 2+2-homo-photocycloaddition resulting in non-UV-absorbing cinnamate dimers [15, 17]. In the case of avobenzone, an equilibrium mixture between the two tautomeric enol and keto forms of the molecule is present [15, 18, 19], the enol tautomer being involved in the irreversible photocycloaddition with octinoxate when the two filters are combined. Further, upon UV irradiation the enol form is photoisomerized into the photoreactive keto isomer that achieves a triplet excited state. This state is responsible for the irreversible photodegradation of the molecule via a Norrish type I cleavage of the CO-C bond, resulting in the formation of two radicals that can further react and form photoproducts [20]. The complete photodegradation process of avobenzone was proposed elsewhere [15, 18]. To slow down the formation of the keto form and subsequent consequences, the simple addition of other UV filters may compete with avobenzone for absorbing light, thus delaying the formation of the excited keto triplet state [21]. This is, however, only a partial protection of avobenzone and cannot avoid the generation of excited state molecules. To overcome this limitation in photoinstability issue, some ingredients were found to show quenching properties of the excited state to prevent from photodegradation of the excited molecule.

For photostable UV filters, the dissipation of absorbed energy occurs through internal conversion, and the absorbed energy is then released in the form of heat due to an intramolecular hydrogen transfer [1]. However, in the case of the photounstable UV filter avobenzone, the molecule can perform an intersystem crossing from the singlet exited state to the triplet excited state, the latter showing a longer lifetime and therefore promoting photodegradation as mentioned above. As a consequence, the stabilization of photounstable UV filters such as avobenzone is possible either by quenching the excited singlet state to avoid the formation of the triplet excited

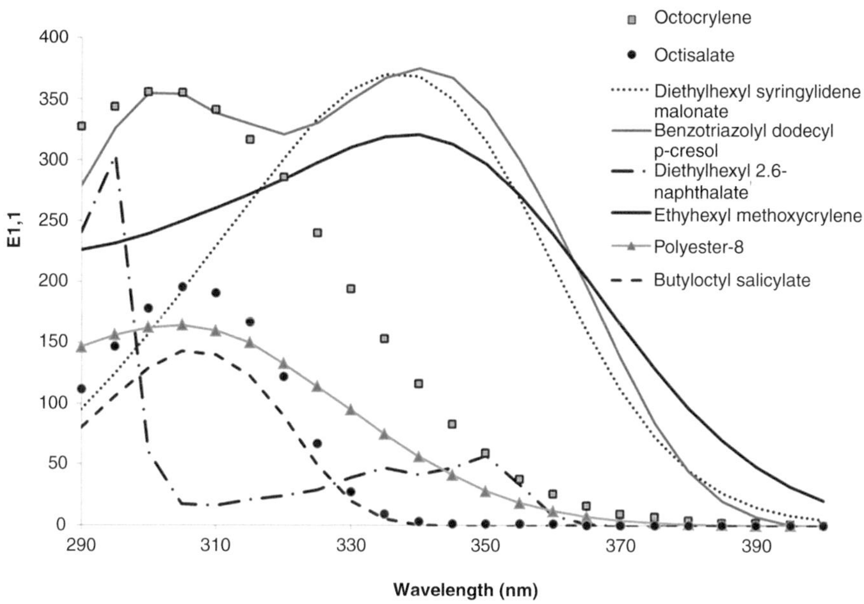

Fig. 13.3 UV absorbance features of emollients promoted as photostabilizers (Data from BASF [29])

state or by quenching the formed triplet excited state. Triplet-triplet energy transfer from the photounstable molecule to the quencher molecule is the most common energy transfer mechanism for photostabilization. To make this process work, the quencher molecule must show a similar energy level to that of the photoexcited state of the photounstable molecule to absorb the excitation energy. The quencher molecule should then ideally return intact to its ground state without self-degradation. As an example, avobenzone shows a triplet energy level close to 60 kcal/mol [22]. Efficient triplet quenchers of avobenzone include other UV filters, particularly bemotrizinol [13] and octocrylene [14], the latter showing a triplet energy level of 55–60 kcal/mol [23] close to that of avobenzone. The two bemotrizinol [13] and octocrylene [14] UV filters were shown to raise significantly the photostability of avobenzone; the recovery of 1 % avobenzone equals 80 % after 10MED when combined with 3 % bemotrizinol compared to a recovery of 25 % only without bemotrizinol [14]. In addition to UV filters, some emollients are promoted to show triplet quenching efficacy as well. Examples of such compounds are diethylhexyl 2,6-naphthalate [24], butyloctyl salicylate, tridecyl salicylate, polyester-8 [25], diethylhexyl syringylidene malonate [26], benzotriazolyl dodecyl p-cresol, and undecylcrylene dimethicone. Recently, the compound ethyhexyl methoxycrylene [27, 28] was introduced for its ability to quench the singlet excited state to avoid the transfer of the molecule from the singlet to its triplet state. To be an effective excited state quencher of avobenzone, these ingredients most often show an inherent UV absorbance as depicted in Fig. 13.3 in terms of specific extinction E1,1. E1,1 is the extinction corresponding to a concentration of 1 % (w/v) solution at an optical thickness of 1 cm of the tested compound. The comparison of the E1,1 values of different compounds over the whole UV range allows a direct comparison of their UV-absorbing performance, the greater the E1,1 value, the greater the UV-absorbing efficacy.

These stabilizers of avobenzone exhibit substantial UV absorbance that goes beyond the UV-absorbing performance of the registered UV filter octisalate or is even as high as the extinction of the well-known UVB filter octocrylene. However, in the contrary to octocrylene and octisalate, they are not registered on the positive list in the annex VI of the cosmetic regulation as UV filters in Europe [30] and have no SCCS opinion. This raises the issue of using compounds referred to as nonofficial registered UV filters. The lack of a registration as official UV filters of the UV-absorbing compounds was already addressed by several cosmetic organizations in Europe and might be also addressed on a European level [31, 32].

To avoid the photoinstability issue of avobenzone, the use of the photostable UVA filter DHHB is a valuable alternative. However, DHHB is not registered as a UV filter in the USA and cannot be used there.

13.2.3 Synergy of Oil- and Water-Dispersed UV Filters

Emulsions are the main formulation type for sunscreen products counting for more than 80 % of the launched sunscreens in 2012–2013 worldwide [33]. Most of the registered UV filters are oil-soluble and will, thus, be formulated into the oil phase of the emulsion. In case of a water-in-oil (W/O) emulsion, the UV filters are distributed in the continuous oil phase directly in contact with the skin during spreading, forming a good coverage and subsequently a uniform protective film. This may explain why W/O sunscreens produce greater SPF values [8, 34]. In the contrary, in oil-in-water (O/W) emulsions, the most popular emulsion type, the filters are distributed in the internal oil phase that hinders the achievement of a uniform distribution of the UV filters after spreading. To visualize this phenomenon, an O/W emulsion containing the oil-dispersed dye Sudan red III pigment (color index 26100) and the water-dispersed blue pigment with the color index 42090 was observed under light microscopy, before (Fig. 13.4a), during (Fig. 13.4b), and after spreading (Fig. 13.4c).

Before spreading, the oil phase is contained inside the droplets (Fig. 13.4a). During spreading, the droplets merge, and the oil phase is released (Fig. 13.4b); finally, after spreading, the water evaporated, and the oil phase is predominant. Nevertheless, a nonvolatile part of the water phase remains in the film, shown as blue spots in Fig. 13.4c. The residual water parts lack UV filters and offer no protection, resulting in unprotected area or “holes” in the protection film and, thus, in reduced UV performance. To overcome this drawback, water- and oil-soluble UV filters may be incorporated in the two phases of the emulsion. This leads to an enhanced efficacy as the nonvolatile water part remaining after water evaporation is protected with the water-dispersed UV filter. The resulting sunscreen film will not

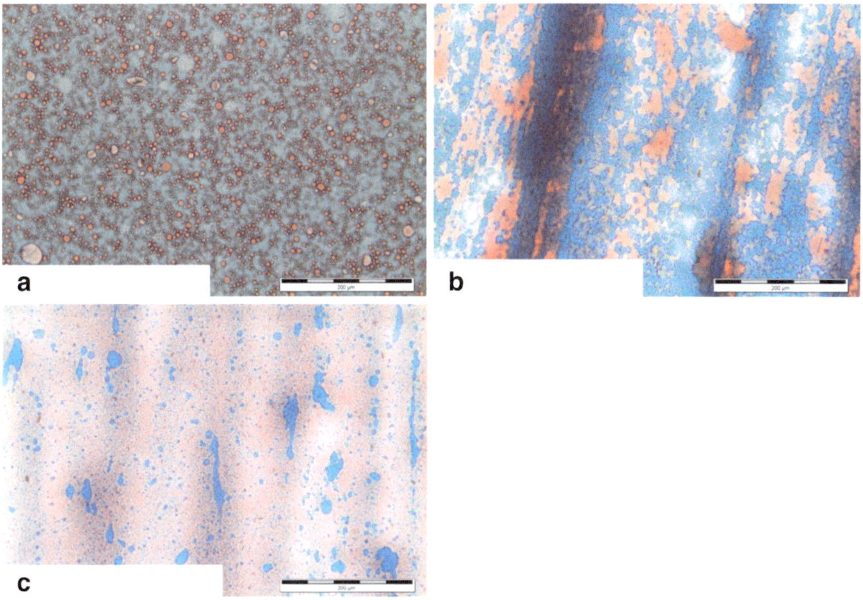

Fig. 13.4 Microscopic evaluation (Olympus CKX41) of an O/W emulsion containing a *red* oil- and a *blue* water-dispersed pigment, (**a**) before spreading, (**b**) during spreading, and (**c**) after spreading. Not protecting the water part (in *blue*) with a water-dispersed UV filter would result in unprotected area or "holes" in the sunscreen film and reduced UV efficacy

show any unprotected area and will end up in a better coverage and optimized UV protection.

Further, the effect of the UV filter distribution in the oil and in the water phase on the UV performance was investigated by Neuenschwander and Herzog [35]. The Colipa P3 standard formulation containing a mixture of oil- and water-dispersed UV filters was used [6]; the ratio between the water filter ensulizole and the oil filter octinoxate was varied to cover a Relative Erythema Active Extinction in the oil phase (REAE) between almost 0 and 1. A REAE of 1 corresponds to a UV filter system based on oil-soluble UV filters exclusively, and to the opposite, a REAE of 0 corresponds to a UV filter system based on water-dispersed UV filters solely. The SPF in vitro of each formulation variant was measured and plotted against its REAE value (Fig. 13.5). In addition, the effect of the water and oil UV filter distribution on the film irregularity, subsequently on the UV performance, was computed. To describe film irregularity, the calibrated quasi-continuous step film model was used [10] and is given in following exponential equation:

$$h(i) = A\exp\left[-B\left(\frac{i}{n}\right)^{c}\right] \tag{13.1}$$

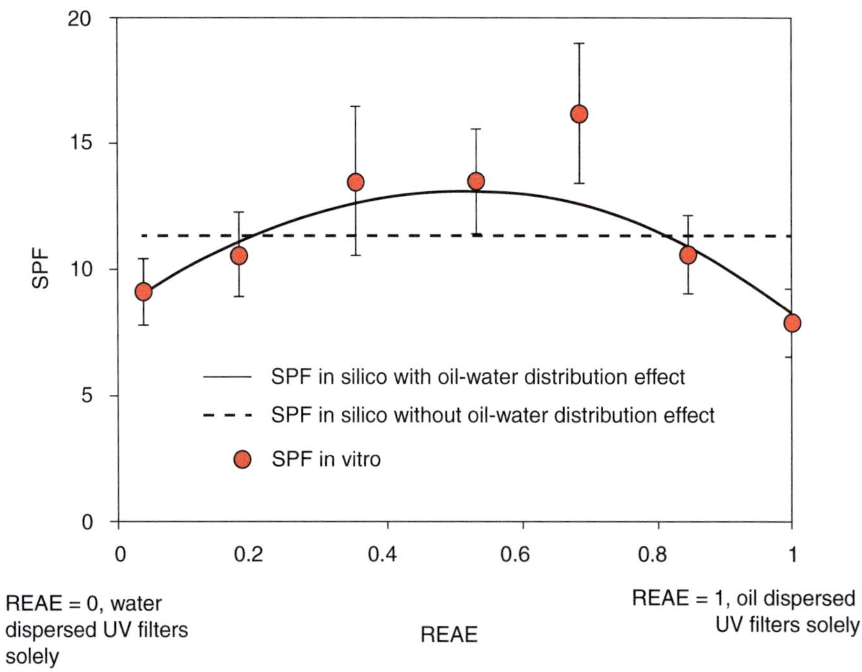

Fig. 13.5 Variation of the SPF in silico (*solid line*) considering the effect of oil-water distribution, SPF in vitro (*circles*, $n = 96$ measurements per formulation) as function of REAE of the UV filter mixture; dashed line is the SPF simulation without consideration of the oil-water distribution effect

where, $h(i)$ is the height of the film at step i, with $i = 1, 2, \ldots, n$, where n is the number of steps the exponential function is divided into, B and C are parameters determining the shape of the film, and A is introduced for normalization. The transmission through the quasi-continuous step film is obtained as the sum of the transmissions through all steps of height $h(i)$.

Using UV filters in the two phases of the sunscreen formulation, REAE between 0.4 and 0.8 appears to enhance the overall UV performance.

13.2.4 Increase of Optical Path Length by Using Scattering Particles

Using particles that exhibit scattering properties is particularly interesting with respect to the boosting of the UV protection. Indeed, such particles are able to increase the optical path length of UV radiation due to their inherent scattering properties, thereby increasing the likelihood of UV radiation to meet a dissolved UV filter molecule before reaching the skin surface, as schematized in Fig. 13.6.

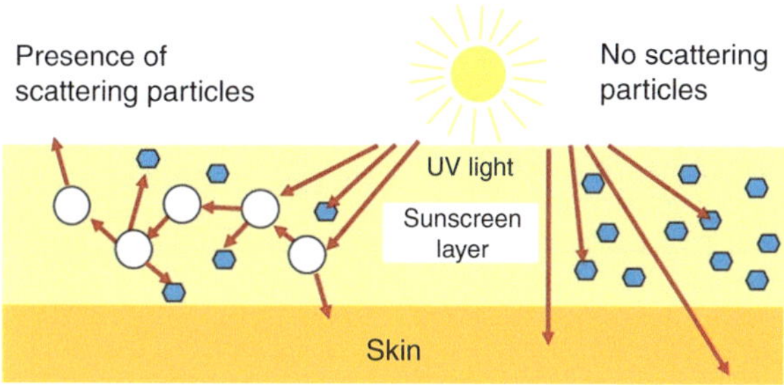

Fig. 13.6 Boosting of UV performance through increase of optical path length using scattering particles. *Blue* objects represent UV filter molecules, and *white circles* represent light scattering particles

The scattering efficiency highly depends on the particle size range relative to the light wavelength. Further, for a particle with a given refractive index, the absorbance and scattering performance of a given particle run inversely, when varying the size if scattering increases then absorbance decreases, and there might be an optimum of particle size for a maximized UV attenuation.

Polymer spheres consisting of styrene/acrylates copolymer act as UV booster material following this principle [36]. In its original product form as well as in the finished formulation, the sphere is filled with water; the water evaporates during spreading leaving an air-filled hollow sphere with an external size of approximately 325 nm. Supplier of this material recommends using about 4–5 % solids of the spheres to achieve SPF boosting.

Interestingly, the particulate UV filters such as the inorganic UV filter titanium dioxide or the organic UV filter bisoctrizole also show scattering properties and are, therefore, able to amplify the UV performance of the used filtering system through this additional characteristic. Since these particulate UV filters are basically selected for their absorbing properties, the additional boosting of efficacy is achieved without the need of a further ingredient that would have merely the scattering activity.

Some authors introduced a method to measure the scattering effect of particulate UV filters using a spectroscopic setup [37, 38]. In these experiments, the impact of scattering particles was shown on the absorbance of a dye having its maximum absorption outside the UV range such as Evans Blue and Patent Blue V. The dye concentration was maintained constant, and the variation of the dye absorbance was monitored while varying the amount of scattering particles. Figure 13.7b displays the example of Patent Blue V dye in combination with the organic particulate UV filter bisoctrizole. The variation of absorbance of a water dispersion of 1.32×10^{-5} M Patent Blue V with increasing volume fraction concentration of the increasing particulate filter bisoctrizole ranging from 0 to 18 % was measured. The λmax of Patent Blue V dye in water at pH 5 lies around 638 nm, outside the absorption range of the particulate UV filter (Fig. 13.7a). The absorbance of the dye could be amplified reaching a sixfold increase with increased concentration of scattering particles; achieving a plateau from the incorporation of 5 % particles (Fig. 13.7b). A similar boosting is produced using the organic particulate UVB filter with INCI tris-biphenyl triazine and titanium dioxide particles.

The boosting effect obtained from ingredients with scattering characteristics can also be shown with SPF in vivo measurements. The combination of 5 % of the

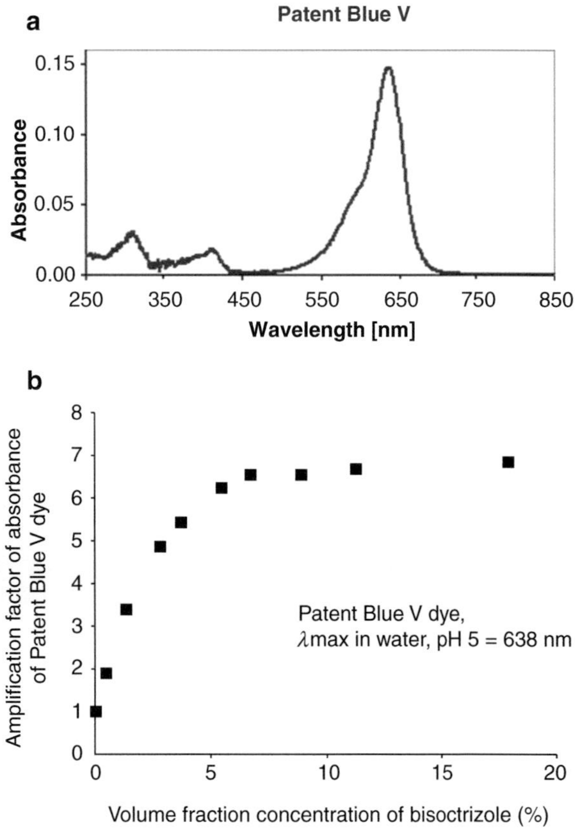

Fig. 13.7 (**a**) Absorbance spectrum of Patent Blue V dyestuff. (**b**) Amplification factor of absorbance of Patent Blue V dye with increasing concentration of the organic particulate broad-spectrum bisoctrizole UV filter

oil-soluble UV filter octinoxate and 4 % of the particulate UV filter bisoctrizole reached an SPF in vivo value of 30 that is much greater than the mere addition of the SPF in vivo values of the two filters tested separately, reaching an SPF value of 9 and 5 for octinoxate and bisoctrizole, respectively [39]. The reason of this boosting is twofold: at first spectral through the synergism between UVB and UVA filters as clarified in Sect. 13.2.1. Further, the boosting is explained through the scattering of bisoctrizole, forward and backward scattering, contributing to about 10 % of the overall effect in the region of absorption band for bisoctrizole [40].

13.3 Improving Film Homogeneity and Distribution of an Applied Sunscreen

The intrinsic absorbing properties of the selected UV filters along with their photocompatibility are primarily responsible for the sunscreen efficacy in terms of SPF, UVA protection, and photostability [8, 41]. Nevertheless, SPF values appear to differ between sunscreens containing the same UV filter composition [8, 42]. Homogeneous distribution of the sunscreen product was shown to contribute to the SPF in vivo value [43]. For optimum performance, the sunscreen film should be of uniform thickness, with an identical thickness over the covered surface area, similarly to a perfect homogeneous distribution of UV filter solution in an optical cell. Understandably, this state can never be attained under in vivo conditions of application due to the skin surface topography that preclude the formation of an even sunscreen film [44]. Furthermore, manual application makes it nearly impossible to reach film uniformity. The sunscreen film is composed of a multitude of different thicknesses, and this irregularity of the film thickness may be the reason for the discrepancy between predictions based on UV transmission of dilute transparent filter solutions and clinical study results [45]. The objective for optimum photoprotection is, therefore, to apply the sunscreen product as uniform as possible.

13.3.1 Use of Specifically Dispersed UV Filters

To be fully effective, UV filters must be properly dissolved and homogeneously distributed on the skin during product application. This might be difficult to reach especially for sunscreens with large SPF values that have high concentration of UV filters. A solution consists to solve and disperse organic UV filters into a matrix. This technology was recently launched for bemotrizinol UV filter dispersed into a polymethylmethycrylate matrix. This dispersed UV filter matrix is promoted to enhance film formation during spreading due to the suppleness of the matrix that spreads over the skin during application resulting into a homogenous distribution of the bemotrizinol molecules into the film and greater SPF values [46].

13.3.2 Use of Film Former Compounds

Many compounds claimed to boost UV performance of sunscreens are found in the market. These excipients are supposed to perform by improving the distribution of the UV actives on the skin. They are often referred to as film formers due to their ability to improve the film forming of a sunscreen formulation during application. Film formers are also often connected to the increase of water resistance. Various classes of film formers exist for sun care application including hydrophobic or water-dispersible ingredients; they may be based on vinylpyrrolidone derivatives, acrylic polymer derivatives, polyester, polyurethanes, maleic derivatives, silicones, etc.

- Waxes were the first ingredients that acted as film formers through their inherent viscosity-building properties. Used to optimize emulsion stability, they also fix the film avoiding its flow downward to the skin furrows. Any viscosity-building ingredient will show this positive effect; however, this precludes the use in spray application.

- The vinylpyrrolidone derivatives such as VP/hexadecane copolymer, VP/eicosene copolymer, and tricontanyl PVP are the most popular, contained in more than 50 % of launched sunscreens over the three last year [47]. Also, the compound with the INCI "aqua (and) hydrolyzed wheat protein/PVP crosspolymer" is a crosspolymer of hydrolyzed wheat protein and polyvinylpyrrolidone that is claimed to optimize film-forming properties of sunscreen emulsions.
- Film formers based on acrylic chemistry such as acrylates copolymer and acrylates/octylacrylamide copolymer are claimed to form a uniform film onto the skin and boost the performance by entrapping the UV filters into the even film matrix due to their hydrophobic nature [48]. The latter is also soluble in ethanol and can serve as film former in the trendy clear lipo-alcoholic sprays or in hydroalcoholic systems upon neutralization with a base.

  Another representative of the acrylic-based chemistry is the acrylate grafted olefin polymer found under the INCI "polyacrylate 15 (and) polyacrylate 17." It combines crystalline and amorphous polymer structures; an amorphous functional acrylic polymer is grafted onto a crystalline polyethylene backbone. The amorphous graft polymer portion is said to slow down the migration of the crystalline wax part resulting in a more uniform distribution of the actives throughout the film [49]. It shows affinity for UV absorbers such as octinoxate and octisalate resulting in more ordered structures during the drying process and a better orientation of the UV segments for photoexcitation. Acrylic based polymers for film forming include further compounds such as C8-22 alkyl acrylate/methacrylic acid crosspolymer or acrylates/C12-22 alkylmethacrylate copolymer.
- The next category of film formers comprises maleic derivatives such as the hydrophobic copolymer with the INCI "C30-38 olefin/isopropyl maleate/MA copolymer." The maleic functionality helps the copolymer in adhering onto the skin for efficient film-forming properties [50]. It needs to be neutralized with a base for O/W emulsions.
- Finally, the silicone ingredients being substantive to the skin offer interesting possibilities for film-forming features. Silicones are particularly known and originally used for their positive effect on the sensory profile, and the use of silicones in sun care increases due to their benefit in film-forming properties [51]. Silicone acrylate copolymers are suitable for this purpose. Indeed, the acrylate backbone is responsible for the film forming on the skin, and the grafted silicone functionalities improve the sensorial behavior. Further, alkylmethylsiloxanes (AMS) based on a silicone backbone grafted with alkyl chains of different lengths are recommended for UV performance boosting. Alkylmethylsiloxanes boost SPF by facilitating the sunscreen spreading and optimizing the formulation rheology. The viscosity is rebuild after spreading enabling to maintain a homogeneous film and distribution of the UV filters. Also silicone elastomers were shown to increase SPF values likely due to the impact on the formulation rheology.

Table 13.1 summarizes the main film former categories and their representatives.

Table 13.1 Nonexhaustive list of film former categories and representative compounds

Main categories of film formers	Compounds (INCI)	Typical use solids (%)	Remarks
Vinylpyrrolidone derivatives	VP/hexadecane copolymer	1–3	First three, most popular film formers, oil-soluble, in waxy or liquid form
	VP/eicosene copolymer		
	Tricontanyl PVP		
	Aqua (and) hydrolyzed wheat protein/PVP crosspolymer	0.5–2.5	Water dispersion (≈45 % solids)
Acrylic based	Acrylates copolymer	1–2	Water dispersion (≈30 % solids), neutralization required
	Acrylates/octylacrylamide copolymer	2	Soluble in ethanol, neutralization required when using water
	Polyacrylate 15 (and) polyacrylate 17	1.5–3.5	Water dispersion (≈30 % solids), no neutralization required
	C8-22 alkyl acrylate/methacrylic acid crosspolymer	0.5–3	Water dispersion (≈47 % solids), no neutralization required
Maleic derivatives	C30-38 olefin/Isopropyl maleate/MA copolymer	1–2	Neutralization required when using water, act also as an anionic emulsifier
Silicone based	Silicone acrylate copolymers	2	≈30–40 % solids
	Alkylmethylsiloxanes	2	Substantive to skin
	Silicone elastomers	4	
	Trifluoropropyldimethylsiloxy/trimethylsiloxy silsesquioxane (and) dimethicone	1–2	≈50 % solids, fluoro-modified silicone resin
Polyamides derivatives	Polyamide-3	1–3	Oil structuring polymers forming cohesive non-water-soluble film
	Polyamide-8		
Polyester based	Polyester-5	1–2	Water dispersible
Polyurethane based	Polyurethane-34	1–3	Water dispersion (≈38–42 % solids) suitable in low viscosity products, no neutralization required

13.3.3 Impact of Emulsion Type and Viscosity

The abovementioned compounds are all claimed to improve film-forming uniformity and subsequently sunscreen performance. The contribution of these compounds on the efficacy had been evaluated by measuring the SPF value with and without the specific ingredient. For most of them, the manufacturers stated that the boosting was achieved through their impact on the formulation rheology and the obtained film that was expected to be more homogeneous. For investigating the film uniformity of an applied sunscreen, several methods were described providing merely qualitative or semiquantitative information. For qualitative assessment, techniques based on fluorescence resulting either from a UV filter present in the sunscreen or from an added fluorescent marker are used to visualize the homogeneity of distribution of the applied product [52]. For quantitative assessment, the use of in vivo fluorescence spectroscopy gave indirect information about the film thickness by converting the fluorescence intensity into an equivalent thickness of an applied product [53].

Recently, some authors introduced a method for determining the precise thickness distribution of an applied sunscreen film on epidermal membrane of pig ear skin based on topographical measurements [34]. The biological pig skin substrate was chosen due to its similarity to human skin that matches the product-to-substrate affinity relevant for in vivo conditions. The film thickness of the applied sunscreen was obtained as the difference of the skin topography data before and after sunscreen application, computed for each single measurement point. The result was expressed as a distribution of frequencies of film thickness over the measured surface area, from which the average film thickness was extracted. In parallel, the SPF in vitro was measured using the same preparations. In that study, the hypothesis that the difference of film thickness may be responsible for the divergence of SPF performance observed between sunscreens containing the same UV filter mixture was examined. The impact of sunscreen vehicle on the SPF in vitro and film thickness distribution both measured on the same pig skin preparations was investigated. The formulations included five different but characteristic vehicles for sun care: an oil-in-water cream (OW-C), an oil-in-water spray (OW-S), a water-in-oil emulsion (WO), a gel (GEL), and a clear lipo-alcoholic spray (CAS). They contained the same UV filter combination and emollient and differed in their emulsifying and thickening system. The authors found a positive correlation between the average film thickness and SPF in vitro measured on pig ear skin within each tested sunscreen underlining the relevance of film thickness for interpreting UV protection differences of formulations with the same filter composition.

Further, the viscosity of the vehicle was found to impact the average film thickness and SPF in vitro. OW-S sunscreen showed a smaller average film thickness and a smaller SPF value than OW-C, film thickness equaled to 2.3 and 1.6 μm and the SPF reached a value of 33 and 16 for OW-C and OW-S, respectively. The thickeners included in OW-C and absent in OW-S appeared to be responsible for the significant difference of film thickness and SPF in vitro between the two sunscreens. The low

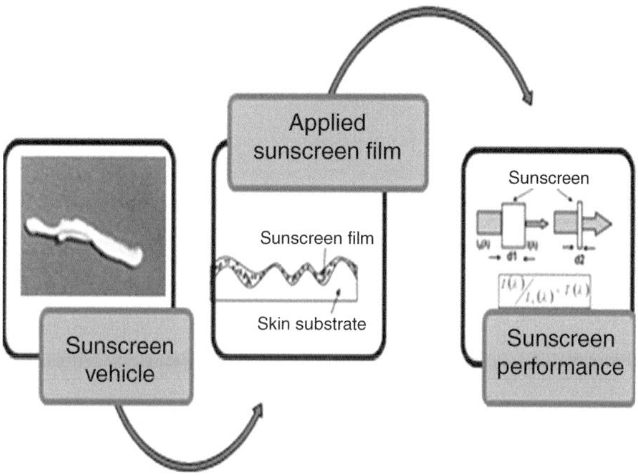

Fig. 13.8 Connection between sunscreen vehicle, film forming, and delivered UV protection

viscosity sunscreens OW-S and CAS which lacked thickeners exhibited the smallest average film thickness values that are connected to a greater occurrence of small film thicknesses. Light transmittance which increases exponentially with decreasing film thickness is inversely proportional to SPF. Subsequently, low viscosity sunscreens OW-S and CAS yielded also the lowest SPF values. They may leave larger areas of ridges virtually uncovered during application while accumulating in the furrows thus leading to an irregular protective film and a lower SPF value. Therefore, the presence of viscosity builder in the formulation seems indeed to be a prevailing prerequisite for UV efficacy.

Further, WO exhibited both the largest average film thickness with a value of 2.9 μm and the highest SPF. In contrast to the other sunscreens, the UV filters of WO are distributed in the continuous phase which does not evaporate, thus assuming to form a uniform protecting film with the help of the thickeners.

This study demonstrated that SPF variation observed between sunscreens containing the same filter system arose from the difference in their film thickness distribution that depended on the sunscreen formulation.

Figure 13.8 shows the significant connections between the sunscreen vehicle-related factor, the film forming, and the measured performance, that is, SPF in vitro of sunscreens.

Finally, Fig. 13.9 summarizes the key parameters emphasized in this chapter that are expected to boost the efficiency of a UV filtering system.

The high expectation of achieving greater UV photoprotection while using reduced amount of UV filters related to economical, ecological-, sensorial, or health-related reasons led to a high interest in understanding the factors and their mechanisms able to influence the efficacy of the UV protection system. Besides the appropriate selection of the UV filters, including adequate absorption profile, photostability, and synergy, also the film thickness distribution on the skin is of high relevance for UV protection. Assessing the effect of individual formulation excipients on the film formation may offer a novel way to optimize sunscreen

Fig. 13.9 Parameters promoting the boosting of the performance of a UV filtering system

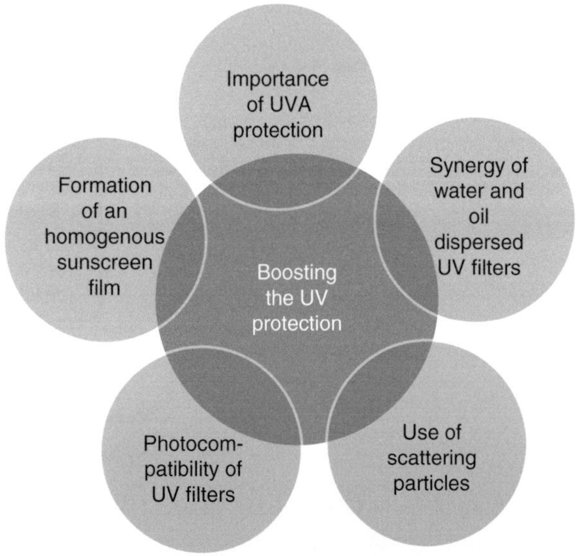

photoprotection during the development step. The effect of the distribution of the UV filters within the applied sunscreen film on the delivered UV protection may be a further factor to be elucidated.

AcknowledgmentsI would like to thank especially Uli Osterwalder of BASF Personal Care and Nutrition GmbH for his great support and his confidence in me, Bernd Herzog and Marcel Schnyder of BASF Grenzach GmbH for their valuable input, and Georgios Imanidis of the Institute of Pharmaceutical Technology, School of Life Sciences, University of Applied Sciences Northwestern, Switzerland, for the fruitful discussions.

References

1. Herzog B, Huglin D, Borsos E, Stehlin A, Luther H (2004) New UV absorbers for cosmetic sunscreens – a breakthrough for the photoprotection of human skin. Chimia 58(7–8):554–559
2. de Groot AC, Roberts DW (2014) Contact and photocontact allergy to octocrylene: a review. Contact Dermatitis 70(4):193–204
3. Avenel-Audran M, Dutartre H, Goossens A, Jeanmougin M, Comte C, Bernier C et al (2010) Octocrylene, an emerging photoallergen. Arch Dermatol 146(7):753–757
4. Matsumoto H, Adachi S, Suzuki Y (2005) Estrogenic activity of ultraviolet absorbers and the related compounds. Yakugaku Zasshi J Pharm Soc Jpn 125(8):643–652
5. Axelstad M, Boberg J, Hougaard KS, Christiansen S, Jacobsen PR, Mandrup KR et al (2011) Effects of pre- and postnatal exposure to the UV-filter octyl methoxycinnamate (OMC) on the reproductive, auditory and neurological development of rat offspring. Toxicol Appl Pharmacol 250(3):278–290
6. ISO 24444:2010 – Cosmetics – sun protection test methods – in vivo determination of the sun protection factor (SPF) (2010). http://www.iso.org/iso/catalogue_detail.htm?csnumber=46523 (accessed 2 February 2016)

7. ISO 24443:2012 – Determination of sunscreen UVA photoprotection in vitro (2012). http://www.iso.org/iso/catalogue_detail?csnumber=46522 (accessed 2 February 2016)
8. Schulz J, Hohenberg H, Pflucker F, Gartner E, Will T, Pfeiffer S et al (2002) Distribution of sunscreens on skin. Adv Drug Deliv Rev 54(Suppl 1):157–163
9. Sayre RM, Dowdy JC, Lott DL, Marlowe E (2008) Commentary on 'UVB-SPF': the SPF labels of sunscreen products convey more than just UVB protection. Photodermatol Photoimmunol Photomed 24(4):218–220
10. Herzog B (2010) Models for the calculation of sun protection factors and parameters characterizing the UVA protection ability of cosmetic sunscreens. In: Colloid stability, Colloids and interface science series. Wiley-VCH Verlag GmbH & Co. KGaA, Weinheim, pp 275–308
11. Anonymous (2010) BASF sunscreen simulator. BASF SE, Ludwigshafen. Available at http://www.basf.com/sunscreen-simulator. Accessed 9 Jan 2015
12. Osterwalder U, Herzog B, Wang SQ (2011) Advance in sunscreens to prevent skin cancer. Expert Rev Dermatol 6(5):479–491
13. Chatelain E, Gabard B (2001) Photostabilization of butyl methoxydibenzoylmethane (Avobenzone) and ethylhexyl methoxycinnamate by bis-ethylhexyloxyphenol methoxyphenyl triazine (Tinosorb S), a new UV broadband filter. Photochem Photobiol 74(3):401–406
14. Herzog B, Wehrle M, Quass K (2009) Photostability of UV absorber systems in sunscreens. Photochem Photobiol 85(4):869–878
15. Dondi D, Albini A, Serpone N (2006) Interactions between different solar UVB/UVA filters contained in commercial suncreams and consequent loss of UV protection. Photochem Photobiol Sci 5(9):835–843
16. Pattanaargson S, Munhapol T, Hirunsupachot N, Luangthongaram P (2004) Photoisomerization of octyl methoxycinnamate. J Photochem Photobiol A Chem 161(2–3):269–274
17. Broadbent JK, Martincigh BS, Raynor MW, Salter LF, Moulder R, Sjoberg P et al (1996) Capillary supercritical fluid chromatography combined with atmospheric pressure chemical ionisation mass spectrometry for the investigation of photoproduct formation in the sunscreen absorber 2-ethylhexyl p methoxycinnamate. J Chromatogr A 732(1):101–110
18. Schwack W, Rudolph T (1995) Photochemistry of dibenzoyl methane UVA filters part 1. J Photochem Photobiol B Biol 28(3):229–234
19. Mturi GJ, Martincigh BS (2008) Photostability of the sunscreening agent 4-tert-butyl-4′-methoxydibenzoylmethane (avobenzone) in solvents of different polarity and proticity. J Photochem Photobiol A Chem 200(2–3):410–420
20. Cantrell A, McGarvey DJ (2001) Photochemical studies of 4-tert-butyl-4′-methoxydibenzoylmethane (BM-DBM). J Photochem Photobiol B Biol 64(2–3):117–122
21. Lhiaubet-Vallet V, Marin M, Jimenez O, Gorchs O, Trullas C, Angel Miranda M (2010) Filter-filter interactions. Photostabilization, triplet quenching and reactivity with singlet oxygen. Photochem Photobiol Sci 9(4):552–558
22. Gonzenbach H, Hill TJ, Truscott TG (1992) The triplet energy-levels of UVA sunscreens and UVB sunscreens. J Photochem Photobiol B Biol 16(3–4):377–379
23. Shaath NA (2007) Chapter 2. Ultraviolet filters. In: The encyclopedia of ultraviolet filters. Allured Publishing Corporation, Carol Stream, pp 9–26
24. Cole CA, Vollhardt J, Mendrok C (2008) Chapter 3. Formulation and stability of sunscreen products. In: Clinical guide to sunscreens and photoprotection, 1st edn. Informa Healthcare, New York, pp 39–52
25. Shaath NA (2007) SPF boosters & photostability of ultraviolet filters. Happi:77–83. http://www.happi.com/contents/view_features/2007-10-01/spf-boosters--photostability-of-ultraviolet-f (accessed 2 February 2016)
26. Chaudhuri RK, Lascu Z, Puccetti G, Deshipande AA, Paknikar SK (2006) Design of a photostabilizer having built-in antioxidant functionality and its utility in obtaining broad-spectrum sunscreen formulations. Photochem Photobiol 82(3):823–828
27. Bonda C (2008) Research pathways to photostable sunscreens. Cosmetics & Toiletries magazine. pp 49–59

28. Bonda C (2009) Sunscreen photostability 101. Happi:72–75. http://shows.happi.com/articles/2009/10/sunscreen-photostability-101 (accessed 2 February 2016)
29. BASF SE, Ludwigshafen, Germany (2014) Determination of molar decadic extinction coefficients of soluble UV-absorbers. Internal method BASF
30. Cosmetic products. Regulation (EC) no 1223/2009 of the European parliament and of the council of 30 November 2009 on cosmetic products. Annex VI (2009). Available at http://eur-lex.europa.eu/LexUriServ/LexUriServ.do?uri=OJ:L:2009:342:0059:0209:en:PDF. Accessed 9 Dec 2014
31. Bundesinstitut für Risikobewertung. 9. Sitzung der BfR-Kommission für kosmetische Mittel, Protokoll der Sitzung vom 3.Mai 2012 (2012). Available at http://www.bfr.bund.de/de/bfr_kommission_fuer_kosmetische_mittel-309.html. Accessed 10 Oct 2014
32. Kantonales Laboratorium Basel. Sonnenschutzmittel und gesichtcremes mit UV-schutz/UV-filter, konservierungsmittel und deklaration. Bericht Nr.45.2009. Available at http://www.gesundheitsschutz.bs.ch/konsum-umwelt/berichte/vor-2010/2009.html. Accessed 14 Jan 2015
33. Osterwalder U, Sohn M, Herzog B (2014) Global state of sunscreens. Photodermatol Photoimmunol Photomed 30(2–3):62–80
34. Sohn M, Hêche A, Herzog B, Imanidis G (2015) Porcine ear skin as a biological substrate for in vitro testing of sunscreen performance. Skin Pharmacol Physiol 28(1):31–41
35. Neuenschwander A, Herzog B (2005) For the prediction of sun protection factors – comparison of in vitro measurements and model calculations. Master thesis, University of Basel, Basel
36. Jones C (2002) Hollow sphere technology for sunscreen formulation. SOFW J 128(9):36–40
37. Herzog B (2011) Influence of particles on the performance of sunscreens. 11th international sun protection conference. Summit Events, London
38. Lademann J, Schanzer S, Jacobi U, Schaefer H, Pflucker F, Driller H et al (2005) Synergy effects between organic and inorganic UV filters in sunscreens. J Biomed Opt 10(1):14008
39. Herzog B (2002) Prediction of sun protection factors by calculation of transmissions with a calibrated step film model. J Cosmet Sci 53(1):11–26
40. Herzog B, Quass K, Schmidt E, Muller S, Luther H (2004) Physical properties of organic particulate UV absorbers used in sunscreens – II. UV-attenuating efficiency as function of particle size. J Colloid Interface Sci 276(2):354–363
41. Herzog B, Sommer K (2000) Investigations on photostability of UV-absorbers for cosmetic sunscreens. In: Proceedings of the XXIth IFSCC international congress, Berlin
42. Chatelain E, Gabard B, Surber C (2003) Skin penetration and sun protection factor of five UV filters: effect of the vehicle. Skin Pharmacol Appl Skin Physiol 16(1):28–35
43. Lademann J, Rudolph A, Jacobi U, Weigmann HJ, Schaefer H, Sterry W et al (2004) Influence of nonhomogeneous distribution of topically applied UV filters on sun protection factors. J Biomed Opt 9(6):1358–1362
44. Gebauer V, Weigmann H-J, Schanzer S, Meinke MC, Vergou T, Sterry W et al (2012) Influence of skin aging effects on the skin surface profile and the correlated distribution of topically applied sunscreens. J Biophotonics 5(3):274–282
45. Oneill JJ (1984) Effect of film irregularities on sunscreen efficacy. J Pharm Sci 73(7):888–891
46. Champ S, Schnyder M (2010) Innovative filter allows water phase dispersion. Personal Care magazine. pp 70–1
47. Global new products database. Personal care portal (2014) Available at http://www.gnpd.com/. Restricted access. Accessed 15 Oct 2014
48. Davis JA, Petersen D, Li D (2007) Use of film-forming polymers for increased efficacy in sunscreens. J Cosmet Sci 58(5):568–569
49. Martin T, Burns T (2006) Novel graft polymer boosts SPF performance. Happi:62–65. http://www.interpolymer.com/stuff/contentmgr/files/8972890e8eaa36ff4fbcab49d351c3d7/miscdocs/Paper-SPF%20Boost%20Happi%20Article-.pdf (accessed 2 February 2016)
50. Hunter A, Trevino M (2004) Film-formers enhance water resistance and SPF in sun care products. Cosmetics & Toiletries magazine. pp 51–5

51. Van Reeth I, Postiaux S, Van Dort H (2006) Silicones bring multifunctional performance to sun care. Cosmetics & Toiletries magazine 121(10):41–54
52. Lademann J, Schanzer S, Richter H, Pelchrzim RV, Zastrow L, Golz K et al (2004) Sunscreen application at the beach. J Cosmet Dermatol 3(2):62–68
53. Rhodes LE, Diffey BL (1997) Fluorescence spectroscopy: a rapid, noninvasive method for measurement of skin surface thickness of topical agents. Br J Dermatol 136(1):12–17

Chapter 14
Sunscreen Photostability

Craig A. Bonda and Dennis Lott

Key Points

- Sunscreens are photochemical systems, and their behavior is best understood through the science of photochemistry.
- Deeper understanding of the complex photochemistry of avobenzone has led to better formulating methods and improved sunscreen performance.
- The photostability of sunscreen products is a function of the photostabilities of the individual UV filters and the photochemical and photophysical interactions between them.
- Photostability will retain a leading role in sunscreen product design as costs and regulatory issues continue to drive sunscreen formulating worldwide.
- Though significant challenges remain, the availability of photostabilizers and, in many areas, new UV filters has allowed the sunscreen industry to make great strides in improving photoprotection.

14.1 A Brief History

Photostability became a genuine concern to the sunscreen industry with the introduction in Europe of avobenzone (butyl methoxydibenzoylmethane or BMDM) in the 1980s and in the USA in the early 1990s. This photolabile

C.A. Bonda (✉)
Inception Partners, LLC, 0s630 Madison Street, Winfield, IL 60190, USA
e-mail: craigbonda@gmail.com

D. Lott
Florida Suncare Testing, Inc, 101 N. Bay Street, PO Box 758, Bunnell, FL, USA
e-mail: lott@live.com

S.Q. Wang, H.W. Lim (eds.), *Principles and Practice of Photoprotection*,
DOI 10.1007/978-3-319-29382-0_14

compound was the first and for years remained the only UV filter to be effective at protecting skin from longer wavelength UVA radiation (320–400 nm), widely believed to be a primary cause of early skin aging and certain skin cancers [1]. Avobenzone degrades rapidly in sunlight [2] and may react chemically with other organic compounds [3]. This spawned an "arms race" among both UV filter suppliers and sunscreen manufacturers to discover ways to photostabilize or replace avobenzone. Scientists in Europe focused on developing photostable UV filters to compete with avobenzone, while other scientists in the USA and Europe focused on discovering new photostabilizers. Both groups were successful: the resulting new UVA filters and photostabilizers are now in widespread use throughout the world.

Several photostable European UVA filters have been submitted for approval to the US Food and Drug Administration for inclusion in the monograph for OTC sunscreen drug products. In 2014, all were deemed by the FDA to have insufficient data on which to base the requisite "generally regarded as safe and effective" (GRASE) determination and were returned to their sponsors for additional information [4]. This signals a continuing role for photostabilizers in sunscreens, especially those to be marketed in the USA but also in other parts of the world where global acceptability is desired and where cost considerations favor the continued use of inexpensive avobenzone as the primary UVA filter.

14.2 Photochemistry of Photostability

The definitive source for general knowledge of organic photochemistry is *Modern Molecular Photochemistry of Organic Molecules* by N.J. Turro, V. Ramamurthy, and J.C. Scaiano (2010, University science Books, Sausolito, CA) [5]. Following is a very brief summary of some of the key aspects as they relate to the subject at hand, sunscreen photostability.

Organic chromophores convert the energy in a quantum of light – a photon – into electronic excitation energy (Turro et al. 2010, p. 27). One photon excites one molecule, and, with rare and obscure exceptions, one and only one of a molecule's electrons is excited to a higher energy state at any one time.

Once excited, a chromophore has several photophysical pathways available to dissipate its excited state energy. These pathways may be "radiative" or "non-radiative." By radiative is meant that the excited chromophore sheds some or all of its energy by emitting a photon; non-radiative pathways expend energy kinetically or vibrationally as heat, or by transferring energy to another molecule (Turro et al. 2010, p. 18–19).

The photostable situation may be represented as follows:

$$R + h\nu \rightarrow {}^{*}R \rightarrow_{\mathrm{pp}} R$$

where R is a chromophore in its ground state, $^*R$ is a chromophore in its excited state, $h\nu$ is the energy in a photon, and $\rightarrow_{pp}$ is energy dissipation purely by photophysical (radiative and non-radiative) processes, thus returning the excited chromophore to the ground state with no changes in its structure or geometry (Turro et al. 2010, p. 40).

Photostable chromophores undergo billions of such cycles – photon absorption, excitation, energy dissipation, and relaxation to the ground state – with a low (not zero!) probability that there will be a net chemical change. In contrast, photolabile chromophores have a relatively high probability that excitation will lead to a net chemical change. The consequence of photolability is photodegradation or photodecomposition, characterized by a loss of absorbance and the appearance of new chemical entities. In sunscreens, photodegradation results in less protection for the skin than would otherwise be expected and exposure of the skin to unwanted photoproducts.

The photolabile situation may be represented as follows:

$$R + hv \rightarrow {}^*R \rightarrow_{\mathrm{pc}} I \rightarrow_{\mathrm{T}} P$$

where $\rightarrow_{pc}$ is a photochemical process, I is a reactive intermediate, $\rightarrow_T$ is a thermal chemical process, and P is a chemical product (Turro et al. 2010, p. 10).

For absorption of a photon and excitation to occur, the energy gap between the electron's ground state orbital, known as the highest occupied molecular orbital or HO, and its initial excited state orbital, known as the lowest unoccupied molecular orbital or LU, must match exactly the energy of the photon. This energy matching requirement is known as the "resonance condition" (Turro et al. 2010, p. 27).

For the UV filters used in sunscreens, the resonance condition requires encounter wavelengths and energies that correspond to the UV portion of the solar spectrum.

The HO of an organic chromophore in the ground state contains a pair of electrons. The electron pairs most commonly involved in excitation of an organic chromophore are those in bonding or π orbitals (e.g., $c{=}c$) and nonbonding or n orbitals such as those found associated with oxygen in carbonyls ($c{=}o$). The transition to the LU by the excited electron is to an anti-bonding orbital, π^*. Thus, the two most common transitions are represented by $\pi \rightarrow \pi^*$ and $n \rightarrow \pi^*$ (Turro et al. 2010, p. 52–55).

In the ground state, the two electrons in the HO are in the singlet state (Fig. 14.1) in which the electrons are "spin-paired," meaning they are spinning about opposite vectors – "up" and "down" – and, in a magnetic field, are precessing 180° out of phase. The ground state is conveniently represented by S_0 and symbolized by 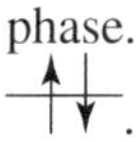. This spin-paired configuration is what allows two negatively charged electrons to overcome their repulsion and occupy the same orbital. The spin-paired configuration is maintained in the initial transition from ground (S_0) to excited state even as the two electrons become orbitally unpaired. Thus, the initial transition after photon absorption is known as the "singlet excited state" which may have more than one energy level and is represented by $S_1, S_2 \ldots S_n$ and symbolized by 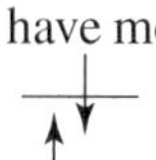.

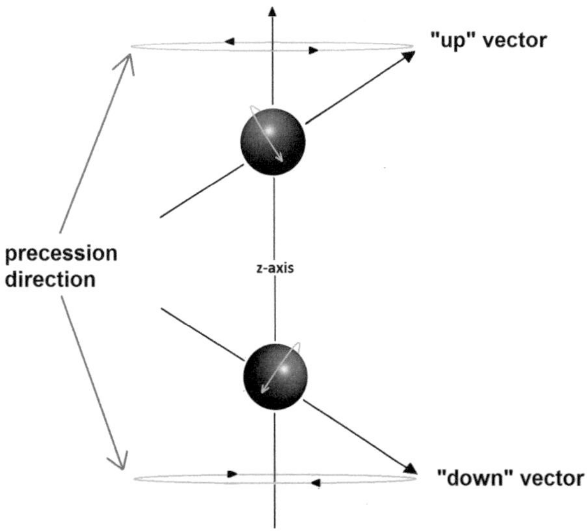

Fig. 14.1 In the singlet state, two paired electrons spin about opposite vectors (“*up*” and “*down*”) and, in a magnetic field, precess 180° out of phase. The *z*-axis is either aligned or opposed to the direction of the magnetic field

Transitions are favored between states that “look like” each other in the sense that their electronic, vibrational, and spin configurations are similar (Turro et al. 2010, p. 45–47, 117). Upon photon absorption, an electron in the singlet ground state naturally transitions to a singlet excited state and almost never to a triplet excited state. For many chromophores, the reverse is also true: an electron in the singlet excited state will tend to relax to the singlet ground state either by dissipating its excess energy as heat (internal conversion) or by emitting a photon (fluorescence).

The return to the ground state from the singlet excited state tends to happen quickly; nanosecond time scales are common. Such a rapid return to the ground state favors photostability since there is little time for chemical processes to compete.

Figure 14.2 depicts the electron configurations of the triplet excited state which is represented by T_1 and symbolized by 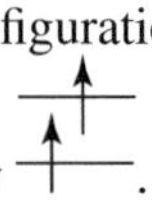. An excited electron reaches a triplet excited state by undergoing a spin flip and phase change usually as the result of a magnetic interaction between the electron’s spin and another electron’s orbital motion (Turro et al. 2010, p. 144). The transition from the singlet excited state to a triple excited state is called “intersystem crossing.” The triplet excited state is metastable; that is, the two electrons are unable to re-pair in their HO unless and until the excited electron undergoes another spin flip and phase change. A chromophore in the triplet excited state behaves as a diradical (i.e., having two unpaired electrons) (Turro et al. 2010, p. 718). This fact coupled with its typically longer lifetime makes the triplet excited state highly reactive and the starting point for most photochemical reactions (Turro et al. 2010, p. 521).

Photochemists use experimental methods to determine the processes a particular chromophore will take in a given set of conditions and record their findings on state

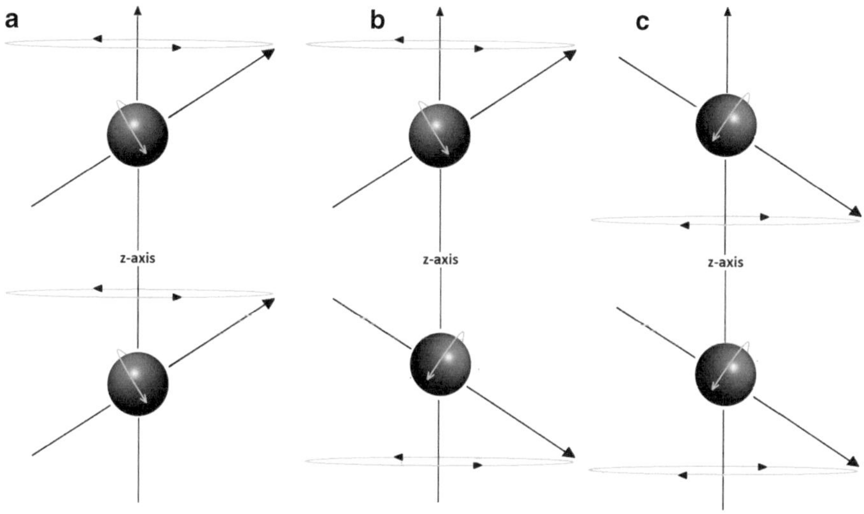

Fig. 14.2 In the triplet state, there are three possible orientations for the electron pair: (**a**) both electron spin about "up" vectors; (**b**) the electrons spin about opposite vectors while precessing in phase; (**c**) both electrons spin about "down" vectors

energy diagrams, also known as Jablonski diagrams, like the one in Fig. 14.3. Key parameters for any photophysical process are its energy (E), its quantum yield (∅), its rate constant (k), and its lifetime (τ). (Since $1/k = \tau$, it is only necessary to measure one: either rate constant or lifetime.) Quantum yield is a measure of the efficiency of a process and is calculated either as the fraction of absorbed photons that produce a specific sequence or by comparing the rate of a specific pathway to the sum of the rates of all competing pathways. For example, if 10 out of 100 excited molecules fluoresce, then the quantum yield of fluorescence is 0.10 (10 %).

Another way for an excited chromophore to return to the ground state is by transferring its energy to another molecule, known as the quencher, Q. Energy transfer can be represented schematically by

$$*R + Q \rightarrow_{\mathrm{ET}} R + *Q$$

where $\rightarrow_{\mathrm{ET}}$ is energy transfer (Turro et al. 2010, p. 390). Thus, the excited chromophore transfers its excited state energy to the ground state quencher which deactivates the chromophore to the ground state and raises the quencher to the excited state. The relative efficiency of a quencher to quench the excited state of a chromophore is characterized by a quenching rate constant, k_{ET}, where ET stands for energy transfer. The actual rate this happens in a solution (or, presumably, in a sunscreen) is the product of the quenching rate constant and the concentration of the quencher, $[Q]$, plus the sum of all other deactivation pathways, k_{D}.

$$k_{\mathrm{q\,obs}} = k_{\mathrm{D}} + k_{\mathrm{ET}} \times [Q]$$

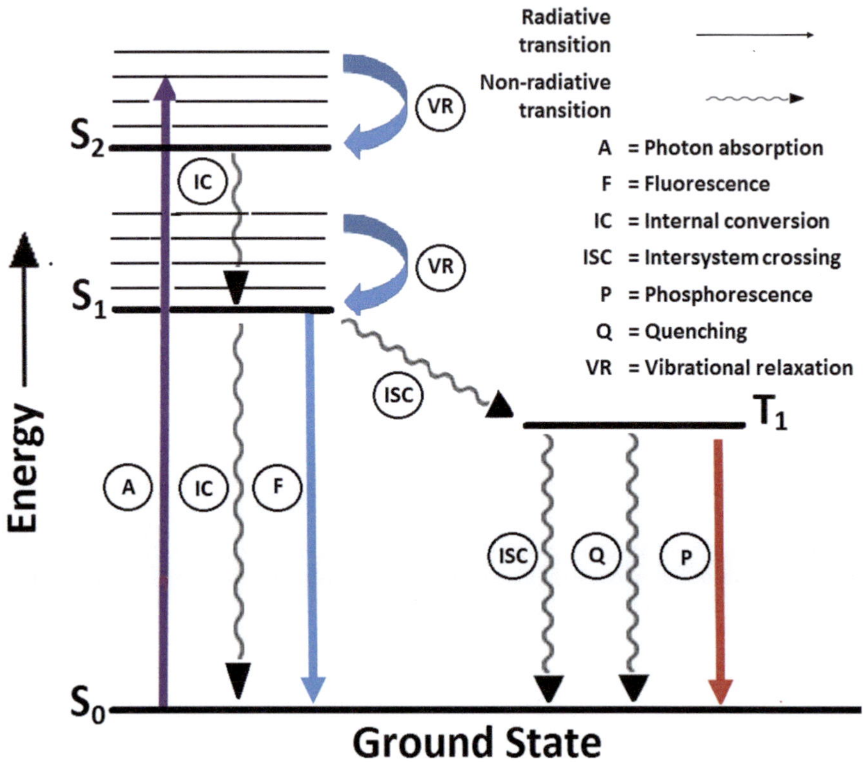

Fig. 14.3 A state energy or "Jablonski" diagram like this is used by photochemists to keep track of an organic chromophore's three most important states: the ground state, S_0; the lowest energy singlet excited state, S_1; and the lowest energy triplet state, T_1. The upward arrow on the left represents photon absorption and excitation. The downward and diagonally pointing arrows represent photophysical processes that drain the chromophore's excited state energy. Key parameters are the energies, quantum yields, and lifetimes of each state and the rates of interstate transitions

where $k_{q\ obs}$ is the quenching rate observed experimentally (Turro et al. 2010, p. 390–391).

This is the basic mechanistic scheme for most of the photostabilizers to be discussed later in this chapter. First, we turn to avobenzone as the exemplar of a photolabile UV filter to find out why photostabilizers are needed in the first place.

14.3 Photochemistry of Avobenzone

Seminal studies published in 1995 by Schwack and Rudolph and in 1997 by Andrae et al. contributed greatly to the early understanding of this important sunscreen ingredient.

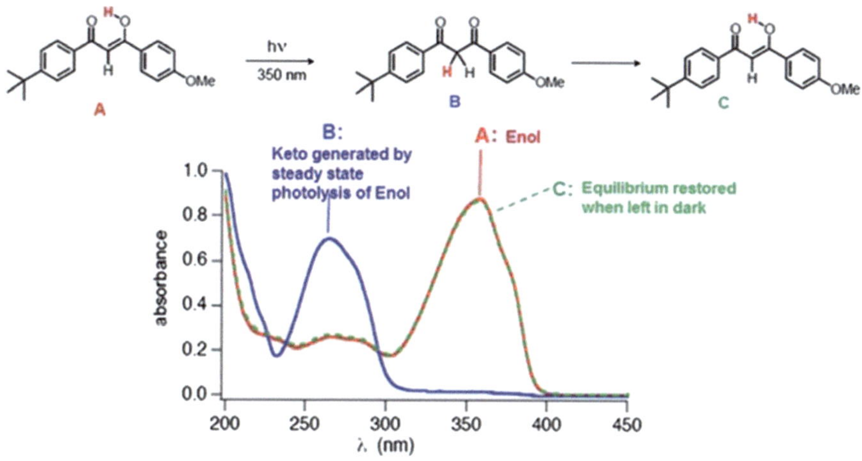

Fig. 14.4 Graph shows that steady-state irradiation of the enol tautomer (*A*) generates the keto tautomer (*B*) which, when left in the dark, spontaneously converts back to the enol form (*C*). (Bonda et al. [2], reprinted with permission)

To investigate the photodegradation of avobenzone, Schwack and Rudolph irradiated 3.5 mmol solutions of avobenzone in non-deaerated cyclohexane, isooctane, isopropanol, and methanol for up to 8 h using a solar simulator filtered to deliver radiation either above 260 nm or 320 nm. Photodegradation progress was monitored by HPLC, and the photoproducts were identified by GC-MS. About 12 photoproducts were identified, all of which originated from one of two radical precursors: a benzoyl radical or a phenacyl radical. Photodegradation proceeded in the nonpolar solvents cyclohexane and isooctane, but not in the polar, protic solvents isopropanol and methanol. In the nonpolar solvents, photodegradation was almost twice as rapid under shorter wave irradiation (>260) than under longer wave irradiation (>320). To find out why avobenzone is photolabile in cyclohexane and isooctane and photostable in isopropanol and methanol, Schwack and Rudolph carried out ^{1}H NMR measurements of avobenzone solutions dissolved in cyclohexane-d_{12} and isopropanol-d_8 (.03 mol). In cyclohexane-d_{12}, avobenzone exhibited 3.5 % keto form, but in isopropanol-d_8, no keto form was detected. Based on these findings, Schwack and Rudolph concluded that avobenzone photodegradation "depends strongly on the presence of the 1,3-keto form" [6]. Therefore, discovering the origins of the keto form and its subsequent behavior under irradiation became of primary interest to researchers.

Andrae et al. showed that photolysis with UV radiation drives the conversion of the enol tautomer to the keto form (Fig. 14.4) [7]. They applied steady-state irradiation to avobenzone in acetonitrile (10^{-5}–10^{-10} M) using both a high-pressure mercury lamp and a xenon light source, observing a decline in peak absorbance at 355 nm and a corresponding increase in peak absorbance at 265 nm. Based on NMR, IR, and HPLC studies, they attributed the spectral change to the light-induced conversion of the enol tautomer to the keto tautomer. Andrae et al. also applied a

14 ns laser pulse of 355 nm to dilute solutions of avobenzone in acetonitrile, observing a transient species with peak absorption at 300 nm. The group attributed the transient absorbance either to an excited *E*-isomer of the enol or to an enol rotamer which were assumed to be intermediates in the conversion to the keto form (see Cantrell and McGarvey and Yamaji and Kida below).

A number of more recent studies published in the literature provide additional guidance to avobenzone's photoinduced behavior under various conditions. Many of the gaps in avobenzone's state energy diagram have now been filled in, providing much needed clarity to its complex photophysics and photochemistry. Following is a sample of the many studies published in the literature.

Cantrell and McGarvey employed nanosecond laser flash photolysis at 355 nm and 266 nm on dilute (10^{-5} M) solutions of avobenzone in acetonitrile [8]. Photolysis at 355 nm produced transient absorbance changes with a new peak at 300 nm and bleaching (loss of absorbance) at 360 nm. No peak at 260 nm was observed, leading to the comment that formation of the keto form must have a low quantum yield (see Yamaji and Kida below). They attributed the transient peak at 300 nm to a non-chelated enol rotamer (NCE), which is a *Z*-isomer. Hill had earlier determined the quantum yield of formation of the 300 nm-absorbing species to be ≈ 0.25 [9]. The lifetime of the NCE rotamer is solvent dependent and ranges from 159 ms in acetonitrile to 0.7 ms in butanol. Upon photolysis at 266 nm, Cantrell and McGarvey observed a permanent loss of absorbance at 360 nm and no increase of absorbance at 260 nm, suggesting that excitation of the keto form leads directly to avobenzone decomposition. Nanosecond excitation at 266 nm of a pre-irradiated solution in deoxygenated acetonitrile generated a transient absorbance spectrum from 300 to 500 nm which was attributed to the triplet state of the keto form. A further experiment found the keto triplet to be quenched by molecular oxygen with a rate constant of 5 $\times$ 10^9 mol^{-1} s^{-1} and a quantum yield of singlet oxygen formation of 0.18.

Huong et al. studied avobenzone photostability in three environments: diluted solutions in laboratory solvents of varying polarity, concentrated solutions in non-volatile solvents, and in commercially available sunscreen products [10]. In dilute solutions irradiated in a xenon test chamber, the study found avobenzone to be photostable or nearly so in dioxane, acetonitrile, ethyl acetate, tetrahydrofuran, ethanol, and isopropanol and photolabile in hexane, heptane, and cyclohexane. The photolability manifested as a rapid decline of absorbance at 350–360 nm and a corresponding increase in absorbance at 260–270 nm. However, in confirmation of work previously reported by Bonda et al. [11], Huong et al. also found that the photodegraded solutions, when left in the dark and monitored for UV absorbance at timed intervals, slowly recovered their initial absorption at 350–360 nm, while their absorption at 260–270 also declined to pre-irradiation levels (Fig. 14.4). They also confirmed another of the findings of Bonda et al. (1997): that as little as 1 % isopropanol in the hexane solution completely inhibited avobenzone's loss of absorption at 350–360 nm upon irradiation. In concentrated solutions of 2 and 4 % (w/w) in various cosmetic oils (mineral oil, isostearyl isostearate, alkyl tartrate, alkyl lactate), photodegradation of avobenzone appeared to be relatively independent of the solvent with as much as 80 % of the avobenzone converted to photoproducts. A total of

11 commercially available European sunscreen products were tested by applying each in a measured amount to a polymethyl methacrylate (PMMA) plate and irradiating it in a xenon test chamber. After irradiation, the sunscreen was extracted with solvent and the resulting solutions analyzed by HPLC. The study found the behavior of avobenzone in these sunscreens to be highly variable, with the loss of compound ranging from 3 % to over 90 %. Loss of SPF ranged from 0 to 50 %.

Mturi and Martincigh employed UV spectroscopy, HPLC, GC-MS, and NMR to investigate avobenzone's photostability in solvents of differing polarity and proticity [12]. As others had, they found avobenzone to be photostable in the polar, protic solvent methanol. In polar, aprotic DMSO, loss of absorbance was attributed to photoisomerization from the enol form to the keto form. However, in nonpolar, aprotic cyclohexane, loss of absorbance was due primarily to photodegradation. In moderately polar, aprotic ethyl acetate, both photoisomerization and photodegradation occurred. However, photoisomerization only occurred in the presence of oxygen, while photodegradation occurred irrespective of oxygen.

In their 2013 paper, Yamaji and Kida reported on their photochemical and kinetic studies of the enol-keto and keto-enol tautomerization processes [13]. Steady-state photolysis of avobenzone in acetonitrile (~10^{-5} mol) produced the characteristic decline in absorbance of the enol form at 356 nm and a corresponding increase in absorbance of the keto form at 265 nm. This happened both in the presence and absence of oxygen. They did not observe generation of the keto form during photolysis of avobenzone in cyclohexane, though production of photodegradation products was observed. Using laser flash photolysis on avobenzone in acetonitrile, Yamaji and Kida were able to determine the quantum yield (Φ_k) of keto tautomer formation to be 0.014 with the value being independent of dissolved oxygen. Laser flash photolysis at 266 nm performed on the keto form produced a new absorption band with a 390 nm peak and a broad band from 450 to 600 nm which was attributed to absorbance of the triplet keto form. The 390 nm signal subsequently decayed at the rate (k) of 1.6×10^6 s^{-1} in the absence of oxygen (lifetime: $\tau_{KT} = 6.25 \times 10^{-7}$ s)[1] and 7.6×10^6 s^{-1} (lifetime: $\tau_{KT} = 1.32 \times 10^{-7}$ s) in aerated acetonitrile solutions. After formation by photolysis of the enol form, the lifetime (τ_K) of the keto form in the dark was determined to be 5.1 h.

Kikuchi, Oguchi, and Yagi studied the excited states of avobenzone and a specially synthesized model of avobenzone's keto form, observing the UV absorption, fluorescence, phosphorescence, and electron paramagnetic resonance spectra (EPR) of both compounds in ethanol at 77° K [14]. From the intersection of the UV absorption and fluorescence spectra, they were able to determine the singlet excited state energy (E_{S1}) of the enol form to be 25,600 cm^{-1} (73.19 kcal mol^{-1}). By similar means, they determined the singlet excited state energy of the keto form analog to be 27,000 cm^{-1} (77.20 kcal mol^{-1}). From the first peak of phosphorescence, they determined the triplet excited state energy (E_{T1}) of the enol form to be 20,400 cm^{-1} (58.33 kcal mol^{-1}) and the triplet excited state energy of the keto form to be 24,400 cm^{-1} (69.76 kcal mol^{-1}). From the decay of the first peak of phosphorescence,

[1] τ_{KT} represents the lifetime of the keto triplet.

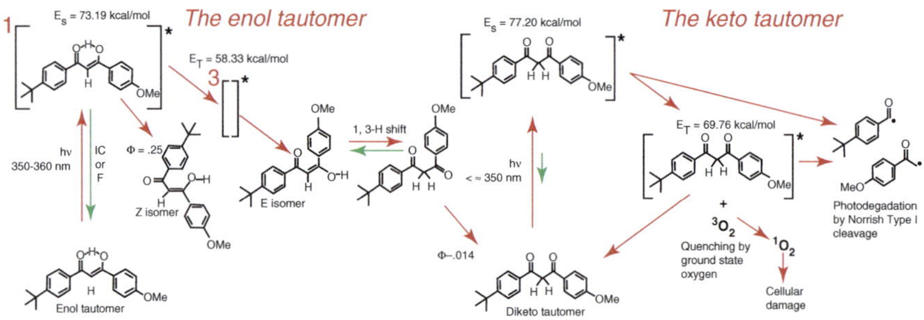

Fig. 14.5 A state energy diagram for avobenzone, compiled primarily from studies conducted at low concentrations in acetonitrile solutions. Photolysis of the enol tautomer drives an increase in the concentration of the keto tautomer, which, when excited by UVR, undergoes a Norrish type I cleavage to produce benzoyl and phenacyl radicals. The *asterisks* signify that the molecule within the brackets is in an excited state (Bonda et al. [2], reprinted with permission)

Kikuchi et al. determined the triplet excited state lifetime (τ_{phos}) of the enol form to be 30 ms and the triplet excited state lifetime of the keto form to be 190 ms.

A compound's fluorescence lifetime puts an upper limit on the lifetime of the singlet excited state. As reported by Bonda et al. (2009), measurements conducted at the University of California-Riverside determined the fluorescence lifetime of the enol form to be 13 ps [15].

From these and other studies, a picture of avobenzone's photophysics and photochemistry has emerged, which is depicted graphically in Fig. 14.5.

14.4 Photostabilities of Other UV Filters

Avobenzone is not the only photolabile UV filter used in sunscreens. In fact, there are no perfectly photostable UV filter, though some are nearly so.

Tarras-Wahlberg et al. irradiated OMC mixed with petrolatum first with 20 MED of UVB radiation and then with 100 J/cm^2 of UVA radiation. They observed slight loss of peak absorption after the UVB dose and a much larger loss of peak absorption after the UVA dose. HPLC analysis of the sample following irradiation revealed formation of a new peak which the researchers attributed to OMC's *cis* isomer, indicating that irradiation drove conversion of the normally dominant *trans* isomer to its *cis* counterpart, which absorbs UV with a similar peak but at a significantly lower molar extinction coefficient [16]. Others have found that when present in high concentrations, OMC can react with itself as two molecules undergo a [2+2] cycloaddition reaction [17].

The photostabilities of 18 UVB filters approved for the use in sunscreens in the EU were studied in vitro by Couteau et al. [18]. Each UV filter was incorporated into its own standardized oil-in-water emulsion. The researchers applied 30 mg of each formulation to roughened PMMA plates. The plates were irradiated in a xenon test

Table 14.1 Photostabilities of UVB Filters [18]

UVB filters (from most to least photostable)	Rate constant of photodecay (k min^{-1})
Iscotriazine (DBT)	.00008
PABA	.0001
Bisoctrizole (MBBT)	.0004
Oxybenzone (OXY)	.0005
Ensulizole (PBSA)	.0005
Benzophenone-5	.0006
Octocrylene (OC)	.0014
Enzacamene (4-MBC)	.0021
Octyl triazine (EHT)	.0022
Homosalate	.0023
3-Benzylidene camphor	.0031
Octinoxate (OMC)	.0031
Polysilicone-15	.0038
Anisotriazine	.0044
Amiloxate	.0059
PEG-25 PABA	.0061
Padimate O	.0062
Octisalate	.0075

Each of the 18 UV filters, listed above from most to least photostable, was incorporated into its own standardized oil-in water emulsion, which was applied to a substrate and irradiated in a xenon test chamber. Measurements were taken at timed intervals and the rate constant of photodecay (k) calculated by the equation $SPF/SPF_0 = e^{-kt}$

chamber filtered to block radiation <290 nm. The SPF was measured at timed intervals with a UV transmittance analyzer. Photodegradation of each formulation was expressed in three ways: as the number of minutes of irradiation required to cause the coated plate to lose 50 % of its SPF ($t_{50\%}$); as the number of minutes of irradiation required to cause the coated plate to lose 10 % of its SPF ($t_{90\%}$); and as the rate constant of photodecay (k) according to the equation $SPF/SPF_0 = e^{-kt}$. Table 14.1 presents the results of the study in rank order from most to least photostable.

Herzog et al. studied the photostabilities of ethylhexyl methoxycinnamate (OMC), ethylhexyl triazine (EHT), avobenzone, BEMT, and OC [19]. They incorporated each UV filter into its own oil-in-water emulsion which they applied to a quartz plate and irradiated in a xenon test chamber. At timed intervals, they used solvent to extract the residual emulsion containing the UV filter from the quartz plate and then analyzed the solution by HPLC. After 50 MED, OC and BEMT were found to be photostable. OMC and avobenzone were strongly degraded (<20 % and <1 % were recovered, respectively), and EHT was less degraded (approximately 50 % was recovered). The researchers noted degradation of OMC is not observed in ethanol solutions at low concentrations. A rapid initial loss of absorption is attributed to a change in the equilibrium between the *trans* and cis isomers (toward the *cis*) which quickly stabilizes and after which no further drop occurs.

14.5 Sunscreen Products and UV Filter Combinations

UV filters are almost never used alone in sunscreen products, which may contain up to six UV filters. Bimolecular interactions between UV filters of the same or different species, or between the UV filters and inactive ingredients with which they are paired, can have a positive, negative, or no effect on the sunscreen's photostability, as illustrated in the studies referenced below.

A major sunscreen manufacturer and marketer in the USA reported studies of the photostabilities of numerous sunscreen products in their comments to the FDA in 2007 [20] and their follow-up supplement in 2008 [21]. In one study, commercially available sunscreen products were applied in measured amounts to microscope slides and exposed to natural sunlight until 7.5 MED was reached as measured by a radiometer. The UV filters were then assayed by HPLC. Independent labs in Sydney, Australia, Winston-Salem, North Carolina, and Ormond Beach, Florida, took part. Some of the products were tested by all three labs, others were tested by two. The 14 products ranged from SPF 30 to SPF 80 and comprised 10 lotions, one lotion spray, two continuous sprays, and one stick product. Four of the products contained OMC in combination with avobenzone, and nine combined OC with avobenzone, two of which also contained OMC. Three contained avobenzone without either OC or OMC. The results may be found in Table 14.2, which groups the products tested by the presence or absence of the three UV filters. Clearly, of the products tested, the most photostable are those that contain OC and avobenzone and no OMC, or do not contain avobenzone at all. In all 12 of the products containing them, the two salicylates, octyl salicylate and homosalate, showed significant photolability, declining on average by about 24 % and 15 %, respectively.

Beasely and Meyer determined the impact of avobenzone photolability on SPF and UVA-PF [22]. They started with a model SPF 50 sunscreen product which contained 3 % avobenzone photostabilized with 7 % OC. They then prepared a

Table 14.2 % UV filters remaining after 7.5 MED of natural sunlight by HPLC

UV Filters	OC + Avo, no OMC (*N*=9)	OC + Avo + OMC (*N*=2)	Avo + OMC, no OC (*N*=2)	OMC, no Avo (*N*=1)
Octocrylene (OC)	100 %	100 %		100 %
Oxybenzone	96.8 %	94.9 %	100 %	97.0 %
Avobenzone (Avo)	91.0 %	59.6 %	25.0 %	
OMC		49.4 %	41.0 %	65.1 %
Octyl salicylate	77.8 %	75.8 %	76.3 %	75.1 %
Homosalate	86.4 %	81.4 %	86.8 %	84.2 %

14 commercially available sunscreen products were applied to microscope slides and exposed to natural 7.5 MED of natural sunlight. The studies were duplicated or triplicated by labs in Australia, North Carolina, and Florida. After exposure, each sunscreen was extracted from the slide by solvent and analyzed by HPLC to determine the amount of each UV filter remaining. The two salicylates showed significant loss in all products. Avobenzone was most photostable when combined with octocrylene (OC) without OMC

series of four new photostable formulations identical in every way to the original except that the avobenzone concentration was reduced by 20 %, 33 %, 67 %, and 100 % (no avobenzone), respectively, in order to simulate corresponding degrees of avobenzone loss due to photodegradation. These products were then tested on human volunteers and the SPF and UVA-PF determined for each and compared to the original. As expected, the researchers found that reducing the avobenzone concentration had the greatest effect on UVA-PF, though SPF suffered significant losses as well. Small losses of avobenzone ($\leq$20 %) had little effect on either SPF or UVA-PF. However, reductions of avobenzone concentrations of 33 % and 67 % resulted in the SPF declining from 51 to about 48 and 45, respectively, and the UVA-PF from about 18 to about 14 and 12, respectively. The formulation containing no avobenzone, which simulated a complete loss of the UVA filter due to photodegradation, achieved SPF 40 and UVA-PF 8.

To approximate the environment in human skin below the surface, Damiani and co-workers prepared liposomes containing pairs of UV filters and suspended them in saline. The suspensions were placed in the wells of cell culture plates and irradiated with UVA delivered by a commercial sun lamp. The total dose was calculated as equivalent to about 90 min of exposure on the French Riviera on a sunny summer day. The irradiated samples were collected, diluted with ethyl acetate, and centrifuged to recover the UV filters, after which UV absorption measurements were made and compared to non-irradiated controls. The photostable combinations paired avobenzone with bis-ethylhexyloxyphenol methoxyphenyl triazine (BEMT), methylene bis-benzotriazolyl tetramethylbutylphenol (MBBT), and diethylamino hydroxybenzoyl hexyl benzoate (DHHB). The combination with OC improved avobenzone's UVA absorption by 35 %, while the combinations with OMC and EHT showed the least photostability, losing most of their absorption throughout the entire UVA range. Combinations of OMC with BEMT, MBBT, DHHB, and EHT were photostable [23].

The oft-used combination of avobenzone and OMC was studied by Herzog and co-workers (2009). They prepared a sunscreen emulsion containing 3.4 % OMC and 2.4 % avobenzone and compared the amount of OMC recovered after irradiation with the amount recovered from the emulsion containing OMC alone. They noted a significant acceleration of OMC photodegradation when avobenzone was added and attributed the increase to the availability of a second pathway to a [2+2] cycloaddition (the first being the reaction of OMC with itself) stemming from the reaction of the enol form of avobenzone with OMC. On the other hand, adding OMC to avobenzone did not affect the amount of avobenzone recovered, indicating that the OMC-avobenzone reaction competed successfully with formation of avobenzone's keto form to reduce the pathway to the Norrish type I cleavage.

As of this writing, the FDA does not permit avobenzone to be combined with either TiO_2 or ZnO in sunscreens marketed in the USA [24]. Both combinations are permitted in many other venues throughout the world however. TiO_2 in particular is widely used in combination with organic UV filters.

Titanium dioxide exists naturally in three crystalline forms: rutile, anatase, and brookite. The TiO_2 grades used in sunscreens are made from rutile or anatase. Both forms are available in a range of particle sizes, from nano to micron. In general, the larger the particle size, the more whitening is the effect on the skin. Both TiO2 and ZnO are semiconductors with band gaps in the solar UV range. Absorption of a photon with energy equal to or greater than the band gap promotes an electron from the valance band to the conduction band, which creates an electron (−)/hole (+) pair. When this happens, molecules close to or adsorbed to the particle surface can interact with these charge carriers to become reduced (gain an electron) or oxidized (lose an electron). Because of this, these metal oxides have photocatalytic properties and can behave as either oxidant or reductant to generate reactive oxygen species (ROS) such as hydroxyl radicals (OH) and superoxide anion (O_2−). These ROS in turn can react with the organic components in sunscreens including UV filters, contributing to their degradation [25]. Of the TiO_2 crystalline forms, anatase is regarded as the more photocatalytically active [26]. For that reason, there have been recent calls to limit the TiO_2 in sunscreens to grades derived from rutile [27]. Commonly, though not always, the TiO_2 and ZnO grades used in sunscreens are passivated (rendered less reactive) by treating the surfaces of the particles with chemically inert substances such as silica, dimethicone, or aluminum hydroxide. Other surface treatments are used to improve the particles' oil or water dispersibility [28].

Kockler et al. studied the influence of TiO_2 particles size on the photostabilities of avobenzone and OC by preparing oil-in-water emulsions in which the avobenzone and OC were dissolved in the oil phase, and various grades of TiO_2 were dispersed in the water phase [29]. TiO_2 grades tested included a silica-coated rutile TiO_2 with a mean particle size of 119 nm, an uncoated anatase nano TiO_2 with mean particle size of 25 nm and an uncoated anatase micro TiO_2 with a mean particle size of 0.6 μm. Measured amounts of the emulsions were applied to glass plates and irradiated for 14.6 h at 400 W/m^2 in a xenon test chamber. After irradiation, solvent was used to extract residual emulsion from the plates, and the solutions were analyzed by HPLC. From the emulsions containing avobenzone alone or combined with coated, micro, and nano TiO2, recovery of avobenzone after irradiation ranged from 0 to 3.81 %. From the emulsion containing OC alone, or combined with coated, micro, and nano TiO2, recovery of OC ranged from 88.33 to 99.98 %. From the emulsions containing avobenzone and OC plus coated, micro, and nano TiO2, recovery of avobenzone was 16.0 %, 12.6 %, and 0.6 %, respectively, and recovery of OC was 98.2 %, 95 %, and 92.5 %, respectively. A separate experiment determined that neither avobenzone nor OC adsorb onto any of the TiO_2 particles' surfaces. The authors concluded that uncoated nano-TiO_2 is more deleterious to both avobenzone and OC than either micro or coated TiO_2.

Nguyen and Schlossman studied avobenzone photostability in dilute solutions in ethanol in the presence of various grades of TiO_2, coated and uncoated, and one untreated and four treated ZnO grades [30]. The ethanol solutions contained 0.04 % avobenzone and 4 % of metal oxide. Each sample was irradiated using a UV lamp for 1 week. Afterwards, each sample was centrifuged to remove the metal oxide from the solution, and the solution's UV absorption and transmittance were measured with a UV/Vis spectrophotometer. Both anatase and rutile forms of TiO_2 were tested. Primary particle sizes ranged from 15 nm to 300 nm. Surface treatments included octyltriethoxysilane, methicone, dimethicone, silica, aluminum stearate, and C9-15 fluoroalcohol phosphate. Among the anatase samples, the one treated with octyltriethoxysilane show the least negative effect, with 19 % of avobenzone's absorbance remaining after irradiation compared to <1 % for the other treatments. Among the first group of rutile samples, the one treated with methicone produced the best result with 38 % of avobenzone's absorbance remaining after irradiation compared to <1 % for the others. Among the second group of rutile samples, the one treated with silica (primary particle size 90 nm) was the best with 76 % of avobenzone's UV absorbance remaining after irradiation compared to 28 % and 3 % for the C9-15 fluoroalcohol phosphate and aluminum stearate treated samples, respectively. Among the ZnO samples tested, the two treated with silica fared the best, with avobenzone retaining 49 % and 18 % of its UV absorbance compared to <1 % and 3 % for the methicone- and silane-treated samples, respectively. The authors concluded that when combining avobenzone with TiO_2, rutile is superior to anatase. Also, surface-treated TiO2 and ZnO are better than uncoated TiO_2 and ZnO for limiting loss of avobenzone's absorbance following irradiation. They also noted that in this study, silica-treated TiO_2 proved to be superior to all other treated metal oxides tested for limiting loss of avobenzone's absorbance following irradiation.

14.6 Photostabilizing Sunscreens

According to an Internet search conducted in November 2014, there are 12 photostabilizers in use in sunscreens somewhere in the world including three UV filters – BEMT, 4-MBC, and OC – that are known to have photostabilizing properties [31]. Of these, only OC is globally approved; the other two are not permitted for use in sunscreens in the United States. The molecular structures of the photostabilizers and other compounds discussed in this chapter may be found in Fig. 14.6.

Herzog et al. showed that one way to increase the photostability of a photolabile UV filter like avobenzone is to increase the optical density of the system, effectively increasing the competition for the same photons. The idea is that the fewer photons absorbed by the photolabile UV filter, the lower will be its photodegradation. They illustrated this by comparing ethanolic solutions of EHT of low and high optical density. After exposure to the same amount of radiation, the solution of lower density displayed a half-life of 61 min compared to 210 min for the solution of higher density. The authors note that this strategy is effective only in cases where increasing the optical density does not also increase the rate of bimolecular chemical reactions, as it does when OMC is added to avobenzone [19].

Herzog et al. also compared and contrasted OC, a photostable UVB filter that is known to quench avobenzone's triplet excited state [32], with BEMT, a broadband (UVA and UVB) UV filter [33]. They determined the quenching rate constants of OC and BEMT for avobenzone, finding that OC is about 2.5 times more efficient than BEMT in stabilizing avobenzone. The authors also concluded that BEMT's stabilizing effect may in part be due to competition with avobenzone for photons.

Another UV filter that has considerable overlap with avobenzone's absorption spectrum is oxybenzone (benzophenone-3). Mendrok-Edinger et al. reported that adding 2 % oxybenzone to 4 % avobenzone increases photostability to 80 % compared to 23 % without [34]. Since it is energetically unlikely that Oxybenzone quenches

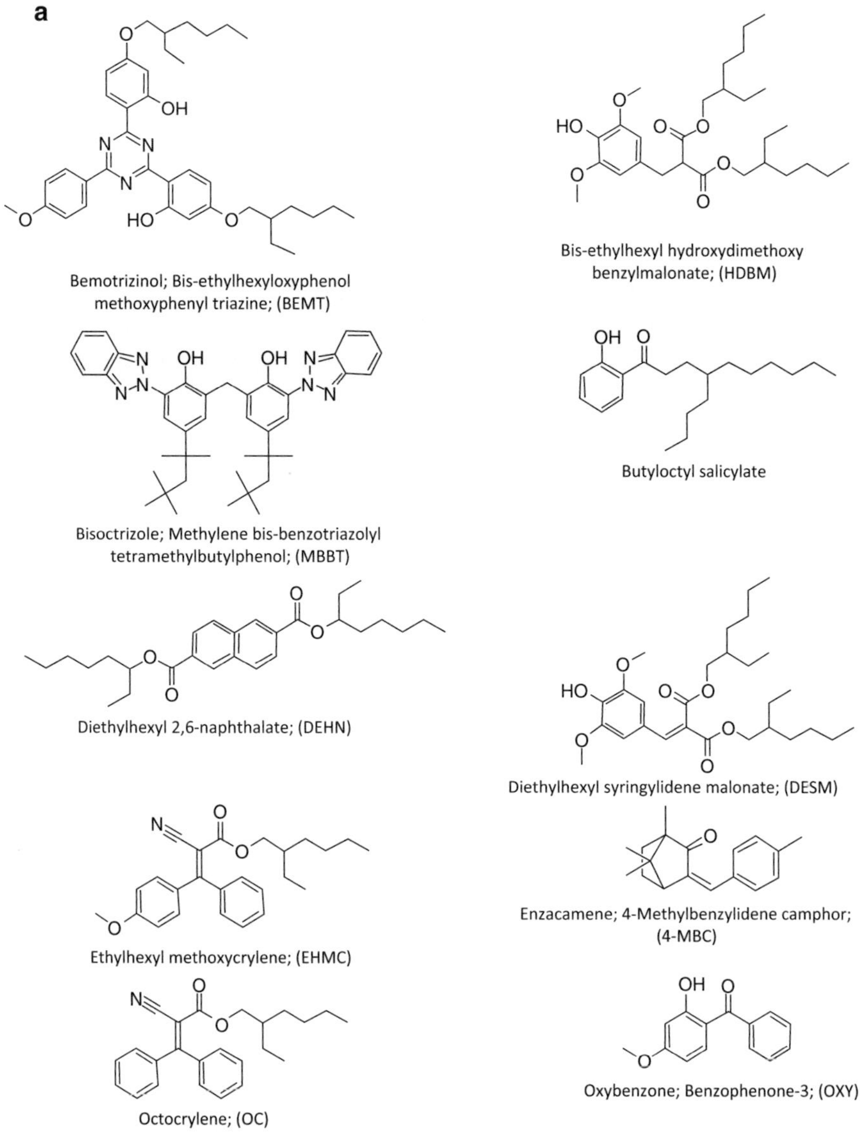

Fig. 14.6 Key chemical compounds discussed in this chapter, identified by their USAN (when relevant), INCI name, and (abbreviation) as used in this chapter. (**a**) Photostabilizers including photostabilizing UV filters, (**b**) Other UV Filters, (**c**) Antioxidants

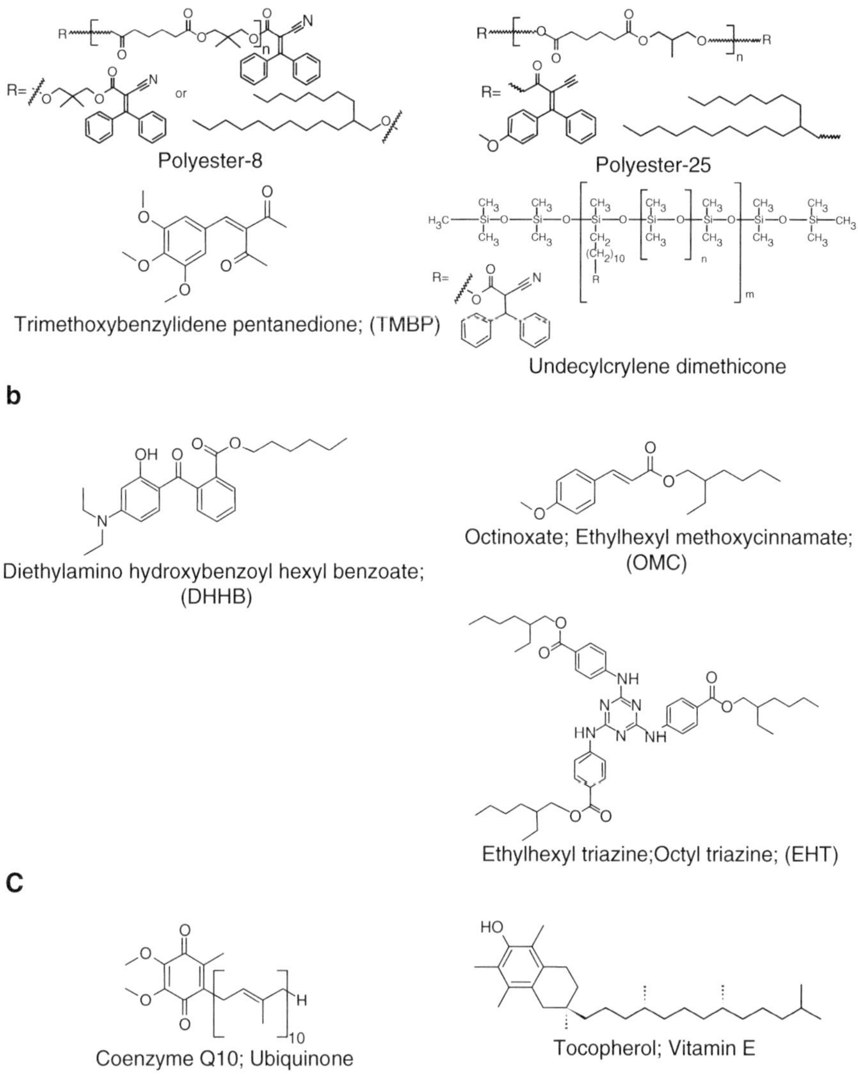

Fig. 14.6 (continued)

avobenzone triplets (using the measured triplet energy of 4-methoxybenzophenone as a proxy) [35], its competition for photons may explain the photostabilizing effect.

For excited state quenching to occur, the transfer of energy from excited UV filter to quencher must be energetically downhill (Turro et al., 2010, p. 385). That is, the excited state energy of the quencher must be lower than the excited state energy of the UV filter *for the same multiplicity* (singlet to singlet, triplet to triplet).

There are two common mechanisms by which an excited state donor (D) transfers energy to a ground state quencher (*Q*). The first is a dipole-dipole interaction (also known as "Coulombic" or "Förster" energy transfer) in which the electric field generated by the excited electron of the donor resonates with an electron of the quencher, essentially transferring the donor's energy *through space* to the quencher (Turro et al., 2010, p. 399). Thus, the donor returns to the ground state, and the quencher is raised to the excited state. This mechanism diminishes with the inverse sixth power of the distance between donor and acceptor (Turro et al., 2010, p. 402). Energy transfer by the dipole-dipole mechanism is the mechanism most often responsible for singlet-singlet quenching.

The second mechanism is known as the electron exchange mechanism (also known as "Dexter" exchange). In this mechanism, the excited donor ($^3D^*$) and quencher (Q) collide such that the donor exchanges its excited state electron for one of the quencher's ground state electrons, returning the donor (D) to the ground state and elevating the quencher ($^3Q^*$) to the excited state. Energy transfer by the Dexter exchange mechanism is easily visualized as follows:

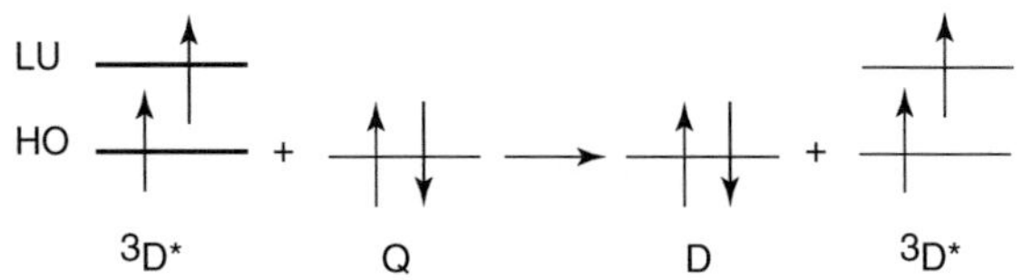

The Dexter exchange mechanism is the most common one for triplet-triplet quenching. The majority of photostabilizers on the market today (2014) function as quenchers of avobenzone's triplet excited state.

OC has long been recognized as a triplet quencher for avobenzone. Mendrok-Edinger et al. (2009) reported that 3.6 % OC added to 4 % avobenzone in a sunscreen emulsion conferred 90 % photostability. Lhiaubet-Vallet et al. tested avobenzone alone and in combination with six other UV filters, measuring by HPLC the amount of avobenzone and UV filter recovered after irradiation for four hours (!) with a solar simulator. The UV filters tested were OMC, OC, BEMT, diethylamino hydroxybenzoyl hexyl benzoate (DHHB), EHT, and dioctyl butamido triazone (DBT). The combination of OC and avobenzone was the clear winner with 84 % of the avobenzone and 100 % of the OC recovered. Next was BEMT and avobenzone, with 72 % of the avobenzone and 96 % of the BEMT recovered. With no photostabilizer, only 41 % of the avobenzone was recovered [36].

Polyester-8 is a low molecular weight (ca. 1900 daltons) organic polymer that is terminated with cyanodiphenyl propenoic acid, the same chromophore as OC. According to its manufacturer, it retains OC's ability to photostabilize avobenzone by a triplet quenching mechanism though with lower efficiency [37]. Undecylcrylene dimethicone (UCD) is a silicone polymer that also incorporates the OC chromophore. The manufacturer's literature states that it "enhances the photostability of the UVA filter avobenzone by quenching its triplet excited state" [38].

Ethylhexyl methoxycrylene (EHMC) is a commercially available cosmetic ingredient that is marketed as a photostabilizer for avobenzone and other photolabile compounds [39]. Kikuchi and co-workers determined EHMC's excited singlet and triplet state energies to be 72.3 kcal mol^{-1} and 55.5 kcal mol^{-1}, respectively [40]. These excited state energies are below those measured by Kikuchi et al. (2009 and 2010) for avobenzone (73.2 kcal mol^{-1} and 58.3 kcal mol^{-1}, respectively) and for OMC (85.49 kcal mol^{-1} and 55.75 kcal mol^{-1}, respectively), making the quenching of the singlet and triplet excited states of both compounds by EHMC energetically feasible. Researchers at the University of California-Riverside confirmed the ability of EHMC to quench avobenzone's singlet excited state. The researchers employed a streak scope (also known as a streak camera) to measure avobenzone's fluorescence lifetime in the absence and presence of varying concentrations of EHMC. At 10 mmol concentration of EHMC, the singlet excited state lifetime of avobenzone was reduced from 1.3×10^{-11} s to 1.86×10^{-12} s, shorter by about an order of magnitude [41].

Bonda et al. (2010) compared EHMC and OC to photostabilize the combination of avobenzone and OMC. The researchers prepared three solutions of 3 % avobenzone and 7.5 % OMC in ethyl acetate. One solution contained 3 % EHMC, one contained 3 % OC, and a third control solution contained no photostabilizer. The solutions were applied to PMMA plates and allowed to dry before they were irradiated with a solar simulator. After 25 MED, the control with no photostabilizer retained 44.5 % of its UVA absorbance compared to 53.9 % with 3 % OC and 83.7 % with 3 % EHMC.

4-Methylbenzylidene camphor (4-MBC; USAN Enzacamene) is a UV filter that functions as an avobenzone photostabilizer, almost certainly by a triplet quenching mechanism. Though not permitted in the USA, it has been used in Europe for decades at concentrations up to 4 %. Mendrok-Edinger et al. (2009) prepared a solution of 4 % 4-MBC and 4 % avobenzone which they applied to a roughened glass plate and then irradiated with 25 MED. Afterward, the plate was washed with solvent, and the resulting solution was analyzed by HPLC. Subsequently, 88 % of the avobenzone was recovered compared to 23 % from the solution containing no photostabilizer.

Another triplet quencher for avobenzone is diethylhexyl 2,6-naphthalate (DEHN) [42]. Mendrok-Edinger et al. (2009) found DEHN to be mildly effective. In their experiment, less than 50 % of avobenzone was recovered after 25 MED. Bonda and Steinberg reported that matched sunscreens containing 3 % avobenzone and either 0 % or 4 % DEHN were exposed to 10 MED of solar-simulated radiation and then analyzed on a UV transmittance analyzer. In the sunscreen without DEHN, UVB and UVA attenuation declined to 77 % and 64 %, respectively, while in the sunscreen with 4 % DEHN, UVB and UVA attenuation remained at 92 % and 91 %, respectively [43].

Polyester-25 is a low molecular weight polymer that is marketed as a photostabilizer for avobenzone [44]. Based on examination of its structural components, it would be expected to function mechanistically in a manner similar to EHMC.

A recent entry to the photostabilizer category is trimethoxybenzylidene pentanedione (TMBP) [45]. The manufacturer tested ethanol solutions containing 3 % avobenzone, 5 % octisalate, and 15 % homosalate to which was added either 4 % OC, 2 % DESM, or 2 % TMBP, measuring UVA absorption before and after irradiation. After 100 J/cm^2, the solution containing TMBP retained about 70 % of its UVA absorption compared to 60 % for OC and about 30 % for DESM.

Another concept is to use antioxidants to photostabilize avobenzone. Afonso et al. investigated this strategy by combining ubiquinone (coenzyme Q-10) and tocopherol (vitamin E) at various ratios with avobenzone in model sunscreen emulsions [46]. They reported a 62.2 % increase in avobenzone photostability when avobenzone was combined with ubiquinone at a 2:1 ratio and a 15.3 % improvement when avobenzone was combined with tocopherol at a 1:2 ratio.

Bis-ethylhexyl hydroxydimethoxy malonate (HDBM) is marketed as an antioxidant that improves avobenzone photostability. According the manufacturer, HDBM's triplet energy is too high to quench avobenzone's triplet excited state. Rudolph et al. tested a solution of 2 % HDBM and 2 % avobenzone in isopropyl myristate which they spread on PMMA plate. The plate was irradiated in a xenon test chamber with the equivalent of 5 MED, after which the sample was extracted with solvent and the absorption of the solution measured. At 355 nm, the avobenzone peak, the sample lost 41 % of its absorbance compared to the control with 2 % avobenzone alone which lost 58 %. A structurally similar compound, DESM, was also tested. DESM is marketed by its manufacturer as both an antioxidant and a triplet quencher for avobenzone. After irradiation, the solution of 2 % DESM and 2 % avobenzone lost 29 % of its absorbance at 355 nm [47].

Butyloctyl salicylate was found by Mendrok-Edinger et al. (2001) to be moderately effective in photostabilizing avobenzone. When butyloctyl salicylate was added at 5 % to a 4 % avobenzone solution then irradiated with 25 MED, 50 % of the avobenzone was recovered compared to 23 % without butyloctyl salicylate. Excited state quenching by butyloctyl salicylate of avobenzone is energetically unfavorable and is therefore ruled out [48]. As a liquid phenol, butyloctyl salicylate, like other salicylate esters, is a protic solvent. Recalling that avobenzone is essentially photostable in protic solvents such as isopropanol, it is likely that the stabilizing effect on avobenzone is due to butyloctyl salicylate's proticity. This effect was previously reported by Bonda et al. (1997).

Sunscreens that combine avobenzone and OMC present a special challenge for photostabilization. Under exposure to UVR, avobenzone and OMC engage in a reaction known as the De Mayo reaction. The De Mayo reaction describes the reaction of an enol with an alkene to produce a [2+2] cycloaddition followed by a retro aldol cleavage [49]. The reaction usually proceeds through the excited enol. However, in the case of avobenzone and OMC, the reaction probably proceeds through the excited alkene, OMC. This view is supported by Kikuchi and Yagi who observed the intermolecular triplet-triplet energy transfer from avobenzone to OMC through measurements of EPR and time-resolved phosphorescence spectra [50]. First they noted that triplet-triplet energy transfer from avobenzone to OMC is energetically favorable because avobenzone's triplet energy ($E_{T1\,enol} = 58.3$ kcal mol^{-1}; $E_{T1\,keto} = 69.8$ kcal mol^{-1}) lies above that of OMC ($E_{T1} = 55.75$ kcal mol^{-1}), while avobenzone's singlet excited state ($E_{S1\,enol} = 73.2$ kcal mol^{-1}) lies below that of OMC ($E_{S1} = 85.5$ kcal mol^{-1}), thus ruling out singlet-singlet energy transfer.

Lhiaubet-Vallet et al. determined the bimolecular quenching rate constant of the methylated avobenzone analog, BM-DBM-Me by OMC to be $7.3 \times 10^9\ M^{-1}\ s^{-1}$. For reference, the researchers also measured the bimolecular quenching rate constant by OC to be $3.8 \times 10^9\ M^{-1}\ s^{-1}$. By inference from

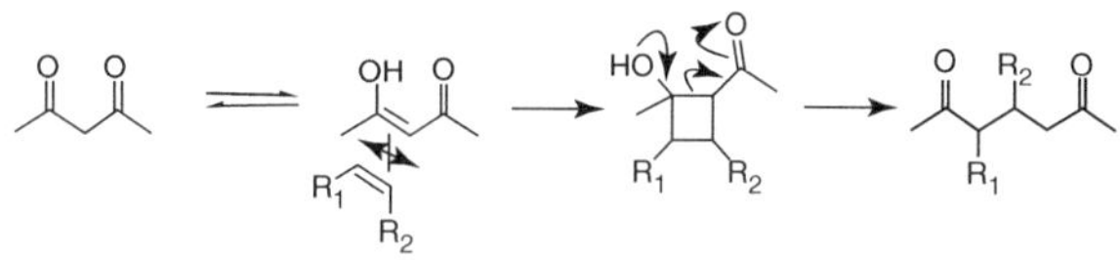

The De Mayo reaction

these findings, avobenzone efficiently transfers its triplet energy to OMC which elevates ground state OMC to its triplet excited state. OMC triplets then become the aggressive species in the previously described De Mayo reaction to photodegrade both compounds and produce photoproducts. OC's quenching rate constant, at only about half of OMC's, is not competitive.

Chatelain and Gabard (2001) studied the ability of BEMT to photostabilize the OMC-avobenzone combination, finding that BEMT exerted a protective effect on both UV filters. In sunscreens containing 5 % each of avobenzone and OMC, adding 5 % BEMT decreased photodegradation of OMC from about 65 % to about 48 % and photodegradation of avobenzone from 45 % to about 35 %. Photostabilizing the combination of OMC and avobenzone remains one of the great challenges in sunscreen formulating.

14.7 Testing Sunscreen Photostability

There are many ways to measure photostability. In this section we are concerned only with methods that measure the photostability of fully formulated sunscreen products as opposed to solvent systems that contain one or two UV filters.

One of the easiest methods to test sunscreen photostability is to monitor the change in transmission of an otherwise transparent plate (e.g., quartz or PMMA) that has been coated with the sunscreen being tested while it is being irradiated by UVR. In this method, the coated plate and suitable controls are placed in the path of the UV beam. Transmission is monitored by a detector in line with the beam but placed on the other side of the plate. The change in UV transmission seen by the detector may be quite rapid for a photolabile product. For example, if the output of the solar simulator is 150 MED/hour, the solar simulator is emitting approximately 0.042 MED per second or about 1 MED every 24 s. Theoretically, the initial output through the product covered plate would be 5 MED/hour for an SPF 30 sunscreen. The MED/hour would rapidly climb for a photolabile product as the sunscreen's ability to absorb UV rapidly declines. The advantage of this method is it is simple and fast. A second advantage is that it somewhat mimics the SPF test. The sunscreen product sees the same spectra in the photostability test as it does in the actual SPF test. If a product is seen to deteriorate rapidly in the photostability test, then essentially the product must be formulated with a heavier load of sunscreen actives than a photostable product would need to obtain the same SPF. The disadvantages of the test are that (1) the photostability of the product may be worse in sunlight than under the solar simulator; and (2) the test does not identify which ingredient or ingredients may be degrading.

A second method involves scanning a spot on a UV-transparent plate such as PMMA or quartz to which a sunscreen has been applied, then irradiating the plate and rescanning in the exact same spot. The scan should be made with a spectrophotometer designed for this application. Most companies in the industry use an instrument called a UV transmittance analyzer for this purpose. It is recommended that several scans in different locations on the plate be made. The irradiation source can be any device that emits UV energy. If a solar simulator is utilized, it is recommended that it has a beam sufficient to cover the entire plate. Of course, natural sunlight can be used as the UV source. In either case a radiometer or spectroradiometer is used to measure the amount of radiation employed. This method also has an advantage in that it is relatively simple. Another advantage is that a variety of irradiation sources can be utilized. Another advantage is that many of the spectrophotometers that are routinely used to test samples like this have software that will automatically calculate such things as SPF, critical wavelength, UVA-PF, etc. Yet another advantage is that the change in absorption at different wavelengths can be seen. This provides some guidance as to which UV filters might be degrading. For example avobenzone is the only UV filter approved in the USA with a maximum absorbance at around 360 nm. If a loss of absorption is greater around this wavelength, then it is reasonable to assume that the avobenzone is degrading. A major disadvantage of this method is, again, it only shows where loss of absorption occurs and does not identify each individual sunscreen.

In the next method, the sunscreen coating the plate is extracted with solvent after exposure to UVR and analyzed by HPLC in order to measure quantitatively the amount off each UV filter that remains. This method is much more precise than the previous two. It also has the advantage that both broad-spectrum UVR sources and natural sunlight can be used for irradiation.

Though this method supplies some of the best information concerning photostability, it does have one distinct disadvantage in that it requires development of a validated analytical method for each different UV filter combination that might be encountered. The difficulty here is that in HPLC the peaks for different compounds often overlap or obscure each other completely, making quantification impossible. To be meaningful, the peaks must be separated, which is a time and resource consuming process.

The fourth method is an in vivo one. As such it is perhaps the most revealing but also the most difficult to perform. It is similar to the previous (HPLC) method in that it involves assaying product to see which individual sunscreens degrade. A measured amount of a sunscreen product is applied to a human volunteer. After irradiation, the application site is washed with a suitable solvent (e.g., ethanol or isopropanol), and the resulting solution is analyzed by HPLC.

The result is a real-world evaluation of how a sunscreen product performs on the skin after UV exposure. A broad-spectrum UV source can be used for irradiation, but even better, natural sunlight can be used.

There are disadvantages. This method is difficult and requires the most skill of several disciplines to accomplish. The analytical method must be validated. The ability to swab most if not all of the available sunscreen from the skin must be validated. The ability to extract the sunscreen from the swab material must be validated. It requires trained clinical personnel to apply the product and monitor the subjects during all phases of the test. Institutional Review Board approval may be required before starting the test.

For additional detail and approaches to measuring sunscreen photostability, the reader is referred to Sayre et al. (2009) [51], Moyal et al. (2002) [52], and Ou-yang et al. (2010) [53].

Before concluding, we offer a few words about light (radiation) sources:

A number of published studies have found that, both theoretically and experimentally, solar simulators differ from each other in the SPF they provide and that even solar simulators that comply with regulatory standards may not provide the same SPF as natural sunlight [54–58]. Whether or not this is due to differences in photostability in natural sunlight compared to artificial sunlight is an open question. Gonzalez et al. (2007) report a case in which photostability of a sunscreen was greater in natural sunlight than in artificial sunlight. On the other hand, Lott contends in his patent titled "Natural Sunlight Photostable Composition" (US 7,309,481) that "…wavelengths present in natural sunlight that are missing in the artificial spectra, or are present in much less relative amounts than in natural sunlight, are responsible (at least in part) for degradation reactions in many sunscreens."

14.8 Summary and Conclusion

The organic UV filters in sunscreens are photochemicals that absorb the energy in ultraviolet radiation (UVR) by converting it to electronic excitation energy. At a molecular level, this is understood as the promotion of a single electron in an outer or valence orbital from its lowest energy state to a previously unoccupied orbital of higher energy, referred to as the excited state. Subsequently if physical processes drain the excess energy so that all of the molecules of the compound return unchanged to the ground state, then the compound is photostable. If, however, the excess energy fuels chemical processes that change some or all of the molecules, the compound is photolabile. Photolabile compounds lose effectiveness as UV absorbers as they are exposed to UVR. So it is with some of the organic chromophores contained in sunscreens and, therefore, with sunscreens themselves.

As recognition of the skin-damaging effects of UVA radiation has grown, sunscreen scientists and photochemists have increasingly turned their attention to understanding avobenzone, still the only effective organic UVA protectant approved worldwide. Today, after 20 years of study, a comprehensive (though still incomplete) picture of avobenzone's complex photochemistry has emerged. In a nutshell, UVR exposure induces fragmentation and radical formation in a dose-related manner. Exactly how this happens is not yet fully understood. What is known is that avobenzone photodegradation is mitigated or curtailed by combining it with compounds that quench its excited states. When combining avobenzone with TiO_2 or ZnO, coated is better than uncoated, and rutile is better than anatase.

All UV filters have been shown to be photolabile to some degree, though under conditions of actual use, many can be considered to be photostable. In contrast, the most widely use UVB filter in the world, OMC, is relatively photostable when tested at low concentration in ethanol, but quite photolabile when tested at realistic concentrations and in formulated products. When OMC and avobenzone are combined, UVR catalyzes a photochemical reaction that degrades both compounds, a result that continues to vex sunscreen formulators and for which no complete "cure" has yet been found though both BEMT and EHMC have been reported to help.

A number of photostabilizers have been developed that are more or less effective at preserving avobenzone from photodegradation. Protic solvents help, as does increasing optical density. The best photostabilizers quench avobenzone's excited states. Most of these are triplet quenchers; one has been shown to quench avobenzone's singlet excited state.

Testing sunscreen photostability is straightforward: a measured amount of product is placed on a substrate and analyzed before and after exposure to UVR and the results compared. Ideally, the sun would serve as the radiation source. As a practical matter, solar simulators must suffice for the foreseeable future.

The saga of sunscreen photostability has already produced a lasting dual legacy: for consumers, the widespread availability in much of the world of photostable sunscreens, and among sunscreen scientists, a new and deeper understanding of sunscreen photochemistry. Just as the former promises better health for millions, the latter portends a future of continual improvement in skin photoprotection.

References

1. Polefka TG, Meyer TA, Agin PP, Bianchini RJ (2012) Effects of solar radiation on the skin. J Cosmetic Dermatol 11:134–143
2. Bonda C, Hu R, Jockusch S (2014) Avobenzone photochemistry: improving photoprotection by stabilizing avobenzone with ethylhexyl methoxycrylene. HPC Today 9:6–10
3. Dondi D, Albini A, Serpone N (2006) Interactions between different solar UVB/UVA filters contained in commercial suncreams and consequent loss of UV protection. Photochem Photobiol Sci 5:835–843
4. http://www.fda.gov/drugs/developmentapprovalprocess/developmentresources/over-the-counterotcdrugs/statusofotcrulemakings/ucm072134.htm
5. Turro NJ, Ramamurthy V, Scaiano JC (2009) Principles of molecular photochemistry: an introduction. University Science Books, Sausalito

6. Schwack W, Rudolph TJ (1995) Photochemistry of dibenzoy methane UVA filters – part 1. Photochem Photobiol B Biol 28:229–234
7. Andrae I, Bringhen A, Bohm F, Gonzenbach H, Hill T, Mulroy L, Truscott TG (1997) A UVA filter (4-*tert*-butyl-4'-methoxydibenzoylmethane): photoprotection reflects photophysical properties. J Photochem Photobiol B Biol 37:147–150
8. Cantrell A, McGarvey DJ (2001) Photochemical studies of 4-*tert*-butyl-4' methoxydibenzoylmethane (BM-DBM). J Photochem Photobiol B Biol 64:117–122
9. Hill TJ (1994) Molecular mechanisms of photoprotection. PhD thesis, Keele University
10. Huong SP, Rocher E, Fourneron J-D, Charles L, Monnier V, Bun H, Andrieu V (2008) Photoreactivity of the sunscreen butylmethoxydibenzoylmethane (DBM) under various experimental conditions. J Photochem Photobiol A Chem 196:106–112
11. Bonda CA, Marinelli PM, Trivedi J, Hopper S, Wentworth G (1997) Avobenzone Photostability in Simple Polar and Non-Polar Solvent Systems. Presentation made to the Society of Cosmetic Chemists Annual Scientific Seminar, Seattle
12. Mturi GJ, Martincigh BS (2008) Photostability of the sunscreening agent 4-*tert*-butyl-4'-methoxydibenzoylmethane (Avobenzone) in solvents of different polarity and proticity. J Photochem Photobiol A Chem 200:410–420
13. Yamaji M, Kida M (2013) Photothermal tautamerization of a UV sunscreen (4-tert-butyl-4'-methoxydibenzoylmethane) in acetonitrile studied by steady-state and laser flash photolysis. J Phys Chem A 117:1946–1951
14. Kikuchi A, Oguchi N, Yagi M (2009) Optical and electron paramagnetic resonance studies of the excited states of 4-tert-butyl-4'-methoxydibanzoylmethane and 4-tert-butyl-4'-methoxydibenzoylpropane. J Phys Chem A 113:13492–13497
15. Bonda C, Pavlovic A, Hansen K, Bardeen C (2009) Singlet quenching proves faster is better for photostability. Cosm Toil 125:40–48
16. Tarras-Wahlberg N, Stenhagen G, Larko O, Rosen A, Wennberg A-M, Wennerstrom O (1999) Changes in ultraviolet absorption of sunscreens after ultraviolet irradiation. J Invest Dermatol 113:547–553
17. Schrader A, Jakupovic J, Baltes W (1994) Photochemical studies on trans-3-methylbutyl 4-methoxycinnamate. J Soc Cosm Chem 45:43–52
18. Couteau C, Faure A, Fortin J, Paparis E, Coiffard LJM (2007) Study of the photostability of 18 sunscreens in creams by measuring the SPF in vitro. J Pharm Biomed Anals 44:270–273
19. Herzog B, Wehrle M, Quass K (2009) Photostability of UV absorber systems in sunscreens. Photochem Photobiol 85:869–878
20. SaNogueira J, Lott DL (2007) Letter to FDA with comments to proposed sunscreen monograph. http://www.regulations.gov/#!documentDetail;D=FDA-1978-N-0018-0652
21. SaNogueira J, Lott DL (2008) Letter to FDA with supplement to comments to proposed sunscreen monograph. http://www.regulations.gov/#!documentDetail;D=FDA-1978-N-0018-0653
22. Beasely DG, Meyer TA (2010) Characterization of the UVA protection provided by avobenzone zinc oxide, and titanium dioxide in broad-spectrum sunscreen products. Am J Clin Dermatol 11(6):413–421
23. Damiani D, Baschong W, Greci L (2007) UV-filter combinations under UV-a exposure: concomitant quantification of over-all spectral stability and molecular integrity. J Photochem Photobiol B Biol 87:95–104
24. Federal Register/Vol. 64, No. 98/Friday, May 21, 1999/Rules and Regulations/Part 352-Sunscreen drug products for over-the-counter human use/subpart B-active ingredients/§352.20 permitted combinations of active ingredients
25. Lewicka ZA (2009) The characteristics of nanoscale sunscreen particles. Thesis submitted for Master of Science degree, Rice University
26. Luttrell T, Halpegamage S, Tao J, Kramer A, Sutter E, Batzill M (2014) Why is anatase a better photocatalyst than rutile? – Model studies on epitaxial TiO2 films. Sci Rep 4:4043
27. Turci F, Peira E, Corazzari I, Fenoglio I, Trotta M, Fubini B (2013) Crystalline phase modulates the potency of nanometric TiO2 to adhere to and perturb the stratum corneum of porcine skin under indoor light. Chem Res Toxicol 26:1579–1590

28. Carlotti ME, Ugazio E, Sapino S, Fenoglio I, Greco G, Fubini B (2009) Role of particle coating in controlling skin damage photoinduced by titania nanoparticles. Free Radic Res 43:312–322
29. Kockler J, Oelgemoller M, Robertson S, Glass BD (2014) Influence of titanium dioxide particle size on the photostability of the chemical UV-filters butyl methoxy dibenzoylmethane and octocrylene in a microemulsion. Cosm 1:128–139
30. Nguyen U, Schlossman D (2001) Stability study of Avobenzone with inorganic sunscreens. Poster Presentation at the Annual Scientific Meeting of the Society of Cosmetic Chemists, New York
31. http://www.justaboutskin.com/sun-protection-guide/how-to-evaluate-uva-protection/sunscreen-active-ingredients/sunscreen-photostabilizers/www.merck-performance-materials.com; www.sytheonltd.com; www.personal-care.basf.com
32. Gonzenbach H, Hill TJ, Truscott TG (1992) The triplet energy levels of UVA- and UVB-sunscreens. J Photochem Photobiol B Biol 16:377–379
33. Chatelain EB, Gabard B (2001) Photostabilization of butyl methoxydibenzoylmethane (avobenzone) and ethylhexyl methoxycinnamate by bis-ethylhexyloxyphenol methoxyphenyl triazine (tinosorb S), a new broadband filter. Photochem Photobiol 74:401–406
34. Mendrok-Edinger C, Smith K, Janssen A, Vollhardt J (2009) The quest for stabilizers and sunscreen photostability. Cosm Toil 124(2):47–54
35. Lin Z-P, Aue WA (1999) Triplet-state energies and substituent effects of excited aroyl compounds in the gas phase. Spectrochimica Acta Part A 56:111–117
36. Lhiaubet-Vallet V, Marin M, Jimenez O, Gorchs O, Trullas C, Miranda MA (2010) Filter-filter interactions. Photostabilization, triplet quenching and reactivity with singlet oxygen. Photochem Photobiol Sci 9(4):552–558
37. HallStar Product Information Sheet PC11030 (2011) http://www.in-cosmeticsasia.com/__novadocuments/15139?v=634826419407530000
38. HallStar Product Information Sheet PC1A054 (2011) http://www.in-cosmeticsasia.com/__novadocuments/15140?v=634826420506970000
39. HallStar Product Information Sheet PC1H044 http://www.hallstar.com/pis.php?product=1h044
40. Kikuchi A, Hata Y, Kumasaka R, Yagi M (2013) Photoexcited singlet and triplet states of a UV absorber ethylhexyl methoxycrylene. Photochem Photobiol 89:523–528
41. Bonda C, Pavlovic A, Hansen K, Bardeen C (2010) Singlet quenching proves faster is better for photostability. Cosme Toil 125:40–48
42. Bonda CA, Marinelli PJ, Hessefort YZ, Trivedi J, Wentworth G (1999) U.S. Patent No 5,993,789
43. Bonda C, Steinberg D (2000) A new photostabilizer for full spectrum sunscreens. Cosm Toil 115:37–45
44. HallStar Product Information Sheet PC11031 (2013) http://www.hallstar.com/pis.php?product=11031
45. Sytheon brochure for Synoxyl HSS. Available online at http://www.in-cosmetics.com/__novadocuments/46438?v=635285132501130000
46. Afonso S, Horita K, Silva e Sousa JP, Almeida IF, Lobao PA, Costa PC, Miranda MS, da Esteves Silva JCG, Sousa Lobo JM (2014) Photodegradation of avobenzone: stabilization effect of antioxidants. J Photochem Photobiol B Biol 140:36–40
47. Rudolph T, Pan J, Scheurich R, Pfluecker F, Graf R, Epstein H (2009) Superior two step approach to completely photoprotect Avobenzone with a designed organic redox pair. SOFW J 135(9):14–19
48. Massaro RD, Blaisten-Barojas E (2011) Theoretical investigation of the photophysics of methyl salicylate isomers. J Chem Phys 135:164306
49. http://www.rocheresearchgroup.com/wp-content/uploads/2011/06/DeMayo_ReactionSR.pdf
50. Kikuchi AM, Yagi M (2011) Direct observation of the intermolecular triplet-triplet energy transfer from UV-a absorber 4-tert-butyl-4'-methoxydibanzoylmethane to UV-B absorber octyl methoxycinnamate. Chem Phys Let 513:63–66

51. Sayre RM, Dowdy JC, Stanfield JW (2009) In vitro sunscreen transmittance measurement with concomitant evaluation of photostability: evolution of a method. Photochem Photobiol 85(4):1038–1040
52. Moyal D, Refregier JL, Chardon A (2002) In vivo measurement of the photostability of sunscreen products using diffuse reflectance spectroscopy. Photodermatol Photoimmunol Photomed 18:14–22
53. Ou-yang HJ, Stanfield JC, Cole CY, Appa Y (2010) An evaluation of ultraviolet a protection and photostability of sunscreens marketed in Australia and New Zealand. Photodermatol Photoimmunol Photomed 26:336–337
54. Sayre RM, Dowdy JC (2010) The FDA proposed solar simulator versus sunlight. Photochem Photobiol Sci 9:535–539
55. Sayre RM, Stanfield JW, Bush A, Lott D (2001) Sunscreen standards tested with differently filtered solar simulators. Photoderm Photoimmunol Photomed 17:278–283
56. Uhlmann B, Mann T, Gers-Berlag H, Sauermann A (1996) Consequences for sun protection factors when solar simulator spectra deviate from the spectrum of the sun. Inter J Cosm Sci 18:13–24
57. Young A, Boles J, Herzog B, Osterwalder U, Baschong W (2010) A sunscreen's labeled sun protection factor may overestimate protection at temperate latitudes: a human in vivo study. J Invest Dermatol 130:2457–2462
58. Lott D (2013) Testing SPF15-100, indoor vs outdoor. Cosm Toil 9:638–647

Chapter 15
Sunscreen Formulation: Optimizing Efficacy of UVB and UVA Protection

Curtis Cole

Key Points

1. Spectral shape of sunscreen products should be designed to best protect against the primary causes of sun damage: sunburn, skin cancer, and skin aging.
2. A spectral absorbance shape with approximately a 3:1 ratio of SPF:UVA-PF will provide equal protection across the UV range for the three main skin damages.
3. Vehicle components are chosen to provide the functional and aesthetic requirements for the use conditions, recreational use in intense sunlight conditions, or daily moisturization for intermittent or incidental sun exposure.
4. UV filters can be "chemical" (organic), "physical" (inorganic) filters, or a mixture of both to provide the desired spectral shape and aesthetic properties.

15.1 Background

Earlier publications [1–3] have outlined the history of development of sunscreen products starting in the 1930s with simple oils or creams to block UVB rays and extend the time one could stay in the sun before sunburning. The original sun filters were phenylbenzimidazole sulfonic acid, benzyl salicylate, and para amino-benzoic acid (PABA) derivatives. World War II soldiers were also familiar with a

C. Cole, PhD
Sun and Skin Consulting, LLC, Ringoes, NJ 08551, USA
e-mail: CurtColePhD@comcast.net

S.Q. Wang, H.W. Lim (eds.), *Principles and Practice of Photoprotection*,
DOI 10.1007/978-3-319-29382-0_15

"red" veterinary petrolatum product that provided sun protection for use in tropical regions. During the 1960s, additional UV filters were developed including the first filters to block (at least partially) in the UVA region, namely, the benzophenones and the metal oxides, titanium dioxide and zinc oxide. In 1972, the US Food and Drug Administration (FDA) initiated the current "Monograph" regulatory system that permitted manufacturers to market certain drug products without pre-market approval from the FDA, as long as the product complied with the stipulations described in the specific drug product monograph publication. The first Proposed Rule for the Over-The-Counter Sunscreen Product monograph was published in 1978 [4] describing the UV-absorbing UV filters that were recognized as safe and effective for use in these sunscreen products, the allowed concentrations and combinations permitted, and a test method to evaluate the sun protection factor (SPF) of the product to be marketed. Only UV filters that were already in market in 1972 and which had sufficient safety toxicology information submitted to the FDA were considered to be "generally safe and effective" (GRAS/E) and permitted in any new sunscreen products. The benzophenones (oxybenzone, sulisobenzone, and dioxybenzone) and titanium dioxide were the only permitted UV filters approved for use in this 1978 Proposed Rule that had any meaningful protection in the UVA portion of the spectrum. Zinc oxide was not considered at the time, either by omission or by lack of submitted supporting safety and efficacy data.

During the 1980s and 1990s, photobiology research focused on the effects of UVA radiation on skin, assessing its ability to cause skin cancer [5–8] by itself or in conjunction with UVB radiation, immune suppression [9–11], and also to contribute to the photoaging [12, 13] processes. While clearly less efficient on a photon vs photon basis compared with UVB radiation, UVA radiation is clearly implicated in virtually all of the same photobiological damage endpoints caused by UVB radiation, although the photochemical process is typically mediated by oxidative pathways rather than direct UV absorbance and lesion/photoproduct induction.

Development of commercial sunscreen products progressed throughout this same period, to provide SPF values beyond the initial envisioned "cap" of SPF 15, and was reaching SPF 30+ by the early 1990s. While immediate sunburn protection was evident via the SPF test for these products, criticism of these "high SPF" sunscreen products became more vocal suggesting that while extending the "safe" exposure time to acute sunburn, these sunscreens were also allowing for extraordinary UVA dose exposure as these sunscreens were primarily protecting only against UVB radiation, with little long-wave UVA protection. The need for broad-spectrum UVA filters was evident. It was however, not until 1996, when zinc oxide and avobenzone were approved as Category I monograph filters that formulators could begin to design truly broad-spectrum protection sunscreens in the USA. But, as formulators quickly discovered, simply adding these two ingredients into formulations was no guarantee of functional broad-spectrum performance or high UVA protection.

15.2 Photobiology Fundamentals for Optimizing Sunscreen Efficacy

In order to design a sunscreen formulation for optimal UV protection, we first have to look at the photobiology occurring in sun-exposed skin and choose the spectral protection distribution of our filters to address the various damages within the skin. The first and most obvious damage to address is sunburn, or erythema, which has a well-characterized action or "sensitivity" spectrum. This action spectrum [14] has been reduced to a mathematical equation used globally for calculations of sunburning effectiveness of light sources, including solar simulators used in sunscreen SPF testing. This action spectrum is similar in shape and magnitude to the action spectrum for DNA absorption and pyrimidine dimmer formation published earlier [15], suggesting that DNA damage may be an initiating chromophore for the sunburn reaction as well. The first definitive action spectra for squamous cell skin cancer [5, 6] showed remarkable similarity to the erythema action spectrum, as did the action spectrum for dermal elastosis [12] as developed by Dr. Kligman and Sayre. These three action spectra are shown graphically in Fig. 15.1. The primary differences are in the UVA range beyond 335 nm, which is the region with the lowest level of certainty on these action spectra. However, the relationship of the UVA to peak UVB sensitivity is on the order of 1:1000 per photon. Factoring in the predominance of UVA in the sun's spectrum (approximately 10:1) and cross multiplying the action spectra with the sun's spectral intensity distribution and summing the contributions in the various regions lead to understanding the importance of each part of the spectrum in causing these three types of damage. The estimates for the

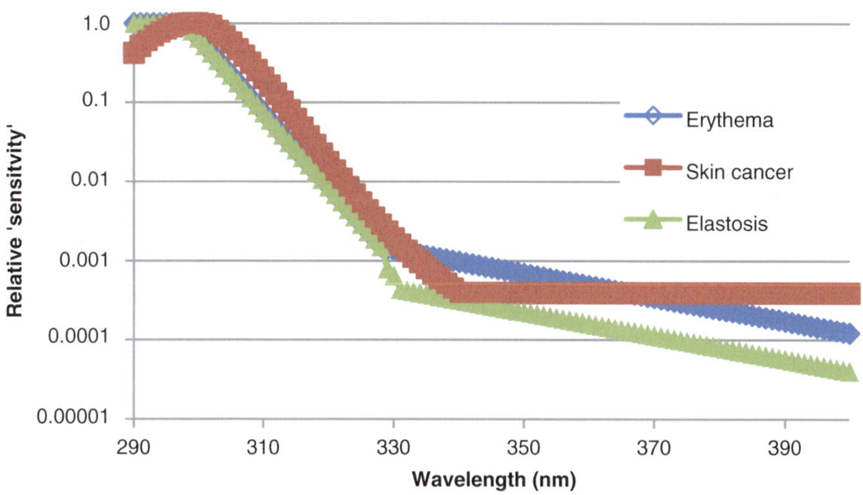

Fig. 15.1 Ultraviolet action spectra describing the sensitivity of the skin for each endpoint as a function of the wavelength of the incident UV photons (Y axis is logarithmic scale)

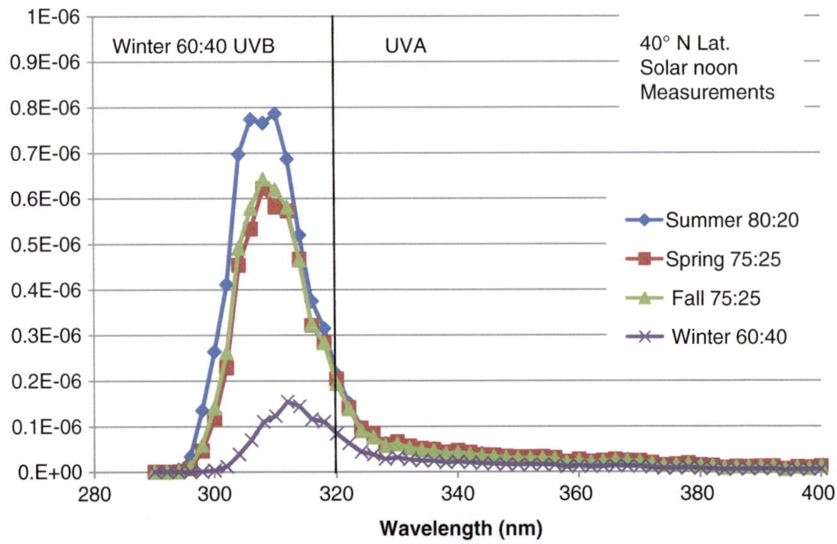

Fig. 15.2 Plot of erythemal energy from sunlight as a function of the time of year. This demonstrates the predominance of UVB in causing sunburn compared to UVA The proportions of UVB:UVA sunburning amounts are shown in the graph legends and range from 80:20 in the summertime to 60:40 in the winter. Based on noon measurements at 40° N. Lat

contributions of UVB and UVA to each of these damages depend primarily on what solar spectrum is used, but the ranges are from 87 % UVB: 13 % UVA if using Australian noontime sun [16] at 19° S latitude to 67 % UVB and 33 % UVA using an "average" lower 48 continental United States solar spectrum (ASTM G173-03 [17] Standard tables for reference solar spectral irradiances: Direct Normal and Hemispherical on 37° Tilted Surface. Book of Standards 14.04 2012). Measurements taken in New Jersey in summertime in the USA indicate approximately 80:20 UVB:UVA split for sunburn potential energy [18] in the summertime and a roughly 60:40 split in winter (see Fig. 15.2). Solar simulators used for sunscreen testing purposes are closer in spectral quality to the Australian sun standard, which is a noontime, low elevation (90 ft. above sea level) observation at the "summer" solstice, representing a high-level solar exposure situation. This solar spectrum yielded an average minimal erythema dose (MED) in just over 9 min of exposure time.

These damage action spectra address some but not all of the known UV damages. Notably missing are action spectra for basal cell skin cancer, malignant melanoma, and immune suppression. A representative model system for studying basal cell skin cancer has not been available for developing action spectra; however it is clearly associated with UV exposures and actinic keratoses [19], as well as squamous cell skin cancer. For many years, the action spectrum for malignant melanoma has been debated and was proposed to be both UVA and UVB based on a fish model [20]. More recently, deFabo has utilized a transgenic mouse model for malignant melanoma and published preliminary action spectrum data indicating that UVB radiation is the initiator of solar induced melanoma [21, 22]. Lastly, immune suppression has been demonstrated to have strong UVB sensitivity per photon as well as sensitivity in the UVA [23], and because of the predominance of UVA in sunlight, UVA has been suggested to be of particular importance in environmental exposures [24]. Sunscreens containing both UVB and UVA protection have been shown to provide protection against immune suppression proportional to the UVA-PF of the sunscreen [25, 26]. The biological data clearly indicate the need for sunscreens to provide UVB and UVA protection for both acute and long-term potential damages.

15.3 How to Design a Sunscreen for "Optimal Protection"

First, we need to decide on what is meant by "optimal" protection. Clearly, protection in both the UVA and UVB portions of the UV spectrum is needed, and metrics need to be chosen to decide when we have reached this "optimal" state of protection.

The breadth of protection has been codified in many geographies to be determined via the critical wavelength test, based on references by Diffey et al. [27], an in vitro spectrophotometric measurement of sunscreen absorbance done in thin film on an artificial substrate. The "critical wavelength" is defined as the wavelength below which 90 % of the area under the absorbance curve of the sunscreen occurs. No considerations are made for the biological activity in the various regions of the spectrum, nor for the spectral distribution of the solar spectrum, nor for the fact that the absorbance scale used in the measurement is a nonlinear logarithmic scale. It is simply an arbitrary calculation to determine how "wide" the "protection" appears in this laboratory test. Used alone, this measure does not fully interpret the UVA biological protection provided by a product, and products with equivalent SPF and equivalent "critical wavelength" can have widely different biological protection as measured with a biologically based UVA-PF test method (with persistent pigment darkening or erythema endpoint) (Fig. 15.3). The critical wavelength test can however be utilitarian in looking at the "breadth" of the "protection," but as a standalone measure, it can be misleading and insufficient to fully describe meaningful UVA "protection."

This now leads to the question: what is a meaningful measure of biological UVA protection and what should be the optimal proportion of protection for the UVB versus the UVA ranges? An acute biological endpoint is needed for a clinical assessment of UVA protection, and several were evaluated as models [28]. The initial test model to evaluate UVA protectiveness of sunscreens employed a photosensitizer, 8-methoxypsoralen [29, 30] (8-MOP), a drug used in the treatment of psoriasis that increases the sensitivity of the skin to UVA radiation via singlet oxygen production. While indicative of protection in the UVA range, the 8-MOP action spectrum does not resemble any known damage spectrum for "normal" (non-photosensitized) skin. Given 8-MOP's status as a known photocarcinogen, it was not found to be a viable test method for routine sunscreen evaluations. The

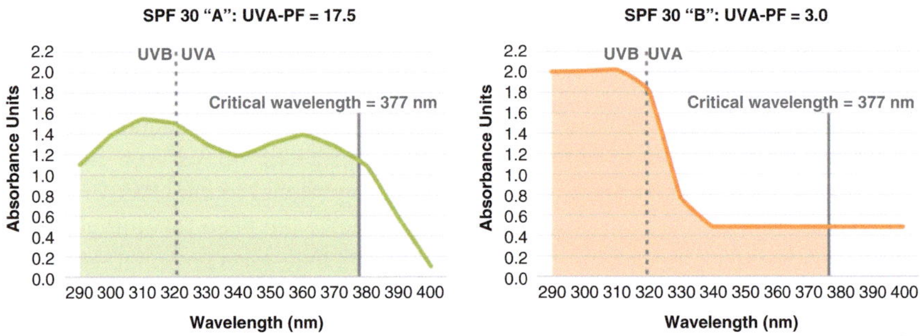

Fig. 15.3 Absorbance measurements for two SPF 30 sunscreens having the same critical wavelength with different absorption distributions and very different UVA protection capabilities as measured by spectrophotometer and UVA-PF assessments

immediate pigment darkening endpoint was investigated; however, the response was found to be dependent on the fluence rate of the light source utilized in the testing as the immediate pigment darkening response is oxygen dependent and the resulting "protection factor" determined for a sunscreen tested with this methodology depended critically on the solar simulator fluence rate [31], which would vary with the laboratory equipment used for the test. Immune response endpoints, while biologically relevant, required complicated exposure protocols and required sensitization of the test subjects, a practice of interest for academic study, but not a viable standard test methodology for routine product evaluations [32, 33].

The use of acute UVA-induced erythema as a test method endpoint was attempted and found to be primarily useful only in phototype I individuals [34], as the initial and most prevalent response to acute UVA exposures is pigment darkening, exhibited in skin phototypes II and higher [35, 36]. A UVA protection factor (UVA-PF) test [37] was developed using only this pigment darkening response as the biological endpoint. This test is analogous to the standard SPF test, but uses only UVA radiation for the exposure source and the minimal dose for persistent pigment darkening as the biological endpoint in place of the minimal erythema dose used in the SPF test. The use of the UVA-PF value has been adopted in many countries, notably Japan, Europe, Australia, as well as some South American countries, as part of regulations to determine "broad-spectrum" classification for labeling [38]. More recently, in vitro methodology has been established that replicate the test results of the human persistent pigment darkening "ultraviolet A protection factor" (UVA-PF) determination [39, 40] alleviating the need to conduct clinical trials involving high fluences of UVA radiation on human subjects. Persistent pigment darkening is a signal of biological harm and is the body's response to "damage" to help prevent further damage. It is a relatively flat spectral indicator with somewhat higher sensitivity in the shortwave UVAII range (320–340 nm), known to be more biologically sensitive relative to UVAI (340–400 nm) for many skin damage endpoints. Notably, only sunscreens having both high SPF *and* high UVA-PF values have been demonstrated to be effective against an endogenous sun sensitivity condition, polymorphous light eruption (PMLE) [41], providing some validation for use of this test methods usefulness for predicting biological protection.

We now have three measures for determining "optimal efficacy," SPF, UVA-PF, and critical wavelength to assess both the height and breadth of the UV protection of sunscreen products. But what should be the proportion of the protection in the various portions of the ultraviolet wavelength region? Should a sunscreen have a flat spectral absorbance profile, or more heavily weighted in the UVB, or maybe in the UVA portion of the spectrum? Do we have enough data to make the determination? Refregier [42] proposed that the ratio of SPF to UVA protection should be approximately 3:1 in order to have equivalent damage distributed into the UVB and the UVA portions of the spectrum, based on fundamental understanding of the relationship between SPF and UVA protection. If a "flat" sunscreen spectrum is used to attenuate the sun's spectrum, then the same proportion of damage (roughly 80 % UVB, 20 % UVA) results as with unattenuated solar UV. If, however the spectrum of the filters used in a sunscreen is weighted in the proportion of SPF: UVA-PF = 3, then the damage is shifted to the right side of the spectrum and distributing the damage equally into the UVB and the UVA portions of the solar spectrum. Having a spectrum with SPF:UVA-PF of >3:1 shifts the spectral damage even more deeper into the UVA range. The choice becomes philosophical at this point as to which distribution of damage is "best," with many regulatory bodies siding with the opinion that a "balanced" distribution is a better approach and adopting the requirement for a SPF:UVA-PF ratio of ≤3.0 in order to make "broad spectrum" or "UVA" protection claims. Coupling this requirement with a critical wavelength measurement of ≥370 nm, there is assurance that a product will have significant breadth and height of UVA protection in addition to the known SPF protection provided by the product.

With these measures established, the formulator can head to the bench to design and "optimal" protection sunscreen product using the tools of the trade.

15.4 Formulating with "Soluble" UV Filters for Optimal Protection

When starting to formulate a new sunscreen product, the formulator must first ascertain the intended use of the product (recreational/water resistant or "daily-wear" moisturization for incidental UV exposure), the target SPF desired, the aesthetic or "feel" characteristics of the product, and the desired delivery system (oil and water emulsions, liquid, alcohol gel, or spray) format, in order to choose the appropriate "soluble" UV filter to be used. The vast majority of products for both recreational and "daily-wear" utilize the oil-soluble UV filters due to their superior ability to absorb UV photons (having a higher extinction coefficient) and deliver good spreading and dry-down characteristics on the skin contributing to SPF and UVA protection efficiency on a % weight basis. In the USA, avobenzone is the only soluble UV filter that can be used to qualify a product for "broad-spectrum" claims, as it is the only soluble UV filter with absorption past the 370 nm "critical wavelength." Thus, it is the most commonly used UV filter in products today in the USA. This limited choice of UVA filters dictates much of the formulation options open to the formulator.

While a highly efficient absorber, avobenzone unfortunately has the tendency to break down upon UVA photon absorption [43] and requires careful formulation. Experience has shown that combinations of avobenzone with octinoxate [44] (and other cinnamate-based filters) or any of the PABA derivative UVB sunscreens leads to rapid photodegradation of both the UVA and the UVB protection due to the interaction of UV photons with these filters, resulting in rapidly diminishing absorption during UV exposure. While capable of delivering the SPF value determined in clinical testing, constant re-application of product with such a non-photostable product is needed to maintain meaningful protection during extended exposures in sunlight. PABA derivative filters have been avoided since the mid-1980s when concerns regarding allergenicity of Padimate A became evident. Padimate-O also known as octyldimethyl PABA has strong UVB absorption characteristics, and an excellent safety profile regarding allergenicity, has, nonetheless, little use in sunscreen products because of its similarity to the Padimate A and because of this destabilizing effect on avobenzone.

For a photostable broad-spectrum product, the formulator must combine other UVB filters with the avobenzone to build a broad-spectrum product. The salicylate filters, homosalate, and octisalate are used to provide UVB protection, despite the fact that their absorbance extinction coefficient is relatively low compared to other filters, such that they are typically used at their maximum permitted concentrations of 15 % and 5 %, respectively. Octocrylene is a good choice to combine with avobenzone for several reasons; it has a relatively strong UVB absorbance compared with the other UVB filters, rapidly increasing SPF values with modest concentrations added, but more importantly, it aids in photostabilization of the avobenzone, helping to transition the triplet state avobenzone molecule back to ground state in a timely manner.

The addition of benzophenone filters to this theoretical formulation provides three additional benefits: it increases the absorbance in the UVB portion of the spectrum, builds protection in the shortwave UVAII region between 320 and 340 nm, and provides additional photostabilization of avobenzone. This UVAII region is not strongly served by either the primary UVB filters or by avobenzone but is still in the biologically sensitive region known to be prone to both direct photon damage and indirect oxidative damage from reactive oxygen species and free radicals.

For all of the above reasons, the vast majority of sunscreen products available on the USA market today consist of combinations of avobenzone, octocrylene, homosalate, octisalate, and oxybenzone filters. US monograph restrictions currently prohibit the use of inorganic filters in combination with avobenzone, the most effective and broadest UVA filter.

If formulating without avobenzone as the primary UVA filter, the only option for a broad-spectrum product requires the use of zinc oxide to provide sufficient breadth of protection to have a critical wavelength of ≥370 nm. Because it is a photostable filter, it can be combined with octinoxate, Padimate-O, or other UVB filters as needed to achieve the desired SPF value.

Water-soluble UV filters become an option when considering daily-wear moisturizer-type products that do not require water resistance. The best water-soluble filter for consideration is ensulizole, which has a high and broad UVB absorbance, but to date, the US monograph currently does not permit marketing of products containing the combination of ensulizole with avobenzone or zinc oxide [45, 46], so that there are no options available to formulate a "broad-spectrum" product in the US market using only water-soluble filters. The only other water-soluble filters permitted to be used are sulisobenzone and trolamine salicylate; however they can be sticky in formulations and are not optimum choice for daily moisturizing products, particularly those used on the face, that require more elegant and pleasant tactile properties.

Ex-USA: Formulation options for sunscreens outside of the USA opens many more options for combinations of soluble UV filters that can provide high SPF and broad-spectrum characteristics. These include the triazine UVB filters, ethyl hexyl triazine (Uvinul T-150) and diethylhexyl butamido triazine (Uvasorb -HEB), that are "triple" UVB chromophores, with extinction coefficients five to ten times higher than other UVB filters. Thus with only a few percent of these filters, significant UVB protection can be provided. Silicone-15 is another novel UVB filter that has a much more modest extinction coefficient but is reported to boost UVB absorption and SPFs in a manner disproportionate to its own absorption properties. Its unique polymeric structure with silicone allows it to provide unique and desirable skin aesthetics to formulations.

Several other UVA1 filters are also available outside of the US market, namely, bis-ethylhexyloxyphenol methoxyphenyl triazine (trade name Tinosorb S™), methylene bis-benzotriazolyl tetramethylbutylphenol (trade name Tinosorb M™), and diethyl amino hydroxybenzoyl hexyl benzoate (Uvinul A$^+$). Tinosorb S™ is an oil-soluble filter with absorption in the mid-UVA range with a secondary peak in the UVB range, and while it does not extend its absorbance as far in the long-wave UVA1 as avobenzone, it has a high extinction coefficient and can provide significant UVA protection with low percentage quantities in formulations. It is very photostable and can provide photostabilization to avobenzone in addition to its UVB protection [47]. Tinosorb M™ is an insoluble particle (nano-size) that has a broad spectral absorbance range that extends beyond 380 nm and is the "broadest" of the UVA filters in spectral absorption.

Ecamsule (Mexoryl SX™) is a mid-range UVA filter (peaking at 340 nm) that is water soluble, and drometrizole trisiloxane (Mexoryl XL™) is an oil-soluble mid-range UVA filter, with a modest extinction coefficient. These two filters have been proprietary filters to L'Oreal. They are typically combined with avobenzone or other UVA1 absorbers for a broad-spectrum profile.

15.5 Formulating with "Insoluble" Filters for Optimum Protection

In the mid-1980s, efforts began to improve the effectiveness and cosmetic attributes of the "insoluble" inorganic UV filters, titanium dioxide and zinc oxide, by reducing the particle size of these materials. Making them "nano"-sized (less than 100 μm for smallest dimension) did two desirable things: it increased the surface area of the molecules per unit weight and providing higher absorption of the UV photons per unit weight and making them more transparent in the visible portion of the spectrum and less visible on the skin. Organic surface coatings added to the molecules eliminated the potential surface reactivity and made them easier to formulate into emulsions in either the water phase or the oil phase, depending on the nature of the surface coating. While never quite achieving ultimate "invisibility," significant progress has been made through careful choices of the suspending excipients and the emulsifiers used.

While reduction in particle size of titanium dioxide shifts the absorption spectrum toward higher UVB protection, and lower UVA protection, and reducing the particle size of zinc oxide can boost the absorbance in the mid UVA1 region [48]. Anderson et al.[46] have a detailed description regarding the inorganic filter characteristics and their formulation. "Nano" titanium dioxide and zinc oxide are typically formulated into lotions and cream emulsion form products, which can be characterized as "oil-in-water" emulsions (oil droplets in a "sea" of water) or as "water-in-oil" emulsion (water droplets in a "sea" of oil). Each form has its own unique advantage depending on the intended use of the product and consumer preference. Different emulsifiers are used for the two forms and with the exterior phase of the emulsion (the "sea" portion) typically constituting the larger proportion of the formulation by weight.

Oil-in-water emulsions with the inorganic sunscreen filters will typically have a more traditional "lotion" feel and use characteristic, with easier spreading, more rapid dry-down time, and a less oily/greasy after-feel when the water has evaporated. This is generally the more consumer preferred form of product. In contrast, the water-in-oil form of this type of product will have a higher oil content and thus take more time to dry down with a heavier and perhaps more oily after-feel. The advantages of this type of emulsion are more moisturization (especially for very dry skin), higher efficiency of the filters to provide UV protection per unit UV filter incorporated into the system, and more inherent water resistance characteristics [49].

As mentioned before, inorganic filters may be combined with all of the soluble filters in the US except avobenzone. This restriction does not apply outside of the USA where the combination of titanium dioxide and zinc oxide with the soluble UV filters is commonly used to augment both the UVB and UVA protection, respectively. Additionally, ex-US, the insoluble UV filter Tinosorb M™ can also be added to provide UVA1 protection beyond the range covered by zinc oxide or avobenzone.

15.6 Summary

Optimizing sunscreen formulations for efficacy with soluble UV filters or insoluble UV filters (be they only insoluble filters, or combinations with soluble UV filters), the objective for the spectral distribution of the protection is to provide proportional protection across the UV spectrum, ideally in such a way as to deliver the SPF:UVA-PF ratio of approximately 2.5:1 to 3:1. This proportion assures proportional UVA protection, with appropriately higher protection weighting in the more damaging UVB portion of the spectrum, distributing the penetrating damage equally across both the UVB and the UVA regions. It should be noted that other opinions suggest that a "flat" or "spectra homeostasis" distribution of protection is "optimal" [50, 51]. This concept ignores the decades of scientific discovery and action spectra determinations that have identified UVB as the more damaging and life-threatening portion of the sun's UV spectrum, notably DNA damage causing skin cancers and, more recently determined, malignant melanoma [21, 22]. Limiting the UVB protection to achieve a "flat" spectral distribution of protection opens the window of skin damage to these more powerful photons, diminishing the overall protection of the product. Consumers in extended sunlight exposure should seek out the highest SPF product available that provides the broad-spectrum protection having an SPF:UVA-PF ration of approximately 3:1 for best protection.

References

1. Urbach F (2001) The historical aspects of sunscreens. J Photochem Photobiol 64(2–3):99–104
2. Roelandts R (2009) History of photoprotection. In: Lim H, Draelos Z (eds) Clinical guide to sunscreens and photoprotection. Informa Healthcare, New York, pp 1–10
3. Cole C (2009) Formulation and stability of sunscreen products. In: Lim H, Draelos Z (eds) Clinical guide to sunscreens and photoprotection. Informa Healthcare, New York, pp 39–51
4. Food and Drug Administration, USA (1978) Sunscreen drug products for over the counter use: proposed safety, effectiveness and labeling conditions. Fed Reg 43(166):38206–38269
5. Cole C, Forbes P, Davies R (1986) An action spectrum for UV photocarcinogenesis. Photochem Photobiol 43:275–284
6. de Gruijl FR, Sterenborg HJ, Forbes PD, Davies RE, Cole C, Kelfkens G, van Weelden H, Slaper H, van der Leun JC (1993) Wavelength dependence of skin cancer induction by ultraviolet irradiation of albino hairless mice. Cancer Res 53:53–60
7. de Gruijl FR (2002) Photocarcinogenesis: UVA vs UVB radiation. Skin Pharmacol Appl Skin Physiol 15:316–320
8. Staberg B, Wulf HC, Klemp P, Brodthagen H (1983) The carcinogenic effect of UVA irradiation. J Invest Dermatol 81:517–519
9. Bestak R, Halliday G (1996) Chronic low-dose UVA irradiation induces local suppression of contact hypersensitivity, Langerhans cell depletion and suppressor cell activation in C3H/HeJ mice. Photochem Photobiol 64:969–974
10. Bestak R, Barnetson R, Nearm M, Halliday G (1995) Sunscreen protection of contact hypersensitivity responses from chronic solar-simulated ultraviolet irradiation correlates with the absorption spectrum of the sunscreen. J Invest Dermatol 105:345–351

11. Iwai I et al (1999) UVA-induced immune suppression through an oxidative pathway. J Invest Dermatol 112:19–24
12. Kligman LH, Sayre RM (1991) An action spectrum for ultraviolet induced elastosis in hairless mice: quantification of elastosis by image analysis. Photochem Photobiol 53:237–242
13. Bissett D et al (1987) An animal model of solar-aged skin: histological, physical, and visible changes in UV irradiated hairless mouse skin. Photochem Photobiol 46(3):367–378
14. McKinley A, Deffey BL (1987) "A reference action spectrum for ultraviolet induced Erythema in human skin". In: Passchier WF, Bosnajakovic BFM (eds) Humen exposure to ultraviolet radiaton: risks and regulations, International congress series. Elsevier, Amsterdam, pp 83–87
15. Setlow R (1974) The wavelengths in sunlight effective in producing skin cancer: a theoretical analysis. Proc Natl Acad Sci U S A 71(9):3363–3366
16. Bernhard G, Mayer B, Seckmeyer G (1997) Measurements of spectral solar UV irradiance in tropical-Australia. J Geophys Res 102(D7):8719–8730
17. ASTM G173-03(2012) Standard tables for reference solar spectral irradiances: Direct Normal and Hemispherical on 37° Tilted Surface. Book of Standards 14.04 2012
18. Cole CA (2001) Measurement of sunscreen UVA protectiveness. Review article. Photomedicine Photoallergy Photodermatology 17(1):2–10
19. Green A et al (1996) Skin cancer in a subtropical Australian population: incidence and lack of association with occupation. AM J Epidemiol 144(11):1034–1040
20. Moan J, Dahlback A, Setlow RB (1999) Epidemiological support for a hypothesis for melanoma induction indicating a role for UVA radiation. Photochem Photobiol 70:243–247
21. DeFabo E (2006) Initial studies on an *in vivo* action spectrum for melanoma induction. Prog Biophys Mol Biol 92(1):97–104
22. De Fabo EC, Noonan FP, Fears T, Merlino G (2004) Ultraviolet B but not ultraviolet a radiation initiates melanoma. Cancer Res 64:6372–6376
23. Ullrich SE, Nghiem DX, Khaskina P (2007) Suppression of an established immune response by UVA: a critical role for mast cells. Photochem Photobiol 83(5):1095–1100
24. Damian DL, Matthews YJ, Phan TA, Halliday GM (2011) An action spectrum for ultraviolet radiation-induced immunosuppression in humans. Br J Dermatol 163(3):657–659
25. Moyal D, Fourtanier A (2002) Effects of UVA radiation on an established immune response in humans and sunscreen efficacy. Exp Dermatol 11(S1):28–32
26. Ngheim DX, Kazimi N, Clydesdale G, Ananthaswamy HN, Kripke ML, Ullrich SE (2001) Ultraviolet a radiation suppresses an established immune response: implications for sunscreen design. J Invest Dermatol 117:1193–1199
27. Diffey BL, Tanner PR, Matts PJ, Nash JF (2000) In vitro assessment of the broad-spectrum ultraviolet protection of sunscreen products. J Am Acad Dermatol 43(6):1024–1035
28. Cole C (2001) Sunscreen protection in the ultraviolet a region: how to measure effectiveness. Photoderm Photoimmunol Photomed 17:2–10
29. Gange R, Soparkar A, Matzinger B, Dromgoole S, Sefton J, DeGryse R (1986) Efficacy of a sunscreen containing butyl methoxydibenzoylmethane against ultraviolet a radiation in photosensitized subjects. J Am Acad Dermatol 15:494–499
30. Lowe N, Dromgoole S, Sefton JH, Bourget T, Weingarten D (1987) Indoor and outdoor efficacy testing of a broad spectrum sunscreen against ultraviolet a radiation in psoralen sensitized subjects. J Am Acad Dermatol 17:224–230
31. Kollias N, Bykowski J (1999) Immediate pigment darkening thresholds of human skin to monochromatic (362 nm) ultraviolet a radiation are fluence rate dependent. Photodermatol Photoimmunol Photomed 15:175–178
32. Fourtanier A, Moyal D, Maccario J, Compan D, Wolf P, Quehenberger F, Cooper K, Baron E, Halliday G, Poon T, Seed P, Walker SL, Young AR (2005) Measurement of sunscreen immune protection factors in humans: a consensus paper. J Invest Dermatol 125(3):403–409
33. Young AR (2004) Methods used to evaluate the immune protection factor of sunscreen: advantages and disadvantages of different in vivo techniques. Cutis 74(5 Suppl):19–23
34. Standfield J, Feldt P, Csortan E, Krochmal L (1989) Ultraviolet a sunscreen evaluations in normal subjects. J Am Acad Dermatol 20:744–778

35. Cole C, Van Fossen R (1992) Measurement of sunscreen UVA protection; an unsensitized human model. J Am Acad Dermatol 26:178–184
36. Cole C (1994) Multicenter evaluation of sunscreen UVA protectiveness with the protection factor test method. J Am Acad Dermatol 30:729–736
37. Chardon A, Moyal D, Hourseau C (1997) Persistent pigment darkening response for evaluation of ultraviolet a protection assays. In: Lowe N, Shaath N, Pathak M (eds) Sunscreens: development, evaluation and regulatory aspects. Marcel Dekker, New York, pp 582–559
38. Japan Cosmetic Industry Association (JCIA) technical bulletin. Measurement standard for UVA protection efficacy, Issued 21 Nov 1995 as effective as of 1 Jan 1996. (The European Cosmetic Toiletry and Parfumery Association)
39. COLIPA In Vitro Photo Protection Methods Task Force (2007) Method for the *in vitro* determination of UVA protection provided by sunscreen products. Guideline 2007, 2nd edn. COLIPA, Brussels
40. ISO 244432012 (2012) Test method: cosmetics-sun protection test method – determination of sunscreen UVA photoprotection *in vitro*
41. Fourtanier A, Moyal D, Selte S (2008) Sunscreens containing the broad-spectrum absorber, Mexoryl SX, prevent the cutaneous detrimental effects of UV exposure; a review of clinical study results. Photoderm Photoimmun Photomed 24(4):164–174
42. Refregier JL (2004) Relationship between UVA protection and skin response to UV light: proposal for labeling UVA protection. Int J Cosmet Sci 26:197–206
43. Tarras-Wahlberg N, Stenhagen G, Larkö O, Rosén A, Wennberg A, Wennerström O (1999) Changes in ultraviolet absorption of sunscreens after ultraviolet irradiation. J Invest Dermatol 113:547–553
44. Sayre MR, Dowdy JC, Gerwig AJ, Williams WJ, Lloyd RV (2005) Unexpected photolysis of the sunscreen octinoxate in the presence of the sunscreen avobenzone. Photochem Photobiol 81(2):452–456
45. Federal Register, 21 CFR Parts 201 and 301 (2011) Labeling and effectiveness testing: sunscreen drug products for over-the-counter human use. 76(117):35623
46. Federal register, 21 CFR Parts 201 and 301 (2007) .Sunscreen products for over-the-counter human use: propose amendment of final monograph. 72(165):49075
47. Chatelain E, Gabard B (2001) Photostabilization of butyl methoxydibenzoylmethane (avobenzone) and ethylhexyl methoxycinnamate by Bis-ethylhexyloxyphenol methoxyphenyl triazine (tinosorb S), a New UV broadband filter. Photochem Photobiol 74(3):401–406
48. Anderson MW, Hewitt JP, Spruce SR (1997) Broad-spectrum physical sunscreens: titanium dioxide and zinc oxide. In: Lowe N, Shaath N, Pathak M (eds) Sunscreens: development, evaluation, and regulatory aspects, 2nd edn. Marcel Decker, New York, pp 353–396
49. Hewitt J (2013) Formulating with nano technologies in skincare: opportunities and challenges. In: Nasir A (ed) Nanotechnology in medicine. Springer Science and Business Media LLC, New York, p 1
50. Osterwalder U, Champ C, Flösser-Müller H, Herzog B (2013) The evoluation of UVA protection. www.skin-care-forum.basf.com. Sept 2013
51. Diffey BL, Brown MW (2012) The ideal spectral profile of topical sunscreens. Photochem Photobiol 88(3):744–747

Chapter 16
Sunscreen Formulation: Optimising Aesthetic Elements for Twenty-First-Century Consumers

Julian P. Hewitt

Key Points

1. Good aesthetic properties (appearance and skin feel) are now seen as an important aspect of sunscreen products, as they encourage greater consumer compliance and also a means of differentiating products from the competition.
2. Sensory panel studies indicate that what is usually desired is a product that spreads easily with a moderately wet feeling during application but feels smooth and dry afterwards with little or no perceivable residue.
3. With organic UV filters, judicious choice of emollients helps to optimise both skin feel and efficacy. Improving the efficacy also enables the formulator to improve aesthetic properties as lower concentrations of UV filters are required to reach the target SPF.
4. With inorganic UV filters, developments in manufacturing and coating technology have produced materials that are transparent on skin while still being effective and also deliver elegant skin feel.

16.1 Introduction

Today's sun care formulator must achieve ever more challenging standards for product efficacy while also making products cosmetically appealing. Performance and aesthetics are in fact dependent on one another. Studies have shown that consumers almost always use less than the "recommended" amount of sunscreen products [1, 2], and this means that the effective "in-use" SPF is considerably less than that tested

J.P. Hewitt
JPH SunCare Technologies Ltd., Durham, UK
e-mail: julian@jphsuncare.com

S.Q. Wang, H.W. Lim (eds.), *Principles and Practice of Photoprotection*,
DOI 10.1007/978-3-319-29382-0_16

and displayed on the label [3, 4]. Among the reasons most frequently cited by consumers for underuse (or complete avoidance) of sunscreens are aesthetic issues, for example, that the products feel too greasy or sticky or they make the skin look shiny or leave a white residue on skin. It can therefore be expected that products with improved aesthetics encourage consumers to apply more product and therefore get closer to the labelled SPF. Conversely, maximising the efficacy of the actives used enables high SPF products to be created with minimal levels of UV filters, which allows the formulator greater freedom to optimise skin feel.

Also, in many parts of the world, efficacy claims for sunscreen products are becoming more regulated and uniform. For example, in Europe, the European Commission Recommendation on labelling and efficacy of sunscreens [5] provides a specific list of SPF claims that can be used: 6, 10, 15, 20, 25, 30, 50 and 50+. Similar restrictions exist in a number of other countries. In terms of UVA claims, many countries now have a single performance criterion for a UVA or broad-spectrum claim, and numerical claims to indicate the degree of UVA protection are either discouraged or explicitly prohibited. This limits the options for manufacturers and marketers to differentiate their products from the competition based on efficacy claims. Improving the cosmetic properties of the product has therefore become an important alternative means of providing differentiating claims. This chapter will discuss how this can be achieved, depending on the type of vehicle and the active ingredients used.

16.2 Desired Aesthetic Properties for Modern Sunscreen Products

Of course, as with any cosmetic or topical product, the "optimum" aesthetic properties depend very much on the personal preferences of the individual consumer and can also be influenced by the environment in which the product is used (e.g. dry or humid, beach or mountain), level of activity (e.g, sunbathing, walking, sports) and area of application (face or body). However, there are some general trends that can be identified.

A study by Vollhardt et al. [6, 2] used descriptive sensory analysis to assess the sensory properties of over 50 different commercial sunscreen lotions with label SPF claims of 30 or 50. Since these were products already on the market, it is reasonable to assume that they give a good representation of the sensory properties that are accepted/desired by consumers. The sensory parameters assessed were grouped into three distinct phases of product application: rub-out, immediate after-feel and after-feel 20 min later. Based on this study, the desirable properties during rub-out can be summarised as:

- "*Wetness*" should be neither too high nor too low.
- *Spreadability* should be high.
- "*Thickness*" should be low.

- "*Whiteness*" should be low, although the data indicate that consumers expect a certain degree of whiteness during rub-out.
- "*Oiliness*" and "*greasiness*" should be relatively low but not excessively so, while "*waxiness*" during rub-out was lower in the products tested. This makes sense, considering the requirement for good spreadability; a product that does not spread well is perceived as more "waxy."
- "*Absorbency*" should be fast but not too fast; if a product absorbs too quickly into the skin, it can be difficult to spread over a wide area.

The key attributes in the after-feel, particularly after 20 min, are:

- Low *gloss*
- Very low *whiteness*; note the contrast here with the rub-out phase – while consumers may accept some whitening during rub-out, they want no visible residue afterwards.
- Very low *stickiness*
- High "*slipperiness*" – in other words consumers are looking for a smooth feeling on skin after application.
- Low *residue*
- Low *oiliness* and *greasiness*, with relatively higher *waxiness*. Again the contrast with the rub-out phase is instructive here; while a perception of high waxiness during rub-out would indicate poor spreadability, in the after-feel phase, it indicates a "dry" after-feel. The prevalence of new sun care products in recent years with claims of "dry skin feel" or "dry touch" shows that this is a desirable property.

In summary, then, what is usually desired is a product that spreads easily with a moderately wet feeling during application but feels smooth and dry afterwards with little or no perceivable (either by touch or sight) residue.

16.3 Sunscreen Vehicles

Sunscreen products can be formulated in a variety of different forms:

- Emulsions
  - O/W or W/O
  - Creams, lotions and sprays
- Anhydrous systems
  - Ointments
  - Sticks
  - Aerosol sprays
  - Oils
- Gels

Emulsions remain the predominant form for sun protection products globally, so this chapter will focus on optimising the aesthetic properties of emulsion-based sunscreen products.

Generally, oil-in-water (O/W) emulsions have a more preferred skin feel than water-in-oil (W/O) systems. This can be intuitively understood; with water as the external phase, there is an immediate sensation of wetness on the skin when an O/W emulsion is applied. Also, as the water begins to evaporate during application, this provides a cooling effect to the skin, which can be a pleasant sensory experience especially for sun care products as they are often applied in hot conditions. This cooling effect can be enhanced by the addition of alcohol or other volatile components to the formulation.

W/O emulsions, on the other hand, with oil as the external phase, tend to feel more "oily" or "greasy" upon application and are generally perceived as "heavier." In some niche applications, this can be welcome, for example, in sun care products for winter sports use, where this more occlusive feel gives a greater sensation of protection in a cold environment. Another application in which the sensory feel of W/O emulsions can be preferred is in baby sun care products, where the "protective" sensation gives parents a sense of reassurance that they have protected their child. In most beach sun care products, though, W/O emulsions have traditionally been seen as the less preferred option in terms of skin feel. However, innovations in W/O emulsifier technology [7, 8] mean that it is now possible to formulate W/O emulsions which have a more elegant skin feel. This allows the sun care formulator to take advantage of the benefits of W/O systems, such as water resistance and increased efficacy of actives while still delivering a formulation that is aesthetically pleasing for the consumer.

16.4 Formulations Based on Organic UV Filters

In discussing the aesthetic properties of formulations containing organic UV filters, it is convenient to classify the filters in four groups:

- Liquid UV filters
- Oil-soluble solid UV filters
- Water-soluble solid UV filters
- Insoluble particulate UV filters

Each of these will be discussed in turn.

16.4.1 Liquid UV Filters

In any cosmetic emulsion, the spreadability of the oil components exerts a significant influence on skin feel, in particular during the application of the product. Bruening et al. [9] described how it is desirable to impart a sensation of smoothness to the skin throughout application. The challenge presented by liquid organic UV filters such as ethylhexyl methoxycinnamate (octinoxate), ethylhexyl salicylate (octisalate), homosalate and especially octocrylene is that these are slow-spreading materials that impart a low degree of smoothness. This therefore needs to be counteracted by the inclusion of fast-spreading emollients that give a much greater and more immediate sensation of smoothness. Ideally, according to Bruening et al., the formulation should include a combination of fast- and medium-spreading emollients which, in combination with the slow-spreading liquid UV filters, create a spreading "cascade" so that a consistent perception of smoothness is maintained throughout the rub-in of the product.

One class of cosmetic emollients that are often included in skin care products to impart a "light", dry skin feel is silicone fluids. However, such materials have a drawback in sun care formulations, which is that they tend to be poor solvents for solid organic UV filters (see next section). However, one sunscreen material allows the formulator to take advantage of the skin feel benefits of silicone chemistry. Polysilicone-15 [10] is a polymeric liquid UVB filter that consists of UV-absorbing chromophores attached to a silicone backbone. This material is not yet approved as a UV filter in the USA but is approved in Europe, Japan, Australia and a number of other countries.

16.4.2 Oil-Soluble Solid UV Filters

When formulating with filters such as butyl methoxydibenzoylmethane (avobenzone), benzophenone-3 (oxybenzone), ethylhexyl triazone (octyl triazone), or bis-ethylhexyloxyphenol methoxyphenyl triazine (bemotrizinol), the formulator's first concern is to ensure good solubility of the active(s) in the oil phase. The UV filters must be effectively dissolved and remain in solution throughout the lifetime of the product and when it is applied on skin. Any recrystallisation has an adverse effect on both efficacy and skin feel. Previous work [11] has shown that, with these oil-soluble sunscreens, SPF efficacy increases with increasing solubility of the active in the oil phase.

One emollient has become virtually an industry standard as a solvent for sunscreens: C_{12-15} alkyl benzoate. This ester is an excellent solvent for most solid organic UV filters and also confers a light, dry emollience with a non-greasy after-feel. However, in recent years a number of new emollients have been developed that offer even better solvency for sunscreens and are claimed to be as good as, if not superior to, C_{12-15} alkyl benzoate in terms of skin feel [12], for example:

- Phenethyl benzoate
- Phenoxyethyl caprylate
- PPG-3 benzyl ether ethylhexanoate
- Ethylhexyl benzoate
- Neopentyl glycol diheptanoate (and) propylene glycol dibenzoate

16.4.3 Water-Soluble Solid UV Filters

There are a number of water-soluble UV filters, but only the following are of significant commercial importance nowadays:

- Benzophenone-4 (UVB/UVA filter)
- Disodium phenyl dibenzimidazole tetrasulfonate (UVA filter)
- Phenylbenzimidazole sulfonic acid (UVB filter)
- Benzylidene camphor sulfonic acid (UVB filter)
- Terephthalylidene dicamphor sulfonic acid (UVA filter)

Of these, the last two are proprietary to L'Oreal, and so for most formulators, the first three in the above list are the only water-soluble filters available. These all require neutralisation with a suitable base in order to render them soluble. In terms of sensory properties, these water-soluble sunscreens tend to have a drying effect on skin feel; this is often advantageous, but the feel can be excessively dry if a high concentration of such filters is used.

16.4.4 Insoluble Particulate Organic Filters

A relatively new class of sunscreen actives are organic UV filters that are not soluble in either oil or water and remain in a particulate form in the final formulation. The first of these was methylene bis-benzotriazolyl tetramethylbutylphenol (MBBT, or bisoctrizole), which is primarily a UVA filter but has a secondary absorption peak in the UVB. In 2014, a second material was added to this class of UV filters when tris-biphenyl triazine (TBPT) was approved in Europe. TBPT gives high absorbance in the UVB and UVA2 (320-340 nm), the latter being a wavelength region that is not well covered by most other UV filters. Both of these materials are supplied as aqueous nanoparticulate dispersions. With regard to sensory properties, both tend to have a drying effect on skin feel (although less so than most water-dispersed inorganic sunscreens). Also, being particulates, both can give rise to an undesirable sensory attribute that is not observed with other organic UV filters, namely, whitening. Both MBBT and TBPT give a low but significant light extinction in the visible region of the spectrum; since they are most typically used at relatively low levels in formulations, this is usually not noticeable, but at higher levels (above 5 % active), a discernible whitening effect may be observed.

16.5 Formulations Based on Inorganic UV Filters

Titanium dioxide (TiO_2) and zinc oxide (ZnO) have been used as sun-protective agents for many years, but it was only with the development of the first "fine particle" (a.k.a. "microfine", "ultrafine") grades of these materials in the late 1980s that they began to achieve significant commercial usage in topical sunscreen products. These fine particle grades provide a high degree of UV attenuation while being substantially transparent to visible light. (NOTE: The term "micronised" is often used as a generic term to describe UV-attenuating grades of TiO_2 and ZnO. This is a misnomer. Micronisation is a specific physical process, involving attrition milling with high gas velocities, typically following a calcination step. Most UV-attenuating grades of TiO_2 and ZnO are produced without this milling step; thermodynamic control of crystal growth is used to obtain the correct fine crystal size.)

TiO_2 is primarily a UVB filter but can also offer significant UVA protection depending on the particle size and size distribution. It is possible to formulate high SPF sunscreen products with TiO_2 as the sole active ingredient. ZnO is less effective than TiO_2 in terms of UVB protection, and hence SPF efficacy, but has a relatively flat extinction profile up to wavelengths of about 360–370 nm and so is typically more effective than TiO_2 in the long-wavelength UVA part of the spectrum. The broad-spectrum protection offered by these materials is one of their major advantages as sunscreen actives. The fact that they do not decay on exposure to UV contributes to their high efficacy. They also have an excellent safety profile [13, 14], making them especially well suited for the formulation of products for sensitive skin and also for babies and children. Another market segment where they predominate is in so-called "natural" sunscreen products; since they are derived from natural mineral sources, they are perceived as being more natural than organic UV filters, which are all synthetic chemicals.

As a result of these advantages, TiO_2 and ZnO have become very widely used in sunscreen products throughout the world. However, products containing only inorganic sunscreens still represent a relatively small share of the market; far more common are those formulations in which inorganic filters are combined with organic actives. In such formulations, the concentration of the inorganic is typically less than 5 %. The fact that inorganics have not achieved even greater market penetration can largely be attributed to aesthetic concerns, both real and perceived.

16.5.1 Improving Transparency of Inorganic Sunscreens

Historically, the biggest problem with inorganic sunscreens was whitening on skin. The original UV-attenuating grades of TiO_2 and ZnO that were developed for personal care use, despite their fine particle size, still often gave a noticeable white film on skin, especially when incorporated at the concentrations required for SPF values above 15. In some applications, this is actually perceived as an advantage; for example, young children tend not to be concerned about the cosmetic appeal of the sun cream applied to them, but their parents like to be able to see that they have protected their child from the sun. Those same parents, however, hate to see an "unsightly" white film on themselves!

Subsequently, further development of inorganic sunscreens resulted in improvements in transparency. Dransfield et al. [15] discussed how advances in the technology of titanium dioxide for sunscreens, relating to both the manufacture and the formulation of fine particle TiO_2, resulted in improved transparency. The theory of light attenuation by titanium dioxide [16] shows that this material becomes progressively more transparent to visible light as the mean particle size is reduced; with a mean particle size of 20 nm (0.02 μm), TiO_2 is essentially completely transparent. However, with a typical particle size distribution, such a product has very low UV attenuation, so it has poor efficacy as a sunscreen. This was demonstrated by Woodruff [17], who compared various grades of titanium dioxide in a standard frame formulation. Included in this study were two aqueous dispersions of TiO_2, one of which had a mean particle size of 40–50 nm and the other a mean particle size of 10–20 nm. While the latter product showed a high degree of transparency, it gave relatively poor SPF performance, with an SPF of only 7.3 from 5 % TiO_2 solids (compared to 22.6 for the other dispersion at the same solids content).

Dransfield et al showed that by using appropriate manufacturing methods for the TiO_2 and by optimising surface treatments (coatings), solids level, dispersants and milling processes, it is possible to produce titanium dioxide dispersions which maintain the optimum mean particle size for UV attenuation but which have a narrower particle size distribution than previously. Such dispersions therefore have greater transparency to visible light, but without any loss of UV performance.

A similar approach has also been applied to zinc oxide, providing high transparency dispersions of this material also. Another approach to making a transparent zinc oxide is by the use of refractive index matching [18]. In this technology, the ZnO particles are actually much larger than conventional sunscreen grades of ZnO (of the order of a micron or more) but have a porous structure that provides closer matching of refractive index between the particles and the emollient in which they are dispersed, thus reducing the scattering of visible light and giving improved transparency.

Even these more transparent materials, however, still need to be formulated correctly in order to realise the improved transparency. The particle size and size distribution need to be maintained, as far as possible, in the final formulation; if the particles agglomerate, they then behave optically as larger particles, and so whitening is increased. The SPF efficacy of inorganic sunscreens, and also transparency, can be influenced by emulsifiers, added emollients, rheological additives and polymers. Each of these can affect the SPF either by influencing the dispersion degree of the active or by affecting the rheology and spreading properties of the formulation. For example, the use of waxes to alter rheological properties has been shown to have a dramatic effect on SPF in W/O emulsions [19]. We can determine, in at least a qualitative fashion, the relative influences of these two mechanisms by looking at changes in the UV/visible spectrum as parameters are altered. If SPF varies solely as a result of changes in rheological/spreading properties, the shape of the spectral curve does not change, indicating that the dispersion degree of the TiO_2 has not changed. If changing a particular ingredient does affect the degree of dispersion, this is reflected in a change in the shape of the UV attenuation curve, as well as a change in SPF. For example, if the dispersion degree of the TiO_2 is improved, the following changes typically occur in the spectrum:

- UVB attenuation increases.
- UVA attenuation decreases.
- Visible attenuation decreases.

As a result, SPF increases, UVA/UVB ratio decreases, and whitening also decreases [20]. In other words, ensuring the optimum dispersion of TiO_2 promotes both high SPF and optimum transparency.

16.5.2 Improving the Skin Feel of Inorganic Sunscreens

The other aesthetic issue to be addressed with inorganic sunscreens is skin feel. The earliest inorganic sunscreen formulations often had less-than-ideal skin feel, giving inorganic filter systems a reputation for being "dry", "draggy", "heavy", or "sticky". Fortunately, considerable progress has been made in improving the skin feel of these systems.

Parameters relating to particulate filters that might be expected to influence skin feel include particle size, surface treatments, and, in the case of dispersions, the carrier medium in which the particles are dispersed. A study of formulations containing oil-dispersed and water-dispersed TiO_2 [21] indicated that variations in particle size – at least within the range of sizes typically seen in UV-attenuating grades of TiO_2 – have little significant influence on skin feel.

The surface properties of the particles, however, do influence skin feel. All modern UV-attenuating grades of TiO_2 are surface-treated with one or more coating materials; the main purpose of these coatings is to prevent photocatalytic activity, but they also aid the dispersibility of the particles and affect sensory properties. The surface treatments can be either hydrophilic or hydrophobic in nature. Hydrophilic coatings are typically other inorganic oxides such as silica, alumina, or zirconia. Hydrophobic surface treatments include organic moieties such as stearate, organometallics such as isopropyl titanium triisostearate, silicones such as dimethicone and silanes such as triethoxycaprylylsilane. Not all zinc oxide grades are coated; ZnO has less photocatalytic activity than TiO_2, so there is less of a requirement for coating in this case. However, many grades do have a surface treatment to aid dispersion and/or feel. The coating materials used are similar to those used for TiO_2.

Inorganics with a hydrophilic surface tend to impart a "dry" skin feel, which can be perceived as "draggy" when the particles are dispersed in the water phase. This effect is lessened when the particles are dispersed in the oil phase, particularly if an effective dispersing agent is included. These dispersing agents are usually surfactants (often polymeric), which bind to the particle surface and effectively change a hydrophilic surface to a hydrophobic one.

Particles in which the primary surface coating is already hydrophobic, however, generally give a more preferred skin feel. One interesting example of this is where hydrophobic TiO_2 particles are incorporated into an aqueous dispersion. A formulation containing such a dispersion was compared to the same formulation containing an aqueous dispersion of hydrophilic TiO_2 [21]. The hydrophobic material was found to give a smoother skin feel, with less drag than the hydrophilic grade. Such aqueous TiO_2 dispersions based on hydrophobic TiO_2 can also be incorporated in W/O emulsions, resulting in a very elegant, light skin feel which is actually more like the typical skin feel of an O/W lotion rather than a W/O system [22].

A recent paper [23] gave a further example of how coating technology can deliver an inorganic sunscreen system with sensory properties that is perfectly suited to modern sunscreen formulations. In this case, a transparent TiO_2 grade similar to that described earlier was surface-treated with a three-part coating system comprising an inorganic silica coating, a hydrolysable bifunctional silane and a hydrophobising agent. A dispersion of this TiO_2 was incorporated into a W/O emulsion, which was then compared against the same formulation prepared with a TiO_2 dispersion of the same particle size distribution, but in which the coating consisted of alumina and aluminium stearate. The two formulations were assessed using a similar descriptive sensory analysis protocol to that used by Vollhardt et al (see Sect. 16.2 of this chapter) [6]; in fact the two studies were carried out by the same company. The formulation containing the silane-coated TiO_2 showed the following characteristics in comparison to the alumina/stearate coated material:

- Higher spreadability during rub-out
- Higher wetness score during rub-out
- Quicker absorbency
- Much lower gloss in the after-feel (both immediate and after 20 min)
- Less oily and more waxy in the after-feel (both immediate and after 20 min)

In summary, referring again to the study by Vollhardt et al, the new coating was superior in all the key characteristics that were identified as being desirable for modern sun care products.

16.6 Combination Formulations

Of course, with the exception of inorganic-only sun care products (e.g. those making "natural" claims or products designed for sensitive skin and/or young children), it is nowadays very unusual for a sun care product to contain only one active ingredient. Even low SPF products usually contain a combination of two or more UV filters, and such combinations are essential for higher SPF products, especially bearing in mind current requirements for UVA protection (both regulatory and market driven). It is here that the skill of the sun care formulator in optimising the SPF efficacy of the formulation also plays a part in optimising the sensory properties.

It is intuitively expected that the higher the SPF, the more oily and/or greasy will be the skin feel of a sun protection product. However, the study by Vollhardt et al. [6] indicated that while this may be the case within a single product line, it is not generally true. The fact that it is not can be attributed at least in part to finding the right combinations of sunscreen actives to maximise efficacy by taking advantage of synergies between different UV filters, allowing, for example, SPF 50 to be achieved with active levels only slightly higher than those needed for SPF 30 [24]. The best synergies are achieved where filters complement each other, for example:

- Combine filters that cover different parts of the UV spectrum, to ensure broad-spectrum protection.
- Combine organic filters with inorganic filters, which has been shown to generate significant synergistic effects [25–29].
- Combine water-based filters with oil-based filters.

The last of these is of particular interest. The use of water-soluble UV filters, or aqueous dispersions of inorganic filters, is often avoided in "beach" products due to concerns over lack of water resistance. However, the addition of low levels of water-based filters to a formulation containing an optimised combination of oil-based filters can give dramatic increases in SPF [24]. Also, the characteristic "dry" skin feel of the water-based filters helps to counteract the oily feel associated with, for example, the liquid organic UV filters.

16.7 The Influence of Formulation Excipients on Skin Feel

Of course, the aesthetic properties of sun care formulations are influenced to a large degree by the other components used as well as by the UV filters themselves. The effects of emollients have been discussed in the preceding sections; the following is a brief discussion of how other excipients can affect sensory properties.

16.7.1 Emulsifiers

What is often not appreciated is the effect that emulsifiers have on the sensory properties of topical skin care products. In fact, it has been demonstrated that during the rub-out phase, emulsifiers actually exert a greater influence on the skin feel than the emollients do [30]. Many traditional O/W emulsifiers produce a skin feeling during rub-out that is more waxy than is ideal for sun care formulations, but nowadays there are plenty of emulsifier systems that give a more suitable feel. One example is potassium cetyl phosphate, which facilitates good spreadability upon application, with a smooth after-feel. It can be combined with co-emulsifiers to deliver a range of textures and viscosities, from viscous lotions to thin sprayable milks.

Another class of emulsifiers that are well suited for sun care are those designed to form liquid crystal networks [31–33]. Liquid crystals, in one form or another, have actually been present in most O/W personal care emulsions for many years, but it is only within the last 25 years or so that they have been recognised as such, and formulators have started to deliberately make use of them to achieve specific effects. Lamellar liquid crystalline phases have been shown to significantly improve emulsion stability. They also have prolonged hydration properties, due to the fact that water is bound into the lamellar structure, making it less prone to immediate evaporation. This helps to give a skin feel that is very well-liked by consumers. For sun care, the most suitable type of liquid crystal systems is hydrosomes, which consist of a delocalised network of lamellar liquid crystal structures. In sun care, the delocalised structure helps to achieve a homogeneous distribution of active ingredients [34], thus increasing SPF efficacy. In terms of sensory properties, such systems typically give a light and silky skin feel with excellent skin play.

16.7.2 Thickeners

There are many different types of rheology modifiers that are used in cosmetic O/W emulsions, including acrylate polymers (e.g. carbomers), natural gums such as xanthan gum, cellulose derivatives, silicate types such as magnesium aluminium silicate and starch-based thickeners. Each has its own sensory characteristics, but the optimum type to use in any given case depends very much on the emulsifier system being used.

In W/O emulsions, waxes are often used as thickeners and as mentioned earlier can have a beneficial effect on SPF in sun care formulations [19]. However, care should be taken to avoid excessive concentrations of wax as this can inhibit the spreading of the formulation, making it difficult and unpleasant to apply. Fine particle silica can also be used as a rheological additive in W/O systems, and this can have a beneficial effect on skin feel, as it counteracts any oiliness or greasiness from the emollients, delivering a drier feel.

16.7.3 Film-Formers

Film-formers, which are often polymers, are frequently added to sun care formulations for one or both of two reasons. Firstly, such ingredients can act as SPF boosters, by giving a more even product film on skin. Secondly, they are used as water-proofing agents. One of the most common types used are PVP copolymers [35, 36], for example, VP/eicosene copolymer. However, these polymers can sometimes give a “sticky” feel to the formulation, so a number of alternatives have been developed that confer water resistance while enabling the formulator to maintain a “light”, smooth skin feel [37].

16.8 Conclusion

There was a time when sun care products would not be very pleasant to apply and would not be as cosmetically elegant as, say, daily skin care products, and consumers would either accept this as a necessary evil of protecting themselves from the sun or would avoid using such products altogether. Nowadays, however, consumers expect a better sensory experience from their sunscreen products, and manufacturers are increasingly using sensory claims as a way of differentiating their products from the competition. Sensory analysis by trained panels enables cosmetic scientists to better understand what consumers want in terms of skin feel, and developments in terms of both active ingredients (UV filters) and formulation excipients are enabling formulators to develop sun care products that are pleasant to apply, encouraging better consumer compliance. This, in turn, makes the products more effective under "real-use" conditions than may have been the case in the past.

References

1. Petersen B, Datta P, Philipsen PA, Wulf HC (2013) Sunscreen use and failures – on site observations on a sun-holiday. Photochem Photobiol Sci 12(1):190–196
2. Saecker C, Janssen A, Vollhardt J (2013) Are we done by preventing sunburn? In: Proceedings of the Florida Sunscreen symposium, Orlando, 18–21 Sept 2013
3. Ou-Yang H, Stanfield J, Cole C, Appa Y, Rigel D (2012) High SPF sunscreens (SPF ≥ 70) may provide ultraviolet protection above minimal recommended levels by adequately compensating for lower sunscreen user application amounts. J Am Acad Dermatol 67(6):1220–1227
4. Bimczok R, Gers-Barlag H, Mundt C, Klette E, Bielfeldt S, Rudolph T, Pflucker F, Heinrich U, Tronnier H, Johncock W, Klebon B, Westenfelder H, Flosser-Muller H, Jenni K, Kockott D, Lademann J, Herzog B, Rohr M (2007) Influence of applied quantity of sunscreen products on the sun protection factor – a multicenter study organized by the DGK Task Force Sun Protection. Skin Pharmacol Physiol 20(1):57–64
5. European Commission (2006) Recommendation of 22 Sep 2006, on the efficacy of sunscreen products and the claims made relating thereto. Official Journal of the European Union L 265/39–L 265/43
6. Vollhardt J, Schoop R, Roos F, Janssen A, Saecker C (2013) The sensory experience of sunscreens – which properties matter? A descriptive sensory analysis of more than 50 sunscreens. In: Proceedings of the sun protection conference 2013: sun protection for the 21st century, London, 4–5 June 2013 (Summit Events Ltd.)
7. Dahms GH (1988) Cosmetic water-in-oil emulsions: application, physical properties and formulations. In: Proceedings of the symposium on "The formulation of cosmetic and topical pharmaceutical products", Bristol, April 1988
8. Tadros ThF et al (1996) Use of a polymeric surfactant (ABA block copolymer) for preparation of stable water-in-oil (W/O) emulsions and water-in-oil-in-water multiple emulsions. In: Proceedings of the 19th IFSCC congress, Sydney, October 1996
9. Bruening S, Leonard M, Kawa R, Issberner U, Tomlinson A (2005) Role of emollients and emulsifiers in sunscreen formulations. In: Shaath NA (ed) Sunscreens: regulations and commercial development, vol 28, 3rd edn, Cosmetic science and technology series. Taylor & Francis, Boca Raton, pp 449–460
10. Schwarzenbach R, Huber U (2003) Optimization of sunscreen efficacy. In: Verlag für chemische Industrie, H. Ziolkowsky GmbH, Augsburg, pp 131–137

11. Wright C (2002) Effects of emollients on efficacy of UV filters. MChem report, York University
12. Hewitt JP (2013) Formulating sun protection products for the 21st century: efficacy, elegance and globality. In: Proceedings of the Florida Sunscreen Symposium, Orlando, 18–21 Sept 2013
13. Nohynek GJ et al (2007) Grey goo on the skin? Nanotechnology, cosmetic and sunscreen safety. Crit Rev Toxicol 37(3):251–277
14. Chen LL, Tooley I, Wang SQ (2013) Nanotechnology in photoprotection. In: Nasir A, Friedman A, Wang SQ (eds) Nanotechnology in dermatology. Springer, New York, pp 9–18
15. Dransfield GP, Hewitt JP, Lyth PL (1998) Advances in titanium dioxide technology. In: Proceedings of the SCS spring conference, London, April 1998
16. Robb JL, Simpson LA, Tunstall DF (1994) Scattering and absorption of UV radiation by sunscreens containing fine particle and pigmentary titanium dioxide. Drug Cosmet Ind 154(3):32–39
17. Woodruff J (1994) Formulating sun care products with micronized oxides. Cosmetics & Toiletries Manufacture Worldwide, London, Aston Publishing Group, pp 179–185
18. McCormick P, Fletcher R, Jones C (2010) Micron-sized zinc oxide dispersion for transparent, high SPF formulas. Cosmet Toil 125(2):50–57
19. Hewitt JP, Dahms GH (1995) The influence of rheology on efficacy of physical sunscreens. In: Proceedings of the IFSCC conference, Montreux, pp 313–323
20. Hewitt JP (1999) Effective use of physical sunscreens: incorporation of physical sunscreens into water-in-oil emulsions. In: Proceedings of the European UV sunfilters conference, Paris, November 1999
21. Hewitt JP, Hine H, Kessell LM (2004) Optimising the sensory properties of physical sunscreen formulations. In: Proceedings of the 23rd IFSCC congress, Orlando, 24–27 Oct 2004
22. Kessell LM, Hewitt JP (2008) Water-in-silicone-oil emulsion for use as a sunscreen product. US patent 2008226727, 18 Sept 2008
23. McNeil K, Sayer R, Miles A (2014) Assessing the sensory performance of novel coating technology. SOFW J 140(7):2–7
24. Hewitt JP, Teague J, Sutcliffe P (2014) Efficacy and elegance in 21st century sun care. Cosmet Toil 129(3):58–65
25. Dahms GH (1994) Compositions containing sunscreens. UK patent 2278055, 23 Nov 1994
26. Dahms GH (1994) Compositions containing sunscreens. UK patent 2279007, 21 Dec 1994
27. Nicoll GA, Scott IR (1991) Cosmetic composition. European patent 0456458, 13 Nov 1991
28. Nearn MR, Redshaw SJ, Burgess G (1995) Sunscreen compositions. US patent 5417961, 23 May 1995
29. Deckner GE (1994) Photostable sunscreen compositions. International patent WO9404131, 3 Mar 1994
30. Wiechers JW, Taelman M-C, Wortel VAL, Verboom C, Dederen JC (2002) Emulsifiers and emollients exert their sensory impact in different phases of the sensory evaluation process but how does one demonstrate the absence of such an influence? IFSCC Magazine 5(2):99–105
31. Dahms GH (1986) Properties of oil-in-water emulsions with anisotropic lamellar phases. Cosmet Toil 101(11):113–115
32. Dahms GH (1990) Optimised formulations for skin care products. SOFW J 1990(10): 388–392
33. Loll P (1994) Liquid crystals in cosmetic emulsions. Cosmetics & Toiletries Manufacture Worldwide, Aston Publishing Group, London, pp 108–120
34. Dahms GH (1992) Formulating with a physical sun block. Cosmet Toil 107(10):87–92
35. Gupta VK, Zatz JL (1999) In vitro method for modelling water resistance of sunscreen formulations. London, J Cosmet Sci 50:79–90
36. Markovic B, Laura D, Rerek M (2001) A laboratory method for measuring the water resistance of sunscreens. Cosmet Toil 116(9):61–68
37. Rigano L (2014) "Very" water-resistant sunscreens. Cosmet Toil 129(3):66–73

Chapter 17
Sunscreen Regulatory Update

Farah K. Ahmed

Key Points

1. Sunscreen active ingredients (or ultraviolet (UV) filters) are regulated globally under a variety of classifications – e.g., over-the-counter drugs, cosmetics, quasi-drugs – and are required to be substantiated for safety and efficacy.
2. Brief overview of the current state of sunscreen regulation around the world, with an expanded focus in the United States, will be provided.
3. Worldwide regulation of sunscreens ensures governmental oversight over the safety and efficacy of sunscreens.

17.1 Introduction

Sunscreen has shown to reduce the risk of developing skin cancer and prevent UV-induced skin aging when used appropriately and in conjunction with other protection modalities. In the United States, sunscreens are regulated by the Food and Drug Administration (FDA) as over-the-counter (OTC) drugs. In many other countries around the world, there are sets of rigorous specifications governing the

Founded in 1894, the Personal Care Products Council is the leading national trade association representing the personal care products industry. Our membership includes approximately 300 active member companies that manufacture or distribute personal care products, including OTC sunscreens. We also represent approximately 300 additional associate members who provide goods and services to manufacturers and distributors of personal care products.

F.K. Ahmed, BS, JD (✉)
Vice President / Chair, Personal Care Products Council—Consumer Healthcare Products Association Joint Sunscreen Task Force, Personal Care Products Council,
Washington, DC, USA
e-mail: ahmedf@personalcarecouncil.org

S.Q. Wang, H.W. Lim (eds.), *Principles and Practice of Photoprotection*,
DOI 10.1007/978-3-319-29382-0_17

safety profile of UV filters and product efficacy and labeling guidelines in place to protect the consumers. To accomplish these tasks, there are regulatory bodies around the world that create and update their individual rules pertaining to the regulation of sunscreen products.

This chapter provides a glimpse to the world of regulation associated with sunscreens. Specifically it will provide (1) a basic background of over-the-counter (OTC) drug product regulation in the United States, (2) specific information on sunscreen regulations, (3) an overview of the Sunscreen Innovation Act (SIA), and (4) a brief summary of global sunscreen ingredient and product regulation.

17.2 Over-the-Counter Drug Product Regulations

In the United States, sunscreens primarily fall within the jurisdiction of the US Food and Drug Administration (FDA or the Agency). FDA regulates all sunscreens as OTC drugs.[1] As such, they must meet standards for safety, efficacy, good manufacturing practices (GMPs), and labeling. The Agency deems any topically applied product claiming a sun protection factor (SPF) to be a sunscreen. Examples of such products include lotions, sprays, daily moisturizers, foundations, lipsticks, etc.

17.2.1 OTC Drug Regulatory Pathways

Two regulatory pathways exist for the legal marketing of OTC drug products: (i) marketing in compliance with an OTC drug monograph, (ii) marketing under the authority of an approved product-specific new drug application (NDA), an abbreviated new drug application (ANDA), or (iii) Rx-to-OTC switch.

17.2.1.1 OTC Monograph

The majority of sunscreen products in the United States are marketed under the OTC sunscreen monograph. An OTC monograph is essentially the recipe for making an OTC drug product and based on ingredients – FDA preapproved (or permitted) active ingredients that support prescribed labeling claims and, in some instances, testing (e.g., SPF). Designated OTC monographs represent regulatory standards for the marketing of nonprescription drug products not covered by new drug applications. These are OTC drugs related to categories that consumers are able to self-diagnose, self-treat, and self-manage. Examples of OTC monograph

[1] An OTC drug product is a drug product marketed for use by the consumer without the intervention of a health care professional in order to obtain the product.

Table 17.1 Over-The-Counter (OTC) drug regulatory pathways

New drug application	Monograph process
Product specific (including formulation)	Ingredient- and category-specific regulations (CFR 330–358)
Confidential filing	Public process – no data
Application submitted for premarket approval	No FDA product-specific premarket application or preapproval
Mandated timelines	No mandated timelines
Application fees (PDUFA)	No user fees
Potential for marketing exclusivity	No potential for marketing exclusivity
Reporting requirements	Limited reporting requirements (serious adverse events)
Comply with good manufacturing practices	Comply with good manufacturing practices

therapeutic categories include both topical and ingested forms such as sunscreens, acne, allergy, diaper rash, cough and cold, antiperspirant, dandruff, skin protectant, external analgesic, psoriasis, etc.

17.2.1.2 New Drug Application (NDA and ANDA)

Currently, there are four specific sunscreen formulations approved in the United States under the new drug application (NDA) process:

Anthelios SX: avobenzone, ecamsule, and octocrylene at 2, 2, and 10 %
Capital Soleil: avobenzone, ecamsule, and octocrylene at 2, 3, and 10 %
Anthelios 20: avobenzone, ecamsule, octocrylene, and titanium dioxide at 2, 2,10, and 2 %
Anthelios 40: avobenzone, ecamsule, octocrylene, and titanium dioxide at 2, 3, 10, and 5%

All four NDAs were filed by L'Oreal.

The term *human drug application* means an application for approval of a new drug (the full formulation and labeling).

The following table (Table 17.1) provides a summary of the differences of these two pathways.

17.2.1.3 Rx-to-OTC Switch

An Rx-to-OTC switch refers to over-the-counter marketing of a product that was once a prescription drug product, for the same dosage form, population, and route of administration. Currently, there is no prescription (or Rx) to OTC sunscreen products in the United States.

17.3 OTC Sunscreen Regulations

On June 14, 2011, FDA released the following sunscreen-related rulemakings: (1) final rule on effectiveness testing and labeling for over-the-counter (OTC) sunscreen products (final rule),[2] (2) proposed rule on SPFs above 50, (3) advance notice of proposed rulemaking (ANPR) on sunscreen dosage forms, (4) draft guidance on OTC sunscreen drug products, and (5) request for comment on the final rule.[3]

17.3.1 Final Rule on Sunscreen Labeling and Efficacy

The final rule outlines permitted and required claims, testing procedures required to substantiate those claims, and claims that are not permitted. It is important to note that these rules amend FDA's drug labeling regulations (i.e., 21 CFR 201) and do not finalize the sunscreen monograph (i.e., 21 CFR 352) nor lift the stay on the implementation of the monograph.

17.3.2 Drug Facts Panel Required

In addition, the final rule lifts the delay of the implementation of the 1999 Drug Facts final rule and requires all sunscreen products to comply with the content and format requirements of that rule. This includes combination cosmetic – sunscreen products such as lipsticks, foundations, and daily moisturizers that are labeled as containing an SPF.

Under the Drug Facts rule, if the information listed under Drug Facts requires more than 60 % of the total available surface area, the Drug Facts labeling can be reduced as specified in the regulation.[4] FDA did not provide for any additional labeling relief under the Final Rule.

---

[2] The final rule (76 FR 35620), codified in § 201.327, establishes labeling and testing requirements for OTC sunscreen products marketed without approved applications and containing only the ingredients specified in the stayed 1999 final rule (aminobenzoic acid (PABA), avobenzone, cinoxate, dioxybenzone, ensulizole, homosalate, meradimate, octinoxate, octisalate, octocrylene, oxybenzone, padimate O, sulisobenzone, titanium dioxide, trolamine salicylate, zinc oxide).

[3] All published in the June 17, 2011 Federal Register.

[4] 21 CFR 201.66(d)(10)

17.3.3 No Ingredient Issues Addressed

The final rule does not address issues related to sunscreen active ingredients, including any new active ingredient combinations, or any sunscreen active ingredients currently under time and extent application (TEA) review.

17.3.4 Effective Date

The final rule effective date was initially set for June 18, 2012, except for products with annual sales less than $25,000 for which the effective date is June 17, 2013. FDA postponed these dates by 6 months to allow companies to comply with the final rule and ensure no shortage of sunscreens on the market. All products labeled on or after the effective date must meet all final rule requirements (see below for additional time/enforcement discretion for SPF testing). Of note, FDA did not require noncompliant products introduced or delivered for introduction into interstate commerce prior to the compliance date, June 18, 2012, to be removed from the market; product delivered to customers, even if in their warehouses, ready to be shipped from manufacturers' warehouses, or imported prior to June 18, 2012, can continue to be shipped and sold; and product imported prior to the compliance date would be protected, as would any product delivered to customers, even if still in customers' warehouses on the effective date.[5]

17.3.5 SPF Testing

The SPF test method was modified to require a smaller number of test subjects to determine a product's SPF (10) compared to the previous methods that required 20–25 test subjects. The reference control formulation was changed from an SPF 4 formulation to an SPF 15 formulation. The finger cot used for sample application no longer requires pre-saturation with test product. The minimum size of the test site for product application was reduced in area, as was the required minimum area for each individual UV exposure. The distance between exposure sites in the test area was reduced. Product application remained at 2 mg/cm^2 with test result read at 16–24 h postexposure. Solar simulator specifications were harmonized with those in the International SPF Method.

[5] Under the general interpretation of "delivered for introduction into interstate commerce," other warehoused product might also be protected but would have to be evaluated on a case-by-case basis.

17.3.6 "Broad-Spectrum" Testing

FDA has abandoned the "four star" rating proposal indicating UVA protection provided on product labels, in favor of a simple "pass/fail" in vitro test for "broad-spectrum" characteristics – known in the industry as the "critical wavelength" test. The proposed test methodology differs from previously published methodology to determine the "critical wavelength" in several attributes and is different from the ISO in vitro UVA test method (in development) as well.

A sunscreen must have a critical wavelength of 370 or higher to be able to make a "broad-spectrum" claim. A "broad-spectrum" claim is necessary in order to make a positive "use" statement regarding prevention of early skin aging and skin cancer on products with an SPF of at least 15; otherwise, a warning statement must be used for the product "uses" (see below).

The FDA "critical wavelength" test method prescribes the use of PMMA plates with a surface roughness from 2 to 7 μm, with a sunscreen application density of 0.75 mg/cm^2, and pre-irradiation of the sample with a fixed 4 MED exposure to solar-simulated radiation. The wavelength at which 90 % of the UV absorbance area under the curve occurs (when summing from 290 toward 400) is defined as the "critical wavelength" and is a measure of the breadth of the protection provided by the product.

17.3.7 The New Label

The FDA also issued new guidance on labeling of sunscreen products as outlined below.

Uses (indications)

- Helps prevent sunburn
- If used as directed with other sun protection measures (see *Directions*), decreases the risk of skin cancer and early skin aging caused by the sun [please note: the sunscreen must be "broad-spectrum" and SPF of at least 15 in order to use this statement]

Warnings

- *Skin cancer/skin aging alert*: Spending time in the sun increases your risk of skin cancer and early skin aging. This product has been shown only to help prevent sunburn, *not* skin cancer or early skin aging [please note: this statement is required for products that are not labeled as "broad-spectrum" or SPF of less than 15]

Directions (for broad-spectrum/SPF $\geq$ 15 and water-resistant)

- Apply liberally (or "generously" and may add "and evenly") 15 min before sun exposure.
- Reapply.
  - After 40 (or 80) minutes of swimming or sweating

  - Immediately after towel drying
  - At least every 2 h

- *Sun protection measures*. Spending time in the sun increases your risk of skin cancer and early skin aging. To decrease this risk, regularly use a sunscreen with broad-spectrum SPF of 15 or higher and other sun protection measures including:
  - Limit time in the sun, especially from 10 a.m. to 2 p.m.
  - Wear long-sleeve shirts, pants, hats, and sunglasses.
- Children under 6 months: Ask a doctor.

Directions (for broad-spectrum and/or SPF $\leq$ 15 and water-resistant)

- Apply liberally (or “generously” and may add “and evenly”) 15 min before sun exposure.
- Reapply.
  - After 40 (or 80) minutes of swimming or sweating
  - Immediately after towel drying
  - At least every 2 h
- Children under 6 months of age: Ask a doctor.

Directions (for broad-spectrum/SPF $\geq$ 15 and not water-resistant)

- Apply liberally (or “generously” and may add “and evenly”) 15 min before sun exposure.
- *Sun protection measures*. Spending time in the sun increases your risk of skin cancer and early skin aging. To decrease this risk, regularly use a sunscreen with broad-spectrum SPF of 15 or higher and other sun protection measures including:
  - Limit time in the sun, especially from 10 a.m. to 2 p.m.
  - Wear long-sleeve shirts, pants, hats, and sunglasses.
- Reapply at least every 2 h.
- Use a water-resistant sunscreen if swimming or sweating.
- Children under 6 months: Ask a doctor.

Directions (for not broad-spectrum and/or SPF $\leq$ 15 and not water-resistant)

- Apply liberally (or “generously” and may add “and evenly”) 15 min before sun exposure.
- Reapply at least every 2 h.
- Use a water-resistant sunscreen if swimming or sweating.
- Children under 6 months of age: Ask a doctor.

Note: FDA is allowing the optional direction heading “for sunscreen use” to appear as the first line under Directions.[6]

---

[6] The agency’s reasoning for this allowance is that consumers who are using these products primarily for cosmetic use may be more likely to understand that they might not receive the intended sun protection if they do not follow the directions in the Drug Facts label.

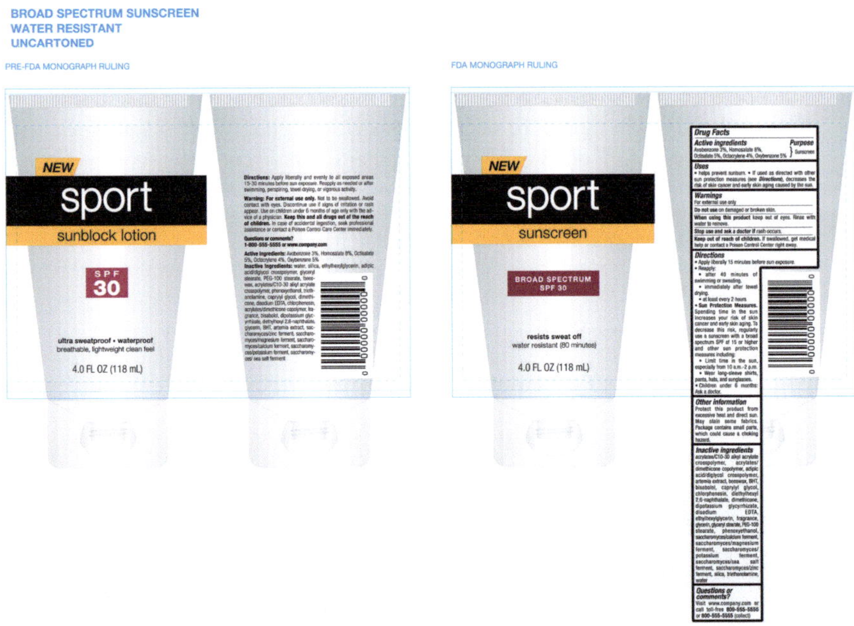

Fig. 17.1 Illustrates the old vs. the new sunscreen labeling requirements

Water resistance claims on the principal display panel must specify either 40 or 80 min of effectiveness while swimming or sweating, based on testing. "Waterproof," "sweatproof," and "sun block" claims are not permitted. FDA did not explicitly allow for a sweat resistance claim (Fig. 17.1).

17.3.8 Proposed Rule on SPFs Above 50

Although FDA acknowledged that SPFs higher than 50 have been substantiated and results are validated and repeatable, it is proposing to limit SPF to "50+" unless the agency receives data demonstrating additional clinical benefit for SFPs above 50.

Sunscreens labeled with SPFs above 50 may remain on the market until this proposed rule becomes final, provided they follow the appropriate SPF test. Depending on how this proposed rule is finalized, these products may/may not be able to continue on the market.

17.3.9 Advance Notice of Proposed Rulemaking on Dosage Forms

FDA published an ANPR requesting additional data on OTC sunscreen products in certain dosage forms. The agency listed those dosage forms that it currently considered potentially eligible for inclusion in the OTC sunscreen monograph (i.e., oils, lotions, creams, gels, butters, pastes, ointments, sticks, and sprays).

For sprays, FDA requested additional data to address remaining questions about effectiveness and safety. The agency also encouraged comments on potential labeling and testing conditions for sunscreens in spray dosage forms, contingent on receiving additional data that would be needed to allow their classification as generally recognized as safe and effective (GRASE.)

FDA also identified certain dosage forms that it does not consider currently eligible for review for potential inclusion in the OTC sunscreen monograph (i.e., wipes, towelettes, powders, body washes, and shampoos).

Sunscreens, such as those in powder form, may remain on the market until this proposed rule becomes final, provided they follow the appropriate testing and labeling. When this ANPR is eventually finalized, we will know which dosage forms may continue on the market.

Although the final rule did not include ingredients, the Agency also noted that it allowed 16 sunscreen active ingredients at the following "up to" concentrations:

- Aminobenzoic acid (PABA), 15 %
- Avobenzone, 3 %
- Cinoxate, 3 %
- Dioxybenzone, 3 %
- Ensulizole, 4 %
- Homosalate, 15 %
- Meradimate, 5 %
- Octinoxate, 7.5 %
- Octisalate, 5 %
- Octocrylene, 10 %
- Oxybenzone, 6 %
- Padimate O, 8 %
- Sulisobenzone, 10 %
- Titanium dioxide, 25 %
- Trolamine salicylate, 12 %
- Zinc oxide, 25 %

However, in FDA's June 14, 2011 rulemakings, the Agency did not address the eight pending sunscreen ingredient applications requesting inclusion into the sunscreen monograph:

- Amiloxate, 10 %
- Bemotrizinol, 10 %
- Bisoctrizole, 10 %
- Diethyl butamido triazone, 3 %
- Drometrizole trisiloxane, 15 %
- Ecamsule, 10 %
- Enzacamene, 4 %
- Octyl triazone, 5 %

As of the date of this publication, FDA has not approved any of the above ingredients; rather, the Agency has requested additional data before it can make its safety and efficacy determination.

17.4 Sunscreen Innovation Act

On November 26, 2014, President Obama has signed the Sunscreen Innovation Act (SIA) into law.[7] The goal of the SIA is to provide an alternative process for review for all ingredient TEAs, including prescribed timelines for review, administrative orders in lieu of rulemaking, and new format for data submissions. The SIA also allows for advisory committees and requires FDA to regularly update congress and the GAO. Of note, FDA's safety evaluations and determinations remain with the Agency.

Key aspects of the Act include:

Determining eligibility: FDA TEA eligibility requirements will be maintained – an ingredient must be used safely for at least five years in at least one country. Eligibility determinations will be made by FDA's Division of Nonprescription Regulation Development (DNRD). Pending ingredient submissions, already deemed eligible by FDA, will be considered eligible for the new review and approval process.

Transparent review: After a finding of eligibility, the ingredient application may be submitted to the existing FDA Nonprescription Drugs Advisory Committee (NDAC) for a safety and effectiveness recommendation or may conduct this review on their own. During the review process, the FDA or the NDAC will receive data from the public and communicate with the application's sponsor to seek clarifying or request additional information. FDA will either concur or deny the NDAC's recommendation or come to its own conclusion.

Predictable and reasonable time frame: The SIA sets time frames for the various stages of the TEA process for both pending and new applications.

Guidance: FDA must issue draft guidance on the implementation of, and compliance with, the requirements with respect to sunscreen TEAs under the Act (e.g., format, data requirements).

---

[7] Sunscreen Innovation Act: http://www.gpo.gov/fdsys/pkg/PLAW-113publ195/pdf/PLAW-113publ195.pdf

Enhancing FDA accountability: FDA is required to submit reports to congress regarding the progress of the program 12 months following enactment and every two years thereafter.

Finalize the sunscreen monograph: Within 5 years of enactment, FDA must finalize the remaining portion of the sunscreen monograph (i.e., the ingredient portion but not necessarily SPF cap or dosage form). If FDA does not finalize SPF cap or dosage form, the Agency must provide its rationale for such provisions not being included in such regulations and a plan and timeline to compile any information necessary to address such provisions through final regulation.

At the time of writing this chapter, the FDA has not approved any of the new UV actives under the TEA review process. Instead as of May 2015, the FDA requested all the manufacturers to submit additional safety and efficacy data for their respective UV actives.

Chronological statutory timeline for all sunscreen TEAs

November 26, 2014: Enactment of the Sunscreen Innovation Act (Public Law 113–195).

January 7, 2015: FDA published notice for comment of feedback letters/proposed sunscreen orders in the Federal Register.

On or before February 6, 2015: FDA meeting request due to FDA from a sponsor of pending application with a feedback letter.

February 23, 2015: Public comment deadline for feedback letters/proposed sunscreen orders for pending applications with feedback letters per January 7th Federal Register notice.

On or before February 24, 2015: Proposed sunscreen orders required for all pending applications without feedback letters at the time of enactment.

On or before March 23, 2015: FDA meeting convened for requests submitted by a sponsor of pending application with a feedback letter.

On or before March 26, 2015: FDA meeting request due to FDA from a sponsor of pending application without a feedback letter at the time of enactment.

On or before April 10, 2015: Public comment deadline for proposed sunscreen orders for pending applications without feedback letters at the time of enactment.

On or before May 10, 2015: FDA meeting convened for requests submitted by a sponsor of pending application without a feedback letter at the time of enactment.

On or before July 9, 2015: Final sunscreen order required for all pending applications without feedback letters at the time of enactment that do not require submission of additional data.

On or before November 26, 2015: Draft guidance regarding the criteria for eligibility and safety and effectiveness determinations.

On or before May 26, 2016: FDA initial report to senate HELP and house energy and commerce committee regarding implementation of the SIA.

On or before November 26, 2016: Final guidance regarding the criteria for eligibility and safety and effectiveness determinations.

On or before November 26, 2017: Initial Government Accountability Office (GAO) report.

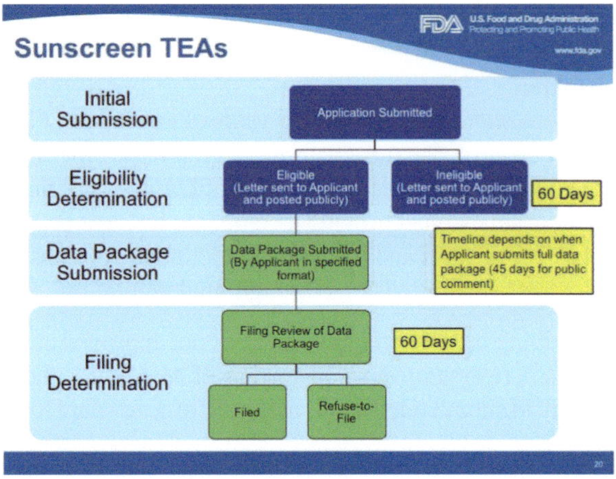

Fig. 17.2 Illustrate the new sunscreen TEA timeline

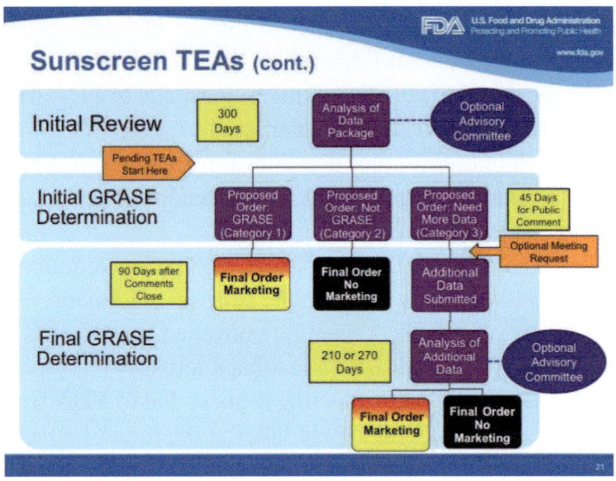

Fig. 17.3 Illustrate the new sunscreen TEA timeline

On or before May 26, 2018: FDA second report to senate HELP and House E&C regarding implementation of the SIA.

On or before November 26, 2019: Final sunscreen monograph published.

On or before May 26, 2020:

- Subsequent Government Accountability Office (GAO) report.
- FDA third report to senate HELP and House E&C regarding implementation of the SIA.

Figures 17.2 and 17.3 illustrate the new TEA timeline[8]

[8] Images by FDA

17.5 Global Sunscreen Regulation

Sunscreens are recognized by global health authorities for their ability to protect consumers from UV exposure and for their role in helping to prevent acute and chronic damage to the skin, including reducing the incidence of skin cancers. These authorities are aligned in that (i) sun protection is a public health priority, (ii) claims regarding efficacy must be proven, and (iii) sunscreen active ingredients are reviewed for safety and require premarket approval. While the above criteria are common among regions, regulatory classifications, available sunscreen active ingredients and concentration limits, testing requirements, labeling, approval process and postmarketing requirements differ. Each of these parameters will be reviewed below for their commonality as well as for their divergence.

17.5.1 Regulatory Classification

Regulatory classifications for sunscreens vary widely from region to region. At first glance, one might believe that differences among these classifications are vast; however, examination of the various definitions reveals common themes. These include the following: a product placed in contact with the various external parts of the human body and a product to protect the skin from UV radiation. These similarities support the common message that sunscreen products, when used as directed, no matter what the regulatory classification, are designed to provide UV protection to consumers and sunscreen active ingredients require premarket approval and supporting preclinical/clinical information.

17.5.2 Available Sunscreen Ingredients, Concentrations, Combinations, and Approval

The area where the greatest differences are most evident is in the wide variety of sunscreen ingredients available to manufacturers and consumers. In the United States, the monograph allows for 16 current sunscreen ingredients with eight pending time and extent applications (TEAs). In other countries, up to 38 sunscreen ingredients are available for manufacturers to formulate sun protection products. Approvals of sunscreen active ingredients require premarket approval and supporting preclinical/clinical information. While some approvals appear to be more stringent, the safety and efficacy of the sunscreen ingredients must be proven prior to use of the ingredient. This is further discussed in an earlier section of this briefing document.

Upon examination, ten sunscreen ingredients are permitted for use globally:

1. Octisalate (ethylhexyl salicylate)
2. Homosalate (3,3,5-trimethylcyclohexyl 2-hydroxybenzoate)
3. Octocrylene (2-cyano-3,3-diphenyl acrylic acid, 2-ethylhexyl ester)
4. Octinoate (octyl methoxycinnamate)
5. Zinc oxide*
6. Oxybenzone (benzophenone-3)
7. Ensulizole (phenylbenzimidazole sulfonic acid)
8. Avobenzone (butyl methoxy dibenzoyl methane)
9. Padimate O (ethylhexyl dimethyl PABA)
10. Titanium dioxide*

*Considered to be light-scattering agents in Japan

17.5.3 Sunscreen Ingredient Safety

Globally, all sunscreen active ingredients require premarket approval, and all have individually been tested in preclinical studies in both short-term and long-term applications. Within limits determined by individual countries, all have demonstrated to have acceptable preclinical and/or clinical safety profiles for human use as directed.

17.5.4 Sunscreen Labeling

While there is no global agreement as to the SPF limits or the regulatory classification of specific product types (recreational vs. every day), all sunscreen products no matter where they are marketed must carry an SPF value. Communication of the level of UVA protection can vary from a "+" marking in Japan, the SPF value and a symbol indicating "UVA" in Europe, to a "broad-spectrum" claim in the United States. All of these statements to the consumer appear on the principal display panel of the sunscreen product.

All products need to provide information to consumers allowing safe use. Warning statements and directions for use should be clear and concise to ensure that even the average consumer can read and understand any risks associated with the product as well as how to properly apply and use.

As discussed in this section, while the regulatory classification of sunscreens varies globally, all major markets agree that sun protection is a public health priority and consider sunscreens a necessary component in preventing both sunburn and skin cancer. These authorities are aligned in that claims regarding efficacy must be proven and that sunscreen active ingredients require premarket approval.

17.6 Conclusions

Both the data and regulatory requirements – in the United States and globally – related to sunscreens substantiate and ensure the safety and efficacy of these products. In part, regulations are meant to protect and enhance public health. They also play a major role in advancing and at time slowing or impeding the technological and scientific progresses that propel companies and industries to develop novel sunscreen products. Needless to say, regulations can impact the state of photoprotection offered by sunscreens.

Chapter 18
Measuring Sunscreen Protection According to the FDA Final Rule

Joseph W. Stanfield, J. William Stanfield, and Eduardo Ruvolo Jr.

Key Points
1. The sun protection factor (SPF) is an in vivo test that estimates the protective efficacy of a sunscreen against erythema.
2. The critical wavelength (CW) test is an in vitro test that has been accepted by the US Food and Drug Administration to measure the broad-spectrum status of sunscreens.
3. Detailed description on the proper steps to conduct SPF and CW tests is provided.
4. Common pitfalls in conducting SPF and CW tests are also outlined.

18.1 Introduction

Historically, the first known studies establishing the basis for sun protection started in the 1930s and were published in the 1940s by H. Blum et al. and in the 1950s by R. Schulze [1, 2]. Professor Franz Greiter invented what is known today as the concept of the sun protection factor (SPF) and introduced sunscreens with SPF labels in 1962 [3, 4]. The original proposed sunscreen monograph, issued in 1978,

J.W. Stanfield, MS (✉)
President, Suncare Research Laboratories, 2518 B Reynolda Road,
Winston Salem, NC 27106-4618, USA
e-mail: jstanfield@suncarelab.com

J.W. Stanfield
General Manager, Suncare Research Laboratories, 2518 B Reynolda Road,
Winston Salem, NC 27106-4618, USA

E. Ruvolo Jr., MS
Senior Research Fellow, Avon Products, One Avon Place, Suffern, NY 10901, USA

S.Q. Wang, H.W. Lim (eds.), *Principles and Practice of Photoprotection*,
DOI 10.1007/978-3-319-29382-0_18

provided the option of an outdoor SPF test using sunlight, as well as a method using indoor ultraviolet lamps [5].

The advantages of using a natural solar light source were cited as a closer approximation of the actual use of sunscreens, including the heat and humidity, use of the full solar spectrum, ability to test several sunscreen products simultaneously, and the ability to estimate tanning efficacy. Disadvantages of using a natural solar light source included the uncontrollable variables of weather, changing cloud cover, changing radiation intensity, changing sun angle, and difficulties of monitoring the constant changes of sun exposure.

The disadvantages of using the indoor solar simulators, such as xenon arc lamps included, were the low output in the visible and infrared wavelengths, the difficulty in measuring the output, and the time-consuming requirement of irradiating only one test site at a time. This last factor became less significant with the introduction of multiport systems. On the other hand, the advantages of using the xenon arc lamp included the constant spectrum and the high UV power output.

It is important to notice that the ratio of UVA (320–400 nm) and UVB (290–320) radiation in sunlight from 9 AM to 3 PM is constant and equal to 21:1 [6]. In solar simulators, the ratio UVA/UVB is around 8:1. This also can be a source of difference when SPF tests are performed indoors using ultraviolet lamps compared to tests performed under natural sunlight.

Eventually the consensus of sunscreen manufacturers favored the xenon arc lamp, especially as SPF values of products began to increase significantly. During the period of the early 1980s, large solar simulators with 1000 and 2500 W were available and utilized in much of the indoor SPF testing. However, they required masking and covering of exposed sites, water cooling, and cumbersome power supplies and large space requirements. These large simulators were eventually replaced by compact xenon arc solar simulators, especially as large-scale SPF testing grew.

The pioneer of the compact xenon arc solar simulator was Daniel S. Berger, from the Department of Medical Physics at Temple University [7]. The original compact xenon arc lamp, known as the Berger solar simulator, employed a continuous 150 W xenon arc with optics and filters that produced a uniform beam, approximately one centimeter in diameter. Its emission spectrum in the UVB region simulated the sun at an elevation of 70°. The goal was to simulate the solar spectrum in the sunburning UVB region, with minimal long wavelength UVA, visible light, and infrared energy. This enabled production of erythema on the backs of volunteer subjects, with relatively short exposure times and minimal discomfort to human volunteer subjects. The compact solar simulator weighed 5 lb and required a 35 lb power supply.

The compact xenon arc lamp rapidly became the mainstay of the SPF test. The output spectrum of the compact xenon arc lamp was considered an acceptable simulation of sunlight, and the FDA and other regulatory agencies worldwide stipulated spectra for indoor sunscreen testing, designed around the compact xenon arc lamp.

A variation of the original Berger solar simulator employs six liquid light guides to irradiate six spots, each 8 mm in diameter. Use of the multiport solar simulator was prohibited until the 2011 US FDA's Final Rule on Labeling and Effectiveness Testing of Sunscreen was issued, because earlier FDA rules required lamp beams at least one centimeter in diameter. Single port and multiport compact xenon arc solar simulators are now available in 300 W versions.

The Berger solar simulator facilitated convenient indoor testing of sunscreen products and made it possible for sunscreen manufacturers to develop products with SPF ratings higher than 15 and eventually as high as 100. Other than the addition of automatic shutters, solid-state power supplies, and 300 W power supplies, the compact xenon arc lamp solar simulator has not changed significantly in the last three decades.

However, the cutoff filters that are required to diminish the heating of the skin by the compact xenon arc lamp solar simulator exaggerate the long wavelength UVB and short UVA and cut away much of the long UVA power [3]. This causes some overestimation of the SPF measured with compact xenon arc lamp solar simulators, compared to that of sunlight (Colipa 1994) [9]. See Fig. 18.1.

To compensate for the shortcomings of the SPF alone, additional tests of sunscreens to demonstrate protection against UVA have been developed. Most notable is the critical wavelength test, devised by Dr. Brian Diffey and published in 1993 [9]. The critical wavelength test will be discussed in Sect. 18.4.

18.2 The SPF Test

18.2.1 Solar Simulators

The FDA Final Rule stipulates the procedures for measuring both the SPF and the critical wavelength [10].

- Continuous emission spectrum from 290 to 400 nm
- Emission spectrum measured at least annually and after replacement of lamp bulb or any change in optical components, using an appropriate spectroradiometer system that is calibrated to a NIST-traceable source

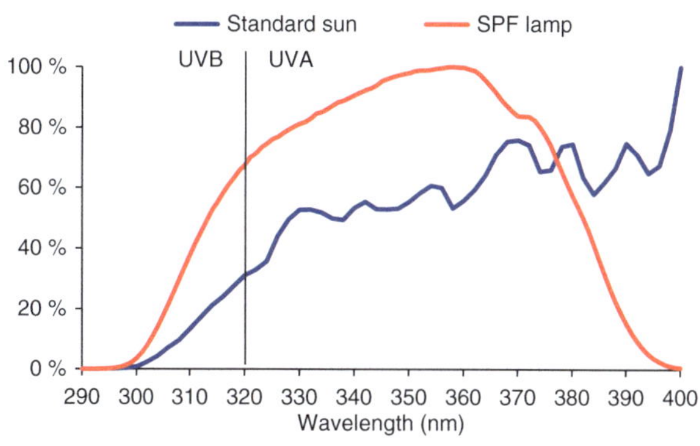

Fig. 18.1 Comparison of the solar simulator and sunlight

- Daily radiation intensity monitored before and after each test, or at least at the beginning and end of each test day using an erythemally weighted radiometer with a calibration consistent with the spectroradiometer system
- No significant time-related fluctuations in the exposure plane (±20 %)
- Good beam uniformity (±20 % from centerline reading)
- UVAII (320–400 nm), ≥ 20 % of total UV irradiance
- UVAI (340–400 nm), ≥ 60 % of total UV irradiance
- Total irradiance from 250 to 1400 nm ≤1500 W/m^2

The permissible ranges of the percent of erythemal dose contributions are shown in Table 18.1.

18.2.2 The Standard Sunscreen

As a positive control, the FDA stipulates use of a standard sunscreen, designated as the padimate O/oxybenzone standard. The active ingredients of the padimate O/oxybenzone standard include 7 % of padimate O and 3 % of oxybenzone. The complete formula of the padimate O/oxybenzone standard is provided in the Final Rule. The padimate/oxybenzone standard must be included in all SPF tests, along with the test products. For the measured value of the test product to be valid, the mean value of the padimate O/oxybenzone standard must fall within the standard deviation range of the expected SPF (i.e., 16±3.43).

18.2.3 Test Subjects

According to the FDA's Final Rule on Labeling and Effectiveness Testing, a panel of ten subjects is required for each test product. Multiple products may be included on the same subjects, and each subject's test must include the padimate O/oxybenzone standard. For each test product, a maximum of three subjects may be rejected due to test failures from the panel and replaced.

Subjects must provide an acceptable written informed consent document and a medical history, including any instance of skin cancer, dysplastic nevi, current use

Table 18.1 Permissible ranges of the percent erythemal dose contributions

Wavelength range	Percent erythemal dose contribution
<290	<0.1
290–300	1.0–8.0
290–310	49.0–65.0
290–320	85.0–90.0
290–330	91.5–95.5
290–340	94.0–97.0
290–400	99.9–100.0

of any medication associated with sun sensitivity, abnormal responses to sunlight, or phototoxic or photoallergic responses. Each subject must be in good general health and have Fitzpatrick skin types I, II, or III. See Table 18.2.

18.2.4 Procedures

Test sites are located on the subject's back, between the shoulder blades and the beltline, and on either side of the midline. Test sites are demarcated using an indelible surgical pen. There are typically four or six horizontally oriented rectangular sites, with typical dimensions of 5 cm by 10 cm. The Final Rule requires an area of at least 30 cm^2 for each product test site. Within each rectangular site, five sub-sites are required, for each UV exposure. Above the rectangular sites, a space is reserved for a horizontal row of two sets of five sub-sites for unprotected minimal erythema doses. Irradiated sites must be separated by at least 0.8 cm. See Fig. 18.2. The person who evaluates the results to determine the SPF should be blinded.

18.2.5 Initial Unprotected MED Dose Administration

On Day 1, after determining that the subject is qualified for participation in the study, the technician will administer a timed series of five UV doses, increasing in 25 % increments.

After determining that the subject has no adverse response, he or she will be instructed to avoid UV exposure and prohibited medications and given an appointment to return to the testing laboratory, within 16–24 h after completion of UV doses.

18.2.6 Initial Unprotected MED Dose Administration

On Day 2, the subject will return to the testing laboratory within 16–24 hours after completion of the unprotected MED doses, for evaluation of responses. The technician will question the subject nondirectively to assess compliance, to identify

Table 18.2 Fitzpatrick skin types

1. Always burns easily; never tans (sensitive)
2. Always burns easily; tans minimally (sensitive)
3. Burns moderately; tans gradually (light brown) (normal)
4. Burns minimally; always tans well (moderate brown) (normal)
5. Rarely burns; tans profusely (dark brown) (insensitive)
6. Never burns; deeply pigmented (insensitive)

Note: Skin type is based on first 30–45 min of sun exposure after a winter season of no sun exposure

Fig. 18.2 Fitzpatrick Skin Types

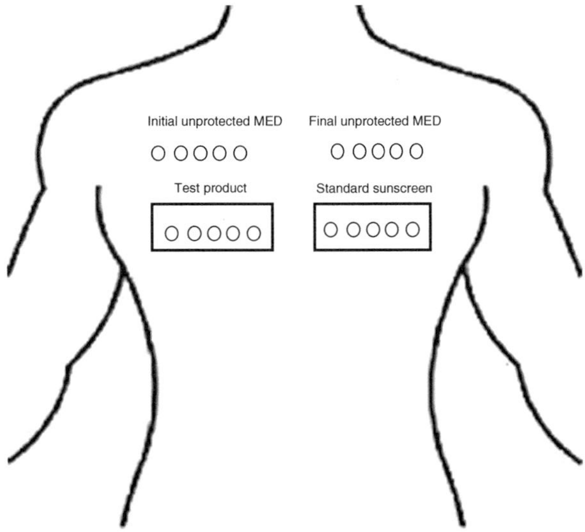

prohibited concomitant medications and UV exposures, and to identify and record any adverse events. If the subject is eligible to continue, a trained evaluator will assess the responses of the UV exposed sites, under warm fluorescent or tungsten illumination of at least 450 lx, to determine the initial unprotected MED. The MED is defined as the smallest UV dose that produces perceptible redness of the skin (erythema) with clearly defined borders at 16–24 h after UV exposure. The progression of intensity of the erythema must be consistent with the UV doses.

18.2.7 Application of Test Products and the Padimate O/ Oxybenzone Standard Sunscreen for SPF Determination

On Day 2, the technician will apply 2 mg per cm^2 of each test product and the standard in its respective designated rectangle. The sunscreens will be applied by "spotting" the material across the area and gently spreading, using a new finger cot for each, until a uniform film is applied to the entire area. The finger cots will not be pre-moistened before the applications.

18.2.8 UV Doses for Test Product MED

After at least 15 min, the technician will administer a series of five progressively increasing, timed UV doses to the sites treated with the test products and standard. The dose series will be determined by the product of the expected SPF of each test product and the subject's initial unprotected MED. See Table 18.3.

18.2.9 UV Doses for Repeat Unprotected Minimal Erythema Dose

On Day 2, the technician will administer a timed series of five UV doses, increasing by 25 % increments, to an unprotected area of the mid-back. The series of five doses will include the initial MED in the center as shown in Table 18.4.

After determining that the subject has no adverse response, he or she will be instructed to avoid UV exposure and prohibited medications and given an appointment to return to the testing laboratory, within 16–24 h after completion of UV doses.

18.2.10 Determination of the SPF

On Day 3, the subjects will return to the testing laboratory within 16–24 h after completion of the unprotected MED doses, for evaluation of responses. The technician will question the subject nondirectively to assess compliance, to identify prohibited concomitant medications and UV exposures, and to identify and record any adverse events. Then a trained evaluator, who did not participate in product applications or administration of UV doses, will evaluate all sites that received UV doses. The technician will determine the repeat unprotected MED as above and compute the SPF values for the test product SPF and standard sunscreen SPF for each subject.

The final unprotected MED used for the SPF computation will be the repeat unprotected MED unless the repeat unprotected MED cannot be determined. In that case, the initial unprotected MED will be used for the SPF computation.

SPF values for individual subjects will be calculated as:

$$\text{SPF} = \text{Protected MED} / \text{Repeat Final Unprotected MED}$$

The mean SPF and standard deviation (SD) will be calculated from valid SPFi values.

Table 18.3 Multiple of expected SPF and subject initial MED for each expected SPF

Expected SPF	Multiple of expected SPF and subject initial MED				
<8	0.64	0.80	1.00	1.25	1.56
≥8–15	0.69	0.83	1.00	1.20	1.44
>15	0.76	0.87	1.00	1.15	1.32

Table 18.4 Multiple of expected SPF and subject initial MED for each expected SPF

Multiple of initial MEDu				
0.64	0.80	1.00	1.25	1.56

The standard error (SE) will be calculated as

$$SE = SD / \sqrt{n}$$

where n equals the number of subjects who provided valid test results.

The t value from student's t distribution table corresponding to the upper 5 % point with $n-1$ degrees of freedom will be obtained.

The labeled SPF value will be determined as the largest whole number less than the following calculation:

$$\text{Labeled SPF} = \text{Mean SPF} - (t * \text{SE})$$

In order for the SPF determination of the test product to be valid, the SPF value of the padimate O/oxybenzone standard should fall within the standard deviation range of the expected SPF (i.e., 16.3 ± 3.43).

18.3 Water Resistance Testing

Water resistance testing will be performed in an indoor fresh water pool, whirlpool, or hot tub maintained at 23°–32° Celsius. The pool and air temperature and the humidity should be recorded.

18.3.1 Water Resistance (40 min)

The labeled SPF will be determined after 40 min of water immersion using the following procedure:

1. Apply the sunscreen as described in Sect. 18.2.7.
2. Perform moderate activity in water for 20 min.
3. Rest out of water for 15 min. Do not towel test site(s).
4. Perform moderate activity in water for 20 min.
5. Rest out of water for 15 min. Do not towel test site(s).
6. Apply the SPF standard as described above.
7. Expose test sites to UV doses as described above.

18.3.2 Water Resistance (80 min)

The labeled SPF will be determined after 80 min of water immersion using the following procedure:

1. Apply the sunscreen as described in Sect. 18.2.7.
2. Perform moderate activity in water for 20 min.

3. Rest out of water for 15 min. Do not towel test site(s).
4. Perform moderate activity in water for 20 min.
5. Rest out of water for 15 min. Do not towel test site(s).
6. Perform moderate activity in water for 20 min.
7. Rest out of water for 15 min. Do not towel test site(s).
8. Perform moderate activity in water for 20 min.
9. Allow test sites to dry completely without toweling.
10. Apply the SPF standard as described above.
11. Expose test sites to UV doses as described above.

18.4 The Broad-Spectrum Protection Test (Critical Wavelength Test)

18.4.1 Background

In 1993, Diffey [8] proposed a spectroscopic method for broad-spectrum classification of sunscreens, based on the absorbance spectrum. The broad-spectrum rating was determined by measuring the absorbance spectrum and integrating the area under the spectral curve from 290 nm to the wavelength at which the area reached 90 % of the total area under the absorbance curve from 290 to 400 nm.

The FDA Final Rule of June 17, 2011 [10] defined the method for evaluating the critical wavelength of sunscreen test products after irradiation with a full-spectrum UV dose of four MEDs (800 effective J/m^2), as follows:

18.4.2 Test Product Application

The amount of test product applied is 0.75 mg/cm^2. The test product is applied to the entire roughened surface of each of at least three PMMA plates, with a roughness value (R_a) of 2–7 μm [11], in a series of small dots. The test product is spread evenly using a gloved finger, with a very light spreading action for approximately 30 s, followed by spreading with greater pressure for approximately 30 s. The plates are then allowed to equilibrate for 15 min in the dark. After equilibration, the plates are irradiated with a full-spectrum UV dose of four MEDs (800 effective J/m^2).

18.4.3 Irradiation

After equilibration, the plates are irradiated with a full-spectrum UV dose of four MEDs (800 effective J/m^2) using a xenon arc solar simulator. The irradiation source must meet the requirements as described in Sect. 18.2.1.

18.4.4 Measurements

After irradiation of the plates, the UV transmission is at wavelengths from 290 to 400 nm at 1 nm intervals using a radiometer equipped with an integrating sphere or an ultraviolet radiation diffuser placed between the sample and the input optics of the spectrometer, to ensure that the radiation received by the spectrometer is not collimated. The spectrometer input slits must be set to provide a bandwidth that is less than one nanometer. In addition, the dynamic range of the spectrometer should be sufficient to measure transmittance accurately through a highly absorbing sunscreen product at all terrestrial solar UV wavelengths (290–400 nm). Finally the UV dose during one measurement cycle must not exceed 0.2 J/cm^2, and a total area of at least 2 cm^2 is measured on each plate. The transmission is measured for five locations on the reference plate coated with 15 µl of glycerin and five locations on the irradiated plates using a lamp that provides continuous full-spectrum radiation from 290 to 400 nm and measuring the transmitted spectral irradiance. The mean transmittance for each wavelength, $T(\lambda)$, is computed as follows:

$$\overline{T(\lambda)} = \frac{\sum_{1}^{5} P(\lambda)/5}{\sum_{1}^{5} C(\lambda)/5}$$

Then

$$\overline{A(\lambda)} = -\log \overline{T(\lambda)}$$

where $\overline{A(\lambda)}$ is the mean absorbance at each wavelength.

The critical wavelength for each plate is then calculated as follows:

$$\int_{290}^{\lambda_c} \overline{A(\lambda)} d\lambda = 0.9 \int_{290}^{400} \overline{A(\lambda)} d\lambda$$

where λ_c = critical wavelength

$\overline{A(\lambda)}$ = mean absorbance at each wavelength

$d\lambda$ = wavelength interval between measurements

Typical results are shown in Figs. 18.3 and 18.4.

18.5 Pitfalls in the SPF Test

18.5.1 Radiometry

Daily radiation intensity measurements and annual calibrations of solar simulator spectra must be conducted properly, using National Institutes of Standards and Technology (NIST)-traceable instruments. Technicians who obtain measurements

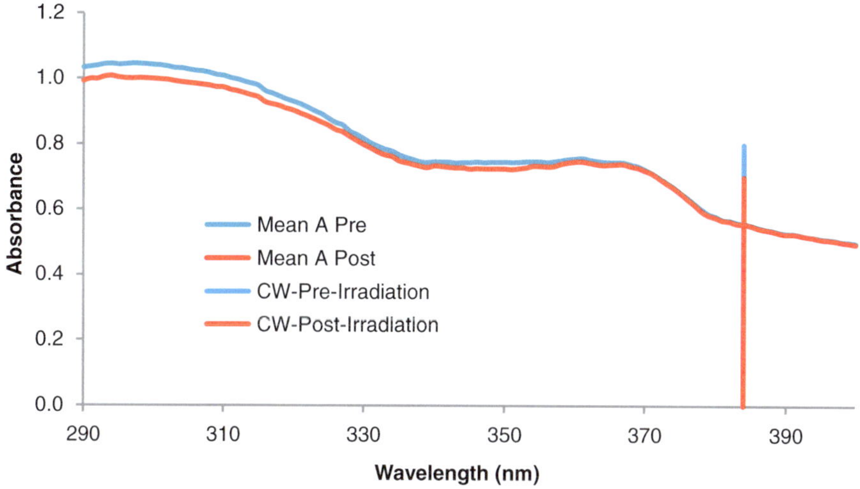

Fig. 18.3 Mean absorbance and mean critical wavelength before irradiation and after a full-spectrum UV dose of four MEDs (800 effective J/m²)

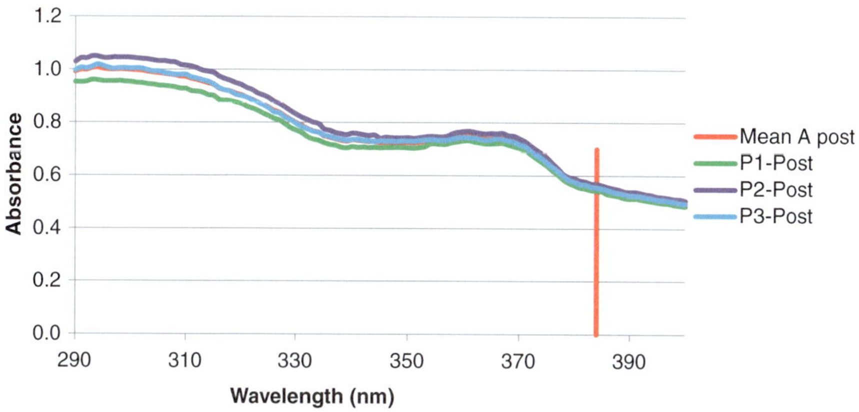

Fig. 18.4 Absorbance spectra, the mean absorbance spectrum, and the critical wavelength for each plate after a full-spectrum UV dose of four MEDs (800 effective J/m²)

must be appropriately trained. One frequent mistake is measuring the output of a UV source using a radiometer detector that is larger than the source. For example, a radiometer detector that is 1 cm in diameter to measure a UV source that is 0.8 cm in diameter. Radiometers must be calibrated according to an appropriate documented interval, and spectroradiometers used to calibrate radiometers must also be calibrated according to an appropriate documented interval, by a qualified expert [12].

18.5.2 Photosensitizing Drugs

Subjects must notify the laboratory of current or recent use of any medication associated with sun sensitivity, abnormal responses to sunlight, or phototoxic or photoallergic responses. Since prospective subjects often forget or overlook photosensitizing drugs they may be taking, it is helpful to read a periodically updated list of potentially photosensitizing drugs to the subject before enrollment in an SPF test. Lists are available on websites such as Medscape (http://emedicine.medscape.com/article/1049648-overview).

18.5.3 Sunscreen Application

Technicians must be properly trained in application procedures for a wide range of sample types, including liquids, lotions, creams, and sticks. Care must be taken to apply a uniform film across the entire test area to ensure the proper concentration of 2 mg per cm^2. Subjects must be monitored to avoid inadvertently removing the sunscreens during the test procedures.

18.5.4 Visual Grading of Responses

An evaluator who is blinded to the application sites must be properly trained to evaluate the erythema response. Inconsistent grading can lead to high variability. In most cases, it is best to have the same evaluator for all subjects in an SPF panel.

18.5.5 Subject Compliance

Subjects that meet the inclusion/exclusion criteria need to be available for testing. Test subjects must be able to meet all study requirements in the appropriate time frames. Noncompliance can lead to unreliable data or missed deadlines.

18.6 Pitfalls in the Broad-Spectrum Test

18.6.1 Measuring the Critical Wavelength in the Broad-Spectrum Test

According to the FDA Final Rule, the spectroradiometer used to measure the critical wavelength must provide a bandwidth less than one nanometer (nm). The Labsphere 2000, which is widely used for ISO 24443 and COLIPA tests for critical wavelength and UVA protection factor determination, has a bandwidth of approximately 4 nm and does not satisfy FDA requirements.

18.6.2 Application of Test Products to PMMA Plates

As with the in vivo test, application can be a factor in unreliable results. The plates are meant to simulate the surface of human skin. Too much or too little rubbing during application can lead to differences in film thickness which can cause high variability.

18.7 Conclusion

The sun protection factor (SPF) is a dimensionless ratio that estimates the protective efficacy of a sunscreen against erythema. The aim of this chapter was, step by step, to describe compliance of UV solar simulators, the assessment of the sun protection factor (SPF) according to the FDA Final Rule, and the determination of the critical wavelength of sunscreens to determine the degree of broad-spectrum protection.

References

1. Blum H, Eicher M, Terus W (1945) Evaluation of protective measures against sunburn. Am J Physiol 146:118–125
2. Schulze R (1956) Einige Versuche und Bemerkungen zum Problem der handelsüblichen Lichtschutzmittel. Parf Kosm 37:310–315
3. Cole C (2014) Sunscreens-what is the ideal testing model? Photodermatol Photoimmunol Photomed 30:81–87
4. Urbach F (1991) Franz Grieter—The man and his work. In: Riklis E (ed) Photobiology. Plenum Press, New York, p 761
5. Department of health, education and welfare, FDA, USA: Sunscreen drug products for over-the-counter human drugs; proposed safety, effective and labeling conditions. Federal register. 43/166, 38206–38269, 25 Aug 1978
6. Kollias N, Ruvolo E Jr, Sayre RM (2011) The value of the ratio of UVA to UVB in sunlight. Photochem Photobiol 87(6):1474–1475
7. Berger D (1969) Specification and design of solar ultraviolet simulators. J Invest Dermatol 53(192):199
8. Diffey BL (1994) A method for broad spectrum classification of sunscreens. Int J Cosmet Sci 16:47–52
9. COLIPA (1994) COLIPA SPF test method. Ref 94/289
10. U.S. Food and Drug Administration, 21 CFR Parts 201 and 310, Federal Register, Vol. 76, No. 117, Friday, June 17, 2011, pp 35620–35665
11. Gadelmawlaa E, SKourab MM, Maksoudc TMA, Elewaa IM, Soliman HH (2002) Roughness parameters. J Mater Process Technol 123(1):133–145
12. Christiaens F, Uhlmann B (2007) Guidelines for Monitoring UV Radiation Sources, Cosmetics Europe

Part III

Chapter 19
Photoprotection in the Era of Nanotechnology

Adnan Nasir

Key Points

- Photoprotection is embedded in the DNA of the human species. It has undergone additional natural and social selection through body hair loss and skin pigment loss.
- Artificial photoprotection predates recorded human history in the form of grooming habits, clothing, and application of tattoos, muds, and clays. Some of these may have been comprised of accidental nanomaterials.
- Early sunscreens were made of organic compounds with ring structures which absorbed ultraviolet light and emitted infrared energy. They thus absorbed UV light, generated heat, and could only be formulated in lipophilic vehicles.
- The modern era of nanoformulation has allowed for these same sunscreens to be incorporated in a variety of cosmetically elegant vehicles, using smaller quantities of active ingredient, for better and more stable photoprotection and enhanced compliance.
- Nanoparticles have also been used to develop inorganic and combination topical sunscreens, as well as entities which combat the effects of photodamage through a variety of other mechanisms, including physical blockade, UV absorption, free radical quenching, antioxidant activity, and delivery of DNA repair enzymes. We are just now witnessing the 'rosy fingered' dawn of the nano-era of photoprotection.

A. Nasir, MD, PhD
Department of Dermatology, UNC Chapel Hill,
3100 Thurston Bowles Bldg, Chapel Hill, NC 27544, USA
e-mail: ANASIR@LIVE.COM

S.Q. Wang, H.W. Lim (eds.), *Principles and Practice of Photoprotection*,
DOI 10.1007/978-3-319-29382-0_19

19.1 Introduction

By some estimates, the number of products employing nanomaterials is doubling annually. Products containing nanomaterials include consumer products such as food and beverages, sporting goods, clothing, coatings for surfaces, personal care products, and medications. Sunscreens also may contain nanomaterials. Some products may be labeled as containing such, and some products may not have labels designating nanomaterial contents.

In dermatology, sunscreen has been a critical area of development of nanomaterials because of its beneficial effects in the prevention of premature aging of the skin, sunburns, prevention of photosensitivity-related drug reactions, prevention of exacerbations of photosensitive diseases, and prevention of skin cancer.

The rate of rise of the incidence of skin cancer over the past several decades has been dramatic. In the early 1930s, the lifetime risk of developing skin cancer was 1 in 5000. By 2004, the rate rose to 1 in 65. If current trends continue, by 2050 the lifetime risk of skin cancer will be 1 in 10. The causes for this rise are multifactorial and may include environmental changes such as global warming, decreased ozone layer protection, increased use of tanning beds, increased outdoor leisure activities, increased travel to temperate and tropical climates, legacy of tobacco use, legacy of radiation exposure, greater awareness, better diagnosis, and as yet undetermined environmental and occupational exposures. Skin cancer accounts for nearly half of all of the diagnosed cancers in United States each year. More than one million cases of skin cancer, melanoma as well as nonmelanoma skin cancer, are diagnosed each year, and one person dies every hour due to skin cancer.

There are a variety of other consequences to photodamage beyond photocarcinogenesis. These include photoaging, photoimmunosuppression, and activation of photosensitive dermatoses. UV light can significantly aggravate certain skin diseases such as cutaneous lupus erythematosus, porphyrias, and some genodermatoses such as xeroderma pigmentosum. Recent studies have shown that strict photoprotection prevents disease-specific lesions from forming by reducing direct damage to the skin lesions and by reducing interferon-driven inflammation [1].

19.1.1 Solar Radiation

Less than 1 % of all of the ultraviolet light reaching the surface of the earth is in the UVC range. About 0.35 % of the total radiation reaching the earth from the sun is in the UVB range, and 6.5 % is in the UVA range. About 43 % of the light reaching the earth is visible, and about 49 % is in the infrared range. The effects of these latter two portions of light spectrum on the skin are not completely understood but are now increasingly believed to be involved in some form photodamage.

While chronic exposure to UVA and UVB has been shown to contribute to sun-induced aging of the skin, recent studies have shown that the skin may also be damaged by wavelengths outside the ultraviolet spectrum. These include photons in the visible and infrared wavelengths. One of the reasons the traditional sunscreens may not be as effective as desired may be the lack of efficacy against visible and infrared light. Photoprotection in the visible and infrared wavelengths may require the development of invisible topical antioxidants or visible and camouflaged photon-blocking agents [2]. Interestingly, broad band light, particularly long-wavelength broadband light, has shown to clinically [3] and genetically [4] improve skin signs of photodamage.

Photoprotection of the skin involves protecting the skin from damage from light of various sources including the sun and artificial light sources. The spectrum of radiation emitted by light is characterized by its wavelength, frequency, and energy. The entire electromagnetic spectrum ranges from gamma rays to a.m. radio waves beginning at wavelengths as short as 0.0001 nm all the way to 100 m or longer. The majority of the sun's energy reaching the surface of the earth is contained in the ultraviolet, visible, and infrared spectrum. Approximately 40 % of the sun's rays are in the visible range, 50 % are in the infrared range, 7 % are in the ultraviolet range, and less than 1 % consist of x-rays, gamma rays, and radio waves.

There is an inverse relationship between frequency and wavelength. Frequency of radiation is an inverse function of wavelength because the speed of light is constant. Photons of longer wavelengths have a lower frequency of radiation and vice versa. By contrast, energy is a direct function of frequency. The higher the frequency of photons, the greater their energy. This energy, when it impinges upon vital structures of the skin, can lead to skin damage. High-energy, or high-frequency, photons can cause considerable damage to the skin, while low-energy, or low-frequency, photons may cause damage but may require a greater total dose, necessitating longer exposures.

The depth of penetration into the skin is an inverse function of the frequency of photon energy. High-energy photons such as those in the UVC range are actually blocked out by the ozone layer of the atmosphere and the stratum corneum. Medium-energy photons such as those in the UVB range penetrate to be level of the epidermis and the dermoepidermal junction. Lower-energy photons in the UVA range can penetrate beyond the dermoepidermal junction into the mid and deep dermis.

19.1.2 Sunscreen History

19.1.2.1 Natural Hominid Photoprotection

Hair covering the body protects against ultraviolet light, trauma, abrasion, and some parasites and microorganisms. One Australian study assessed the protective effects of beards and mostaches under ultraviolet radiation [6]. Facial hair was found to give the skin an ultraviolet protection factor of 2–21, depending upon the solar zenith angle and beard-mostache length. Hair also can insulate and camouflage the skin. Adaptations of hairlessness include less drag while swimming, less snagging in dense undergrowth, and reduced risk of overheating. Dark skin may have developed hand in hand with the loss of body hair. Lack of hair and abundant and highly active eccrine glands give hominids an advantage in cooling capacity.

Through the process of natural selection, melanin levels have been optimized to minimize ultraviolet light damage, in order to protect folic acid and DNA from solar rays while permitting enough light to penetrate the skin to stimulate adequate vitamin D synthesis and photo conversion. Research has recently shown that sun protection is probably not the primary driver of skin pigmentation. Common ancestors shared among humans and chimpanzees have light pigmentation of their skin covered by dark hair. This lightly pigmented skin is capable of tanning. This type of response to sun exposure is far more effective at combating skin cancer and far more adaptive than albinism.

Approximately one million years ago, early humans lost body hair and acquired pigmented exposed skin in order to adapt to a hot sunny climate. Several lines of evidence, including analysis of the MC1R gene, suggest that dark pigmentation was acquired soon after loss of body hair [7]. Tightly curled hair on the head allowed photoprotection and cooling, allowing air to breeze through, but blocking out sunlight. Contemporaneously with MC1R gene changes, modifications in the stratum corneum improved the epidermal barrier against abrasion and microbes. Stratum corneum keratinocyte response to sun exposure includes immediate dark pigmentation, which may be due to rearrangement of melanosomes and photo oxidation of eumelanin.

Individuals with darker Fitzpatrick skin types tend to have a more intense immediate pigmentary response. The delayed tanning response develops from hours to days following UV exposure. Because skin cancer, even in sunny climates, tends to occur after the age of reproduction, selective pressure for dark skin probably was not designed to reduce the risk of skin cancer. Nonmelanoma skin cancer is typically not fatal, and its incidence increases with age. Melanoma, while potentially fatal and tending to occur more frequently in younger individuals, especially young women, is rare compared to nonmelanoma skin cancer. For millennia, the Inuit have carved snow goggles from caribou antlers and sinew, creating form-fitting curved eye masks with narrow slits to limit light exposure to the eyes and prevent photokeratitis.

19.1.2.2 Folic Acid and Vitamin D as Selective Pressures

Folic acid (vitamin B_9) is used for DNA repair in and to prevent neural tube defects. Low levels of folic acid induced by photolysis can also lead to reduced fertility because of potentially fatal birth defects [8]. Folic acid is also important in spermatogenesis, and reduced levels may also potentially contribute to male infertility. Ultraviolet light exposure reduces folic acid levels. Diminished folic acid levels are detrimental to DNA repair and embryogenesis. Selective pressure would promote tend to promote melanogenesis to preserve optimum folic acid levels. It has been speculated that hunters and gatherers received significant amounts of vitamin D through their diets of fish and animal livers. With the advent of agriculture, early Europeans required vitamin D supplementation, and those with less pigment in their skin were able to synthesize it with suboptimal ultraviolet light exposure. Vitamin D receptors occur in 36 different tissues, and studies show the importance of vitamin D in the immune system, the musculoskeletal system, the intestine, the kidney, and the reproductive system. Vitamin D deficiencies have been associated with rickets and multiple sclerosis. Because of its effect on reproduction, preservation of folic acid levels may have exerted more selective evolutionary pressure than preservation of vitamin D levels.

19.1.2.3 Photoprotection History

Evidence suggests that recent changes in the skin, eye, and hair pigmentation have been due to social and sexual selection. The ancient Egyptians considered light skin more attractive than dark skin. In the desert environment, it was difficult to maintain fair skin. Translations of hieroglyphics from Egyptian tombs have revealed ingredients such as rice bran extract, jasmine, and lupine extract for treating damage to the skin and reducing the likelihood of a tan or of a sunburn. One of the components of rice bran extract, oryzanol, has been shown to have UV-absorbing properties [9].

Examples of low-cost photoprotectants using local materials can be found in Southern Africa. African clays have been used for cosmetic purposes, ceremonial purposes, ritual coming-of-age ceremonies, local hygiene practices, social signaling, camouflage, and photoprotection. Aboriginal peoples of South Africa have used two types of clay for photoprotection: red and white. The Xhosa tribes in the Amathole Mountain area use red clay for face painting [10]. Clays are composed of fine grains containing traces of metals such as nanoparticulate aluminum silicates, organic matter, bound together by water in a mineral structure. In general particle sizes of clays range from 1000 to 2000 nm. This permits tight aggregation and packing of clay components. These clays have been studied for their photoprotective properties [10]. Overall, it has been determined that clays from the Amathole Range have a low sun protection factor but a broad spectrum of activity.

Before the modern era of photoprotection, sunburn was believed to the caused by heat rather than ultraviolet light. In 1801, Johann Wilhelm Ritter discovered ultraviolet rays. He described properties of light with wavelengths shorter than those in blue and referred to light in this region as infraviolet (which we now term ultraviolet). While Hippocrates and Aristotle developed early theories of skin color and climate, it wasn't until 1820 that Everard Home of England dispelled the notion that heat led to sunburns. He began exploring why inhabitants of temperate climates have darker skin than inhabitants of northern climates. He found the correlation surprising given the fact that darker skin tends to absorb more heat and lighter skin less heat. He would have expected dark skin in colder climates as one means of capturing as much ambient heat as possible. Home observed this directly when he covered one of his pale hands with a dark cloth and left the other hand exposed to sunlight. Even though the hand covered with the dark cloth registered a warmer temperature, it did not sunburn compared to the exposed hand. He surmised that skin pigment protected against sunburn and that sunburn was not due to heat. Home concluded that it was the dark pigment in skin, or melanin, which protected the skin from ultraviolet light-induced damage.

In 1878, Otto Veiel had shown the benefits of tannin in protecting against ultraviolet light. The usefulness of tannin was limited by its tendency to stain the skin. In 1922, it was demonstrated that the wavelengths of light most likely to induce sunburn were in the 280–315 nm wavelength range. By developing filters which specifically targeted this wavelength, the first sunscreens containing para-aminobenzoic acid, benzyl salicylate, and benzyl cinnamate were developed.

Sunscreens were initially developed, and their use proliferated during the Second World War in order to protect soldiers deployed in the Pacific tropics and the African desert from sunburn causing rays. Early sunscreens blocked rays in the UVB portion of the solar spectrum. Traditional measurements of sunscreen effectiveness have focused on this portion of the light spectrum and have not addressed protection against UVA or UBC or visible or infrared light.

The stigma of dark skin has led to a plethora of skin-lightening products. The impact of these products has been greatest in countries like South Africa and India. Some of these products contain mercury and have been the target of FDA regulation and United States. In India, controversial skin whiteners have also been developed for the vaginal area. Skin lighteners, when permanently depleting cutaneous melanocytes, can lead to increased vulnerability to UV light and can mask the appearance of melanoma. Nanoparticles can be formulated in a broad range of hues and can be manufactured to make sunscreens which blend in with a variety of skin types. They may prove useful for individuals who have undergone temporary or permanent lightening procedures.

19.1.3 Sunscreen Composition

Sunscreens are typically suspensions of active ingredients which may be organic or inorganic. Organic sunscreens are typically composed of molecules containing carbon, hydrogen, oxygen, and nitrogen structured to absorb ultraviolet light in the UVB and UVA range. Organic sunscreen molecules are typically small, from a few to several dozen Angstroms in size. Organic sunscreens typically have a ring structures with free electrons which capture ultraviolet light energy and become activated to a higher-energy level. This excess energy is then released at a longer wavelength and lower energy such as infrared energy. In order to conserve energy, multiple infrared (IR) wavelength photons may be released to balance the energy of a single incoming high-energy ultraviolet (UV) photon. Thus, organic sunscreens can be thought of as UV to IR converters, absorbing UV light and releasing heat.

19.1.3.1 Organic Sunscreens

The ring structures of organic sunscreens can be configured to have different wavelength peaks and ranges of absorption. Combining a variety of organic molecules can give rise to a broad spectrum of UV absorption. The majority of sunscreen organic compounds that are approved by the FDA are excellent UVB blockers. A smaller number of UVA blockers has been approved and is under consideration for future approval.

19.1.3.2 Inorganic Sunscreens

Inorganic sunscreens typically are clusters of ions such as zinc, iron, or titanium coupled to oxygen. These clusters are manufactured in particles ranging in size from 10 to 300 nm. The mechanism of action of inorganic sunscreens differs from organic sunscreens. Inorganic sunscreen effectively blocks and absorbs UV from the 200 to 380 nm size range with a steep drop-off after 380 nm. Thus, inorganic sunscreens have a high utility for UVC, UVB, and UVA light.

Macromolecular clusters of inorganic sunscreens are not generally accepted by the public because of their opacity. They leave a white residue on the skin and, if they are used at all, tend to be under used to minimize this effect. The opacity is due to the light scattering effect of the large clusters of inorganic sunscreens. Typical clusters of zinc oxide and titanium dioxide tend to be 200 nm or greater. Clusters of this size are effective at scattering light of a wavelength twice their diameters. Thus, large clusters of 200 mm or greater tend to scatter light in the visible range, 400–700 nm. Scattering of visible light when reflected to the eyes appears quite. Organic sunscreens do not scatter visible light because of their small size. Compared to a 200 nm particle of titanium dioxide capable of scattering light in the 400–700 nm range, a one nanometer particle of methoxycinnamate is unable to scatter visible light.

Small particles are small obstacles to longer wavelengths of light. Objects much smaller than visible light rays (100 nm or smaller) do not scatter visible light effectively. Therefore, nanoparticulate sunscreens in the 100 nm size range or smaller appear essentially invisible. Light scatter as a function of wavelength demonstrates this phenomenon clearly.

19.1.3.3 Nanoformulation

Formulation of sunscreens in nanocarriers may offer advantages over traditional formulation.

Increased Spectrum Bandwidth

For example, butyl methoxy dibenzoylmethane and octocrylene in combination confer broad-spectrum ultraviolet light protection. These are trapped in high densities in lipid nanocarriers made from rice bran oil and raspberry seed oil. Sunscreens made in this fashion reflect 91–93 % of UVA and UVB rays, respectively, in cream formulations containing only 3.5 % of active ingredient and 10.5 % of vegetable oils. The carriers have been shown to be stable with very slow release kinetics after application (4–17.5 % over 24 h). This ability to combine and concentrate broad-spectrum sunscreen components in small biocompatible and biodegradable lipid carriers leads to greater efficacy, greater flexibility in combinatorial formulation, reduced manufacturing costs from reduced amount of active ingredient required, and superior efficacy.

Increased Stability

Naturally occurring photoprotectants in plants are unstable and rapidly degraded once the plant is destroyed. The peels of apples are rich in photoprotective antioxidant compounds. These can be extracted to yield apple peel ethanolic extracts (APETE). The inherently unstable contents of these extracts can be stabilized when incorporated into PLGA nanocarriers. In vitro studies have shown photoprotective effects of nano-APETE carriers on cultured dermal fibroblasts.

Enhanced Release Kinetics

Some synthetic compounds are also subject to instability and aggregation as well as potential percutaneous absorption. One example is 4-methylbenzylidine camphor. When incorporated into microspheres, 4-MBC particles showed the same photoprotective capacity as the free chemical compound, greater stability, and significantly slower release kinetics.

Enhanced Compliance

This is discussed in more detail below but occurs as a result of the combination of benefits and reduced risks of nanoformulation.

19.2 Sunscreen Analysis

Standard methods for evaluating sunscreens include the use of photometers and animal and human studies to evaluate minimal erythema-inducing doses. Alternatives to human and animal testing are constantly being developed to assess the protective efficacy of sunscreens. One nanotechnology-based methodology involves a so-called cell dosimeter [11]. This in vitro method measures specific DNA repair enzymes as well as cell viability after exposure to radiation with UV light. In addition, the assay is made more sensitive through the use of xeroderma pigmentosum cells. This assay was able to demonstrate protection of cells using sunscreens against UVB light, but not against UVA light or natural sunlight. Skin equivalence has also been used to measure photodamage from ultraviolet light. The results can be assessed by cyclopyrimidine dimer formation and sunburn cell formation. Studies using skin equivalents have shown reduced cyclopyrimidine dimer formation and sunburn cell formation when sunscreen was applied prior to dosing with ultraviolet light.

19.3 Topical Agents

Topical sun protective agents include metallic physical blockers such as zinc oxide, titanium dioxide; organic chemical filters such as cinnamates, benzophenones, Mexoryl SX, XL, and Tinosorb M, S; antioxidants such as hydroxycinnamic acids, polyphenols including flavonoids-genistein, silymarin, equol, quercetin, apigenin, green tea extract, resveratrol, staxanti, anthocyanins, tannins, pycnogenol, and others (DHA, caffeine, polygonum multiflorum)-fullerenes, N-(4-pyrodoxylmethylene)-1-serine, creatine, and idebenone; nonsteroidal anti-inflammatory compounds such as COX-2 inhibitors; and "after-exposure" compounds which affect DNA repair, such as the enzymes photolyase, T4 endonuclease, and DNA oligonucleotides.

19.3.1 Fabrics

Other obvious sources of sun protection include hats, umbrellas, and shade structures (natural, such as terrain and foliage; as well as artificial, such as awnings and roofs). The term umbrella derives from the Latin *umbra*, meaning shade or shadow. Originally, umbrellas were developed in ancient Egypt and contained palm fronds for sun protection. Modifications made their way to Europe through the Greeks. The Chinese developed waterproof umbrellas for rain protection. Sunglasses and photochromic contact lenses and intraocular lenses provide eye protection; however, these have proved dangerous in the sudden dark of bridges and tunnels [22]. As already mentioned, prehistoric circumboreal inhabitants have carved slits in bones and antlers to develop snow goggles to prevent photokeratitis. Photoprotective glass can be found on vehicles and on industrial and residential windows. Nanomaterials are making inroads in modifying the fabric of umbrellas and the photoprotective properties of lenses and building materials for consumer use.

19.3.1.1 Traditional Cotton

Studies of fabrics have shown that the sun protective factor (UPF) attributable to clothing is directly proportional to the structure of the fabric and the tightness of the weave in the fabric [12]. UPF numbers consistently increase after repeated washing of cotton garments because of shrinkage and reduction in fabric aperture diameter. For example, for pure cotton T-shirts, UPF increased from a baseline of 19–40.6 after weekly washing for 10 weeks. After repeated washing, fabric shrinkage, and knit hole size reduction, fabric hole area decreased from 8 to 3.9 %. Simple advice for increasing the sun protective properties of clothing is to wear only after repeated washing. Darker fabrics may also confer slightly greater photoprotection.

19.3.1.2 Electrospun Fibers

Modification of the fiber with nanomaterials may further enhance photoprotective properties. Magnesium L-ascorbic acid 2-phosphate (MAAP) and α-tocopherol acetate (α-TAC) are stable derivatives of vitamin C and E. In one study, using the coaxial electrospinning technique, polyacrylonitrile nanofibers were coupled with magnesium ascorbic acid phosphate and tocopherol acetate. Core-shell blended nanofibers showed stable release and retention of their contents over 6 h. These fibers have the potential for incorporation into textiles or sprays for long-lasting topical application [13].

19.3.1.3 Optical Fabrics

Incorporation of light conducting nanofibers into woven material is the basis for nanofibers using distributed optics [14–18]. Distributed optics can be used for conduction and redirection of light of a desired wavelength. Distributed optical fabrics may be used for biomedical monitoring of the wearer. They may be used to camouflage the wearer. They may be used for delivery of phototherapy to the wearer's skin. They may also prove useful for photoprotection using optical interference.

19.3.1.4 Radioprotective Fabrics

Rubberlike fabrics containing ultrafine powders of heavy atoms in a polyurethane, polyvinylchloride matrix have been studied for scattering X-rays and gamma rays [19]. These fabrics may be useful for radiation protection in the military and in medicine. Medical uses could include protection of health care workers working with radioactive materials and devices, as well as demarcating fields of the skin for protection from radiotherapy [20].

In one Canadian study, Pb-free shielding materials containing barium, bismuth, and gadolinium were compared in fabrics of single layers, bilayers, and in cream formulations [21]. The ability of bismuth containing shielding materials to attenuate radiation in the 60–130 kV range compared favorably to Pb-based compounds. The benefit of bismuth fabric is lighter weight.

19.3.2 Liposome

19.3.2.1 Definition

These are micro- and nanoparticulate vesicles with lipid bilayers consisting of charged ionic phospholipids and cholesterol. The amphipathic phospholipids typically consist of a polar head bound by phosphate and glycerol to two fatty acids with chains of 10–24 carbon atoms and 0–6 double bonds. Cholesterol is interspersed in this lipid bilayer. Liposomes can be small (20–100 nm) or up to 1000 nm. They can be unilamellar, oligolamellar, and multilamellar.

19.3.2.2 Background

Liposomal nanoparticulate sunscreens have been investigated for their durability in the presence of plain water and salt water as well as during profuse perspiration. In one study, four separate preparations of SPF 50, 30, 25, and 15 were applied at the recommended concentration of 2 mg/cm^2 to the skin of 30 healthy adult volunteers with Fitzpatrick skin type II [23]. Study subjects were then exposed to plain water or salt water or made to perspire heavily. For all treated groups, the SPF 25 preparation showed a decreased protection factor 83–91 % of baseline, while the remaining sunscreens maintained a 96 % or higher relative protection compared to baseline. Liposomal formulations of sunscreens offered persistent sun protection after exposure of skin to plain water, salt water, and profuse perspiration in healthy adult volunteers with Fitzpatrick skin type II.

19.3.2.3 Daylong actinica

In a pilot study of 20 patients with cutaneous lupus erythematosus, subjects treated with a very high SPF broad-spectrum nanoformulated liposomal sunscreen (*Daylong actinica*) noted significant protection from radiation with artificial UVA/UVB light [24]. The findings were confirmed histologically on skin biopsy.

19.3.2.4 DNA Repair Enzymes

These are so-called morning-after creams because they are designed to repair damage to cells after maximal threshold ultraviolet light exposure. One drawback to these types of agents is that—by giving users an exaggerated sense of confidence—they may promote, rather than prevent, excessive sun exposure.

Photolyase

Polymorphic light eruption is a common photodermatosis which may be due to a combination of aberrant UV-induced immunosuppression and augmented immune reactivity to haptens converted into antigens under the influence of UV light. In a small randomized double-blind placebo-controlled trial, the protective effects of a DNA repair enzyme containing topical lotion (containing photolyase from *Anacystis nidulans* and *Micrococcus luteus*) were compared to placebo and SPF 30 sunscreen after exposure to ultraviolet light in subjects prone to polymorphic light eruption [25]. These "after-exposure" topical studies demonstrated reduced polymorphic light eruption symptoms and scores in patients treated with the repair enzymes. These studies suggest that liposomal preparations containing DNA repair enzymes may prevent or blunt the effects of UV light on PLE.

T4 Endonuclease

Liposomes containing T4 endonuclease V or the heat-inactivated version of the enzyme have been shown to reduce the incidence of basal cell carcinoma by 30 % and actinic keratosis by 68 % in small studies of patients with xeroderma pigmentosum [26]. In more recent studies, liposomal formulations were placed on the skin of human subjects with a prior history of skin cancer 2, 4, and 5 h after exposure to ultraviolet light [27]. Skin biopsies were taken and confirmed the presence of the enzyme in the tissue of treated subjects. Histology did not show significant changes in the UV-induced erythema response or microscopic sunburn cell formation. However there was nearly complete attenuation of IL − 10 and TNF − α mRNA and protein production.

T4N5 liposome containing lotions have been shown to reduce UV-induced DNA damage in the skin of patients with xeroderma pigmentosum. The heat-inactivated enzyme is highly stable, can refold, and can recover enzymatic activity. Because these DNA repair liposomes can eliminate damaged DNA within a few hours of treatment, they may prove useful for combating the effects of ultraviolet light-induced damage to the skin.

19.3.2.5 Disaccharides

Modification of ocular UV protectors with liposomes has shown some benefit for their use in the skin. Trehalose is a naturally occurring disaccharide which is typically used as a protein stabilizer to reduce ultraviolet light-induced damage to the eye when topically applied to cornea. Liposomal formulations of trehalose were evaluated for their photoprotective effects on human keratinocyte cell lines against L-carnosine, ergothioneine, L-ascorbic acid, and DL-α-tocopherol [28]. The trehalose-laden liposomes showed the greatest protection against the formation of UV-induced cyclobutane pyrimidine dimers, 8-hydroxy 2-deoxy guanosine, and protein carbonylation products.

19.3.2.6 Octyl Methoxycinnamate

Sunscreens made of liposomes encapsulating octyl methoxycinnamate showed superior efficacy and delayed release kinetics compared to non-liposomal formulations [29]. They had a higher sun protection factor, but did not show increased water resistance compared controls.

19.3.2.7 Lipoic Acid

Liposomes containing magnesium ascorbyl phosphate, α-lipoic acid, and kinetin were tested for photoprotection in UV-irradiated hairless mice [30]. On mouse skin, daily application for 4 weeks resulted in reduced transepidermal water loss and sustained skin hydration and viscoelasticity. Free radical scavenging activity and UV-induced damage protection were noted in mice. The viscoelastic and hydration properties of the skin were found to be similar after 4 weeks of application on human skin.

19.3.2.8 Resveratrol

Resveratrol is a botanical polyphenol with antioxidant and free radical scavenging properties. Oligolamellar liposomes of a varicty of compositions were loaded with resveratrol and evaluated for their properties and stability over 60 days [31]. In tests of photoprotection after UVB irradiation, HEK 293 cell lines were tested for viability in the presence of free or encapsulated resveratrol. Free resveratrol was less toxic and more UV protective then its free counterpart.

19.3.2.9 CDBA

CDBA, 4-cholesterocarbonyl-4′-(N,N′-diethylaminobutyloxy) azobenzene, is an azobenzene compound which has shown enhanced UVA and UVB photoprotection and stability in nanoliposomal formulations [32].

19.3.3 Elastic Liposome

A subset of liposomes are the deformable variety known as elastic liposomes. These are able to interdigitate between keratinocytes in the stratum corneum and epidermis to allow for better penetration persistence and distribution upon topical application. Elastic liposomes loaded with benzophenone-3 in the 100 nm size range at a concentration of 20.34 % (M/M) showed significant protective effects against ultraviolet radiation [33].

19.3.4 *Niosome*

19.3.4.1 Definition

Niosomes are vesicle carriers with an aqueous core surrounded by one or more layers of phospholipids, typically cholesterol and one or more nonionic surfactants such as alkyl ethers, alkyl esters, alkyl amides, long chain fatty acids, and amino acids. Thus, the surfaces of niosomes are *nonionic surface active agents*, from which the name is derived. They range in size from 100 to 200 nm. Niosomes tend to be made from biocompatible and biodegradable agents. They tend to be nontoxic and non-immunogenic. They are stable and highly resistant to hydrolytic degradation. They are amphiphilic and can accommodate contents of a wide range of solubilities. Niosomes are difficult and complex to formulate and may suffer from aggregation, leaching, or dispersion, which can limit shelf life.

19.3.4.2 Background

Niosomes tend to have greater penetration capability than standard emulsions and are typically more stable than standard liposomes. Thin film hydration is a common manufacturing technique and has been used to make niosomes containing minoxidil. Niosomes and liposomes containing avobenzone and arbutin are under development to create sunscreens which have added pigment-reduction capacity [34].

19.3.4.3 Polyphenols

Polyphenols from black tea extract have been packaged in multilamellar niosomes [35]. These were applied topically onto the skin of nude mice and shown to have enhanced penetration of caffeine and gallic acid than comparable controls dispersed in aqueous solutions. Black tea extract may be useful in the future as a topical sunscreen when delivered in a niosome vehicle.

19.3.5 *Ethosome*

19.3.5.1 Definition

Ethosomes have been developed as transdermal drug delivery systems. They are a type of soft vesicle composed of phospholipids (such as phosphatidylcholine, phosphatidylserine, and phosphatidic acid) in a high concentration of *ethanol* (20–50 %) and *water* (from which they derive their name). Ethanol acts as a permeation enhancer, and its content can be varied to accommodate a broad range of active ingredients. Ethosome size can be controlled from the nm to sub-mm range. Ethosomes are non-toxic and can be formulated in creams, lotions, gels, and patches. Ethosomes can be formulated for pilosebaceous targeting (minoxidil), transdermal hormone delivery (testosterone), and transdermal drug delivery (i.e., trihexyphenidyl hydrochloride for Parkinson disease, zidovudine for HIV, acyclovir for HSV, cyclosporine for psoriasis, bacitracin for reduced toxicity, and cannabidiol for inflammation and edema).

19.3.5.2 Background

Ethosomes tend to be associated with enhanced drug penetration. They may therefore have greater utility in photoprotection at the dermal level, such as delivery of antioxidants, or repair enzymes.

19.3.5.3 Cucurma Longa

Turmeric extract from *Cucurma longa* was formulated in liposomes, ethosomes, and transferosomes [36]. Alcoholic extracts prepared and ratios of 0.5–2 % W/W were evaluated for their interaction with the skin. Entrapment efficiency was the highest with transferosomes, in between with ethosomes, and least with liposomes. This study suggested that nano-vesicles are maybe useful vehicles for optimal delivery of turmeric extracts to the skin for their antioxidant, astringent, antimicrobial, and moisturizing properties.

19.3.5.4 Apigenin

Apigenin is a bioflavonoid which has been shown to have antioxidant activity and a number of cellular targets involving GTPase activation, membrane transport, and mRNA metabolism/alternative splicing [37]. It has been studied as a potential topical and systemic anti-inflammatory and antitumor agent. In one trial, optimization studies were conducted to determine ideal formulations for delivery of apigenin to the skin. Comparisons were made of ethosomes, liposomes, and elastic liposomes. It was found that increasing phospholipid content in ethosomes (especially Lipoid S75), propylene glycol content, and ethanol content enhanced skin deposition and transdermal delivery. Optimized ethosomes showed the greatest reduction of cyclooxygenase-2 levels in mouse skin after exposure to UVB light.

19.3.6 Solid Lipid Nanoparticle

19.3.6.1 Background

These are colloidal vehicles comprised of solid lipid cores mixed in defined ratios with water or an aqueous surfactant. The lipids tend to be biocompatible, biodegradable, and nontoxic, making them ideal for cosmetics and cosmeceutical preparations. Because of their small size, they pack tightly, have high occlusivity, promote skin hydration, and limit transepidermal water loss. They are relatively easy to manufacture, easy to scale up, and easy to sterilize, and don't require special solvents. Some solid lipid nanoparticles, for example, crystalline cetylpalmitate nanoparticles (CCP-NP), have inherent photoprotective activity [38]. Native CCP-NP have about 2–3-fold greater UV-absorbing properties compared to traditional emulsions. This effect has been shown to give synergistic and additive photoprotective effects to sunscreen contents. For example, CCP-NP containing 2-hydroxy-4-methoxybenzophenone (Eusolex 4360) were threefold more photoprotective compared to reference emulsions.

19.3.6.2 Definition

Solid lipid nanoparticles are designed to disperse and solubilize lipophilic compounds in their cores. Lipids found in solid lipid nanoparticles can be mono-, di-, and triglycerides, cholesterol, and waxes. These can be stabilized by emulsifiers such as amphiphilic surfactants.

19.3.6.3 Benzophenone-3

Solid lipid nano- and microparticles prepared by the solvent-free spray-congealing technique have been tested for durability of photoprotection and percutaneous absorption [39]. Solid lipid nanoparticles of benzophenone-3 have also been created by hot high-pressure homogenization and shown to be more stable and less cytotoxic and phototoxic than nanopolymer [poly(ε-caprolactone)] encapsulated benzophenone-3.

19.3.6.4 Zinc Oxide and Octocrylene

In order to broaden the spectrum of photoprotection, combination agents are sometimes indicated. Solid lipid nanoparticles can accommodate the formulation of two otherwise immiscible ingredients. In one study, crystalline solid lipid nanoparticles containing water-soluble zinc oxide and lipophilic octocrylene were shown to be stable, photoprotective in the 290–400 nm bandwidth, and shown to have synergistic protection with the nanoparticle's endogenous UV-blocking properties. The synergy allowed for reducing the concentration of active ingredients to 0.6 %.

19.3.6.5 Lutein

Lutein has antioxidant and blue light-blocking properties. Because of its poor solubility, it is an ideal candidate for lipid nanoparticle delivery to the skin. In one study, lutein was incorporated into nanocarriers such as nanoemulsions (NE), solid lipid nanoparticles (SLN), and nanostructured lipid carriers (NLC) using high-pressure homogenization [41]. All three were found to be stable. The SLN had the lowest release (0.4 %) of content after 24 h, compared to NE which had the highest release (19.5 %). None of the lutein in SLN permeated pig skin after 24 h. Only a small fraction (0.06 %) of the lutein was degraded after exposure to 10 MED, compared to 6–8 % in the NLC, 14 % in the NE, and 50 % for lutein powder suspended in corn oil.

19.3.6.6 Tocopherol

Synthetic solid lipid nanoparticles were shown in one study to have inherent UV protective activity. This effect was synergistically augmented with the incorporation of tocopherol acetate. Solid lipid nanoparticles containing tocopherol were twice as effective at UV blockade than reference emulsions containing identical lipid content [5, 40, 42, 45].

19.3.6.7 Titanium

SLN prepared using conventional and hybrid methodologies were able to enhance the photoprotectivity of titanium dioxide compared to reference emulsions [43]. They were also able to allow lower concentrations of titanium dioxide for equivalent photoprotection.

19.3.6.8 Chitin

Chitin is poorly soluble in most aqueous formulations and emulsions. Preparations of SLN containing 3,4,5-trimethoxybenzoylchitin were shown to act as effective sunscreens [44]. The effect was synergistic with the endogenous UV-blocking activity of the SLN and could be augmented with the incorporation of tocopherol.

19.3.7 Nanostructured Lipid Carrier

19.3.7.1 Background

These are second-generation solid lipid nanoparticles. The core of nanostructured lipid carriers is a blended mixture of solid lipid and liquid lipid as a hybrid carrier. The solid lipid is a long chain fatty acid, and the liquid lipid is a short chain fatty acid. The ratios of the blends are 70:30 (long/short) to 99.9:0.01 (long/short). Nanostructured lipid carriers are used to overcome unfavorable solid lipid nanoparticle tendencies such as particle growth, unpredictable gelation, poor drug/active ingredient loading, and drug/active expulsion during storage. Typical solid lipids used include bees wax, carnauba wax, Dynasan, precifac, stearic acid, apifil, and Cutina CP. Typical liquid lipids include Cetiol V, Miglyol, castor oil, oleic acid, davana oil, palm oil, and olive oil. Sometimes emulsifiers are added to optimize the blend. These can include Miranol Ultra, PlantaCare, Tween 80, Pluronic F68, Poloxamer 188, and Phospholipon 90G. In dermatology, nanostructure lipid carrier preparations have been used for sunscreens and topical drugs (minoxidil, tacrolimus, miconazole nitrate).

19.3.7.2 Definition

Solid lipid nanoparticles typically have a crystalline matrix with little room for active ingredients. This often leads to drug expulsion out of the particles over time and a rapid drop-off in efficacy. Nanostructured lipid carriers are a hybrid of a solid lipid surrounding a liquid lipid drug carrier space. This leads to enhanced drug loading and stable storage.

19.3.7.3 Tocopherol

Tocopherol has more potent antioxidant activity than its conjugate tocopherol acetate; however, it is viscous, poorly soluble, and photo-unstable and can cause irritant dermatitis. In one small study, the high-pressure homogenization technique was used to create nanostructured lipid carriers and nanoemulsions of tocopherol. Particle sizes of 67 nm NLC and 586 ± 210 nm NE were formed. About 30 % tocopherol was released from the NLC within 2 h, while only 4 % was released from the NE. Both formulations were shown to retain antioxidant activity, to be non-irritating, and to protect tocopherol from UV degradation.

19.3.7.4 Chemical Sunscreens

Ethylhexyl triazone (EHT), diethylamino hydroxybenzoyl hexyl benzoate (DHHB), Bemotrizinol (Tinosorb S), octyl methoxycinnamate (OMC), and avobenzone (AVO) are chemical sunscreens which offer a broad spectrum of photoprotection into the UVA range [46]. These agents differ in their solubility, spectrum of activity, and stability. They were incorporated into nanostructured lipid carriers and nanoemulsions formulated to optimize topical application and their properties evaluated. When these agents were incorporated into nanostructured lipid carriers, their permeability into the skin was dramatically reduced, and they remained on the stratum corneum. OMC and AVO were not as photo-stable as predicted, while the remaining compounds retained their photostability. No significant difference was seen in the photoprotection between nanoemulsions and nanostructured lipid carriers.

19.3.7.5 Wax Carriers

Formulations composed of three molecules (ethylhexyl triazone, bis-ethylhexyloxyphenol methoxyphenyl triazine, and ethylhexyl methoxycinnamate) in a carnauba wax nanostructured lipid carrier and beeswax nanostructured lipid carrier were synthesized in one study using hot high-pressure homogenization [47]. Particle sizes were 200 nm. The carnauba wax preparations had 45 % higher SPF values compared to beeswax nanostructured lipid carriers, showing that the photo-protective effects of the nanostructured lipid carrier depended as much on their lipid composition as on their structure.

19.3.7.6 Ethylhexyl Methoxycinnamate

Ethylhexyl methoxycinnamate (EMC) is typically used as a UVB blocker; however, it is poorly soluble and photolabile. Micro- and nanoparticles in one study were made from rice bran wax, ozokerite, and glyceryl behenate and formulated to contain 70 % EMC by lipid mass [48]. Nanoparticles were found to have twice the absorbance of light at 310 nm compared to the microparticles, regardless of composition. Native EMC lost 30 % of its efficacy after 2 h of UV exposure, compared to 10–21 % loss for the NLC formulations. No significant penetration of EMC was shown for the NLC preparations.

19.3.7.7 Lycopene

Nanostructured lipid carriers composed of biocompatible lipids from rice oil and cholesterol were manufactured to be loaded with lycopene. Particle sizes of nanostructured lipid carriers ranged from 287 to 405 nm. Cholesterol was found to reduce stability of particles and its exclusion as well as storage at 4 °C or room temperature led to the greatest stability [49, 50].

19.3.8 Microsphere

These are powders consisting of natural materials or biodegradable polymers. Natural materials can include proteins (albumin, gelatin, collagen) or carbohydrates (starch agarose, carrageenan, chitosan). Polymers can include PMMA, epoxy polymers, lactides, glycolides, block copolymers, polyalkyl cyanoacrylates, and polyanhydrides. Particle sizes tend to be less than 200 μm. Microspheres can be microcapsules, with active ingredients in the interior, or micromatrices, where the active ingredient is dispersed evenly throughout the particle.

The UV filter 4-methylbenzylidene camphor (4-MBC), while offering excellent photoprotection, suffers from photo-instability, rapid drop-off in efficacy, undesirable percutaneous absorption, and potential effects on the thyroid gland. Microspheres containing 4-MBC formulated in oil/water emulsions have been demonstrated to have the same photoprotective activity as native 4-BMC preparations, but with longer duration of activity and slower release from emulsions [51].

19.3.9 Gold

Gold metal particles are emerging it has excellent candidates for nanomaterials with biologic uses. Gold nanoparticles are biocompatible, easy to synthesize, and easy to conjugate with a number of other compounds. They have been used for cancer diagnosis and therapy, drug delivery, and as biologic probes. Phytolatex synthesized gold nanoparticles have been shown to enhance the sun protection factor of sunscreen when added to native sunscreen at 2–4 % concentrations [52].

19.4 Safety

19.4.1 Hazards of Traditional Sunscreens

19.4.1.1 Dermatitis

Contact dermatitis from topical and cosmetic agents accounts for up to 4 % of dermatology visits, and more than half of these are due to allergic contact dermatitis [53, 54]. Irritant and allergic contact dermatitis and photo-contact dermatitis need to be considered when dispensing sunscreen. Contact dermatitis studies in children have shown that more than 6 % are photoallergic to traditional UV filters or vehicles. The most common allergies are to benzophenone-3, octyl methoxycinnamate, and *para*-aminobenzoic acid.

19.4.1.2 Absorption

A number of sunscreen ingredients have been detectable in the plasma following topical administration [55]. These are largely organic compounds such as benzophenone, octyl methoxycinnamate, and 4-MBC. Nanoparticulate and microsphere versions of these compounds have a reduced tendency to be absorbed and can be used in lower concentrations for the same degree of photoprotection.

19.4.1.3 Endocrine Disruption

It is generally recommended that oxybenzone and octocrylene be avoided in children [56–58]. Vitamin D deficiencies can occur from application of sunscreen, but these are more likely when 2 mg/m^2 are applied, which is the recommended dose. Applications of 1.5 mg/m^2, which are more in the range of typical applications in most subjects, do not significantly inhibit production of vitamin D_3.

19.4.1.4 Instability

Sunscreen ingredients can degrade upon UV exposure, chlorinated water exposure, oxidation, or exposure to high temperatures [59]. Nanoparticulate formulations of sunscreens tend to be more stable to heat, light, and reactive oxygen species.

19.4.1.5 Narrow Spectrum of Activity

Individual components of sunscreen typically have narrow ranges of protection in either the UVB or UVA portion of the electromagnetic spectrum. Broad-spectrum sunscreens require mixtures of two or more ingredients to achieve adequate photoprotection. Nanoformulations of metallic physical blockers can offer broad protection blockage with a single ingredient.

19.4.1.6 Lack of Compliance Due to Formulation

Traditional organic sunscreen components are lipophilic and require an oil-based vehicle for dissolution. These formulations can have a greasy feel, can be comedogenic, and can be difficult, especially for male patients, to adopt on a regular basis. One reason for the higher incidence of skin cancer in men, particularly over the age of 50, may be the lack of regular sunscreen use, possibly due to formulations which do not appeal to this segment of the population [60].

19.4.2 Benefits of Nanoformulations

19.4.2.1 Less Ingredient Required

Because of their greater efficacy, their high surface-to-volume ratio, their high occlusivity, and their controlled stability, nanoformulations of sunscreens tend to require lower total concentrations of active ingredient (organic or inorganic) than their traditional counterparts. This can lead to lower manufacturing costs and potentially lower overall exposure to chemical agents. Some studies have shown that high concentrations of physical blockers can cause perioral dermatitis [61].

19.4.2.2 Detoxification

Concern about hazards associated with metallic nanoparticles stems from in vitro studies showing the generation of free radicals. Some studies showed that the level of clastogenicity increased upon UV exposure. However, comparisons of zinc oxide nanoparticles to known photoclastogens such as 8-MOP [62] showed substantially minimal effects (2–4× increase in vitro for zinc oxide, and >15,000× increase for 8-MOP). The Ames test showed no increased mutagenicity for zinc oxide. Human studies have shown no evidence of phototoxicity. Commercial nanoparticulate sunscreens have been coated to detoxify them. Coating of nanometallic sunscreens with inert oxides of silica has been shown to eliminate the risk of reactive oxygen species generation. Furthermore, aggregation of nanoparticles reduces their surface-to-volume ratio and reactivity. A number of studies have now shown very little to no dermal penetration of metallic sunscreen nanoparticles following application to the skin. This includes studies of intact, flexed, and stripped skin. Minimal penetration has been noted on abraded skin. One study of hairless mice showed slight differences in absorption of nanoparticulate zinc when compared to larger particle size zinc, but no toxicity and no effect on zinc homeostasis [63–65]. Furthermore, permeability comparisons demonstrate that pig and rat skin are 4- and 9–11-fold more permeable than human skin. Most of the recent studies show minimal or no absorption.

19.4.2.3 Vehicle Flexibility

Because nanoformulation allows for the precise selection of particle size, shape, charge, and chemical composition, nanophotoprotective agents can be manufactured in a wide variety of formats and vehicles to allow for optimal stability, UV protection, composition, and texture to permit the widest possible range of adoption and compliance.

19.5 Compliance

19.5.1 Cosmetic Elegance

One of the greatest hurdles to sunscreen uses compliance. Optimal application requires at least 2 mg/cm^2 be applied evenly and smoothly across the intended surface with frequent reapplication to account for rubbing, perspiration, and immersion-related loss. In one study of vacationers interviewed at an airport on their way to and returning from a vacation, many were found to have the misconception that tanning prior to departure for a tropical vacation would lead to sunburn, and nearly 44 % were found to be sunburned upon return [66]. Furthermore, while many travelers understood the need to use sunscreen, many did not factor the use of protective clothing, hats, and eyewear into their vacation plans. Studies have shown that patients are more likely to comply with sunscreen use when using an emollient of their choice. Typically, patients tend to prefer less greasy vehicles to greasier ones. This is a realm in which nanoformulation enjoys a distinct advantage.

19.5.2 Viscous Fingering

Studies have shown that patient education on application technique is important in improving the efficacy of sunscreen. A well-studied problem in the application of sunscreen is known as viscous fingering. This is the formation of stripes and grooves along the pattern of fingers use to apply sunscreen. This nonuniform but widely practiced application method leads to reduced efficacy. A technique of application developed in France in which subjects dose sunscreen, apply it, and then spread it was shown to be readily adopted and understood by subjects and to result in more evenly applied sunscreen and a greater quantities, more in line with what is considered adequate. Some researchers have suggested regulations for the education material associated with sunscreens in order to assure proper application technique [67].

References

1. Zahn S, Graef M, Patsinakidis N, Landmann A, Surber C, Wenzel J, Kuhn A (2014) Ultraviolet light protection by a sunscreen prevents interferon-driven skin inflammation in cutaneous lupus erythematosus. Exp Dermatol 23(7):516–518
2. Chiarelli-Neto O, Ferreira AS, Martins WK, Pavani C, Severino D, Faião-Flores F, Maria-Engler SS, Aliprandini E, Martinez GR, Di Mascio P, Medeiros MH, Baptista MS (2014) Melanin photosensitization and the effect of visible light on epithelial cells. PLoS One 9(11):e113266
3. Alexiades-Armenakas M (2011) Aging facial skin: infrared broad band light technologies. Facial Plast Surg Clin North Am 19(2):361–370
4. Chang AL, Bitter PH Jr, Qu K, Lin M, Rapicavoli NA, Chang HY (2013) Rejuvenation of gene expression pattern of aged human skin by broadband light treatment: a pilot study. J Invest Dermatol 133(2):394–402
5. Vandelinder V, Bachand GD (2014) Photodamage and the importance of photoprotection in biomolecular-powered device applications. Anal Chem 86(1):721–728
6. Parisi AV, Turnbull DJ, Downs N, Smith D (2012) Dosimetric investigation of the solar erythemal UV radiation protection provided by beards and moustaches. Radiat Prot Dosimetry 150(3):278–282

7. Jablonski NG, Chaplin G (2014) The evolution of skin pigmentation and hair texture in people of African ancestry. Dermatol Clin 32(2):113–121
8. Jablonski NG, Chaplin G (2010) Colloquium paper: human skin pigmentation as an adaptation to UV radiation. Proc Natl Acad Sci U S A 107(Suppl 2):8962–8968
9. Shaath NA (2010) Ultraviolet filters. Photochem Photobiol Sci 9(4):464–469
10. Dlova NC, Nevondo FT, Mwangi EM, Summers B, Tsoka-Gwegweni J, Martincigh BS, Mulholland DA (2013) Chemical analysis and in vitro UV-protection characteristics of clays traditionally used for sun protection in South Africa. Photodermatol Photoimmunol Photomed 29(3):164–169
11. Schuch AP, Moraes MC, Yagura T, Menck CF (2014) Highly sensitive biological assay for determining the photoprotective efficacy of sunscreen. Environ Sci Technol 48(19):11584–11590
12. Wang SQ, Kopf AW, Marx J, Bogdan A, Polsky D, Bart RS (2001) Reduction of ultraviolet transmission through cotton T-shirt fabrics with low ultraviolet protection by various laundering methods and dyeing: clinical implications. J Am Acad Dermatol 44(5):767–774
13. Wu XM, Branford-White CJ, Yu DG, Chatterton NP, Zhu LM (2011) Preparation of core-shell PAN nanofibers encapsulated α-tocopherol acetate and ascorbic acid 2-phosphate for photoprotection. Colloids Surf B Biointerfaces 82(1):247–252
14. D'Angelo LT, Weber S, Honda Y, Thiel T, Narbonneau F, Luth TC (2008) System for respiratory motion detection using optical fibers embedded into textiles. Conf Proc IEEE Engl Med Biol Soc 2008:3694–3697
15. De Jonckheere J, Narbonneau F, Kinet D et al (2008) Optical fibre sensors embedded into technical textile for a continuous monitoring of patients under magnetic resonance imaging. Conf Proc IEEE Engl Med Biol Soc 2008:5266–5269
16. Eden JG, Park S-J, Ostrom NP, Chen K-F (2005) Recent advances in microcavity plasma devices and arrays: a versatile photonic platform. J Phys D Appl Phys 38:1644–1648
17. Sorin F et al (2009) Exploiting the collective effects of optoelectronic devices integrated into a single fiber. Nano Lett 9:2630–2635
18. Sorin F et al (2007) Multimaterial photodetecting fibers: a geometric and structural study. Adv Mater 19:3872–3877
19. Ashley S (2003) X-ray proofing. To save himself, a physician enters the rag trade. Sci Am 288(5):34–35
20. Jones MA, Cocker M, Khiani R, Foley P, Qureshi N, Wong KC, Rajappan K, Betts TR (2014) The benefits of using a bismuth-containing, radiation-absorbing drape in cardiac resynchronization implant procedures. Pacing Clin Electrophysiol 37(7):828–833
21. McCaffrey JP, Tessier F, Shen H (2012) Radiation shielding materials and radiation scatter effects for interventional radiology (IR) physicians. Med Phys 39(7):4537–4546
22. Allen MJ (1979) Highway tests of photochromic lenses. J Am Optom Assoc 50(9):1023–1027
23. Korting HC, Schöllmann C (2011) Resistance of liposomal sunscreen formulations against plain water as well as salt water exposure and perspiration. Skin Pharmacol Physiol 24(1):36–43
24. Patsinakidis N, Wenzel J, Landmann A, Koch R, Gerß J, Luger TA, Metze D, Surber C, Kuhn A (2012) Suppression of UV-induced damage by a liposomal sunscreen: a prospective, open-label study in patients with cutaneous lupus erythematosus and healthy controls. Exp Dermatol 21(12):958–961
25. Hofer A, Legat FJ, Gruber-Wackernagel A, Quehenberger F, Wolf P (2011) Topical liposomal DNA-repair enzymes in polymorphic light eruption. Photochem Photobiol Sci 10(7):1118–1128
26. Zahid S, Brownell I (2008) Repairing DNA damage in xeroderma pigmentosum: T4N5 lotion and gene therapy. J Drugs Dermatol 7(4):405–408
27. Wolf P, Maier H, Müllegger RR, Chadwick CA, Hofmann-Wellenhof R, Soyer HP, Hofer A, Smolle J, Horn M, Cerroni L, Yarosh D, Klein J, Bucana C, Dunner K Jr, Potten CS, Hönigsmann H, Kerl H, Kripke ML (2000) Topical treatment with liposomes containing T4

endonuclease V protects human skin in vivo from ultraviolet-induced upregulation of interleukin-10 and tumor necrosis factor-alpha. J Invest Dermatol 114(1):149–156
28. Emanuele E, Bertona M, Sanchis-Gomar F, Pareja-Galeano H, Lucia A (2014) Protective effect of trehalose-loaded liposomes against UVB-induced photodamage in human keratinocytes. Biomed Rep 2(5):755–759
29. Mota Ade C, de Freitas ZM, Ricci Júnior E, Dellamora-Ortiz GM, Santos-Oliveira R, Ozzetti RA, Vergnanini AL, Ribeiro VL, Silva RS, dos Santos EP (2013) In vivo and in vitro evaluation of octyl methoxycinnamate liposomes. Int J Nanomedicine 8:4689–4701
30. Campos PM, de Camargo Júnior FB, de Andrade JP, Gaspar LR (2012) Efficacy of cosmetic formulations containing dispersion of liposome with magnesium ascorbyl phosphate, alpha-lipoic acid and kinetin. Photochem Photobiol 88(3):748–752
31. Caddeo C, Teskac K, Sinico C, Kristl J (2008) Effect of resveratrol incorporated in liposomes on proliferation and UV-B protection of cells. Int J Pharm 363(1–2):183–191
32. Xu Q, Geng S, Dai Y, Qin G, Wang JY (2013) CDBA-liposome as an effective sunscreen with longer UV protection and longer shelf life. J Photochem Photobiol B 129:78–86
33. Severino P, Moraes LF, Zanchetta B, Souto EB, Santana MH (2012) Elastic liposomes containing benzophenone-3 for sun protection factor enhancement. Pharm Dev Technol 17(6):661–665
34. Liu JJ, Nazzal S, Chang TS, Tsai T (2013) Preparation and characterization of cosmeceutical liposomes loaded with avobenzone and arbutin. J Cosmet Sci 64(1):9–17
35. Yeh MI, Huang HC, Liaw JH, Huang MC, Huang KF, Hsu FL (2013) Dermal delivery by niosomes of black tea extract as a sunscreen agent. Int J Dermatol 52(2):239–245
36. Kaur CD, Saraf S (2011) Topical vesicular formulations of Curcuma longa extract on recuperating the ultraviolet radiation-damaged skin. J Cosmet Dermatol 10(4):260–265
37. Shen LN, Zhang YT, Wang Q, Xu L, Feng NP (2014) Enhanced in vitro and in vivo skin deposition of apigenin delivered using ethosomes. Int J Pharm 460(1-2):280–288
38. Wissing SA, Müller RH (2001) Solid lipid nanoparticles (SLN)--a novel carrier for UV blockers. Pharmazie 56(10):783–786
39. Martins RM, Siqueira S, Fonseca MJ, Freitas LA (2014) Skin penetration and photoprotection of topical formulations containing benzophenone-3 solid lipid microparticles prepared by the solvent-free spray-congealing technique. J Microencapsul 31(7):644–653
40. Berkman MS, Yazan Y (2012) Solid lipid nanoparticles: a possible vehicle for zinc oxide and octocrylene. Pharmazie 67(3):202–208
41. Mitri K, Shegokar R, Gohla S, Anselmi C, Müller RH (2011) Lipid nanocarriers for dermal delivery of lutein: preparation, characterization, stability and performance. Int J Pharm 414(1-2):267–275
42. Wissing SA, Müller RH (2001) A novel sunscreen system based on tocopherol acetate incorporated into solid lipid nanoparticles. Int J Cosmet Sci 23(4):233–243
43. Cengiz E, Wissing SA, Müller RH, Yazan Y (2006) Sunblocking efficiency of various TiO(2)-loaded solid lipid nanoparticle formulations(1). Int J Cosmet Sci 28(5):371–378
44. Song C, Liu S (2005) A new healthy sunscreen system for human: solid lipid nanoparticles as carrier for 3,4,5-trimethoxybenzoylchitin and the improvement by adding Vitamin E. Int J Biol Macromol 36(1-2):116–119
45. Abla MJ, Banga AK (2014) Formulation of tocopherol nanocarriers and in vitro delivery into human skin. Int J Cosmet Sci 36(3):239–246
46. Puglia C, Damiani E, Offerta A, Rizza L, Tirendi GG, Tarico MS, Curreri S, Bonina F, Perrotta RE (2014) Evaluation of nanostructured lipid carriers (NLC) and nanoemulsions as carriers for UV-filters: characterization, in vitro penetration and photostability studies. Eur J Pharm Sci 51:211–217
47. Nikolić S, Keck CM, Anselmi C, Müller RH (2011) Skin photoprotection improvement: synergistic interaction between lipid nanoparticles and organic UV filters. Int J Pharm 414(1-2):276–284

48. Durand L, Habran N, Henschel V, Amighi K (2010) Encapsulation of ethylhexyl methoxycinnamate, a light-sensitive UV filter, in lipid nanoparticles. J Microencapsul 27(8):714–725
49. Riangjanapatee P, Müller RH, Keck CM, Okonogi S (2013) Development of lycopene-loaded nanostructured lipid carriers: effect of rice oil and cholesterol. Pharmazie 68(9):723–731
50. Okonogi S, Riangjanapatee P (2014) Physicochemical characterization of lycopene-loaded nanostructured lipid carrier formulations for topical administration. Int J Pharm 478(2):726–735
51. Centini M, Miraglia G, Quaranta V, Buonocore A, Anselmi C (2014) Improving photoprotection: 4-methylbenzylidene camphor microspheres. Pharm Dev Technol 22:1–9
52. Borase HP, Patil CD, Salunkhe RB, Suryawanshi RK, Salunke BK, Patil SV (2014) Phytolatex synthesized gold nanoparticles as novel agent to enhance sun protection factor of commercial sunscreens. Int J Cosmet Sci 36(6):571–578
53. de Groot AC, Roberts DW (2014) Contact and photocontact allergy to octocrylene: a review. Contact Dermatitis 70(4):193–204
54. Haylett AK, Chiang YZ, Nie Z, Ling TC, Rhodes LE (2014) Sunscreen photopatch testing: a series of 157 children. Br J Dermatol 171(2):370–375
55. Janjua NR, Kongshoj B, Andersson AM, Wulf HC (2008) Sunscreens in human plasma and urine after repeated whole-body topical application. J Eur Acad Dermatol Venereol 22(4):456–461
56. Gilaberte Y, Carrascosa JM (2014) Sun protection in children: realities and challenges. Actas Dermosifiliogr 105(3):253–262
57. Dewalque L, Pirard C, Charlier C (2014) Measurement of urinary biomarkers of parabens, benzophenone-3, and phthalates in a Belgian population. Biomed Res Int
58. Frederiksen H, Aksglaede L, Sorensen K, Nielsen O, Main KM, Skakkebaek NE, Juul A, Andersson AM (2013) Bisphenol A and other phenols in urine from Danish children and adolescents analyzed by isotope diluted TurboFlow-LC-MS/MS. Int J Hyg Environ Health 216(6):710–720
59. Crista DM, Miranda MS, Esteves da Silva JC (2015) Degradation in chlorinated water of the UV filter 4-tert-butyl-4′-methoxydibenzoylmethane present in commercial sunscreens. Environ Technol 36(9–12):1319–1326
60. Buller DB, Andersen PA, Walkosz BJ, Scott MD, Maloy JA, Dignan MB, Cutter GR (2012) Compliance with sunscreen advice in a survey of adults engaged in outdoor winter recreation at high-elevation ski areas. J Am Acad Dermatol 66(1):63–70
61. Abeck D, Geisenfelder B, Brandt O (2009) Physical sunscreens with high sun protection factor may cause perioral dermatitis in children. J Dtsch Dermatol Ges 7(8):701–703
62. Dufour EK, Kumaravel T, Nohynek GJ, Kirkland D, Toutain H (2006) Clastogenicity, photo-clastogenicity or pseudo-photo-clastogenicity: genotoxic effects of zinc oxide in the dark, in pre-irradiated or simultaneously irradiated Chinese hamster ovary cells. Mutat Res 607(2):215–224
63. Osmond-McLeod MJ, Oytam Y, Kirby JK, Gomez-Fernandez L, Baxter B, McCall MJ (2014) Dermal absorption and short-term biological impact in hairless mice from sunscreens containing zinc oxide nano- or larger particles. Nanotoxicology 8(Suppl 1):72–84
64. Leite-Silva VR, Le Lamer M, Sanchez WY, Liu DC, Sanchez WH, Morrow I, Martin D, Silva HD, Prow TW, Grice JE, Roberts MS (2013) The effect of formulation on the penetration of coated and uncoated zinc oxide nanoparticles into the viable epidermis of human skin in vivo. Eur J Pharm Biopharm 84(2):297–308
65. Adachi K, Yamada N, Yoshida Y, Yamamoto O (2013) Subchronic exposure of titanium dioxide nanoparticles to hairless rat skin. Exp Dermatol 22(4):278–283
66. Køster B, Thorgaard C, Philip A, Clemmensen IH (2011) Vacations to sunny destinations, sunburn, and intention to tan: a cross-sectional study in Denmark, 2007-2009. Scand J Public Health 39(1):64–69
67. Fujikake K, Tago S, Plasson R, Nakazawa R, Okano K, Maezawa D, Mukawa T, Kuroda A, Asakura K (2014) Problems of in vitro SPF measurements brought about by viscous fingering generated during sunscreen applications. Skin Pharmacol Physiol 27(5):254–262

Chapter 20
The Role of Topical Antioxidants in Photoprotection

Mary S. Matsui

Key Points

- There many reasons for interest in the photoprotective potential of topical antioxidant botanical extracts. These include consumer demand for non-sunscreen photoprotective ingredients, the understanding that longwave (UVA) ultraviolet radiation in particular induces considerable oxidative stress, and an interest in supplementing sunscreen formulations to increase stability and protection while decreasing the use of chemical and physical sunscreens.
- The botanical product most studied for topical photoprotection is derived from *Camellia sinensis*, the tea plant. Topical application of the most potent constituent, EGCG, has been shown to inhibit UV-induced leukocyte infiltration, DNA damage, immune suppression, dermal degradation, and erythema.
- Other botanicals that have been demonstrated to have photoprotective properties include genistein, resveratrol, grape seed proanthocyanidins, *Polypodium leucotomos* (fern) extract, and certain combinations of ferulic acid, vitamin C, and vitamin E.
- Sunscreens formulated with antioxidants/botanical extracts may have additive or synergistic photoprotective effects when compared with either of these agents alone.
- Variables that impact the benefits of botanical extracts or other antioxidants include unknown optimal concentrations, possible interactions between ingredients, and the instability of antioxidants. At present, there is no labeling information requirement for ingredient concentration, and at least one study showed that the levels of antioxidants in some "off the shelf" sunscreen products were below that required for efficacy.

M.S. Matsui, PhD
Executive Director, External Research R&D Basic Science and Technology,
The Estee Lauder Companies, Inc., 125 Pinelawn Rd., Melville, NY 11747, USA
e-mail: mmatsui@estee.com, msm1@columbia.edu

S.Q. Wang, H.W. Lim (eds.), *Principles and Practice of Photoprotection*,
DOI 10.1007/978-3-319-29382-0_20

For several reasons, there is great popular interest in the use of topical antioxidants for skin photoprotection and antiaging therapies. Many consumers, influenced particularly by numerous Internet sources giving nonmedical advice, information, and testimonials, believe that "naturally derived" ingredients, plant extracts, and food components are superior or healthier than "chemical" sunscreens. Other factors contributing to the popularity of these types of alternative products include dissatisfaction with the aesthetic properties of current sunscreen/sunblock products, the perception that the chemicals in OTC products are unhealthy, unsafe, or damage the environment and the belief that natural ingredients provide additional benefits not found in sunscreens. Finally, there is interest in supplementing sunscreen products by manufacturers, as there is some evidence that it is possible to stabilize sunscreens with antioxidants [2]. This chapter will discuss the topical use of antioxidants, primarily but not exclusively in the form of botanical extracts and will review the scientific evidence for their efficacy against the damaging effects of ultraviolet radiation (UVR) on human skin.

Endogenous antioxidants that scavenge for ROS include superoxide dismutase, glutathione peroxidase, ascorbate, alpha-lipoic acid, and catalase. Excessive ROS generated during UV exposure depletes endogenous antioxidants and causes a state of oxidative stress in cells that can damage cellular proteins, lipids, and DNA, trigger apoptosis, and contribute to photocarcinogenesis. A review of endogenous antioxidant strategies and oxidant-induced cellular damage and mechanisms can be found in Khan et al. [22]. Also, in particular, Table 1 and Fig. 1 contained in an earlier review [1] are recommended for a concise summary of botanicals and their mechanisms of action.

Sunscreen/sunblock ingredients protect skin from solar radiation through three basic mechanisms: reflection, dispersion, and absorption (for review, see Schalka and Silva dos Reis [34]). In contrast, antioxidants generally have little to no ability to physically block UVR and act to protect the skin by other mechanisms. The efficacy of sunscreens to protect skin against UVR is virtually universally measured and regulated by specific, in vivo (UVB) and in vitro (UVA) assays such as "sun protection factor" (SPF) which is based on UVR-induced erythema, immediate pigment darkening, and "critical wavelength." Because erythema is primarily driven by direct DNA damage and repair and less by oxidative stress, UVR protection provided by antioxidants is best measured by endpoints other than SPF. In addition, it should be noted that significant damage, including DNA mutations, immune suppression, and collagen breakdown can occur in the absence of sunburn.

There is some epidemiological evidence that higher dietary or systemic levels of antioxidants are associated with a lower risk of nonmelanoma skin cancers and photoaging signs in humans [3, 7, 15, 33], and there are animal/rodent studies showing this efficacy for oral supplementation of antioxidants. There is extensive experimental evidence that exogenous antioxidants are anti-inflammatory and suppress oxidative stress pathways in in vitro cell culture and that topical antioxidants are photoprotective in acute and chronic animal models of UVR-induced skin damage. Reviews of these data can be found in Afaq and Mukhtar [1], Khan et al. [22], and Passantino et al. [32]. This chapter will focus on the most recent data

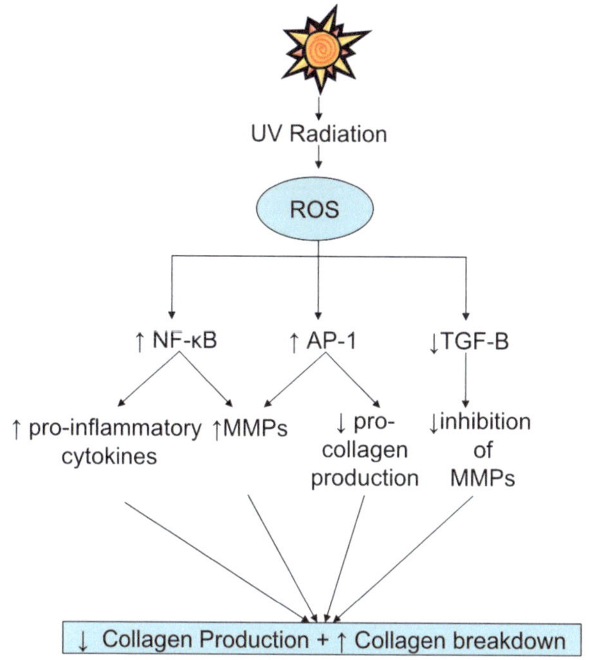

Fig. 20.1 UV radiation initiates production of reactive oxygen species (*ROS*), which is followed acutely by secondary messengers and increased expression of proinflammatory cytokines. Long-term, exposure results in decreased collagen production and increased collagen breakdown, leading to signs of skin photoaging (Reproduced from Zussman et al. [44])

obtained from topical application of antioxidants/botanical extracts in human, in vivo clinical models.

In practice, antioxidants in topical products are supplied largely as botanical extracts, including those from green, black, white, and red teas, pomegranate, cabbage, broccoli, soybeans, grapes, tomatoes, turmeric, ginger, algae, and chocolate. They can include polyphenols, carotenoids, tocopherols, tocotrienols, glutathione, ascorbic acid, flavonoids, proanthocyanidins, stilbenes, coumarins, lignans, omega-3 polyunsaturated fatty acids, and enzymes with antioxidant activity. There are a few antioxidants that are supplied "as is," most notably vitamins C and E. For the most part, topical antioxidant constituents overlap oral or systemic non-sunscreen botanical ingredients that provide photoprotection, which are reviewed in Chap. 22.

The detrimental effects of solar exposure include sunburn, UV-induced immune suppression, skin cancer, and photoaging. Ultraviolet A (UVA) (320–400 nm) exposure induces the generation of reactive oxygen species (ROS) such as superoxide, hydrogen peroxide, lipid peroxyl, nitric oxide, singlet oxygen, and hydroxyl radicals which damage proteins and cellular structures. UVA-induced oxidative stress is considered responsible for increased prostaglandin E_2 and activation of the epidermal growth factor receptor, both of which are involved in causing epidermal hyperproliferation and inflammation [24, 25]. It has also been shown that ultraviolet B wavelengths (290–320 nm), in addition to being directly absorbed by DNA bases and causing mutagenic lesions such as cyclobutane pyrimidine dimers (CPDs) and pyrimidine(6-4)pyrimidine photoproducts (6-4PPs), are also capable of initiating oxidative stress [35]. Increased ROS generation can overwhelm endogenous antioxidant defense mechanisms, resulting in oxidative stress and oxidative photodamage of proteins and other macromolecules in the skin. These ROS are believed to be critical mediators of the photoaging and photocarcinogenesis processes. Exposure to either UVA or UVB can result in oxidation of amino acid residues such as lysine, arginine, and proline, which leads to the formation of carbonyl derivatives that affect the structure and function of proteins. Other protein-related damage includes tyrosine cross-links, amino acid interconversions, and peptide bond cleavages. Lipid peroxidation also damages cell membranes, and a major oxidative lesion in DNA is 8-hydroxy-2′-deoxyguanosine (8-OHdG). The cascade of events leading to clinical signs of photoaging is shown in Fig. 20.1. Repeated exposure to ROS leads to an accumulation of cellular damage and visible signs of photoaging. Considering the extent of potential damage, the most important attribute of antioxidants is their capacity to quench reactive oxygen species (ROS) and prevent the resulting cascade of protein, lipid, and DNA oxidation, which leads to inflammation, mutation, and structural/functional damage.

Four main categories of research models are available to study the effects of antioxidants on prevention of photodamage to human skin: in vitro chemical antioxidant properties, in vitro cell-based assays, animal (mouse) in vivo, and human in vivo models. As to the first category, chemical analytical methods, basic antioxidant properties have been compiled for edible plants and foodstuff in vitro [6, 13, 23]. Screening for active ingredients to include in topical photoprotective products can be facilitated by assays as the "ferric-reducing ability of plasma" (FRAP), the oxygen radical absorbance capacity assay (ORAC) assay," and the DPPH radical scavenging efficacy. Tissue culture work has provided considerable understanding of basic mechanisms, and animal studies have shown the benefits of topical antioxidants against UVR-induced carcinogenesis. These have been reviewed elsewhere, and so in vivo human studies will be emphasized in this chapter.

The botanical product most studied for topical photoprotection is derived from *Camellia sinensis*, the tea plant. Tea is one of the most widely consumed beverages in the world, second only to water, and has been long regarded for its antioxidant, anti-inflammatory, and anticancer properties. Tea is commercially available mainly in three forms: green, black, and oolong tea, but white and red can also be found. Of the total commercial tea consumption worldwide, about 78 % is consumed in the form of black tea (primarily Europe, Russia, the Middle East, India, and North America), and about 20 % is consumed in the form of green tea (primarily Asian countries like, Japan, China, Korea, parts of India, and a few countries in North Africa and the Middle East). Tea contains variable amounts of three main types of polyphenols (flavonoids, stilbenes, and lignans). Flavonoids are divided into six subclasses: flavonols, flavones, isoflavones, flavanones, anthocyanidins, and flavanols. Of the flavonoids, the majority are monomeric flavanols called catechins.

The four main catechin compounds are (−)-epigallocatechin-3-gallate (EGCG), (−)-epigallocatechin (EGC), (−)-epicatechin-3-gallate (ECG), and (−)-epicatechin (EC). The most extensively studied catechin with potent antioxidant, anticancer, and anti-inflammatory properties is EGCG (reviewed in OyetakinWhite et al. [31]; Nichols and Katiyar [30]).

The benefits of tea polyphenols (TP) against UV-induced effects were first demonstrated in human skin by [19]. This report showed that topical application to human skin of (−)-epigallocatechin-3-gallate (EGCG), the major polyphenolic constituent in green tea, was able to inhibit UVB-induced infiltration of leukocytes (macrophage/neutrophils) and generation of prostaglandin (PG) metabolites, particularly PGE_2. This is important because infiltration of leukocytes is a major source of ROS in skin exposed to UVR, and PG metabolites play a critical role in free radical generation and skin tumor promotion in multistage skin carcinogenesis.

In this and subsequent related papers, the overriding goal was to compare, in humans, the impact of topical tea extracts against markers of UVR damage associated with immune suppression, carcinogenesis, and photoaging. It is important to distinguish the mechanisms of action possible for botanical photoprotection and to exclude the possibility that green tea extracts (as well as other botanicals) act merely as a sunscreen. Unlike sunscreens, GTPs do not appear to absorb significantly in the terrestrial solar spectrum, as their UV absorption maxima occurs at 273 nm. Because the tea extract (particularly at the concentrations used in vivo) does not appreciably absorb UVB wavelengths, it does not effectively filter out erythemogenic UVR wavelengths. One implication of this is that TPs, when combined with topical formulations that contain traditional sunscreens, may have additive or synergistic photoprotective effects when compared with either of these agents alone.

In a 2001 study, skin on the back of human subjects was pretreated for 30 min with solutions of 0.25–10 % GTPs in ethanol [8]. The skin was then irradiated with a solar simulator at twice the individual's minimal erythema dose (MED). At 24, 48, and 72 h postexposure, erythema was quantified with a chromameter, and biopsies were taken from the exposed sites. Even though erythema is not the most sensitive endpoint measurement of antioxidant photoprotection, it was found to be reduced in a dose-dependent manner at 24, 48, and 72 h postirradiation. Figure 20.2 illustrates the clinical appearance of skin 24 h after having been treated with green TPs followed by solar-simulated light (ssUVR). GTPs were also shown to reduce sunburn cells and to protect against UVR-induced Langerhans cell depletion, endpoints linked to keratinocyte programmed cell death/apoptosis, and cutaneous cell-mediated immune responses, respectively. EGCG and ECG, the two polyphenols that contain a galloyl group at the 3 position, were the two constituents that were most effective against UVR damage, whereas (−)-epicatechin (EC) and (−)-epigallocatechin (EGC) were ineffective. In the same report, human skin was treated with 5 % GTP, irradiated with 2 MEDs solar-simulated light, and a significant decrease in DNA damage in the sites treated with GTPs was demonstrated by P^{32}-postlabeling analysis.

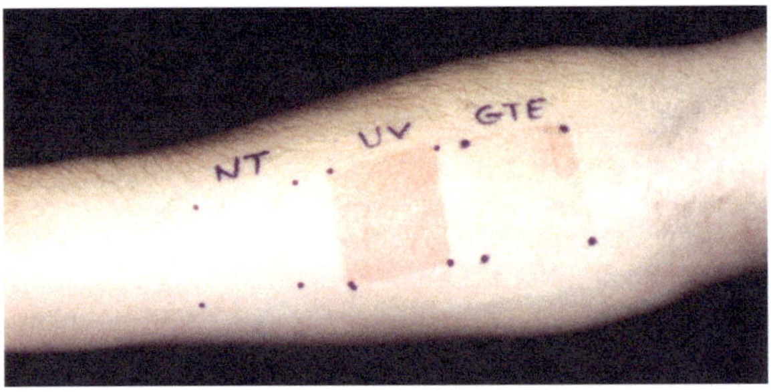

Fig. 20.2 Clinical appearance of skin 24 h after having been treated with GTP followed 30 min later by a 2-MED dose of solar-simulated light. At left is skin treated with vehicle alone. Middle is skin treated with UVR and vehicle. Right is skin treated with both GTP and UVR. Photo supplied by SK Katiyar and CA Elmets

A further study sought to examine the protective effects of topical white tea or green tea against markers of UVR damage that are associated with immune suppression and carcinogenesis [5]. This was accomplished by performing: (1) immunohistochemical analysis for oxidative DNA damage and for epidermal Langerhans cells (LCs) from biopsies obtained after in vivo irradiation of human skin in the presence or absence of the topical tea formulations; (2) assessments of in vivo contact hypersensitivity using the contact sensitizer dinitrochlorobenzene (DNCB); and (3) an analysis of UVR-induced epidermal LC depletion in vitro, using a skin explant model. In this study, the SPF for the tea extracts was determined to be 1. Ten volunteers participated in the study that assessed skin biopsies by immunohistochemical analyses and found that both green tea and white tea partially prevented UV-induced depletion of CD1a+ cells and ssUVR-induced generation of 8-OHdG, as illustrated in Fig. 20.3a, b. Ninety subjects were used to assess the ability of tea extracts to prevent ssUVR-induced immune suppression using 0.75 and 2MED. The results showed a trend (in the face of large interindividual variability) toward preservation of the ability to sensitize subjects to DNCB, suggesting that tea-treated subjects had greater preservation of their CHS response after ssUVR exposure, relative to untreated subjects. In a separate study, CPDs were found to be significantly reduced after 2MED ssUVR exposure by pretreatment with either 0.2 % white tea or 0.5 % green tea extracts. In summary, GTPs in general and EGCG in particular, have, in human clinical studies, been shown to reduce UVB-induced erythema, sunburn cell formation, leukocyte infiltration, and protect against ssUVR-induced Langerhans' cell depletion, generation of 8-OHdG, and immune suppression (CHS). Animal studies support this human evidence that topical GTP protects from UVR-induced immunosuppression [20–21]. In addition, UVR alteration of IL-10 and IL-12, critical cytokines involved in UVR-induced inflammation and immune suppression, has been shown to be modified by pretreatment with GTPs. For example, the reduction in UV-induced DNA damage by GTPs appears to be mediated via induction of interleukin (IL)-12 [36], previously shown to induce NER DNA repair. Katiyar [18] has reviewed the evidence for this additional mechanism of action for GTPs in particular that these phytochemicals induce DNA repair and thereby counteract the effect of UVR exposure on photoaging and carcinogenesis.

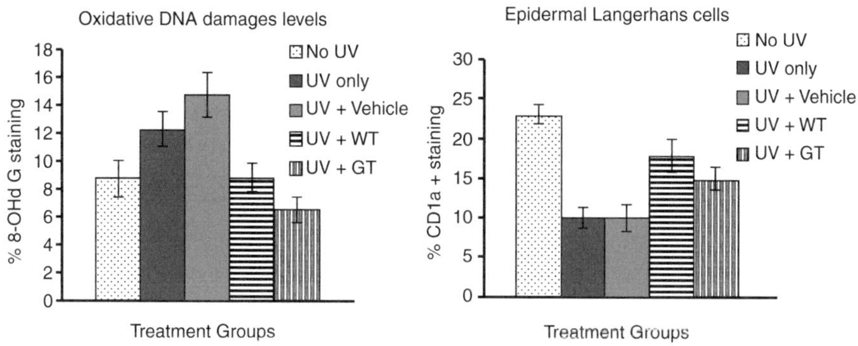

Fig. 20.3 (**a**) Oxidative damage was measured via levels of 8-hydroxy-2′-deoxyguanosine (OhdG) staining in skin biopsies obtained 72 h after a single 2-MED dose of ssUVR. Untreated and vehicle-treated skin showed increased 8-OhdG, whereas 8-OhdG levels in white tea (*WT*)-treated and green tea (*GT*)-treated skin were not different from control unirradiated skin. (**b**) Biopsies obtained 72 h after a single ssUVR dose of 2 MED showed decreased epidermal CD1a+ Langerhans cells (LC) in untreated and vehicle-treated skin. White tea (*WT*) and green tea (*GT*) application 15 min prior and immediately after irradiation partially prevented SSR-induced LC depletion

Other flavonoids, the isoflavones found in plants such as red clover, soybean, *Psoralea corylifolia*, and additional legumes, have been reported to possess significant antioxidant, estrogenic, and tyrosine kinase inhibitory activity. Genistein is an isoflavone and phytoestrogen typically derived from soybeans or red clover and is a popular nutraceutical. Like GTPs, more work has been done on oral benefits (as opposed to topical) and on other health issues such as breast and prostate cancers, postmenopausal syndrome, diabetes, osteoporosis, and cardiovascular diseases. Some promising work, primarily in animal and cell culture models, has been performed showing genistein is also capable of providing photoprotection [14].

Hairless mice were protected against UVR-induced inflammation, edema, and immunosuppression by topical applications of genistein, equol, isoequol, or dehydroequol [39]. A study published in 2003 demonstrated that topical genistein potently inhibited UVB-induced photocarcinogenesis, decreased the levels of UVR-induced CPDs, and blocked signs of photoaging in hairless mice [38]. Another 2003 publication examined the possible molecular signaling mechanisms for the genistein beneficial effect on mediators of photoaging in human subjects [17]. UVR-induced ROS are critical for MAP kinase activation, which leads to increased expression of the transcription factor AP-1 (cFos/cJun), which in turn upregulates MMP gene expression and degradation of the dermal extracellular matrix. This second report showed that UVR-induced induction of EGF-R phosphorylation, cJun protein, JNK MAP kinase, ERK MAP kinases, and MMP-1 was reduced by genistein in human skin in vivo, thus strongly suggesting its value in prevention of photoaging.

In a further study, genistein ameliorated the detrimental effects of UVB irradiation in a human reconstituted skin model, namely, proliferating cell nuclear antigen (PCNA) and CPDs [28]. It has been suggested that specific ratios of genistein and another isoflavone, daidzein, when combined and administered at specific ratios and concentrations, exert a synergistic photoprotective effect that is greater than the effect obtained with each isoflavone alone [16]. Indeed, the idea that these redox-active compounds, which cooperate in an integrated manner in plants cells, also may cooperate in animal cells has been reviewed before [13]. A network of antioxidants with different chemical structures and properties may be needed for optimal protection against oxidative damage.

Other botanical extracts that have some human experimental evidence to show potential for topical photoprotection include resveratrol [9], grape seed [43], and fern extract [10]. Resveratrol is a chemopreventive phytochemical found in grape skin and seeds, red wine, peanuts, and fruits. Most works on the benefits of resveratrol have used it as an oral supplement, but there is an array of animal studies that support the exploration of topical resveratrol for photoprotection which have been summarized previously [32]. Topical application of resveratrol in hairless mice has been shown to reduce signs of oxidative stress and inflammation induced by UVB exposure. In human subjects, daily topical application of a stabilized resveratrol derivative, resveratrate, prior to irradiation with solar-simulated UVR for four consecutive days, provided significant protection against erythema, melanin synthesis, tanning, and sunburn cell formation compared to unprotected skin [40]. Under the experimental conditions used, a typical "antioxidant blend" containing primarily ascorbate and tocopherol was not as effective against these endpoints. The unique model used in this study, of repetitive irradiation, and further, the use of solar-simulated UVR rather than UVB alone, has additional relevance and power to demonstrate the value of this botanical material. Although not specifically on photoprotective capabilities of resveratrol, an interesting report recently suggested that the combination of topical resveratrol, baicalin, and vitamin E was able to reverse the signs of skin photoaging by virtue of the blends' antioxidant properties and its ability to upregulate endogenous antioxidant defense systems [9].

The photoprotective properties of grape seed proanthocyanidins has been demonstrated in human volunteers, also using a repetitive irradiation protocol, with three UVR exposures (one per day) in which subjects received topical applications of grape seed extract (GSPE) in solution or vehicle on sites that were then subjected to 2MED solar-simulated radiation 30 min after treatment [43]. There was a significant decrease in SBCs and p53+ cells in the GSPE+ UV group compared with the UV group and the vehicle+ UV group. There was also significant protection against UV-induced Langerhans cell depletion, illustrated in Fig. 20.4. Virtually all of the very extensive research on the photoprotective properties of fern extract (*Polypodium leucotomos*) have used the oral route of administration; however, there is at least one report that it is efficacious when applied topically [10].

Ferulic acid, vitamin C, and vitamin E are not usually thought of as botanicals but of course do exist in plants—ferulic acid can be found in wheat, corn, and legumes, among other sources. Human studies have been conducted with a topical formulation of 15 % L-ascorbic acid, 1 % α-tocopherol, and 0.5 % ferulic acid (CEFer). In a study using subjects with Fitzpatrick skin type II or III and a protocol in which CEFer was applied to skin over a 4-day period, skin was exposed to 2, 4,

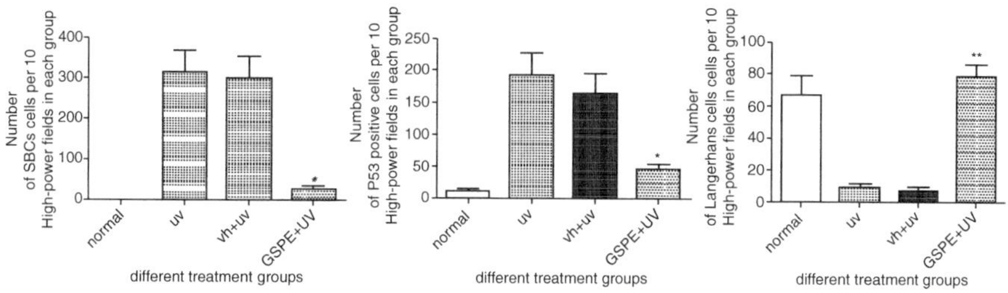

Fig. 20.4 Characterization of normal skin or skin treated with 2-MED simulated solar radiation (SSR) only or skin treated with vehicle or GSPE followed 30 min later by 2-MED SSR. Specimens were taken 24 h after UV exposure. Skin biopsies were analyzed for sunburn cells (SBCs), p53 positive cells, and density of Langerhans cells (Modified from Yuan et al. [43])

6, 8, and 10MED on sites treated with CEFer and evaluated 1 day later [29]. CEFer was very effective at reducing thymine dimer mutations. It also provided substantial protection against erythema and upregulation of the immune suppressive cytokine IL-10 and significantly decreased sunburn cells, p53 expression, and proinflammatory cytokine mRNA expression. In another study using Chinese subjects, a single, 5-MED dose of ssUVR substantially induced large amounts of sunburn cell formation, thymine dimer formation, overexpression of p53 protein, and depletion of CD1a+ Langerhans cells [41]. The antioxidant complex containing vitamins C and E and ferulic acid conferred significant protection against these endpoints.

Interestingly, the ferulic acid papers lead to another aspect of topical antioxidant use that has been addressed more than once, following conflicting data on tumor incidence after long-term antioxidant application and tissue culture experiments showing a prooxidant effect of (usually high concentrations of) antioxidants. In at least one study, topical 5 % alpha-tocopherol promoted carcinogenesis when applied on chronically UVB-irradiated mouse skin [4]. However, a stabilized formulation of vitamin E combined with vitamin C and ferulic acid decreased tumor number and tumor burden and prevented the development of malignant skin tumors in female mice with UVB-irradiated skin.

It has recently become apparent that human skin may be at increased risk of photoaging from infrared radiation as well as UVA and UVB. The biological significance and mechanisms of action for visible and IR wavelengths in human skin is discussed in Chap. 3. The relevance to this chapter is that the mechanism by which infrared radiation (IR), in particular near-infrared radiation (IRA radiation, 760-1,440 nm), causes damage is through oxidative stress [11]. In a recent study, an SPF 30 sunscreen was tested versus the same sunscreen supplemented with an antioxidant cocktail containing grape seed extract, vitamin E, ubiquinone, and vitamin C to evaluate protection against IRA [12]. Exposure to IRA radiation significantly upregulated MMP-1 expression, and treatment with the SPF30 sunscreen alone did not provide significant protection, but the MMP-1 response was significantly reduced if the SPF30 sunscreen plus the antioxidant cocktail was applied prior to IRA radiation.

The IRA study introduces another issue that needs to be addressed when speaking of topical antioxidants for photoprotection, which is the addition of topical antioxidants to UVA/UVB sunscreens, a scenario already taking place in the consumer landscape. Few studies have addressed the effects of this combination, although some have suggested that because the mechanism of action is different from sunscreens they would be expected to add to protection provided by sunscreens. Ideally, topical antioxidants would improve protection against photoaging and carcinogenesis caused by UV irradiation even in the presence of broad-spectrum UVA+ UVB sunscreens.

Two separate studies using the same formulation of antioxidants and sunscreens were published that show additional protection is possible even when an SPF 25 broad-spectrum sunscreen is used. A sunscreen containing benzophenone, avobenzone, and octyl methoxycinnamate was compared to the same product plus ascorbyl phosphate, tocopherol acetate, *Echinacea pallida* extract, chamomile extract, and caffeine. Because MMP1 is the major enzyme implicated in collagen damage and photoaging of UV-irradiated human skin, the first study asked whether the addition of antioxidants to an SPF 25 sunscreen would improve protection against solar-simulated UVR-induced activation of MMP1 after one exposure [26]. Both sunscreen alone and sunscreen plus antioxidants reduced the expression of MMP1 relative to unprotected ssUVR-irradiated control skin (Fig. 20.5). With no protection, the average increase in MMP1 was 4.75-fold; with sunscreen alone, the increase was 2.4-fold; and in skin treated with sunscreens plus antioxidants, the increase was only 1.75-fold. The difference in protection between the sunscreen alone and the sunscreen plus antioxidants was significant and suggests that additional benefit against sun damage can be gained by adding antioxidants to sunscreens. In another clinical study with the same sunscreen and sunscreen plus antioxidants formulas but using a repetitive irradiation model [42] with exposure to 1.5 MED for 4 consecutive days, additional protection provided by antioxidants was also shown. Antioxidants alone did not reduce erythema,

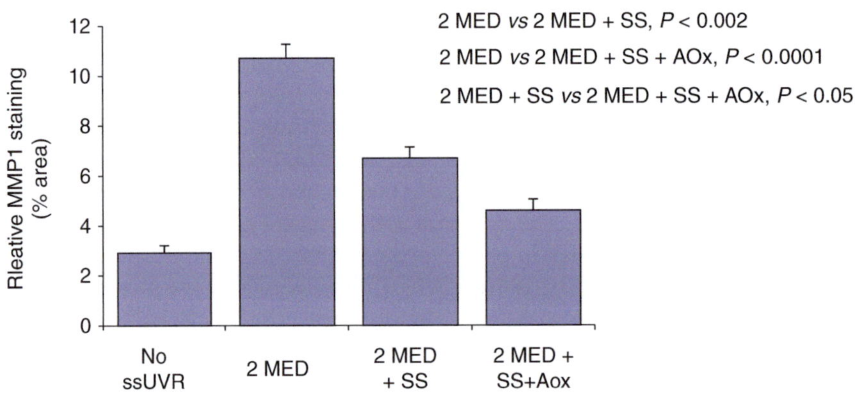

Fig. 20.5 The effect of ssUVR, sunscreens, and sunscreens plus antioxidants on MMP1 expression in human skin in vivo. The skin of human subjects was treated as indicated: (a) no ssUVR, (b) 2-MED ssUVR, (c) 2 MED plus SSþAOx, and (d) 2 MEDþSS alone. Biopsies were analyzed by immunohistochemistry using a monoclonal antibody to MMP1

reduced pigmentation by 30 %, and completely protected against Langerhans cell depletion. Antioxidants plus sunscreens protected better against pigmentation than sunscreens alone (for a summary of erythema and pigment data, see Fig. 20.6). Antioxidants alone protected against UV-induced hyperproliferation, as shown by epidermal thickness and cytokeratins 16 and 5/6 biomarkers, and did so better than sunscreens alone. Most interesting, although protection against a marker of photoaging, MMP-9, did not reach significance when either sunscreens or antioxidants were applied separately, when they were combined, there was complete protection against MMP-9 induction. This study demonstrates that non-sunscreen materials such as antioxidants can contribute significant value when added to an SPF 25 sunscreen and applied topically to human skin in vivo.

In contrast to these in vivo studies on specific formulations of sunscreens plus antioxidants, which show that antioxidants can provide additional protection against in vivo UVR-induced effects, a recent study using in vitro and ex vivo methods was unable to demonstrate any additional benefit to sunscreens by supplementing them with antioxidants [37]. Twelve sunscreens were tested using two methods: electron spin resonance spectroscopy to evaluate the formulations after application to ex vivo pig skin for their ability to reduce UVR-induced free radicals and the antioxidant potential using the DPPH assay. The sunscreens had SPFs from 15 to 55 and had UVA-PF values of 2.4–28.2. The sunscreen products contained tocopheryl acetate, tocopheryl glucoside, ascorbyl palmitate, ubiquinone, ascorbyl tetraisopalmitate, and plant extracts. The sunscreens themselves offered significant protection against free radicals generated by UVR, and it was determined that the radical protection in the tested products was derived mainly from the sunscreens' UVA filters. The antioxidants in these products appeared to offer no contribution to radical protection. These findings would seem to indicate that broad-spectrum sunscreen will not benefit from the addition of botanical or other antioxidant ingredients; however, these results may not truly reflect the potential for "sunscreen plus antioxidant" products. As mentioned by the authors and in the caveats below, the sunscreens tested were "off the shelf," and the concentrations of added antioxidants were not given on the product label (and could have been very low). In addition, UVR

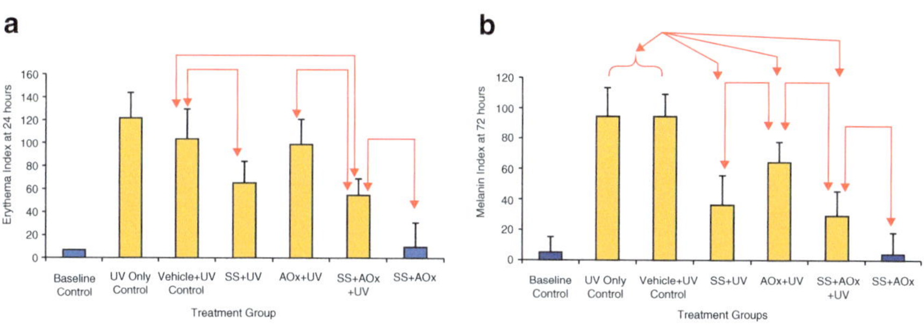

Fig. 20.6 Effect of sunscreens (*SS*) with or without antioxidants (*AOx*) on (**a**) erythema or (**b**) melanin formation after repetitive ultraviolet (*UV*) radiation exposure. *Yellow bars*, irradiated sites; *blue bars*, nonirradiated sites (Modified from [42])

exposure levels may not have been sufficiently challenging, or entirely relevant, as the model was ex vivo pig skin.

Therefore, one of the caveats for phytochemical photoprotection includes the lack of regulatory standards by which this additional protection can be measured and then articulated on product labels. In fact, in most of the world, no concentration needs to be given, and they must be listed as "inactive ingredients." More credible testing of finished product using relevant endpoints on human subjects should be undertaken, the optimal concentration should be determined for individual components and mixtures of ingredients, and the stability of ingredients need to be carefully monitored (as antioxidants are notoriously unstable). In addition, the bioavailability/delivery of active supplements to the skin needs to be better understood, as both water- and oil-soluble materials can protect lipids against UVR-induced peroxidation; however, the bioactive portion must be able to partition into the lipid bilayers to be protective [27]. There also exists potential synergy or antagonism between ingredients, which under certain conditions such as high concentrations, can act as prooxidants. Finally, in part because antioxidants are frequently supplied as semicharacterized botanical extracts, the risk of adverse reactions such as allergic or irritant sensitization must be considered.

In conclusion, there is ample evidence that certain antioxidants and botanical extracts have potential to contribute to photoprotection when used topically. While not to be recommended as alternatives to sun avoidance, broad-spectrum sunscreens, and protective clothing, they should be considered valuable adjuvants in the prevention of photoaging and skin cancer. Supplemental photoprotection will benefit those who have heightened personal and professional risk factors such as Fitzpatrick skin types I–II; environmental risk factors such as occupational exposure, geographic location, and elevation; extended outdoor recreational activities; patients with previous skin cancer, photosensitive dermatological conditions, or patients on medication that renders them photosensitive; and immunosuppressed patients. However, caution must be taken when communicating the benefits of topical antioxidants to consumers, who may already be bombarded with misinformation, such as the statements taken from Internet sites and which include phrases such as "research says antioxidants work better than sunscreen," "our skin is so well designed that when the solar rays hit it the antioxidants that are in the body actually move up and form a protective shield and act just like sunscreen," and "antioxidants are the exact answer—they act just like sunscreens." Ideally, any product with a claim to enhance photoprotection with antioxidants would have been clinically tested under relevant and scientifically rigorous conditions.

Abbreviations

6-4PPs	Pyrimidine(6-4)pyrimidine photoproducts
CPDs	Cyclobutane pyrimidine dimers
EC	(−)-Epicatechin

ECG	(−)-Epicatechin-3-gallate
EGC	(−)-Epigallocatechin
EGCG	(−)-Epigallocatechin-3-gallate
GTPs	Green tea polyphenols
IR	Infrared radiation
LCs	Langerhans cells
ROS	Reactive oxygen species
SPF	Sun protection factor
ssUVR	Solar-simulated light
TPs	Tea polyphenols
UVR	Ultraviolet radiation

References

1. Afaq F, Mukhtar H (2006) Botanical antioxidants in the prevention of photocarcinogenesis and photoaging. Exp Dermatol 15(9):678–684
2. Afonso S, Horita K, Sousa E, Silva JP, Almeida IF, Amaral MH, Lobão PA, Costa PC, Miranda MS, Esteves da Silva JC, Sousa Lobo JM (2014) Photodegradation of avobenzone: stabilization effect of antioxidants. J Photochem Photobiol B 140:36–40
3. Black HS, Rhodes LE (2006) The potential of omega-3 fatty acids in the prevention of non-melanoma skin cancer. Cancer Detect Prev 30(3):224–232
4. Burns EM, Tober KL, Riggenbach JA, Kusewitt DF, Young GS, Oberyszyn TM (2013) Differential effects of topical vitamin E and C E Ferulic® treatments on ultraviolet light B-induced cutaneous tumor development in Skh-1 mice. PLoS One 8(5):e63809
5. Camouse MM, Domingo DS, Swain FR, Conrad EP, Matsui MS, Maes D, Declercq L, Cooper KD, Stevens SR, Baron ED (2009) Topical application of green and white tea extracts provides protection from solar-simulated ultraviolet light in human skin. Exp Dermatol 18(6):522–526
6. Carlsen MH, Halvorsen BL, Holte K, Bøhn SK, Dragland S, Sampson L, Willey C, Senoo H, Umezono Y, Sanada C, Barikmo I, Berhe N, Willett WC, Phillips KM, Jacobs DR Jr, Blomhoff R (2010) The total antioxidant content of more than 3100 foods, beverages, spices, herbs and supplements used worldwide. Nutr J 9:3–11
7. Cosgrove MC, Franco OH, Granger SP, Murray PG, Mayes AE (2007) Dietary nutrient intakes and skin-aging appearance among middle-aged American women. Am J Clin Nutr 86(4):1225–1231
8. Elmets CA, Singh D, Tubesing K, Matsui M, Katiyar S, Mukhtar H (2001) Cutaneous photo-protection from ultraviolet injury by green tea polyphenols. J Am Acad Dermatol 44(3):425–432
9. Farris P, Yatskayer MS, Chen N, Yevgeniy K, Oresajo C (2014) Evaluation of efficacy and tolerance of a nighttime topical antioxidant containing resveratrol, baicalin, and vitamin E for treatment of mild to moderately photodamaged skin. J Drugs Dermatol 13(12):1467–1472
10. Gonzalez S, Pathak MA, Cuevas J, Villarubia VG, Fitzpatrick TB (1997) Topical or oral administration with an extract of Polypodium leucotomos prevents acute sunburn and psolaren-induced phototoxic reactions as well as depletion of Langerhans cells in human skin. Photodermatol Photoimmunol Photomed 13:50–60
11. Grether-Beck S, Marini A, Jaenicke T, Krutmann J (2014) Photoprotection of human skin beyond ultraviolet radiation. Photodermatol Photoimmunol Photomed 30(2-3):167–174
12. Grether-Beck S, Marini A, Jaenicke T, Krutmann J (2015) Effective photoprotection of human skin against infrared a radiation by topically applied antioxidants: results from a vehicle controlled, double-blind, randomized study. Photochem Photobiol 91(1):248–250

13. Halvorsen BL, Carlsen MH, Phillips KM, Bøhn SK, Holte K, Jacobs DR Jr, Blomhoff R (2006) Content of redox-active compounds (ie, antioxidants) in foods consumed in the United States. Am J Clin Nutr 84:95–135
14. Huang CC, Hsu BY, Wu NL, Tsui WH, Lin TJ, Su CC, Hung CF (2010) Anti-photoaging effects of soy isoflavone extract (aglycone and acetylglucoside form) from soybean cake. Int J Mol Sci 11(12):4782–4795
15. Ibiebele TI, van der Pols JC, Hughes MC, Marks GC, Williams GM, Green AC (2007) Dietary pattern in association with squamous cell carcinoma of the skin: a prospective study. Am J Clin Nutr 85(5):1401–1408
16. Iovine B, Iannella ML, Gasparri F, Monfrecola G, Bevilacqua MA (2011) Synergic effect of genistein and daidzein on UVB-induced DNA damage: an effective photoprotective combination. J Biomed Biotechnol 2011:692846
17. Kang S, Chung JH, Lee JH, Fisher GJ, Wan YS, Duell EA, Voorhees JJ (2003) Topical N-acetyl cysteine and genistein prevent ultraviolet-light-induced signaling that leads to photoaging in human skin in vivo. J Invest Dermatol 120(5):835–841
18. Katiyar SK (2011) Green tea prevents non-melanoma skin cancer by enhancing DNA repair. Arch Biochem Biophys 508(2):152–158
19. Katiyar SK, Matsui MS, Elmets CA, Mukhtar H (1999) Polyphenolic Antioxidant (-)-epigallocatechin-3-gallate from Green Tea Reduces UVB-induced Inflammatory Responses and Infiltration of Leukocytes in Human Skin. Photochem Photobiol 69:148–153
20. Katiyar SK, Challa A, McCormick T, Cooper K, Mukhtar H (1999) Prevention of UVB-induced immunosuppression in mice by the green tea polyphenol ())-epigallocatechin-3-gallate may be associated with alterations in IL-10- and IL-12 production. Carcinogenesis 20:2117–2124
21. Katiyar SK, Elmets CA, Agarwal R, Mukhtar H (1995) Protection against ultraviolet-B radiation-induced local and systemic suppression of contact hypersensitivity and edema responses in C3H/HeN mice by green tea polyphenols. Photochem Photobiol 62:855–861
22. Khan N, Afaq F, Mukhtar H (2008) Comprehensive invited review cancer chemoprevention through dietary antioxidants: progress and promise. Antioxid Redox Signal 10(3) doi:10.1089/ars.2007.1740, © Mary Ann Liebert, Inc
23. Maia Campos PMBG, Gianeti MD, Kanashiro A, Lucisano-Valim YM, Gaspar LR (2006) In vitro antioxidant and in vivo photoprotective effects of an association of bioflavonoids with liposoluble vitamins. Photochem Photobiol 82:683–688
24. Matsui MS, DeLeo VA (1990) Longwave ultraviolet radiation and promotion of skin cancer. Cancer Cells 3:8–12
25. Matsui MS, Scheide S, Laufer L, DeLeo VA (1989) Ultraviolet B radiation inhibits epidermal growth factor binding to mammalian cells. J Invest Dermatol 92:617–622
26. Matsui MS, Hsia A, Miller JD, Hanneman K, Scull H, Cooper KD, Baron E (2009) Non-sunscreen photoprotection: antioxidants add value to a sunscreen. J Investig Dermatol Symp Proc 14(1):56–59
27. Mishra AK, Mishra A, Chattopadhyay P (2011) Herbal cosmeceuticals for photoprotection from ultraviolet B radiation: a review. Trop J Pharm Res 10(3):351–360
28. Moore JO, Wang Y, Stebbins WG, Gao D, Zhou X, Phelps R, Lebwohl M, Wei H (2006) Photoprotective effect of isoflavone genistein on ultraviolet B-induced pyrimidine dimer formation and PCNA expression in human reconstituted skin and its implications in dermatology and prevention of cutaneous carcinogenesis. Carcinogenesis 27(8):1627–1635
29. Murray JC, Burch JA, Streilein RD, Iannacchione MA, Hall RP, Pinnell SR (2008) A topical antioxidant solution containing vitamins C and E stabilized by ferulic acid provides protection for human skin against damage caused by ultraviolet irradiation. J Am Acad Dermatol 59(3):418–425
30. Nichols JA, Katiyar SK (2010) Skin photoprotection by natural polyphenols: anti-inflammatory, antioxidant and DNA repair mechanisms. Arch Dermatol Res 302(2):71–83

31. OyetakinWhite P, Tribout H, Baron E (2012) Protective mechanisms of green tea polyphenols in skin. Oxid Med Cell Longev 2012:Article ID 560682
32. Passantino L, Costa M and Matsui MS (2013). Skin Cancer Prevention Strategies. In: Highlights in Skin Cancer, Dr. Pierre Vereecken (Ed.), ISBN: 978-953-51-1073-6, InTech, Available from: http://www.intechopen.com/books/highlights-in-skin-cancer/skin-cancer-prevention-strategies
33. Perner D, Vierkötter A, Sugiri D, Matsui M, Ranft U, Esser C, Ethève S, Goralczyk R, Kaneko N, Yamamoto A, Morita A, Krutmann J, Krämer U (2011) Association between sun-exposure, smoking behaviour and plasma antioxidant levels with the different manifestation of skin ageing signs between Japanese and German women – a pilot study. J Dermatol Sci 62(2):138–140
34. Schalka S, Manoel Silva dos Reis V (2011) Sun protection factor: meaning and controversies. An Bras Dermatol 86(3):507–515
35. Schneider LA, Bloch W, Kopp K, Hainzl A, Rettberg P, Wlaschek M, Horneck G, Scharffetter-Kochanek K (2006) 8-Isoprostane is a dose-related biomarker for photo-oxidative ultraviolet (UV) B damage in vivo: a pilot study with personal UV dosimetry. Br J Dermatol 154(6):1147–1154
36. Schwarz A, Maeda A, Gan D, Mammone T, Matsui MS, Schwarz T (2008) Green tea phenol extracts reduce UVB-induced DNA damage in human cells via interleukin-12. Photochem Photobiol 84(2):350–355
37. Wang SQ, Osterwalder U, Jung K (2011) Ex vivo evaluation of radical sun protection factor in popular sunscreens with antioxidants. J Am Acad Dermatol 65(3):525–530
38. Wei H, Saladi R, Lu Y, Wang Y, Palep SR, Moore J, Phelps R, Shyong E, Lebwohl MG (2003) Isoflavone genistein: photoprotection and clinical implications in dermatology. J Nutr 133:3811S–3819S
39. Widyarini S, Spinks N, Husband AJ, Reeve VE (2001) Isoflavonoid compounds from red clover (Trifolium pratense) protect from inflammation and immune suppression induced by UV radiation. Photochem Photobiol 74(3):465–470
40. Wu Y, Jia LL, Zheng YN, Xu XG, Luo YJ, Wang B, Chen JZ, Gao XH, Chen HD, Matsui M, Li YH (2013) Resveratrate protects human skin from damage due to repetitive ultraviolet irradiation. J Eur Acad Dermatol Venereol 27(3):345–350
41. Wu Y, Zheng X, Xu XG, Li YH, Wang B, Gao XH, Chen HD, Yatskayer M, Oresajo C (2013) Protective effects of a topical antioxidant complex containing vitamins C and E and ferulic acid against ultraviolet irradiation-induced photodamage in Chinese women. J Drugs Dermatol 12(4):464–468
42. Wu Y, Matsui MS, Chen JZ, Jin X, Shu CM, Jin GY, Dong GH, Wang YK, Gao XH, Chen HD, Li YH (2011) Antioxidants add protection to a broad-spectrum sunscreen. Clin Exp Dermatol 36(2):178–187
43. Yuan XY, Liu W, Hao JC, Gu WJ, Zhao YS (2012) Topical grape seed proanthocyandin extract reduces sunburn cells and mutant p53 positive epidermal cell formation, and prevents depletion of Langerhans cells in an acute sunburn model. Photomed Laser Surg 30(1):20–25
44. Zussman J, Ahdout J, Kim J (2010) Vitamins and photoaging: do scientific data support their use? J Am Acad Dermatol 63(3):507–525

Chapter 21
The Role of DNA Repair in Photoprotection

Nevena Karaman-Jurukovska and Daniel B. Yarosh

21.1 DNA Damage Induced by Light

21.1.1 Light Sources

Life on earth evolved utilizing solar electromagnetic energy, but at the same time, this energy has adverse biological effects. The extent of the effects on the skin depends greatly on the wavelength of light absorbed by its biomolecules. The most damaging are the shorter wavelengths in the ultraviolet (UV) region because they are most readily absorbed by the skin.

By convention, UV wavelengths are designated as UVA (320–400 nm), UVB (290–320 nm), and UVC (200–290 nm). The shorter the wavelength, the greater absorption of the UV energy by earth's atmosphere. UVC, the shortest wavelength band, is effectively absorbed by atmosphere stratospheric gases and therefore fails to reach the surface of the earth. The ozone molecules and atmosphere efficiently filter UVB, so that only a small fraction actually reaches the earth surface (around 5 %). Its local intensity may vary with the solar zenith angle, which differs by the time of day, the year, the latitude, and the local cloud density. For the long UV wavelengths, 95 % of UVA energy reaches the earth with its steady presence during the day, making it the most abundant [35].

Artificial light from incandescent light bulbs and compact fluorescent lamps present an additional source of UV exposure, mostly UVA. The International Commission on Illumination recommends maximal UV radiation of 30 J/m^2 within 8 h. While the average daily exposure from outdoors is much lower, the cumulative effects might be significant due to prolonged and continual daily exposures [41].

N. Karaman-Jurukovska, PhD • D.B. Yarosh, PhD (✉)
R&D Division, Basic Science Research Department, Estee Lauder Companies,
Melville, NY, USA
e-mail: dyarosh@danyarosh.com

S.Q. Wang, H.W. Lim (eds.), *Principles and Practice of Photoprotection*,
DOI 10.1007/978-3-319-29382-0_21

21.1.2 Direct DNA Damage

DNA directly absorbs the energy of UVC and UVB irradiation. The adsorbed energy causes intranucleotide cross-linking by dimerization of pyrimidines and formation of *cis-syn* cyclobutane pyrimidine dimers (CPDs) and pyrimidine (6–4) pyrimidone photoproducts (6-4PP) [30, 49]. To a much lesser extent, purine dimers and pyrimidine photohydrates are formed as well. The cyclobutane rings of CPDs are formed between the 5,6 bonds of two adjacent pyrimidine bases (thymine, cytosine, or 5-methylcytosine). CPD formation is influenced by sequence context [42] and formed exclusively at dipyrimidines and preferentially at TT sites. The efficiency of CPD formation at different dipyrimidine sequences is estimated at a ratio of 55:33:11:1 for TT>TC>CT>CC [10]. In addition to the nucleotide sequences, the chromatin structure and its environment have a significant impact on the distribution of CPDs and the rate of their repair. Efficient repair in regions of DNA damage requires nucleosomal rearrangements to allow DNA repair complex initiation.

The formation of (6–4)PPs arise through a complex electron rearrangement resulting in generation of a single covalent bond between position 6 and position 4 of two adjacent pyrimidine bases [27]. The frequency of (6–4)PPs formation by UVB is at the same level as the formation of CPDs but is repaired at much faster rate [49].

For a while it was assumed that UVA could not induce CPDs due to the inability of DNA to efficiently absorb in the UVA range. However, CPDs were readily detected upon UVA exposures [2, 33]. After exposure of cultured cells and the skin to large doses of UVA, higher ratios of oxidized purines to CPDs are found than in naked DNA [4]. Analysis of the CPDs produced by UVA revealed that the predominant site for CPD formation is at TT compared to TC and CT sites and that (6–4)PPs are almost undetectable.

The exact mechanism of CPD formation upon UVA irradiation is still subject of debate. Some data suggests involvement of yet undetermined UVA chromophore that is capable of transferring energy to DNA by photosensitization – a triplet energy transfer mechanism [13]. Other evidence supports direct DNA absorption, with much lower efficiency than that of UVB. This absorption has a very distinctive signature – exclusive TT dimer formation [15].

Recently, a new pathway for formation of CPDs has been described wherein fragments of melanin are excited by UV-induced reactive oxygen and nitrogen species and then transfer the energy to DNA to form CPDs [32] This process is remarkable in that CPDs continue to form even in the dark. The relative importance of this photochemical reaction in the overall yield of DNA damage in intact human skin is an exciting new area of research.

21.1.3 Indirect DNA Damage

Indirect DNA damage is a result of UV energy absorption by either proteins or DNA-bound chromophores through photosensitization. As a result of photooxidation, the generated superoxide radicals or singlet oxygens react with nucleotides and form several kinds of base lesions. The *8-oxo-7,8-dihydro-2′-deoxyguanosine* (8-oxo-dGua) is the most frequent and therefore most studied UVA-induced oxidative base lesion. If not repaired prior to the DNA replication, 8-Oxo-dGua mispairs with 2′-deoxyadenosine (dA) and induces $G \rightarrow T$ transversion mutations which are considered the fingerprint mutations of UVA-induced oxidized guanines in human skin carcinogenesis [4]. UVA induces DNA strand breaks and oxidized pyrimidines at a much lower frequency.

Melanocytes that secrete UV-absorbing melanin provide localized protection from the sun's electromagnetic energy. Just in the recent decade, the accumulated evidence reveals that the melanin, an optical absorber, free radical scavenger, and antioxidant, can also form melanin radicals in the presence of metal ions. In such a way, the melanin becomes a strong oxidant and might be involved in a UV-mediated DNA damaging events [38] and as noted above perhaps even CPD formation. Partially polymerized melanin is particularly effective in photooxidation in that it promotes 8-oxo-dGua formation in presence of singlet oxygen [29]. In an animal model, the incidence of UVA-induced melanoma was associated with oxidative DNA damage, and the increase in production of 8-oxo-dGua required both UVA and melanin [28].

21.2 DNA Repair

The knowledge of DNA repair pathways has gone from an arcane corner of nucleic acid biochemistry to the subject of a college textbook [11]. The molecular details of the reactions that lead to reversal, or removal and resynthesis, of damaged DNA can be found there. Here we discuss the particular aspects of DNA repair that can prevent photodamage and their sequelae.

DNA damage induced either directly or indirectly by sunlight is roughly randomly distributed among the target nucleotides in the genome. However, because the information content of the nucleotides is not randomly distributed within the genome, the biological consequences of DNA lesions are not of equal importance. As a result, repair of a minority of lesions, such as in the exons or on the transcribed strand, has much greater biological importance than repair of others in the introns or non-transcribed strands. DNA repair systems, both endogenous and therapeutic, have indeed focused on repairing some regions, such as transcribed strands, faster than others, in order to relieve phototoxic effects.

Here we will focus only on the main DNA repair pathways for photodamage.

21.2.1 Nucleotide Excision

Nucleotide excision employs a complex of enzymes to recognize gross distortions in the double helix and cut out a strip of approximately 30 nucleotides surrounding the lesion causing the distortion. The bulkier the lesion, the more readily nucleotide excision repair recognizes it, and conversely, the more subtle the nucleotide modification, the longer it takes to find and remove them. The great advantage of this system is that it is not lesion specific, so that nucleotide excision repair can remove damage that the organism has never experienced before, including modern chemical carcinogen adducts that were invented in the last 100 years.

This pathway has many substrates, but it is not fast. It may take only 10 min to incise UV-induced lesions [18], but following a sunburn it may take 12 h to remove half the cyclobutane pyrimidine dimers in exposed skin [43].

21.2.2 *Base Excision*

Base excision repair uses one lead glycosylase enzyme that recognizes a small class of modified bases and releases them from the phosphodiester backbone to create vacant (abasic) sites in DNA. These sites are then repaired by a common set of enzymes that remove the damaged regions on one strand and replace only about 4 nucleotides. The lead enzymes have narrow substrate specificity, but fortunately, several are custom fit for DNA damage induced by sunlight. Important oxidation photoproducts, particularly 8-oxo-dGua, are quickly and efficiently repaired by base excision repair in about 6 h.

One strategy for enhancing DNA repair is to introduce into skin cells glycosylases specific for cyclobutane pyrimidine dimers. This shifts the repair pathway from nucleotide to base excision repair. Not only does it speed up repair but it also reduces the frequency of mutagenic mistakes [46].

21.2.3 *Photoreactivation*

Photoreactivation is a direct reversal of DNA damage mediated by a light-activated enzyme that uses the energy captured from light to reverse aberrant covalent bonds formed in DNA by photon absorption from sunlight. These enzymes are found ubiquitously in plants, reptiles, and marsupials but not mammals including humans. It seems our photolyase gene has been hijacked by evolution to become a blue light sensor for the circadian rhythm!

Photolyases have been found for both CPD and (6–4)PPs, the two most common direct forms of photodamage. Despite being derived from another kingdom, these enzymes perform a quick and efficient repair inside human cells [39].

21.2.4 *Lesion Bypass by Polymerase*

Human cells harbor a fail-safe mechanism for handling DNA photodamage. They have polymerase η (eta) that, during replication of a photodamaged DNA template, quickly and efficiently inserts the correct nucleotide opposite a pyrimidine lesion.

Although this doesn't remove the damage, it preserves the genome integrity until an excision mechanism can recognize and remove it. A genetic defect in this fail-safe mechanism produces the cancer-prone xeroderma pigmentosum variant phenotype.

21.2.5 Cellular Regulation of DNA Repair

DNA repair enzymes and pathways are closely coordinated with the rest of the cell's functions. Foremost among these coordinators is the p53 protein. Loss of its function is a perquisite for many skin cancers. DNA damage triggers release of p53 protein from its inhibitor, which frees it to form a transcription activator for its target genes. Most of these genes code for cell cycle checkpoints, inhibitors of proliferation and activators of DNA repair. Sustained activation of p53 protein leads to apoptosis and cell death. In this way, p53 gives the cell a greater opportunity to repair its DNA and, failing that, a road to suicide to avoid mutations and oncogenic transformation.

A large number of DNA Damage Response (DDR) proteins, many of them activated by p53, work together to signal that cell cycling should stop [7]. DNA repair activity is further tied to the health status of the cell through AMPK (5'-AMP-activated protein kinase), which senses energy levels in cells and whose activation increases DNA repair [44]. Furthermore, single-stranded breaks in DNA produced during repair can activate poly(ADP-ribose) polymerase to consume NAD, which saps the cell of molecules essential to production of ATP and lower cellular energy.

DNA repair is tied not only to the cell cycle but also to the circadian rhythm. This should not be surprising since the risk of photodamage to skin DNA is directly related to the presence of the sun in the sky. The genes and proteins in human cells that produce a feedback loop to create the circadian clock (BMal1, Clock, Cryptochrome, and Period) also regulate the cell cycle and DNA repair [34]. The peak of DNA repair capacity is late afternoon, just as the accumulation of daytime sun damage to skin DNA is reaching its maximum.

The DDR genes, including p53, work through regulation of transcription. Downstream of transcription, miRNA (micro-RNA) are also modulated following UV, and they further regulate the DDR genes by increasing or decreasing gene silencing complexes [31]. Cell survival after UV is dependent on the proper functioning of the gene silencing apparatus.

Many of the steps of the DDR pathways involve protein modification of the downstream target. These modifications include classical phosphorylation, acetylation, and, as we have discussed, poly(ADP-ribosyl)ation, which serve to activate or inhibit enzyme activity. Another form of modification is ubiquitin and/or SUMO (small ubiquitin-related modifier) additions to protein, which may coordinate assembly of protein complexes or designate them for destruction to make way for a repair response [40].

21.2.6 Therapeutic Intervention with DNA Repair

The simplest way to intervene in DNA repair is to accelerate the first step of DNA repair, the recognition and incision of damaged bases. This has been accomplished by encapsulating various enzymes in liposomes for delivery into skin cells, including T4 endonuclease V [47] and *M. luteus* UV endonuclease [8] for CPDs, OGG1 for 8-oxo-dGua [45], and photolyase for direct reversal of CPDs [39]. These exogenous but small enzymes are indeed able to enter the nucleus and recognize and then repair DNA damage in mammalian skin.

The hormone α-MSH protects the skin not only by inducing protective pigment but also by inducing p53 and subsequent reduction in cell cycling and initiation of DNA repair [14], a property that may be shared with the α-MSH analog afamelanotide, now undergoing clinical testing.

Induction and synchronization of the circadian rhythm by delivery of peptides to skin cells has been reported to amplify DNA repair [25]. Application of such peptides at night may therefore accelerate repair of DNA damage accumulated during the day.

Binding of certain ligands to receptors activates DNA repair even in the absence of a DNA damage inducing signal. IL-12 binding to its receptor increases repair of UV-induced cyclobutane pyrimidine dimers [36]. The toll-like receptors TLR-3 and TLR-4 mediate damage-associated pattern recognition (DAMP). Agonists of these receptors modulate DNA repair after UV [1, 12]. They may act in part by activating p53 [26]. Since extracellular DNA is recognized as DAMP and bound by TLRs, this may explain the observations that dTpT and small oligonucleotides activate DNA repair through a p53-dependent mechanism [22]. TLRs also distinguish pathogenic from benign surface bacteria, and this may also explain the long-standing observation that extracts of probiotic bacteria enhance DNA repair [3].

HMGB1 (high-mobility group protein B1) is a component of histones but also participates in intercellular communication and recruitment of stem cells to the skin from bone marrow. It is able to activate DNA repair and increase survival after UV [21]. This may provide a new use for compounds modulating HMGB1 levels in the skin.

21.2.7 Botanical Induction of DNA Repair

Antioxidants naturally block oxidation of DNA and are discussed in Chap. 20. There are recurrent reports of antioxidants inhibiting the formation of cyclobutane pyrimidine dimers by UV (e.g., [23]). One explanation might be that antioxidant polyphenols, such as from green tea or polypodium leucotomos, induce IL-12, which then activates the DNA repair pathways to remove cyclobutane pyrimidine dimers [17]. Another may be that antioxidants inhibit energy transfer by oxidized melanin fragments [32].

Topically applied ginseng saponin and silymarin reduce UV toxicity in part by increasing nucleotide excision repair [5, 16]. Interestingly, topically applied caffeine may improve skin health after UV by *inhibiting* DNA repair and forcing more skin cells into apoptosis [20].

The depletion of ATP by poly(ADP-ribose) polymerase may be countered by oral niacin intake and thereby prevent the energy crisis and reduction in DNA repair following UV [19].

21.3 Clinical Consequences of Unrepaired Photodamage to DNA

DNA damage contributes to many of the sequelae of UV exposure, as evidenced by animal studies, by DNA repair deficiency diseases, and by enhancing DNA repair in human skin.

Within a few days after sufficient UV exposure, mouse and human skin develop a reduced ability to properly respond to specific sensitizing antigens [50]. DNA damage, especially CPDs, contribute to this immunosuppression by inducing the release of immunosuppressive soluble mediators and impairing antigen-presenting cells. This reduced ability to respond may allow highly antigenic precancerous skin cells to escape immune surveillance and form a tumor. Enhancing DNA repair reduces the immunosuppressive effect of UV in humans [24, 39].

Chronic UV exposure accelerates the appearance of aging. Especially in lightly pigmented people, this appears as an increase in skin wrinkling and uneven pigmentation. DNA damage contributes to destruction of collagen by inducing the expression of the collagenase MMP-1 [9]. DNA damage is also a trigger for skin pigment production, since one of the purposes of the pigment is to absorb UV and block additional DNA damage [6].

Finally, DNA damage is a central element in the development of skin cancers, including squamous and basal cell carcinoma and melanoma. Mutations in tumor suppressor genes are frequently identified in all these cancers that have the changes characteristic of UV-induced DNA damage [37]. In animal models of DNA repair deficiency and the human genodermatosis xeroderma pigmentosum (XP), with defective DNA repair, the rates of UV-induced skin cancer are greatly increased. Enhancing DNA repair in normal or XP patients reduced their development of new actinic keratoses and basal cell carcinomas [8, 48].

References

1. Ahmad I, Simanyi E, Purushotham G et al (2014) Toll-like receptor-4 deficiency enhances repair of UVR-induced cutaneous DNA damage by nucleotide excision repair mechanism. J Invest Dermatol 134:1710–1717

2. Besaratinia A, Yoon JI, Schroeder C, Bradforth SE, Cockburn M, Pfeifer GP (2011) Wavelength dependence of ultraviolet radiation-induced DNA damage as determined by laser irradiation suggests that cyclobutane pyrimidine dimers are the principal DNA lesions produced by terrestrial sunlight. FASEB J 25(9):3079–3091
3. Born A, Born W (1987) Replicative and repair DNA synthesis after solar damage. Acta Dermatol Venerol 134:40–42
4. Cadet J, Douki T (2011) Oxidatively generated damage to DNA by UVA radiation in cells and human skin. J Invest Dermatol 131(5):1005–1007
5. Cai B-X, Jin S-L, Luo D et al (2009) Ginsenoside Rb1 suppresses ultraviolet radiation-induced apoptosis by inducing DNA repair. Biol Pharm Bull 32:837–841
6. Chen H, Weng Q, Fisher D (2014) UV signaling pathways within the skin. J Invest Dermatol 134:2080–2085
7. Cotta-Ramusino C, McDonald E, Hurov K et al (2011) A DNA damage response screen identifies RHINO, a 9-1-1 and TopBP1 interacting protein required for ATR signaling. Science 332:1313–1317
8. DeBoyes T, Kouba D, Ozog D et al (2010) Reduced number of actinic keratoses with topical application of DNA repair enzyme creams. J Drug Dermatol 9:11519–11521
9. Dong K, Damaghi N, Picart S, Markova N, Obayashi K, Okano Y, Masaki H, Grether-Beck S, Krutmann J (2008) UV-induced DNA damage initiates release of MMP-1 in human skin. Exp Dermatol 17:1037–1044
10. Douki T, Cadet J (2001) Individual determination of the yield of the main UV-induced dimeric pyrimidine photoproducts in DNA suggests a high mutagenicity of CC photolesions. Biochemistry 40(8):2495–2501
11. Friedberg E, Walker G, Siede W, Wood R, Schultz R, Ellenberger T (eds) (2006) DNA repair and mutagenesis. ASM Press, Washington DC
12. Harberts E, Gaspari AA (2013) TLR signaling and DNA repair: are they associated? J Invest Dermatol 133:296–302
13. Ikehata H, Kawai K, Komura J, Sakatsume K, Wang L, Imai M, Higashi S, Nikaido O, Yamamoto K, Hieda K, Watanabe M, Kasai H, Ono T (2008) UVA1 genotoxicity is mediated not by oxidative damage but by cyclobutane pyrimidine dimers in normal mouse skin. J Invest Dermatol 128(9):2289–2296
14. Kadekaro A, Chen J, Yang J et al (2012) Alpha-melanocyte-stimulating hormone suppresses oxidative stress through a p53-mediated signaling pathway in human melanocytes. Mol Cancer Res 10:778–786
15. Kappes UP, Luo D, Potter M, Schulmeister K, Runger TM (2006) Short- and long-wave UV light (UVB and UVA) induce similar mutations in human skin cells. J Invest Dermatol 126(3):667–675
16. Katiyar S, Mantena S, Meeran S (2011) Silymarin protects epidermal keratinocytes from ultraviolet radiation-induced apoptosis and DNA damage by nucleotide excision repair mechanism. PLoS One 6, e21410
17. Katiyar S, Elmets CA, Katiyar SK (2007) Green tea and skin cancer: photoimmunology, angiogenesis and DNA repair. J Nutr Biochem 18:287–296
18. Kaufmann W, Briley L (1987) Reparative strand incision in saponin-permeabilized human fibroblasts. Mutat Res 184:237–243
19. Kirkland JB (2012) Niacin requirements for genomic stability. Mutat Res 733:14–20
20. Koo S-W, Hirakawa S, Fujii S et al (2007) Protection from photodamage by topical application of caffeine after ultraviolet irradiation. Br J Dermatol 156:957–964
21. Lange S, Mitchell D, Vasquez K (2008) High mobility group protein B1 enhances DNA repair and chromatin modification after DNA damage. Proc Natl Acad Sci U S A 105:10320–10325
22. Lee MS, Yaar M, Eller MS et al (2009) Telomeric DNA induces p53-dependent reactive oxygen species and protects against oxidative damage. J Dermatol Sci 56(3):154–162
23. Lin JY, Selim MA, Shea CR et al (2003) UV photoprotection by combination topical antioxidants vitamin C and vitamin E. J Am Acad Dermatol 48:866–874
24. Lucas D, Ke M, Matsui M, Maes D, Cooper K, Stevens S, Baron E (2008) Immune protective effect of a moisturizer with DNA repair ingredients. J Cosmet Dermatol 7:132–135

25. Maes D, Pernodet N, Mammone T et al (2010) Skin repair compositions comprising circadian gene activators and a synergistic combination of sirt 1 gene activators. US Patent Appl 20100028317
26. Menendez D, Shatz M, Azzam K et al (2011) The toll-like receptor gene family is integrated into human DNA damage and p53 networks. PLoS Genet 7:e1001360. doi:10.1371/journalpgen.1001360
27. Mitchell DL, Nairn RS (1989) The biology of the (6–4) photoproduct. Photochem Photobiol 49(6):805–819
28. Noonan FP, Zaidi MR, Wolnicka-Glubisz A, Anver MR, Bahn J, Wielgus A, Cadet J, Douki T, Mouret S, Tucker MA, Popratiloff A, Merlino G, De Fabo EC (2012) Melanoma induction by ultraviolet A but not ultraviolet B radiation requires melanin pigment. Nat Commun 3:884
29. Pellosi MC, Suzukawa AA, Scalfo AC, Di Mascio P, Martins Pereira CP, de Souza Pinto NC, de Luna Martins D, Martinez GR (2014) Effects of the melanin precursor 5,6-dihydroxy-indole-2-carboxylic acid (DHICA) on DNA damage and repair in the presence of reactive oxygen species. Arch Biochem Biophys 557:55–64
30. Pfeifer GP (1997) Formation and processing of UV photoproducts: effects of DNA sequence and chromatin environment. Photochem Photobiol 65(2):270–283
31. Pothof J, Verkaik N, van Ijcken W et al (2009) MicroRNA-mediated gene silencing modulates the UV-induced DNA-damage response. EMBO J 28:2090–2099
32. Premi S, Wallisch S, Mano C, Weiner A, Bacchiocchi A, Wakamatsu K, Bechara E, Halaban R, Douki T, Brash D (2015) Chemiexcitation of melanin derivatives induces DNA photoproducts long after UV exposure. Science 347:842–847
33. Rochette PJ, Therrien JP, Drouin R, Perdiz D, Bastien N, Drobetsky EA, Sage E (2003) UVA-induced cyclobutane pyrimidine dimers form predominantly at thymine-thymine dipyrimidines and correlate with the mutation spectrum in rodent cells. Nucleic Acids Res 31(11):2786–2794
34. Sancar A, Lindsey-Boltz L, Kang T-H et al (2010) Circadian clock control of the cellular response to DNA damage. FEBS Lett 584:2618–2625
35. Schuch AP, Yagura T, Makita K, Yamamoto H, Schuch NJ, Agnez-Lima LF, Macmahon RM, Menck CF (2012) DNA damage profiles induced by sunlight at different latitudes. Environ Mol Mutagen 53(3):198–206
36. Schwarz T, Schwarz A (2009) DNA repair and cytokine responses. J Investig Dermatol Symp Proc 14:63–66
37. Shah P, He Y (2014) Molecular regulation of UV-induced DNA repair. Photochem Photobiol. doi:10.1111/php.12406
38. Simon JD, Peles D, Wakamatsu K, Ito S (2009) Current challenges in understanding melanogenesis: bridging chemistry, biological control, morphology, and function. Pigment Cell Melanoma Res 22(5):563–579
39. Stege H, Roza L, Vink A et al (2000) Enzyme plus light therapy to repair DNA damage in ultraviolet-B-irradiated human skin. Proc Natl Acad Sci U S A 97:1790–1795
40. Thomson T, Guerra-Rebollo M (2010) Ubiquitin and SUMO signaling in DNA repair. Biochem Soc Trans 38:116–131
41. Tian Y, Liu W, Niu T, Dai C, Li X, Cui C, Zhao X, Yaping E, Lu H (2014) The injury and cumulative effects on human skin by UV exposure from artificial fluorescence emission. Photochem Photobiol 90(6):1433–1438
42. Tornaletti S, Rozek D, Pfeifer GP (1993) The distribution of UV photoproducts along the human p53 gene and its relation to mutations in skin cancer. Oncogene 8(8):2051–2057
43. Tung B, McGregor W, Wang Y, Maher V, McCormick J (1996) Comparison of the rate of excision of major UV photoproducts in the strands of the human HPRT gene of normal and xeroderma pigmentosum variant cells. Mutat Res 2:65–74
44. Wu C, Qiang L, Han W et al (2013) Role of AMPK in UVB-induced DNA damage repair and growth control. Oncogene 32:2682–2689
45. Wulff B, Schick J, Thomas-Ahner J et al (2008) Topical treatment with OGG1 enzyme affects UVB-induced skin carcinogenesis. Photochem Photobiol 84:317–321

46. Yarosh D (2002) Enhanced DNA repair of cyclobutane pyrimidine dimers changes the biological response to UV-B radiation. Mutat Res 509:221–226
47. Yarosh D, Alas L, Yee V et al (1992) Pyrimidine dimer removal enhanced by DNA repair liposomes reduces the incidence of UV skin cancer in mice. Cancer Res 52:4227–4231
48. Yarosh D, Klein J, O'Connor A, Hawk J, Rafal E, Wolf P (2001) Effect of topically applied T4 endonuclease V in liposomes on skin cancer in xeroderma pigmentosum: a randomized study. Lancet 357:926–929
49. Yoon JH, Lee CS, O'Connor TR, Yasui A, Pfeifer GP (2000) The DNA damage spectrum produced by simulated sunlight. J Mol Biol 299(3):681–693
50. Yu SH, Bordeaux JS, Baron ED (2014) The immune system and skin cancer. Adv Exp Med Biol 810:182–191

Chapter 22
Oral and Systemic Photoprotection

Salvador González, Yolanda Gilaberte, and Angeles Juarranz

Key Points

- Oral photoprotective agents could potentially be a suitable complement to topical sunscreen photoprotection.
- The effect of oral photoprotective agents is mainly systemic, by reducing photoinduced oxidation, skin photodamage, and photoaging.
- In addition to their photoprotective effect, some of these agents also have anticancer properties.
- Many botanical agents and formulations have antioxidant activity/properties that provide photoprotection through different mechanisms.
- Evaluation of the photoprotective effect of oral agents includes photoimmunoprotection, antimutagenic, and antioxidant activities.

S. González, MD, PhD (✉)
Medicine and Medical Specialities Department, Alcalá University, Madrid, Spain

Dermatology Service, Memorial Sloan-Kettering Cancer Center, New York, NY, USA

Instituto Ramón y Cajal de Investigación Sanitaria (IRYCIS), Madrid, Spain
e-mail: salvador.gonzalez@ifc.es; gonzals6@mskcc.org

Y. Gilaberte, MD, PhD
Dermatology Service, Hospital San Jorge, Huesca, Spain

A. Juarranz, PhD
Instituto Ramón y Cajal de Investigación Sanitaria (IRYCIS), Madrid, Spain

Biology Department, Universidad Autónoma de Madrid, Madrid, Spain

S.Q. Wang, H.W. Lim (eds.), *Principles and Practice of Photoprotection*,
DOI 10.1007/978-3-319-29382-0_22

22.1 Oral Photoprotective Agents

Photoprotection typically involves applying a thin layer of barrier agents to the skin prior to sun exposure. There are practical limitations with this approach, e.g., uneven and/or cumbersome application, short half-life on skin, potential side effect of the agents, lack of systemic efficiency, etc.

Oral photoprotectives do not protect the skin directly from high-energy photons; hence, they are not very efficient against solar-induced erythema. However, they are simple to take (usually as pills), their half-life can be determined pharmacologically, and they do have systemic effects. These products may contain one or several active substances that promote different mechanisms of photoprotection, particularly related to antioxidant activities [6, 7]. These mechanisms reload the antioxidant activities of the body after systemic loss of endogenous antioxidants during UV exposure [8, 9]. In many cases, oral photoprotective agents also downregulate UV-induced immunosuppression [10]. In the next sections, we provide an update on the best characteristics of these substances (Table 22.1).

22.1.1 Vitamin Derivatives

22.1.1.1 Carotenoids

They are plant pigments present in a wide array of vegetables and fruits, most notably tomato. Carotenoids are endowed with antioxidant activity. Although one study did not support their efficacy on skin photoprotection [11], a modest, dose-dependent photoprotective effect has been reported upon oral administration in another study [12].

The most represented carotenoid in tomato is lycopene. Lycopene displays a significant activity as a singlet oxygen scavenger. One study reported that 10–12-week treatment with oral lycopene (16 mg daily) renders subjects less prone to develop erythema in response to UV [13]. In addition, oral administration of a mixture of 2.5 mg lycopene, 4.7 mg beta-carotene, and 5×10^8 *Lactobacillus johnsonii* protected the development of UVA-induced polymorphous light eruption [14].

Other carotenoids, globally named xanthophylls, include astaxanthin, lutein, and zeaxanthin. These have been shown to prevent sun-induced erythema when administered orally, particularly in combination with topical administration of the same compounds [15]. Combined oral and topical administration of lutein and zeaxanthin provided higher degree of antioxidant protection that either one alone. Astaxanthin has been shown to inhibit the production of lipid peroxides and decrease the accumulation of polyamines induced by UVA photons [16].

Table 22.1 Oral and systemic photoprotective agents

Carotenoids
Lycopene
Xanthophylls
Nicotinamide
Combination of antioxidants:
Mixture of tocopherol and ascorbate
Mixture of lycopene, beta-carotene, alpha-tocopherol, and selenium
Seresis: carotenoids (β-carotene and lycopene), vitamins C and E, selenium, and proanthocyanidins
Dietary botanicals: Dietary flavonoids and phenolics
Green tea polyphenols
Polypodium leucotomos extract
Isoflavones
Genistein
Equol
Silymarin
Quercetin
Apigenin
Pomegranate
Citrus + rosemary extract
Cocoa extract
Resveratrol
Ferulic and caffeic acids
Pycnogenol
Sulforaphane
Forskolin
Cat's claw (*Uncaria tomentose)* extract
Fo-Ti (*Polygonum multiflorum*)
Dietary non-botanicals, and others:
ω-3 Polyunsaturated fatty acid
Probiotics
Idebenone
N-(4-pyridoxylmethylene)-l-serine
Cyclooxygenase 2 inhibitors
Afamelanotide (melanotan I)
Melanotan II

22.1.1.2 Nicotinamide

It is the amide version of vitamin B_3. It has proven useful for the management of acne, photoaging, and photoimmunosuppression. The underlying mechanism involves modulation of inflammatory cytokine expression and other enzymatic mechanisms related to DNA repair [17]. Oral administration of nicotinamide or niacin decreases photoinduced skin carcinogenesis and photoaging in mice and prevents photoimmunosuppression and development of actinic keratoses in humans [18, 19].

22.1.2 Antioxidant Combinations

22.1.2.1 Ascorbate + Tocopherol

These two vitamins with potent antioxidant properties are not photoprotective when used separately [20–22]. However, they enhance the photoprotective effects of each other [23, 24]. Furthermore, T opical application of combinations of both vitamins with melatonin also enhanced the photoprotective response against UV-induced erythema [25]. The mechanism of this synergy is unclear, but it may depend on the ability of ascorbate to reduce tocopherol, transferring the free radicals captured by the latter to the medium, where they are quenched by other antioxidant systems present in the skin [26].

22.1.2.2 Other Antioxidant Combinations

Daily oral administration of two tablets containing an antioxidant complex for 7 weeks reduced UV-induced lipoperoxide levels, sunburn, inflammation, and p53 expression; however, this combination increased pigmentation. Each tablet contains a combination of 3 mg of tomato lycopene, 3 mg of natural alpha and beta-carotene, 5 mg of alpha-tocopherol, and 37.5 mg of organic selenium incorporated in *Saccharomyces cerevisiae* in dry state [27].

22.1.2.3 Seresis®

It is a proprietary combination of natural antioxidants made from grape proanthocyanidins, carotenoids (β-carotene and lycopene), vitamins C and E, and selenium. Oral uptake of Seresis® retards the onset of UVB-mediated erythema and increased expression of matrix metalloproteinases [28].

22.1.3 Dietary Botanicals

This general term includes antioxidant and anti-inflammatory flavonoids and other phenolics found in vegetable foodstuffs. Flavonoids are the most important natural antioxidants due to their chemical nature, which contains phenolic rings that can absorb free radicals to form phenoxy radicals [29]. There are different subfamilies of flavonoids according to their chemical structure, including flavonols, flavones, flavanones, isoflavones, catechins, anthocyanidins, and chalcones. In the next pages, we discuss the merits of each of the major members of these subfamilies in terms of oral photoprotection [30].

22.1.3.1 Green Tea Polyphenols (GTPPs)

The major antioxidant moiety of green tea (*Camellia sinensis*) is a mixture of polyphenols derived from epicatechins, epicatechin (EC), epigallocatechin (EGC), epicatechin gallate (ECG), and epigallocatechin gallate (EGCG). The latter constitutes approximately 40 % of total GTPPs at the source (green tea leaves). Oral administration of GTPPs decreases UVB-induced tumorigenesis in normal and hairless mice [31, 32]. This effect is mainly based on their antioxidant properties: EGCG significantly reduces the production of lipid peroxides [33]. However, it also has additional protection mechanisms, including production of IL-12 and the subsequent activation of IL-12-dependent DNA repair machinery. This pathway undoes DNA damage in skin cells and skin-associated immune cells, e.g., Langerhans cells. GTPPs not only prevent the onset of DNA damage-related tumorigenesis but also enhance several active mechanisms of tumor rejection, e.g., they impair angiogenesis required for tumor cell feeding and also activate the cellular arm of adaptive immunity (CTL) to destroy tumor cells [31].

GTPPs also delay photoaging by preventing the UV-induced activation of the inflammatory transcription factors AP-1 and NF-κB [34]. They also inhibit MMP expression and reduce UV-mediated collagen cross-linking [34, 35].

There are several major limitations preventing the widespread use of GTPPs preparations. They are very sensitive to oxidation, quickly losing their activity. In fact, their half-life in the bloodstream is <3 h [36]. Another limitation is that they are poorly soluble in lipid preparations, which greatly limits their penetration through the skin [37], although it favors its oral uptake and absorption. Mixing GTPPs with nontoxic organic solvents, e.g., oleic acid, improves their stability and penetrance [38, 39]. However, its toxicity at high doses needs to be investigated [40].

22.1.3.2 *Polypodium leucotomos* Extract (Fernblock®)

Extracts made from leaves of the fern *Polypodium leucotomos* are rich in polyphenols. These antioxidant compounds are the molecular basis for the common use of *Polypodium leucotomos* extracts to treat inflammatory skin conditions in indigenous Central American cultures. In addition, these extracts can modulate immune phenomena in response to inflammatory insult, e.g., UV-induced sunburn. Fernblock® is active topically and orally. At a molecular level, it scavenges free radicals, e.g., singlet oxygen, hydroxyl, and superoxide, and prevents lipid peroxidation [41, 42]. Fernblock® enhances the function of endogenous antioxidant systems such as glutathione S-transferase (GST) [43], and it inhibits the isomerization and inactivation of *trans*-urocanic acid [44]; it also prevents oxidant DNA damage (8-hydroxyguanine) and accelerates the repair of damaged DNA, particularly T-T dimers [45], which underlies its ability to prevent immunosuppression [46]. Finally, Fernblock® prevents inflammation by inhibiting UV-induced expression of TNF-alpha and inducible nitric oxide synthase [47] and COX-2 [45].

The role of Fernblock® has been assessed in psoralen-UVA (PUVA) and UVB-induced changes [48–50]. In both cases, oral Fernblock® administration elevated the threshold of UV-induced tanning (melanogenic dose) and the minimum UV dose to cause erythema (erythematogenic dose) [28] . Beyond the new threshold, Fernblock® decreased the degree of erythema (i.e., the erythema vs. time slope was less steep), reduced the number of sunburn cells, and ameliorated skin immune cell depletion [51, 52]. A recent study described that oral administration of Fernblock® in a hairless mouse model delayed the onset of skin tumors and increases p53 expression in UV-irradiated skin [53].

Topical treatment with Fernblock® had comparable effects in skin sensitivity to UV radiation and immune depletion, with similar mechanisms involved, i.e., inhibition of oxidation and inflammation and immune protection. In addition, topical application assays have indicated anti-photoaging capability and long-term immune protection, including reduced elastosis and development of skin tumors in response to chronic exposure to UVB [54]. It has also been shown to decrease the development of polymorphous light eruption and solar urticaria [50].

22.1.3.3 Isoflavones

These are a subfamily of flavonoids molecularly similar to mammalian estrogen. Their ability to act as photoprotectors is a current topic of interest. Some isoflavones or isoflavone-rich compounds are:

Genistein: It is an isoflavone obtained from fermented soy, fava, and coffee beans. It is a potent tyrosine kinase inhibitor, and it is endowed with strong antioxidant capability [55]. A specific mechanism that involves the transcription factor Nrf2 is activated by low doses of oral genistein and is likely involved in its high oral tolerance [56, 57]. As a photoprotector, oral genistein inhibits UVB-mediated skin photoaging and skin tumor formation in a rodent model [58].

Equol: It is a metabolite from the genistein analog daidzein. It is naturally enriched in red clover (*Trifolium pratense*) [59]. Topically, equol confers protection against UV photons and decreases UV-induced tumorigenesis [60] and photoaging [61]. Although not tested as an oral photoprotector, a recent report indicates high oral tolerance [62], indicating its suitability for oral photoprotection assays.

Silymarin: It is a flavonoid enriched in the seeds of milk thistle (*Silybum marianum).* Silymarin contains three species: silybin, silydianin, and silychristin. Whereas its topical use confers photoprotection due to the silybin contained in the preparation [63], its oral use in photoprotection has not been assessed explicitly. Silymarin is an inhibitor of P-glycoprotein efflux pump [64] and modulates the bioavailability of other drugs [65], which may compromise its usefulness in oral photoprotection schemes.

Quercetin: It is a flavonoid mainly found in oak bark and many other vegetables and seeds. It is a very potent antioxidant with topical photoprotective effect [66], but it has not been assessed as an oral photoprotection agent. Similar to silymarin, it may affect the bioavailability of other drugs, e.g., paclitaxel [67], and it has an effect on DNA cleavage [68]. Hence, its potential as an oral photoprotector is controversial.

Apigenin: It is a flavonoid endowed with antitumor capability [69]. Topically, it decreases tumor emergence upon exposure to UV photons in a rodent model. This effect seems to be caused, at least in part, by inhibition of COX2 expression [70].

22.1.3.4 Pomegranate (*Punica granatum*, fam. Punicaceae)

The flesh, peel, and seeds of pomegranate contain high amounts of polyphenols, including catechins, anthocyanidins (e.g., delphinidin, cyanidin, and pelargonidin), and tannins. Pomegranate has a strong reputation as a natural antioxidant [71]. As an oral photoprotector, the Mukhtar group has described its efficacy in preventing photocarcinogenesis in a UVB-irradiated mouse model [72, 73].

22.1.3.5 Citrus + Rosemary Extract

Citrus contains a significant amount of flavonoids, whereas rosemary is high in polyphenols and diterpenes. Oral administration of a combination of citrus and rosemary extracts increased the minimal erythema dose in human patients [74]. Together with their lack of toxicity, this is a promising dietary complement with photoprotective ability.

22.1.3.6 Cocoa Extract

Cocoa (chocolate) extracts are rich in polyphenols, mainly flavanols. These molecules act as ROS scavengers, inhibitors of lipid peroxidation and endogenous oxidative enzymes, e.g., NADPH oxidase, and inducers of proteins involved in protection against stress such as Nrf2 (reviewed in [75]). Its efficacy in oral photoprotection has been demonstrated in humans. In controlled conditions, oral administration chocolate with high flavanol content decreased UV-mediated erythema appearance and other immediate effects of UV exposure [76].

22.1.3.7 Resveratrol

It is a polyphenolic phytoalexin found in the peels and seeds of grapes, nuts and fruits, and red wine. Its topical photoprotective effects are well documented [77]. Oral administration of resveratrol in a p53-sensitive mouse tumor model decreases the onset of UV-mediated tumorigenesis [78], and this effect is related to its ability to modulate TGF-beta [78] and NF-kB [79]. In addition, resveratrol boosts the response to radiation therapy in hyperproliferative, precancerous, and neoplastic conditions [80].

22.1.3.8 Ferulic and Caffeic Acids

Caffeic acid is a precursor of ferulic acid. Both belong to the family of hydroxycinnamic acids. They are generated during the biosynthesis of aromatic amino acids phenylalanine and tyrosine, and they are crucial intermediates of lignin synthesis that bind to complex polysaccharides, e.g., pectins, in plant surfaces.

Their topical use in photoprotection is well documented, particularly that of ferulic acid because it is more lipophilic than caffeic acid [81]. Ferulic acid not only exerts a direct antioxidant effect, but it also synergizes with vitamins C and E to double their photoprotective effect [82]. Their photoprotective effects by oral route have not been addressed explicitly. Previous evidence indicates that oral administration of plant extracts enriched in ferulic acid delays the onset of cancer [83], suggesting its efficacy in oral schemes.

22.1.3.9 Pycnogenol®

Pycnogenol is an extract of the bark of *Pinus pinaster Ait.* It is endowed with potent antioxidant, anti-inflammatory, and anticarcinogenic properties, but it has only been used topically to confer photoprotection [84].

22.1.3.10 Sulforaphane

It is an organosulfur compound from the isothyocyanate family commonly found in cruciferous vegetables, e.g., broccoli. Its role in oral chemoprevention is supported by its effect on the expression of phase II enzymes [85]. Oral treatment with sulforaphane decreases the appearance of skin tumors in a high-susceptibility rodent model [86] likely by inhibition of AP-1 activation [87], suggesting its potential in photoaging and the prevention of photoinduced carcinogenesis [88].

22.1.3.11 Forskolin

It is a terpene obtained from Indian coleus (*Coleus forskohlii*). It is a classic activator of the cAMP signaling pathway, and it also restores pigmentation in individuals suffering from missense mutations in the melanocortin-1 receptor, MC1R [89]. Long-term topical application is possible without significant side effects [90]. Forskolin also exerts its photoprotective effect by increasing epithelial thickening due to increased keratinocyte proliferation in a cAMP-dependent manner [91]. In vitro, forskolin protects keratinocytes from UV-induced apoptosis [92]. Oral administration of forskolin has been assessed for non-skin-related therapeutic uses, e.g., asthma [93] and cardiovascular disease [94].

22.1.3.12 Cat's Claw *(Uncaria tomentosa)* Extract

Cat's claw is a climbing plant indigenous from the Andes region. Water-soluble extracts from its leaves have displayed high efficacy in topical photoprotection assays, with a remarkable ability to enhance cyclobutyl pyrimidine dimer repair [95]. Orally, cat claw extracts have not been assayed for photoprotection, but it is well tolerated and decreases experimental endometriosis in a rodent model [96].

22.1.3.13 Fo-Ti (*Polygonum multiflorum*)

It is an extract from the root of *Polygonum multiflorum* (PM), with a long history in Traditional Chinese Medicine. It displays antibacterial, antifungal, and antiaging properties and has topical photoprotective effect [97]. However, its efficacy as an oral photoprotector remains to be determined.

22.1.4 Dietary Non-botanicals and Other Oral Photoprotective Agents

22.1.4.1 ω-3 Polyunsaturated Fatty Acid

Omega-3 fatty acids have limited photoprotective properties. They modestly decreased the appearance of sunburn cells and inflammation upon UV treatment as well as longer-term effects of UVA exposure [98]. Its main limitation as an oral photoprotector is that the dose required for this effect is likely larger than the gastric tolerance threshold; plus it has an unpleasant taste.

22.1.4.2 Probiotics

Probiotics are live microorganisms that when administered in adequate amounts confer a health benefit on the host. A nutritional supplement containing lycopene, beta-carotene, and *Lactobacillus johnsonii* reduced early UV-induced skin damage caused by simulated or natural sun exposure in humans; moreover, it provides protection against the development of UVA-induced polymorphous light eruption [99]. Oral administration of *Lactobacillus rhamnosus* GG significantly delays skin tumors appearance in mice chronically irradiated with ultraviolet radiation [100].

22.1.4.3 Idebenone

Idebenone is a more lipophilic analog of coenzyme Q10, which has higher skin penetrance. Idebenone alleviates the onset of UV-induced photoaging [101], although this is controversial [102]. Its efficacy as an oral photoprotector has not been addressed, but its oral administration increases nerve growth factor (NGF) production [103], and it is beneficial in patients with Leber's hereditary optic neuropathy [104].

22.1.4.4 N-(4-pyridoxylmethylene)-l-Serine (PYSer)

It is an iron quencher that inhibits metal-dependent ROS generation with significant effect in photoaging [105] but untested as an oral photoprotection agent.

22.1.4.5 Cyclooxygenase 2 (COX-2) Inhibitors

Chemical COX-2 inhibitors have potential as oral photoprotectors due to their strong anti-inflammatory effects, which include decreasing erythema and dermal neutrophil infiltration and activation, prostaglandin E2 (PGE_2) levels, and the appearance of sunburn cells [106]. However, their specific use as photoprotectors is unlikely due to their wide-ranging pharmacologic effects.

22.1.4.6 Afamelanotide (Melanotan I) and Melanotan II

These are synthetic analog of alpha-melanocyte-stimulating hormone (α-MSH), administered by subcutaneous injections. They promote melanogenesis [107]. Afamelanotide (melanotan I) (Nle4-D-Phe7), a linear molecule, has been shown to have photoprotective effects in clinical trials, including excellent photoprotective properties for erythropoietic protoporphyria and solar urticaria [108, 109]. Melanotan I should be distinguished from melanotan II, a cyclic variant which increases pigmentation at lower cumulative doses than melanotan I, but it also resulted in decreased appetite and increased libido. This is not part of any commercial or investigational formulation for human use, but it can be obtained illegally on the Internet and other sources [110] for tanning and cosmetic and recreational purposes [111]. Very recent studies report anecdotal coincidence of melanotan II use with the emergence of melanoma [112, 113].

22.2 Evaluating Oral Photoprotection

Non-topical forms of photoprotective agents cannot be evaluated using the SPF or erythema protection factor scales. However, other parameters used for topical sunscreens can be applied for oral photoprotection agents, including:

(i) Photoimmunoprotection: The oral treatment under evaluation can be assessed for UV-induced suppression of contact- or delayed-type hypersensitivity responses. This can be done using a unique sub-erythemal dose of UV radiation, which enables direct comparison with SPF, but it requires a large number of volunteers and is not cost-effective [114]. Alternatively, it can be done by using prior contact with specific chemical irritants. The major drawback is that this is not directly comparable to the effect of UV radiation, but it indicates whether the treatment modulates the ability of the immune system to respond to the insult.
(ii) Antimutagenic activity: This is being developed in nonhuman models. This parameter is assessed as the ability of the oral treatment to prevent mutations in key genes involved in the photocarcinogenic process, e.g., p53 [115].
(iii) Antioxidant activity: In vitro schemes including UVB irradiation of keratinocytes and subsequent staining for T-T dimers and sunburn cells could become the new standard in measuring the photoprotective ability of a new compound. Such measurements could be extended to in vitro antioxidant testing. Again, the major issue is that this cannot be extrapolated to the effect of oral administration directly (but it could be after appropriate in vivo measurements of bioavailability, tissue distribution, and half-life).

22.3 Future Perspectives

Non-topical photoprotection is a rapidly expanding field that still lacks gold standards and is vulnerable to counterfeit and fraud (e.g., the current situation with the distribution and effect of melanotan II). But the premise of non-topical, especially oral, photoprotection holds undeniable promise. Of course, oral photoprotective agents are not meant to completely substitute topical photoprotection. Although some substances, e.g., forskolin, increase epidermal thickening, UV irradiation of the skin will always damage unprotected cells. Oral supplementation is aimed at countering the long-term effects of sun exposure, which are more related to immunosuppression, chronic inflammation, and photocarcinogenesis. Our current view is that the field strongly needs standardization for the assessment of the effectiveness of oral photoprotection, particularly measurements of antioxidant activity. Active involvement of regulatory agencies, e.g., FDA, will help with the establishment of gold standards and more research on the myriad of new substances and combinations of substances that will likely change the landscape of photoprotection in the next 20 years.

References

1. Seite S, Colige A, Piquemal-Vivenot P, Montastier C, Fourtanier A, Lapiere C et al (2000) A full-UV spectrum absorbing daily use cream protects human skin against biological changes occurring in photoaging. Photodermatol Photoimmunol Photomed 16(4):147–155
2. Moyal D (1998) Immunosuppression induced by chronic ultraviolet irradiation in humans and its prevention by sunscreens. Eur J Dermatol 8(3):209–211
3. van der Pols JC, Xu C, Boyle GM, Parsons PG, Whiteman DC, Green AC (2006) Expression of p53 tumor suppressor protein in sun-exposed skin and associations with sunscreen use and time spent outdoors: a community-based study. Am J Epidemiol 163(11):982–988
4. Al Mahroos M, Yaar M, Phillips TJ, Bhawan J, Gilchrest BA (2002) Effect of sunscreen application on UV-induced thymine dimers. Arch Dermatol 138(11):1480–1485
5. Bernerd F, Vioux C, Asselineau D (2000) Evaluation of the protective effect of sunscreens on in vitro reconstructed human skin exposed to UVB or UVA irradiation. Photochem Photobiol 71(3):314–320
6. Fernandez-Garcia E (2014) Skin protection against UV light by dietary antioxidants. Food Funct 5(9):1994–2003
7. Chen AC, Damian DL, Halliday GM (2014) Oral and systemic photoprotection. Photodermatol Photoimmunol Photomed 30(2–3):102–111
8. Pattison DI, Davies MJ (2006) Actions of ultraviolet light on cellular structures. EXS 96:131–157
9. DeBuys HV, Levy SB, Murray JC, Madey DL, Pinnell SR (2000) Modern approaches to photoprotection. Dermatol Clin 18(4):577–590
10. Pilkington SM, Gibbs NK, Friedmann PS, Rhodes LE (2014) Nutritional abrogation of photoimmunosuppression: in vivo investigations. Photodermatol Photoimmunol Photomed 30(2–3):112–127
11. Garmyn M, Ribaya-Mercado JD, Russel RM, Bhawan J, Gilchrest BA (1995) Effect of beta-carotene supplementation on the human sunburn reaction. Exp Dermatol 4(2):104–111
12. Biesalski HK, Obermueller-Jevic UC (2001) UV light, beta-carotene and human skin – beneficial and potentially harmful effects. Arch Biochem Biophys 389(1):1–6
13. Stahl W, Heinrich U, Aust O, Tronnier H, Sies H (2006) Lycopene-rich products and dietary photoprotection. Photochem Photobiol Sci 5(2):238–242
14. Marini A, Jaenicke T, Grether-Beck S, Le Floc'h C, Cheniti A, Piccardi N et al (2014) Prevention of polymorphic light eruption by oral administration of a nutritional supplement containing lycopene, beta-carotene, and Lactobacillus johnsonii: results from a randomized, placebo-controlled, double-blinded study. Photodermatol Photoimmunol Photomed 30(4):189–194
15. Palombo P, Fabrizi G, Ruocco V, Ruocco E, Fluhr J, Roberts R et al (2007) Beneficial long-term effects of combined oral/topical antioxidant treatment with the carotenoids lutein and zeaxanthin on human skin: a double-blind, placebo-controlled study. Skin Pharmacol Physiol 20(4):199–210
16. Goto S, Kogure K, Abe K, Kimata Y, Kitahama K, Yamashita E et al (2001) Efficient radical trapping at the surface and inside the phospholipid membrane is responsible for highly potent antiperoxidative activity of the carotenoid astaxanthin. Biochim Biophys Acta 1512(2):251–258
17. Surjana D, Damian DL (2011) Nicotinamide in dermatology and photoprotection. Skinmed 9(6):360–365

18. Gensler HL, Williams T, Huang AC, Jacobson EL (1999) Oral niacin prevents photocarcinogenesis and photoimmunosuppression in mice. Nutr Cancer 34(1):36–41
19. Surjana D, Halliday GM, Martin AJ, Moloney FJ, Damian DL (2012) Oral nicotinamide reduces actinic keratoses in phase II double-blinded randomized controlled trials. J Invest Dermatol 132(5):1497–1500
20. Fuchs J, Kern H (1998) Modulation of UV-light-induced skin inflammation by D-alpha-tocopherol and L-ascorbic acid: a clinical study using solar simulated radiation. Free Radic Biol Med 25(9):1006–1012
21. McArdle F, Rhodes LE, Parslew R, Jack CI, Friedmann PS, Jackson MJ (2002) UVR-induced oxidative stress in human skin in vivo: effects of oral vitamin C supplementation. Free Radic Biol Med 33(10):1355–1362
22. McArdle F, Rhodes LE, Parslew RA, Close GL, Jack CI, Friedmann PS et al (2004) Effects of oral vitamin E and beta carotene supplementation on ultraviolet radiation-induced oxidative stress in human skin. Am J Clin Nutr 80(5):1270–1275
23. Eberlein-Konig B, Ring J (2005) Relevance of vitamins C and E in cutaneous photoprotection. J Cosmet Dermatol 4(1):4–9
24. Zussman J, Ahdout J, Kim J (2010) Vitamins and photoaging: do scientific data support their use? J Am Acad Dermatol 63(3):507–525
25. Dreher F, Gabard B, Schwindt DA, Maibach HI (1998) Topical melatonin in combination with vitamins E and C protects skin from ultraviolet-induced erythema: a human study in vivo. Br J Dermatol 139(2):332–339
26. Wefers H, Sies H (1988) The protection by ascorbate and glutathione against microsomal lipid peroxidation is dependent on vitamin E. Eur J Biochem 174(2):353–357
27. Cesarini JP, Michel L, Maurette JM, Adhoute H, Bejot M (2003) Immediate effects of UV radiation on the skin: modification by an antioxidant complex containing carotenoids. Photodermatol Photoimmunol Photomed 19(4):182–189
28. Greul AK, Grundmann JU, Heinrich F, Pfitzner I, Bernhardt J, Ambach A et al (2002) Photoprotection of UV-irradiated human skin: an antioxidative combination of vitamins E and C, carotenoids, selenium and proanthocyanidins. Skin Pharmacol Appl Skin Physiol 15(5):307–315
29. Graf E (1992) Antioxidant potential of ferulic acid. Free Radic Biol Med 13(4):435–448
30. Agati G, Brunetti C, Di Ferdinando M, Ferrini F, Pollastri S, Tattini M (2013) Functional roles of flavonoids in photoprotection: new evidence, lessons from the past. Plant Physiol Biochem 72:35–45
31. Katiyar S, Elmets CA, Katiyar SK (2007) Green tea and skin cancer: photoimmunology, angiogenesis and DNA repair. J Nutr Biochem 18(5):287–296
32. Elmets CA, Singh D, Tubesing K, Matsui M, Katiyar S, Mukhtar H (2001) Cutaneous photoprotection from ultraviolet injury by green tea polyphenols. J Am Acad Dermatol 44(3):425–432
33. Lee SR, Im KJ, Suh SI, Jung JG (2003) Protective effect of green tea polyphenol (−)-epigallocatechin gallate and other antioxidants on lipid peroxidation in gerbil brain homogenates. Phytother Res 17(3):206–209
34. Rutter K, Sell DR, Fraser N, Obrenovich M, Zito M, Starke-Reed P et al (2003) Green tea extract suppresses the age-related increase in collagen crosslinking and fluorescent products in C57BL/6 mice. Int J Vitam Nutr Res 73(6):453–460
35. Vayalil PK, Mittal A, Hara Y, Elmets CA, Katiyar SK (2004) Green tea polyphenols prevent ultraviolet light-induced oxidative damage and matrix metalloproteinases expression in mouse skin. J Invest Dermatol 122(6):1480–1487
36. Kim S, Lee MJ, Hong J, Li C, Smith TJ, Yang GY et al (2000) Plasma and tissue levels of tea catechins in rats and mice during chronic consumption of green tea polyphenols. Nutr Cancer 37(1):41–48
37. Farris P (2007) Idebenone, green tea, and Coffeeberry extract: new and innovative antioxidants. Dermatol Ther 20(5):322–329
38. Dvorakova K, Dorr RT, Valcic S, Timmermann B, Alberts DS (1999) Pharmacokinetics of the green tea derivative, EGCG, by the topical route of administration in mouse and human skin. Cancer Chemother Pharmacol 43(4):331–335

39. Nwuha V, Nakajima M, Tong J, Ichikawa S (1999) Solubility study of green tea extracts in pure solvents and edible oils. J Food Eng 40(3):161–165
40. Hsu S (2005) Green tea and the skin. J Am Acad Dermatol 52(6):1049–1059
41. Gonzalez S, Pathak MA (1996) Inhibition of ultraviolet-induced formation of reactive oxygen species, lipid peroxidation, erythema and skin photosensitization by *Polypodium leucotomos*. Photodermatol Photoimmunol Photomed 12:45–56
42. Gomes AJ, Lunardi CN, Gonzalez S, Tedesco AC (2001) The antioxidant action of Polypodium leucotomos extract and kojic acid: reactions with reactive oxygen species. Braz J Med Biol Res 34(11):1487–1494
43. Mulero M, Rodriguez-Yanes E, Nogues MR, Giralt M, Romeu M, Gonzalez S et al (2008) Polypodium leucotomos extract inhibits glutathione oxidation and prevents Langerhans cell depletion induced by UVB/UVA radiation in a hairless rat model. Exp Dermatol 17:653–658
44. Capote R, Alonso-Lebrero JL, Garcia F, Brieva A, Pivel JP, Gonzalez S (2006) Polypodium leucotomos extract inhibits trans-urocanic acid photoisomerization and photodecomposition. J Photochem Photobiol B 82(3):173–179
45. Zattra E, Coleman C, Arad S, Helms E, Levine D, Bord E et al (2009) Oral polypodium leucotomos decreases UV-induced Cox-2 expression, inflammation, and enhances DNA repair in Xpc +/− mice. Am J Pathol 175:1952–1961
46. Siscovick JR, Zapolanski T, Magro C, Carrington K, Prograis S, Nussbaum M et al (2008) Polypodium leucotomos inhibits ultraviolet B radiation-induced immunosuppression. Photodermatol Photoimmunol Photomed 24(3):134–141
47. Janczyk A, Garcia-Lopez MA, Fernandez-Penas P, Alonso-Lebrero JL, Benedicto I, Lopez-Cabrera M et al (2007) A Polypodium leucotomos extract inhibits solar-simulated radiation-induced TNF-alpha and iNOS expression, transcriptional activation and apoptosis. Exp Dermatol 16(10):823–829
48. Nestor M, Bucay V, Callender V, Cohen JL, Sadick N, Waldorf H (2014) Polypodium leucotomos as an adjunct treatment of pigmentary disorders. J Clin Aesthet Dermatol 7(3):13–17
49. Gonzalez S, Gilaberte Y, Philips N (2010) Mechanistic insights in the use of a Polypodium leucotomos extract as an oral and topical photoprotective agent. Photochem Photobiol Sci 9(4):559–563
50. Choudhry S, Bhatia N, Ceilley R, Hougeir F, Lieberman R, Hamzavi I, Lim HW (2014) Role of oral polypodium leucotomos extract in dermatologic diseases: a review of the literature. J Drugs Dermatol 13(2):148–153
51. Middelkamp-Hup MA, Pathak MA, Parrado C, Garcia-Caballero T, Rius-Diaz F, Fitzpatrick TB et al (2004) Orally administered Polypodium leucotomos extract decreases psoralen-UVA-induced phototoxicity, pigmentation, and damage of human skin. J Am Acad Dermatol 50(1):41–49
52. Middelkamp-Hup MA, Pathak MA, Parrado C, Goukassian D, Rius-Diaz F, Mihm MC et al (2004) Oral Polypodium leucotomos extract decreases ultraviolet-induced damage of human skin. J Am Acad Dermatol 51(6):910–918
53. Rodriguez-Yanes E, Cuevas J, Gonzalez S, Mallol J (2014) Oral administration of Polypodium leucotomos delays skin tumor development and increases epidermal p53 expression and the anti-oxidant status of UV-irradiated hairless mice. Exp Dermatol 23(7):526–528
54. Alcaraz MV, Pathak MA, Rius F, Kollias N, González S (1999) An extract of *Polypodium leucotomos* appears to minimize certain photoaging changes in a hairless albino mouse animal model. Photodermatol Photoimmunol Photomed 15:120–126
55. Messina MJ, Persky V, Setchell KD, Barnes S (1994) Soy intake and cancer risk: a review of the in vitro and in vivo data. Nutr Cancer 21(2):113–131
56. Zhang T, Wang F, Xu HX, Yi L, Qin Y, Chang H et al (2013) Activation of nuclear factor erythroid 2-related factor 2 and PPARgamma plays a role in the genistein-mediated attenuation of oxidative stress-induced endothelial cell injury. Br J Nutr 109(2):223–235
57. Zhai X, Lin M, Zhang F, Hu Y, Xu X, Li Y et al (2013) Dietary flavonoid genistein induces Nrf2 and phase II detoxification gene expression via ERKs and PKC pathways and protects against oxidative stress in Caco-2 cells. Mol Nutr Food Res 57(2):249–259

58. Wei H, Saladi R, Lu Y, Wang Y, Palep SR, Moore J et al (2003) Isoflavone genistein: photoprotection and clinical implications in dermatology. J Nutr 133(11 Suppl 1):3811S–3819S
59. Widyarini S, Spinks N, Husband AJ, Reeve VE (2001) Isoflavonoid compounds from red clover (Trifolium pratense) protect from inflammation and immune suppression induced by UV radiation. Photochem Photobiol 74(3):465–470
60. Widyarini S, Husband AJ, Reeve VE (2005) Protective effect of the isoflavonoid equol against hairless mouse skin carcinogenesis induced by UV radiation alone or with a chemical cocarcinogen. Photochem Photobiol 81(1):32–37
61. Reeve VE, Widyarini S, Domanski D, Chew E, Barnes K (2005) Protection against photoaging in the hairless mouse by the isoflavone equol. Photochem Photobiol 81(6):1548–1553
62. Schwen RJ, Nguyen L, Plomley JB, Jackson RL (2012) Toxicokinetics and lack of uterotropic effect of orally administered S-equol. Food Chem Toxicol 50(5):1741–1748
63. Pinnell SR (2003) Cutaneous photodamage, oxidative stress, and topical antioxidant protection. J Am Acad Dermatol 48(1):1–19; quiz 20–22
64. Crocenzi FA, Basiglio CL, Perez LM, Portesio MS, Pozzi EJ, Roma MG (2005) Silibinin prevents cholestasis-associated retrieval of the bile salt export pump, Bsep, in isolated rat hepatocyte couplets: possible involvement of cAMP. Biochem Pharmacol 69(7):1113–1120
65. Park JH, Park JH, Hur HJ, Woo JS, Lee HJ (2012) Effects of silymarin and formulation on the oral bioavailability of paclitaxel in rats. Eur J Pharm Sci 45(3):296–301
66. Casagrande R, Georgetti SR, Verri WA Jr, Dorta DJ, dos Santos AC, Fonseca MJ (2006) Protective effect of topical formulations containing quercetin against UVB-induced oxidative stress in hairless mice. J Photochem Photobiol B 84(1):21–27
67. Choi JS, Jo BW, Kim YC (2004) Enhanced paclitaxel bioavailability after oral administration of paclitaxel or prodrug to rats pretreated with quercetin. Eur J Pharm Biopharm 57(2):313–318
68. Robinson MJ, Corbett AH, Osheroff N (1993) Effects of topoisomerase II-targeted drugs on enzyme-mediated DNA cleavage and ATP hydrolysis: evidence for distinct drug interaction domains on topoisomerase II. Biochemistry 32(14):3638–3643
69. Torkın R, Lavoie JF, Kaplan DR, Yeger H (2005) Induction of caspase-dependent, p53-mediated apoptosis by apigenin in human neuroblastoma. Mol Cancer Ther 4(1):1–11
70. Tong X, Van Dross RT, Abu-Yousif A, Morrison AR, Pelling JC (2007) Apigenin prevents UVB-induced cyclooxygenase 2 expression: coupled mRNA stabilization and translational inhibition. Mol Cell Biol 27(1):283–296
71. Afaq F, Mukhtar H (2006) Botanical antioxidants in the prevention of photocarcinogenesis and photoaging. Exp Dermatol 15(9):678–684
72. Afaq F, Saleem M, Krueger CG, Reed JD, Mukhtar H (2005) Anthocyanin- and hydrolyzable tannin-rich pomegranate fruit extract modulates MAPK and NF-kappaB pathways and inhibits skin tumorigenesis in CD-1 mice. Int J Cancer 113(3):423–433
73. Afaq F, Khan N, Syed DN, Mukhtar H (2010) Oral feeding of pomegranate fruit extract inhibits early biomarkers of UVB radiation-induced carcinogenesis in SKH-1 hairless mouse epidermis. Photochem Photobiol 86(6):1318–1326
74. Perez-Sanchez A, Barrajon-Catalan E, Caturla N, Castillo J, Benavente-Garcia O, Alcaraz M et al (2014) Protective effects of citrus and rosemary extracts on UV-induced damage in skin cell model and human volunteers. J Photochem Photobiol B 136:12–18
75. Scapagnini G, Davinelli S, Di Renzo L, De Lorenzo A, Olarte HH, Micali G et al (2014) Cocoa bioactive compounds: significance and potential for the maintenance of skin health. Nutrients 6(8):3202–3213
76. Heinrich U, Neukam K, Tronnier H, Sies H, Stahl W (2006) Long-term ingestion of high flavanol cocoa provides photoprotection against UV-induced erythema and improves skin condition in women. J Nutr 136(6):1565–1569
77. Flamini R, Mattivi F, De Rosso M, Arapitsas P, Bavaresco L (2013) Advanced knowledge of three important classes of grape phenolics: anthocyanins, stilbenes and flavonols. Int J Mol Sci 14(10):19651–19669
78. Kim KH, Back JH, Zhu Y, Arbesman J, Athar M, Kopelovich L et al (2011) Resveratrol targets transforming growth factor-beta2 signaling to block UV-induced tumor progression. J Invest Dermatol 131(1):195–202

79. Adhami VM, Afaq F, Ahmad N (2003) Suppression of ultraviolet B exposure-mediated activation of NF-kappaB in normal human keratinocytes by resveratrol. Neoplasia 5(1):74–82
80. Reagan-Shaw S, Mukhtar H, Ahmad N (2008) Resveratrol imparts photoprotection of normal cells and enhances the efficacy of radiation therapy in cancer cells. Photochem Photobiol 84(2):415–421
81. Saija A, Tomaino A, Trombetta D, De Pasquale A, Uccella N, Barbuzzi T et al (2000) In vitro and in vivo evaluation of caffeic and ferulic acids as topical photoprotective agents. Int J Pharm 199(1):39–47
82. Lin FH, Lin JY, Gupta RD, Tournas JA, Burch JA, Selim MA et al (2005) Ferulic acid stabilizes a solution of vitamins C and E and doubles its photoprotection of skin. J Invest Dermatol 125(4):826–832
83. Nair SC, Panikkar B, Akamanchi KG, Panikkar KR (1991) Inhibitory effects of Ixora javanica extract on skin chemical carcinogenesis in mice and its antitumour activity. Cancer Lett 60(3):253–258
84. Sime S, Reeve VE (2004) Protection from inflammation, immunosuppression and carcinogenesis induced by UV radiation in mice by topical Pycnogenol. Photochem Photobiol 79(2):193–198
85. Cheung KL, Kong AN (2010) Molecular targets of dietary phenethyl isothiocyanate and sulforaphane for cancer chemoprevention. AAPS J 12(1):87–97
86. Dinkova-Kostova AT, Jenkins SN, Fahey JW, Ye L, Wehage SL, Liby KT et al (2006) Protection against UV-light-induced skin carcinogenesis in SKH-1 high-risk mice by sulforaphane-containing broccoli sprout extracts. Cancer Lett 240(2):243–252
87. Dickinson SE, Melton TF, Olson ER, Zhang J, Saboda K, Bowden GT (2009) Inhibition of activator protein-1 by sulforaphane involves interaction with cysteine in the cFos DNA-binding domain: implications for chemoprevention of UVB-induced skin cancer. Cancer Res 69(17):7103–7110
88. Dinkova-Kostova AT (2008) Phytochemicals as protectors against ultraviolet radiation: versatility of effects and mechanisms. Planta Med 74(13):1548–1559
89. D'Orazio JA, Nobuhisa T, Cui R, Arya M, Spry M, Wakamatsu K et al (2006) Topical drug rescue strategy and skin protection based on the role of Mc1r in UV-induced tanning. Nature 443(7109):340–344
90. Spry ML, Vanover JC, Scott T, Abona-Ama O, Wakamatsu K, Ito S et al (2009) Prolonged treatment of fair-skinned mice with topical forskolin causes persistent tanning and UV protection. Pigment Cell Melanoma Res 22(2):219–229
91. Scott TL, Christian PA, Kesler MV, Donohue KM, Shelton B, Wakamatsu K et al (2012) Pigment-independent cAMP-mediated epidermal thickening protects against cutaneous UV injury by keratinocyte proliferation. Exp Dermatol 21(10):771–777
92. Passeron T, Namiki T, Passeron HJ, Le Pape E, Hearing VJ (2009) Forskolin protects keratinocytes from UVB-induced apoptosis and increases DNA repair independent of its effects on melanogenesis. J Invest Dermatol 129(1):162–166
93. Gonzalez-Sanchez R, Trujillo X, Trujillo-Hernandez B, Vasquez C, Huerta M, Elizalde A (2006) Forskolin versus sodium cromoglycate for prevention of asthma attacks: a single-blinded clinical trial. J Int Med Res 34(2):200–207
94. Bristow MR, Ginsburg R, Strosberg A, Montgomery W, Minobe W (1984) Pharmacology and inotropic potential of forskolin in the human heart. J Clin Invest 74(1):212–223
95. Emanuel P, Scheinfeld N (2007) A review of DNA repair and possible DNA-repair adjuvants and selected natural anti-oxidants. Dermatol Online J 13(3):10
96. Nogueira Neto J, Coelho TM, Aguiar GC, Carvalho LR, de Araujo AG, Girao MJ et al (2011) Experimental endometriosis reduction in rats treated with Uncaria tomentosa (cat's claw) extract. Eur J Obstet Gynecol Reprod Biol 154(2):205–208
97. Hwang IK, Yoo KY, Kim DW, Jeong SJ, Won CK, Moon WK et al (2006) An extract of Polygonum multiflorum protects against free radical damage induced by ultraviolet B irradiation of the skin. Braz J Med Biol Res 39(9):1181–1188

98. Rhodes LE, O'Farrell S, Jackson MJ, Friedmann PS (1994) Dietary fish-oil supplementation in humans reduces UVB-erythemal sensitivity but increases epidermal lipid peroxidation. J Invest Dermatol 103(2):151–154
99. Bouilly-Gauthier D, Jeannes C, Maubert Y, Duteil L, Queille-Roussel C, Piccardi N et al (2010) Clinical evidence of benefits of a dietary supplement containing probiotic and carotenoids on ultraviolet-induced skin damage. Br J Dermatol 163(3):536–543
100. Weill FS, Cela EM, Paz ML, Ferrari A, Leoni J, Gonzalez Maglio DH (2013) Lipoteichoic acid from Lactobacillus rhamnosus GG as an oral photoprotective agent against UV-induced carcinogenesis. Br J Nutr 109(3):457–466
101. McDaniel D, Neudecker B, Dinardo J, Lewis J 2nd, Maibach H (2005) Clinical efficacy assessment in photodamaged skin of 0.5% and 1.0% idebenone. J Cosmet Dermatol 4(3):167–173
102. Tournas JA, Lin FH, Burch JA, Selim MA, Monteiro-Riviere NA, Zielinski JE et al (2006) Ubiquinone, idebenone, and kinetin provide ineffective photoprotection to skin when compared to a topical antioxidant combination of vitamins C and E with ferulic acid. J Invest Dermatol 126(5):1185–1187
103. Takeuchi R, Murase K, Furukawa Y, Furukawa S, Hayashi K (1990) Stimulation of nerve growth factor synthesis/secretion by 1,4-benzoquinone and its derivatives in cultured mouse astroglial cells. FEBS Lett 261(1):63–66
104. Klopstock T, Yu-Wai-Man P, Dimitriadis K, Rouleau J, Heck S, Bailie M et al (2011) A randomized placebo-controlled trial of idebenone in Leber's hereditary optic neuropathy. Brain 134(Pt 9):2677–2686
105. Kitazawa M, Ishitsuka Y, Kobayashi M, Nakano T, Iwasaki K, Sakamoto K et al (2005) Protective effects of an antioxidant derived from serine and vitamin B6 on skin photoaging in hairless mice. Photochem Photobiol 81(4):970–974
106. Fischer SM, Lo HH, Gordon GB, Seibert K, Kelloff G, Lubet RA et al (1999) Chemopreventive activity of celecoxib, a specific cyclooxygenase-2 inhibitor, and indomethacin against ultraviolet light-induced skin carcinogenesis. Mol Carcinog 25(4):231–240
107. Dorr RT, Lines R, Levine N, Brooks C, Xiang L, Hruby VJ et al (1996) Evaluation of melanotan-II, a superpotent cyclic melanotropic peptide in a pilot phase I clinical study. Life Sci 58(20):1777–1784
108. Fabrikant J, Touloei K, Brown SM (2013) A review and update on melanocyte stimulating hormone therapy: afamelanotide. J Drugs Dermatol 12(7):775–779
109. Biolcati G, Marchesini E, Sorge F, Barbieri L, Schneider-Yin X, Minder EI (2014) Long-term observational study of afamelanotide in 115 patients with erythropoietic protoporphyria. Br J Dermatol 172(6):1601–1612
110. Langan EA, Nie Z, Rhodes LE (2010) Melanotropic peptides: more than just 'Barbie drugs' and 'sun-tan jabs'? Br J Dermatol 163(3):451–455
111. Wessells H, Fuciarelli K, Hansen J, Hadley ME, Hruby VJ, Dorr R et al (1998) Synthetic melanotropic peptide initiates erections in men with psychogenic erectile dysfunction: double-blind, placebo controlled crossover study. J Urol 160(2):389–393
112. Hjuler KF, Lorentzen HF (2014) Melanoma associated with the use of melanotan-II. Dermatology 228(1):34–36
113. Ong S, Bowling J (2012) Melanotan-associated melanoma in situ. Australas J Dermatol 53(4):301–302
114. Fourtanier A, Moyal D, Maccario J, Compan D, Wolf P, Quehenberger F et al (2005) Measurement of sunscreen immune protection factors in humans: a consensus paper. J Invest Dermatol 125(3):403–409
115. Maier T, Korting HC (2005) Sunscreens – which and what for? Skin Pharmacol Physiol 18(6):253–262

Chapter 23
Photoprotection from Sunless Tanning Products and Colored Cosmetics

Zoe Diana Draelos

Photoprotection is traditionally associated with the use of sunscreens and physical objects, such as clothing, sunglasses, hats, umbrellas, scarves, etc., together with behavioral modification by seeking shade, While these are some of the most effective methods of protecting the skin from the damaging UV radiation produced by the sun, there are other creative methods of obtaining sun protection from products that are not traditionally considered. These alternatives include sunless tanning products and colored cosmetics. While these are not a substitute for sunscreens and protective clothing, they might be a useful addition to a sun-protective regimen and are worth discussing for their additive effect. Both products are used primarily to adorn the body through creating a colored cover over the skin and are classified as cosmetics from a regulatory standpoint in the USA.

This chapter will examine the use of sunless tanning products and cosmetics as sun protection adjuvants, discussing their history, chemistry, safety, and utility for photoprotection.

23.1 Photoprotection and Sunless Tanning Products

Sunless tanning products are an interesting cosmetic category because application of the cream simulates the tan achieved with sun exposure. While the primary reason to use sunless tanning products is to achieve tan without exposure to the sun, the active agent in sunless tanning products, known as dihydroxyacetone (Fig. 23.1), was an active listed on the sunscreen monograph for many years.

Z.D. Draelos, MD
Department of Dermatology, Duke University School of Medicine,
2444 North Main Street, Durham, NC 27262, USA
e-mail: zdraelos@northstate.net

S.Q. Wang, H.W. Lim (eds.), *Principles and Practice of Photoprotection*,
DOI 10.1007/978-3-319-29382-0_23

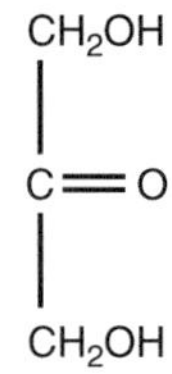

Fig. 23.1 Chemical structure of dihydroxyacetone (DHA) is structurally a sugar

Dihydroxyacetone, abbreviated DHA, was originally synthesized in the 1920s but rediscovered by Eva Wittgenstein, MD, in 1957 while she was studying orally administered DHA on childhood glycogen storage diseases. She observed that the children developed skin browning where the brown saliva contacted the skin. She subsequently applied the liquid to her own skin and noticed the "tanned" color. The product was commercialized in 1959 as a successful shaving lotion, known as "Man-Tan" [1].

23.1.1 Chemistry of DHA

DHA is the active agent in all presently marketed sunless tanning products and is a 3-carbon sugar appearing as a white, crystalline hygroscopic powder. DHA is formed when glycerol is fermented by *Gluconobacter oxydans*. It interacts with amino acids, peptides, and proteins to form chromophores known as melanoidins [2]. Melanoidins structurally have some similarities to skin melanin, but are not able to function as electron donors to reactive oxygen species [3]. Tanning occurs when melanin becomes oxidized, a reaction that cannot occur with DHA.

DHA interacts with the stratum corneum to form the melanoidins as the entire brown color can be removed by tape stripping the skin. No DHA is found in the viable epidermis or dermis after topical application accounting for its systemic safety profile. Thus, the thicker the stratum corneum, the more deeply the skin will pigment. For this reason, the brown is less intense on the face where the stratum corneum is thin and more intense on the elbows and knees where the stratum corneum is thicker. It also produces a much darker stain on the palms and the soles, areas that do not normally tan.

In addition to the thickness of the stratum corneum, the color produced by DHA is controlled by skin pH and the pH of the sunless tanning product. If the skin or the formulation is alkaline, the DHA color will be more orange. Conversely, if the skin or the formulation is acidic, the DHA color will be pinkish yielding a more natural appearance. For this reason, manufacturers typically formulate their products at a pH of 5–6 to yield the best color development.

The amount of water in the formulation can also affect the sunless tanning product color. If too much water is present, the DHA color development will be less as the water inhibits the melanoidin formation. For this reason, DHA products are not formulated with glycerin, which is a humectant capable of attracting water. Instead the DHA is placed in a propylene glycol and sorbitol vehicle to increase melanoidin formation and the intensity of the stain produced.

23.1.2 Melanoidins and the Maillard Reaction

The reaction that occurs on the skin surface creating the melanoidins, which yield the simulated tan color, is known as the Maillard reaction (Fig. 23.2). The Maillard reaction occurs when a protein binds to a sugar. Thus, the keratin protein of the skin reacts with the sugar DHA to create the browning reaction [4]. DHA is technically categorized as a colorant or colorless dye. It reacts with amines, peptides, and free amino acids in the stratum corneum. The first step is the conversion of DHA to pyruvaldehyde with the elimination of water. Then the ketone or aldehyde interacts with skin keratin to form an imine [5]. The remaining specifics of the reaction are still unknown, but the resulting products are cyclic and linear polymers that have a yellow or brown color.

The chemical reaction is usually visible within 1 h after DHA application, but maximal darkening may take 8–24 h [6]. Many sunless tanning products contain a temporary dye to allow the user to note the sites of application and to promote even application, but this immediate color should not be confused with the Maillard reaction.

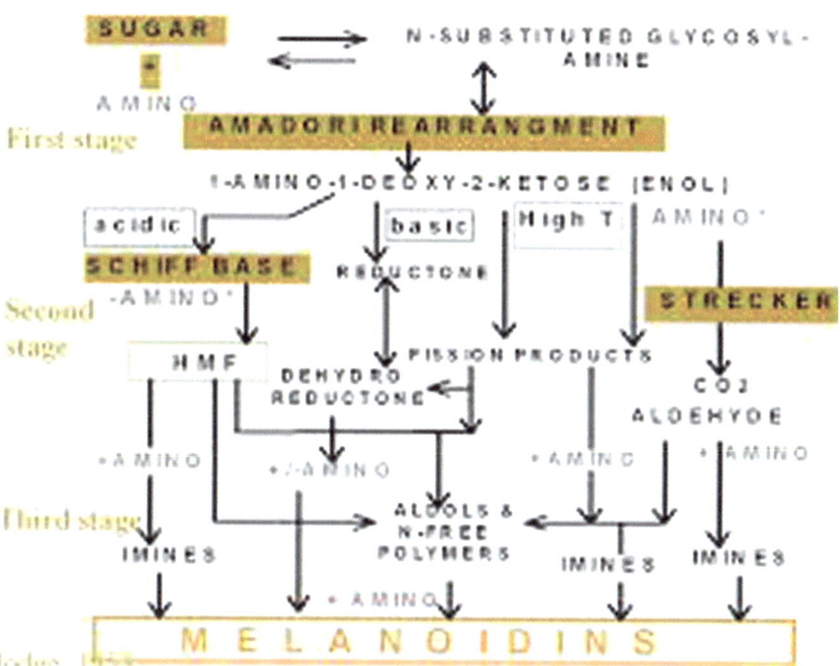

Fig. 23.2 The Maillard reaction. The Maillard reaction involves the interaction of the DHA sugar with the stratum corneum keratin protein to produce a pigmented substance known as a melanoidin

23.1.3 Sunless Tanning Product Formulation

As mentioned previously, sunless tanning product formulation is challenging, as water inhibits the Maillard reaction, meaning that all DHA-containing products need to be oil based. DHA is usually added to a creamy base in concentrations of 3–5 % [7]. Lower concentrations of DHA produce mild tanning, while higher concentrations produce greater melanoidin formation [8]. Formulators can vary the depth of color production by controlling the DHA concentration allowing the sale of sunless tanning products in light, medium, and dark shades. The depth of color can also be increased by adding another source of protein to the product. For example, applying a sulfur-containing amino acid, such as methionine sulfoxide, to the skin first followed by the application of DHA will result in higher melanoidin formation and a deeper simulated tan. It is important to understand this chemical reaction, as the deeper simulated tan does not necessarily equate to increased sun protection.

One of the major cosmetic drawbacks of sunless tanning products is their distinct and somewhat unpleasant odor, which is difficult to mask. A variety of fragrances have been added to modern formulations in an attempt to mask the odor, but once the fragrance evaporates from the skin surface, the characteristic DHA odor returns.

The staining reaction that occurs with DHA is limited strictly to the stratum corneum and can be readily removed with tape stripping and exfoliation. Thus, the product must be reapplied daily to maintain the optimal skin darkening. The color will fade as the stratum corneum sloughs over 14 days. There are no known side effects, except for possible irritation, from frequent application; allergic contact dermatitis may occur, as discussed next.

23.1.4 DHA Safety

DHA is a nontoxic ingredient both for ingestion and topical application. It has a proven safety record with only a few reported cases of allergic contact dermatitis [9]. In the 1920s, it was determined that large quantities of oral DHA did not produce toxicity, and the LD50 in rats is over 16 g/kg. It is interesting to note that the phosphate of DHA is one of the intermediates in the Krebs cycle known as dihydroxyacetone monophosphate. Topically applied DHA reacts immediately upon contact with the stratum corneum amines and is not absorbed for this reason. DHA has not been detected in the urine or serum of volunteers following topical application [7].

Patients who are allergic to one sunless tanning product may be allergic to all sunless tanning products as DHA is a common ingredient. While the reported instances of allergic contact dermatitis to DHA are few, practical experience indicates a much higher incidence. The author personally sees two patients per month with allergic contact dermatitis to sunless tanning products. To confirm the allergy, it is best to patch test the patient to the product the patient purchased under an occlusive bandage for 48 h followed by removal and evaluation 24 and 48 h later.

23.1.5 DHA Photoprotection

The final question remains the ability of DHA to provide photoprotection. DHA was listed on the sunscreen monograph at one time but has since been replaced by better agents with superior UV-absorbing qualities; therefore, it is no longer considered a sunscreen ingredient. DHA absorbs long wavelength UV in the 300–380 nm range [10]. It has an SPF of 3–4 [11].

What does this mean? It means that no SPF rating can be assigned to DHA, as it now has become simply a cosmetic and not an over-the-counter drug. Nevertheless, there is some photoprotective value to DHA. It was originally used in a 3 % concentration in combination with 0.25 % lawsone. The advantage to DHA is that an irreversible reaction occurs when the DHA sugar binds to the keratin protein that cannot be removed by rubbing. This is not the case with modern sunscreen formulations. While it is important to remind patients that the simulated tanned appearance created by sunless tanning creams requires additional sunscreen use, a sunless tanning preparation applied first several days before an extended outdoor outing with additional sunscreen applied on top 30 min before sun exposure might be helpful.

In addition, there are some formulations of sunless tanning products that contain monographed sunscreen ingredients. DHA can be combined with organic sunscreens that do not contain amino groups, such as octyl methoxycinnamate, homosalate, octocrylene, and benzophenone. It also can be combined with inorganic sunscreens (zinc oxide and titanium dioxide). The challenge with inorganic sunscreen combinations is that the zinc oxide and titanium dioxide can discolor brown in the bottle if 5 % DHA is combined with 5 % inorganic sunscreen after only a few days. Nevertheless, the use of sunless tanning creams containing sunscreens may encourage application compliance.

23.2 Photoprotection and Colored Cosmetics

In addition to novel uses of sunless tanning products for photoprotection, colored cosmetics can also be used creatively to enhance the efficacy of traditional sunscreens. This discussion evaluates the formulation of facial powders, facial foundations, and lipsticks presenting ideas as to how these three popular colored cosmetics can assist in sun protection.

23.2.1 Facial Powders

Facial powder is traditionally used to provide coverage of complexion imperfections, oil control, a matte finish, and tactile smoothness to the skin. However, facial powder can also increase photoprotection longevity when dusted on top of a sunscreen film after it has completely dried; it can also increase the SPF of a sunscreen by providing an additional layer of organic sunscreen ingredients (Fig. 23.3). In addition, there are some pigmented powder sunscreen formulations that have become very popular for patients with multiple allergies and sensitive skin, since the powder formulations have ewer ingredients than cream or spray sunscreens with similar SPF values.

Facial powders are composed of talc, also known as hydrated magnesium silicate, combined with pigments that camouflage the underlying skin. The pigments used in face powder listed in order of increasing opaqueness are: titanium dioxide, kaolin, magnesium carbonate, magnesium stearate, zinc stearate, prepared chalk, zinc oxide, rice starch, precipitated chalk, and talc. It is generally accepted that the optimum opacity is achieved with a particle size of 0.25 μm. This is important because the opacity of a facial powder directly correlates with its ability to shield the skin from UV radiation. Opaque facial powders that are used as stand-alone sunscreens rely on higher concentrations of titanium dioxide, a monographed inorganic sunscreen ingredient, to achieve their SPF rating. Adding various concentrations of iron oxides, to match the various brown tones representative of the human population, minimizes the cosmetically unattractive whiteness of the powder. In addition to iron oxides as the main pigment, other inorganic pigments such as ultramarines, chrome oxide, and chrome hydrate may be used. All of the additional pigments may increase the product SPF, even though they are not monographed sunscreen ingredients.

Facial powders are available in two formulations: opaque and transparent. The opaque powders, previously discussed, mitigate the penetration of UV radiation and can be applied on top of a spray, lotion, or cream sunscreen to augment the ability of the sunscreen to shield the skin or used alone as an SPF-rated powder sunscreen. It also prevents the transmission of visible light. Transparent powders are more natural appearing due their ability to allow some light to reach the skin surface,

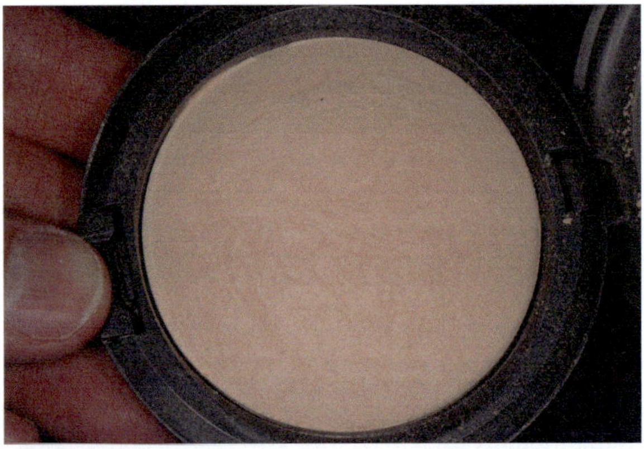

Fig. 23.3 Facial powder. Titanium dioxide and talc that form the basis for facial powder are also used as inorganic sunscreens

but their sun-protective ability is diminished. Transparent powders have the same formulation as full coverage powders except they contain less talc, titanium dioxide, or zinc oxide, since coverage is not a priority. Transparent facial powders commonly have a light reflective shine, produced by nacreous pigments, such as bismuth oxychloride, mica, titanium dioxide-coated mica, or crystalline calcium carbonate. They are not used as stand-alone sunscreens but can be dusted over a sunscreen for added protection.

While facial powders contain ingredients that function as sunscreens, powder can also increase the ability of the sunscreen film to remain in place on the skin surface. One of the most common causes of sunscreen failure is removal of the product due to rubbing, wiping, and water contact. The sunscreen film is also degraded as it mixes with sweat and sebum. Magnesium carbonate can be added to facial powders to absorb sebum, thus minimizing the ability of sebum to destroy the sunscreen emulsion. Kaolin, also known as hydrated aluminum silicate, may also function to absorb oil and perspiration [12]. Other specialty additives in more expensive boutique powders include partially hydrolyzed ground raw silk, corn silk, treated starch, and synthetic resins for increased oil and perspiration absorption.

Powder can be applied to the face over sunscreen with a brush, pad, or fingers. Brushing the powder is least effective as the particles sit on top of the sunscreen, but represents the easiest application method. Pressing the powder into the sunscreen film with a pad or fingers is more effective as the powder becomes embedded in the sunscreen, increasing the longevity of both products on the face. In general, a transparent powder can increase the SPF of a sunscreen by 2 SPF points, for example, from an SPF of 7 to an SPF of 9, while an opaque powder can increase the sunscreen SPF by five numerical points. It is important to remember that the powder does not improve the water resistance of the sunscreen film to abundant sweat, precipitation, or submersion in water. Nevertheless, facial powders are a valuable sunscreen adjuvant for some patients.

23.2.2 *Facial Foundations*

Facial foundations are another important category of cosmetic that can supplement facial photoprotection. If you take the facial powder formulation discussed previously and add a moisturizer, you end up with a facial foundation. Older nomenclature labeled facial foundation a liquid powder. Facial foundations are available in a variety of formulations to include liquid, mousse, water-containing cream, soufflé, anhydrous cream, stick, cake, and shake lotion [13]. Each of these formulations offers a different degree of facial protection, partly due to the ingredients in the facial foundation and to the addition of monographed sunscreen ingredients. Thus, a more modern name for facial foundations might be a pigmented sunscreen. The role of facial foundations in photoprotection will be explored.

The most popular facial foundations are liquid formulations containing water, oils, titanium dioxide, and iron oxides. The liquid formulations can be further subdivided into water-based, oil-based, oil-free, and water-free forms. Water-based formulations contain water as the highest concentration ingredient with the oil-soluble ingredients emulsified into the water. This is important because most organic sunscreens are oil soluble. Water-based formulations occupy the majority of the facial foundation market because they are easy to apply and dry down quickly, can be removed with water, and are nonocclusive making them comfortable to wear. Water-based facial foundations are oil-in-water emulsions containing a small amount of oil in which the pigment is emulsified with a relatively large quantity of water. The primary emulsifier is usually a soap such as triethanolamine or a nonionic surfactant. The secondary emulsifier, present in smaller quantity, is usually glyceryl stearate or propylene glycol stearate. These popular foundations are appropriate for dry to normal skin. Organic sunscreens can be added in addition to the inorganic titanium dioxide already present in the formulation. The most popular organic sunscreen added to the oil phase of water-based facial foundation is octyl methoxycinnamate, a UVB filter, yielding an SPF between 8 and 30, depending on the concentration.

The second most popular formulations are oil-based foundations where a water-in-oil emulsion is created. These foundations are usually employed for high coverage and camouflaging purposes because pigments are usually suspended in the oil phase allowing a higher concentration to be easily achieved. The oil phase may be composed of mineral oil, lanolin alcohol, vegetable oils (coconut, sesame, safflower), and synthetic esters (isopropyl myristate, octyl palmitate, isopropyl palmitate). The water evaporates from the foundation following application, leaving the pigment in oil on the face. This provides facial skin with a moist feeling, especially desirable in dry complected patients. It is also easier to achieve a higher SPF in oil-based formulations because the sunscreen is dissolved in the oil phase along with the pigment.

The third most popular foundation formulations are oil-free, so named because they contain no animal, vegetable, or mineral oils. They do contain other oily substances, such as the silicone derivatives dimethicone or cyclomethicone. Silicone derivates behave just like oils on the skin are usually added as the oil emulsified into water in water-based facial foundations. These foundations are usually designed for oily complected individuals with acne, since silicone is a noncomedogenic oil. Again, monographed sunscreen actives can be added to the oil phase.

There are some special facial foundation formulations that are not very popular but provide unique benefits for patients unable to use traditional organic sunscreens yet require excellent photoprotection. These individuals may present to the dermatologist complaining of rashes, breakouts, irritation, etc., associated with sunscreen application. It is sometimes difficult to determine which monographed sunscreen ingredient is the cause and whether true allergic or irritant contact dermatitis is present. For these complex patients, it may be worthwhile to consider opaque facial foundations. These are high-coverage formulations that contain waxes to create a thicker, occlusive, more moisturizing formula with the ability to dissolve larger quantities of pigment. If the cream is completely without water and only composed of oils, it is known as an anhydrous cream and possesses waterproof characteristics. The cream can be applied to the face as dipped from a jar, wiped from a compact, or stroked from a rod packaged in a roll-up tube [14]. For patients with exquisite sun sensitivity, superior photoprotection is achieved by first applying a traditional sunscreen followed by application of an anhydrous waterproof cream foundation. For patients with the inability to use traditional sunscreens, the anhydrous waterproof cream foundation can be used alone.

In summary, the ability of a facial foundation to provide sun protection is directly proportional to its ability to conceal or cover the underlying skin, a quality known as "coverage." Further, the coverage of a foundation is directly related to the amount of titanium dioxide, zinc oxide, talc, and kaolin in the formulation. Sheer coverage foundations with minimal titanium dioxide are almost transparent and have an SPF around 2, moderate coverage foundations are translucent and have an approximate SPF of 4–5, anhydrous high-coverage foundations with large amounts of titanium dioxide may be opaque, acting as a total physical sunblock which protects against UV and visible light. Thus, facial foundations can be important tools for photoprotection.

23.2.3 Lipsticks

The final colored cosmetic that has important photoprotective qualities is lipstick. Lipsticks contain pigments that can function as sun-protective ingredients but can also contain monographed sunscreen ingredients allowing them to possess an SPF rating. The lips are a common site of actinic cheilitis and may also be afflicted with squamous cell carcinoma. Lipsticks are an excellent cosmetic for preventing lip photodamage.

Lipsticks are mixtures of waxes, oils, and pigments in varying concentration to yield the characteristics of the final product (Fig. 23.4). Several different lipstick formulations are currently marketed. Lipsticks labeled as "long wearing" are excellent for photoprotection and are designed to remain on the lips for a prolonged period of time. They are composed of high wax, low oil, and high pigment concentrations, which accounts for their intrinsic SPF of 4–5 even though they do not contain monographed sunscreen ingredients [15]. The waxes incorporated into lipstick formulations are white beeswax, candelilla wax, carnauba wax, ozokerite wax, lanolin wax, ceresin wax, and other synthetic waxes. Lipsticks combine these waxes to achieve a desired melting point that controls the hardness of the lipstick and the ability of the lipstick to coat the lips when applied. Oils are then selected, such as castor oil, white mineral oil, lanolin oil, hydrogenated vegetable oils, or oleyl alcohol, to form a film suitable for application to the lips. The thickness of the film over the lips determines the degree of photoprotection provided and the ability of the film to remain in place on the lips, but the photoprotection is due to the pigments dispersed in the oil and the suspended in the waxes.

A variety of coloring agents are used in lipsticks to achieve the wide variety of shades available in the marketplace. Since lipsticks are removed by eating, speaking,

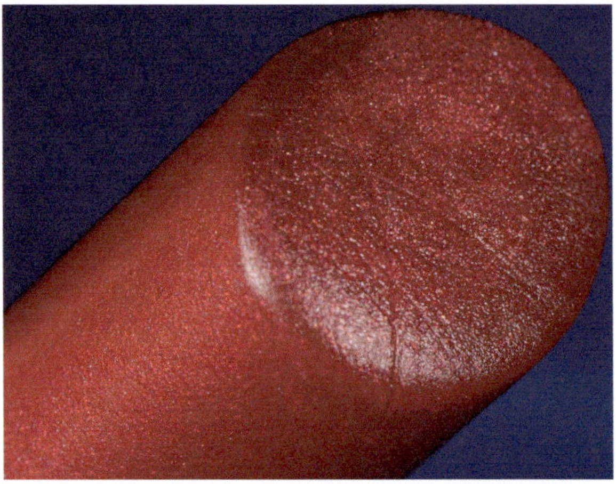

Fig. 23.4 Lipstick. Opaque lipstick confers excellent photoprotection to the lips

and lip licking, they commonly are ingested. Thus, the US Food and Drug Administration controls the coloring agents that can be used in lipsticks, which also provide photoprotection. The Food and Drug Administration divides certified colors into three groups: Food, Drug, and Cosmetic (FD&C) colors, Drug & Cosmetic (D&C) colors, and External Drug & Cosmetic colors. Only the first two groups can be used in lipsticks [16]. While these pigments can provide some photoprotection, they are not monographed sunscreen ingredients. Additional monographed ingredients can be added, converting the lipstick into an OTC drug. Most lipsticks do not have an SPF over 30 because the addition of higher concentrations of monographed sunscreen ingredients will give the product a bitter unpalatable taste. The best lipsticks are those with a high titanium dioxide and pigment load that are completely opaque when applied to the lips.

One unique type of lipstick that provides long-lasting protection contains a lip stain [17]. These lip stains contain indelible coloring agents known as bromo acids, consisting of fluoresceins, halogenated fluoresceins, and related water-insoluble dyes [18]. These lipsticks are colored red and stain the lips a reddish color. The stain produces some minimal photoprotection but is best combined with a sunscreen-containing lip balm. The lip stain is applied first followed by the lip balm slightly boosting the lip balm SPF.

23.3 Summary

Dermatologists typically think of sunscreen sprays, lotions, and creams when body and facial photoprotection is required. This chapter expands the number of products that should be considered. While sunless tanning creams offer minimal photoprotection with an SPF of 3–4, they can be used as a safer tanning alternative than sun exposure. Increased compliance might be achieved in some patients by using a sunscreen-containing sunless tanning preparation. Superior facial photoprotection can be achieved either by using an opaque facial powder sunscreen or applying a facial powder over a sunscreen. Even greater facial photoprotection can be achieved by applying a traditional sunscreen followed by a facial foundation and then topped with a dusting of facial powder. Combine this facial photoprotection with an opaque pigmented lipstick and the patient is now ready for an attractive day at the beach. The creative use of sunless tanning creams and colored cosmetics can enhance photoprotection.

References

1. Maibach HI, Kligman AM (1960) Dihydroxyacetone: a sun-tan-simulating agent. Arch Dermatol 82:505–507
2. Wittgenstein E, Berry KH (1961) Reaction of dihydroxyacetone (DHA) with human skin callus and amino compounds. J Invest Dermatol 36:283–286
3. Meybeck A (1977) A spectroscopic study of the reaction products of dihydroxyacetone with aminoacids. J Soc Cosmet Chem 28:25–35
4. Wittgenstein E, Berry KH (1960) Staining of skin with dihydroxyacetone. Science 132:894–895
5. Chaudhuri RK, Hwang C (2001) Self-tanners: formulating with dihydroxyacetone. Cosmet Toilet 116:87–96
6. Faurschou A, Wulf HC (2004) Durability of the sun protection factor provided by dihydroxyacetone. Photodermatol Photoimmunol Photomed 20(5):239–242
7. Kurz T (1994) Formulating effective self-tanners with DHA. Cosmet Toilet 109(11):55–61
8. Maes DH, Marenus KD (1994) Self-tanning products. In: Baran R, Maibach HI (eds) Cosmetic dermatology. Martin Dunitz, London
9. Morren M, Dooms-Goossens A, Heidbuchel M et al (1991) Contact allergy to dihydroxyacetone. Contact Dermatitis 25:326–327
10. Johnson JA, Fusaro RM (1987) Protecton against long ultraviolet radiation: topical browning agents and a new outlook. Dermatologica 175:53–57
11. Muizzuddin N, Marenus KD, Maes DH (1997) UVA and UVB protective effect of melanoids formed with dihydroxyacetone and skin. Poster presentation, AAD meeting, San Francisco
12. Wetterhahn J (1988) Loose and compact face powder. In: de Navarre MG (ed) The chemistry and manufacture of cosmetics, vol IV, 2nd edn. Allured Publishing Corporation, Wheaton, pp 921–946
13. Fiedler JG (1972) Foundation makeup. In: Balsam MS, Sagarin E (eds) Cosmetics, science and technology, vol 1, 2nd edn. Wiley-Interscience, New York, pp 317–334
14. Flick EW (1989) Cosmetic and toiletry formulations, 2nd edn. Noyes, Park Ridge, pp 124–125
15. Cunningham J (1992) Color cosmetics. In: Williams DF, Schmitt WH (eds) Chemistry and technology of the cosmetics and toiletries industry. Blackie Academic & Professional, London, pp 143–149
16. de Navarre MG (1975) Lipstick. In: The chemistry and manufacture of cosmetics, 2nd edn. Allured Publishing Corporation, Wheaton, p 778
17. Boelcke U (1961) Requirements for lipstick colors. J Soc Cosmet Chem 12:468
18. Poucher WA (1984) Perfumes, cosmetics and soaps, vol 3, 8th edn. Chapman and Hall, London, pp 196–207

Chapter 24
Photoprotection by Clothing and Fabric

Thilo Gambichler, Isabelle Rooms, and Lisa Scholl

Key Points

- Clothing provides simple and effective broad-spectrum photoprotection.
- Photoprotection by clothing is affected by several factors, including the material, thickness, and color.
- Ultraviolet protection factor (UPF) is the in vitro assessment of photoprotection of fabric. Similar to SPF, it is weighted toward the assessment of protection against erythema, the predominant effect of UVB.
- Clothing with UPF of at least 40 is preferred.

24.1 Background

Skin cancer is the most common type of cancer in the United States. In 2006, more than one million people were diagnosed with basal cell carcinoma (BCC) or squamous cell carcinoma (SCC). Malignant melanoma (MM), the third and most often fatal type of skin cancer, is expected to be diagnosed in approximately 60,000 people and hold into account for over 8000 deaths in 2007. Between 1975 and 2004, the annual age-adjusted incidence rate for MM (new cases diagnosed per 100,000 people) nearly tripled, from about 7 to 19 cases per 100,000 [1–3]. Solar UV radiation is ubiquitous during daylight hours. Ambient ground-level UV is comprised mainly of UVA (320–400 nm) plus a small proportion (<10 %, variable by time of day, season, and location) of UVB (290–320 nm). Within-person and between-person UV doses vary greatly, depending on location, time of day and season, clothing habits, and skin pigmentation [4]. Exposure to UV radiation on the skin results in demonstrable

T. Gambichler, MD (✉) • I. Rooms, MD • L. Scholl, MD
Department of Dermatology, Ruhr-University Bochum,
Gudrunstr. 56, Bochum 44791, Germany
e-mail: t.gambichler@klinikum-bochum.de

S.Q. Wang, H.W. Lim (eds.), *Principles and Practice of Photoprotection*,
DOI 10.1007/978-3-319-29382-0_24

mutagenic effects. The *p53* suppressor gene, which is frequently mutated in skin cancers, is believed to be an early target of UV radiation inducing neoplasms such as SCC [5]. Fair-skinned individuals, who are more sensitive to the effects of exposure at these wavelengths, are at higher risk of developing skin cancer. The amount of average annual UV radiation correlates with the incidence of skin cancer. There is a direct relationship between the incidence of nonmelanoma skin cancer and latitude. The closer an individual is to the equator, the greater the UV energy to which they are exposed [6, 7]. MM mortality in the United States and Canada has also been shown to directly correlate with ambient UV exposure. The correlation of MM incidence to UV radiation exposure is greater when ambient UVA radiation is also included [6–9].

Apart from sun avoidance, the most frequently used form of UV protection is the application of sunscreens. The use of textiles as a means of sun protection has been underrated in previous education campaigns, even though suitable clothing potentially offers usually simple and effective broad-spectrum protection against sunlight [10–14]. In Australia, Cancer Council education campaigns have long urged the use of clothing in conjunction with hats, sunglasses, and sunscreens as UV protection [15]. However, a number of studies have recently shown that, contrary to popular opinion, some textiles provide insufficient UV protection [16]. In addition to skin cancer formation, photoaging and photosensitive disorders (e.g., polymorphous light eruption, lupus erythematosus, porphyrias, solar urticaria, and phototoxic/photoallergic reactions) may also be prevented by UV protective clothing. Consequently, the use of suitable textiles, which block UVB as well as UVA radiation, has been recommended for photosensitive patients [17–21]. Most of the photosensitive diseases are provoked by wavelengths in the UVA range [19]. In some of these disorders (e.g., solar urticaria, chronic actinic dermatitis), even very small UV doses can lead to exacerbation. The data of several studies indicate that some aspects of sun protection are being practiced consistently, while others, such as the use of UV protective clothing, are not [10, 22, 23].

24.2 Ultraviolet Protection Factor Assessed In Vitro and In Vivo

Direct and diffuse UV transmittance through fabric is the crucial factor determining the grade/amount of UV protection of textiles. Spectroradiometers and spectrophotometers are suitable for the assessment of the spectral irradiance. These measurements are usually performed in the wavelength range of 290–400 nm and operated in five or fewer nm steps. They are generally made under "worst-case" conditions, with collimated radiation beams at a right angle to the fabric [10, 24]. To determine the in vitro ultraviolet protection factor (UPF), the spectral irradiance (both source * and transmitted $^{\#}$ spectrum) is weighted against the erythemal action spectrum § [25]. The UPF is calculated as follows:

$$\mathrm{UPF} = \int E_\lambda \cdot S_\lambda \cdot d_\lambda \,/ \int E_\lambda \cdot S_\lambda \cdot T_\lambda \cdot d_\lambda$$

[E_λ = relative erythemal spectral effectiveness §; S_λ = solar spectral irradiance in W/m^2 (Albuquerque, New Mexico, 37.8° S, 17 January 1990) *; T_λ = spectral transmission of the sample #; d_λ = bandwidth in nm; λ = wavelength in nm; the integrals ($\int$) are calculated over the wavelength range of 290–400 nm]

The UPF is defined as the ratio of the average effective UV radiation irradiance calculated for unprotected skin to the average effective UV radiation irradiance calculated for skin protected by the test fabric [26]. Intra- and interlaboratory comparative trials indicate that spectrophotometry is a precise test method to determine the UPF, in particular for samples with UPFs below 50 minimal erythema doses (MEDs) [27–29]. UPFs greater than 50 are only of theoretical interest as even in Australia, the maximum daily UV exposure is less than 40 MEDs.

UV dosimetry has been used to measure erythemal UV exposures underneath and above textile materials. Similarly, polysulfone films have been employed in in vivo simulated studies as small portable badges monitoring UV doses on mannequins and mobile subjects [10, 30–33]. Ravishankar and Diffey [33] concluded that the protection provided by textiles worn in sunlight is, on average, 50 % higher than obtained by conventional in vitro testing using collimated radiation beams. In contrast to polysulfone films, the sensitivity curve of biological UV dosimeters such as DLR biofilm (*B. subtilis*) provides good similarity to the action spectrum for UV-induced erythema in human skin.

The DRL biofilm is a wavelength and time integrating biological UV dosimeter weighting the UV radiation according to its DNA-damaging potential [34]. It was shown that cycling jerseys have comparable UPF values when tested spectrophotometrically according to the Australian/New Zealand standard or under stationary sun exposure with DRL biofilms [36, 31]. In accordance with results reported by Ravishankar and Diffey, however, the jerseys revealed a much higher UPF when tested under "real" conditions during cycling. We also conducted a field-based study with biofilms and found that the UPF of a garment worn during outdoor activities was significantly higher than the UPF measured in the laboratory [10, 35].

Analogous to SPF testing of sunscreens, in vivo measurements in human volunteers with the sun as UV source are extremely impracticable for the determination of the UPF. In general, xenon arc solar simulators with collimated radiation beams are used with filters to absorb wavelength below 290 nm and to reduce visible and infrared radiation. In most studies, the in vivo method has been conducted by in vivo checking of the UPF values measured in vitro [36, 37, 18, 38–41]. Based on the skin phototype, the MED is determined with incremental UVB doses on the upper back of a subject and is read after 24 h. To measure the MED of the protected skin, the textile is placed on the skin of the other side of the back [36]. The incremental UVB doses for determination of the MED of unprotected skin are multiplied with UPF determined in vitro, resulting in incremental UVB doses for the MED testing of the protected skin. If the in vitro method is in agreement with the in vivo method, the ratio of the MED of protected skin to the MED of unprotected skin results in the original in vitro UPF. Several studies [10, 36, 39, 41], however, have shown that the UPFs determined with the in vivo method are significantly lower than the UPF values obtained in vitro when the fabric samples were tested "on skin." The inconsistency of the data in previous studies is certainly due to different methodologies (e.g., different test protocols, UV sources, and textile materials).

24.3 Fabric Parameters: Type, Construction, Dyes, and Ultraviolet Absorbers

For undyed fabrics, there are differences in the UV-absorbing properties of the fiber. Summer clothing is usually made of cotton, viscose, rayon, linen, and polyester or combinations thereof. Other materials such as nylon or elastane are also found in bathing suits and nylon stockings (Table 24.1). Usually, consumers consider lightweight non-synthetic fabrics, e.g., cotton, viscose, and linen, the most comfortable for summer textiles [10, 42]. Comparing different types of material in relation to the UPF is difficult and is only possible in a limited number of cases. In the case of synthetic fibers (e.g., polyester, polyamide), the analysis is even more difficult because the UV protection of these materials depends on the type and amount of additives to the fiber (e.g., antioxidants or UV stabilizers). In particular, polyester usually has good UV-blocking properties, since this fabric provides relatively low UVB transmission. This is most likely due to a large conjugated system in the polymer chains [43, 44]. Polyester or polyester blends may be the most suitable type of fabric for UV protective garments. However, its permeability for wavelength in the UVA range is frequently higher compared to other types of fiber [18]; this is of crucial significance for many patients suffering from photosensitive disorders. Bleached cotton and viscose rayon provide relatively low UV protection. This was confirmed by a study of Crews et al. who reported that bleached cotton print clothing had a UV transmission of 23.7 %, whereas unbleached cotton print cloth showed a UV transmission of 14.4 %.

The influence of bleaching was also evident among silk fabrics in their study. Compared to bleached textiles, unbleached fabrics such as cotton and silk have better UV protective properties due to natural pigments absorbing UV radiation and

Table 24.1 Summary of parameters significantly influencing the UPF of apparel textiles

Fabric material	UPF of cotton, viscose, rayon < linen, nylon, wool, silk < polyester[a]
Fabric porosity, weight, and thickness	UPF increases with small yarn-to-yarn spaces, fabric weight, and thickness
Fabric color	UPF increases with darker colors
UV absorbers	UPF is improved by UV absorbers
Stretch	UPF decreases under stretch
Wetness	UPF decreases for wet cotton
Wash	UPF increases for cotton fabrics

[a]When other parameters are kept constant

other impurities. Very few studies have considered the "fiber-fabric construction processing" history of fabrics to fully elucidate the UV protection abilities of fabrics. Sarkar [45] recently reported the effect of fabric processing treatments, both chemical and biochemical, on the transmission of UV radiation through selected white and undyed fabrics. He reported that chemical processing methods such as desizing and bleaching have a deleterious effect on UV transmission through fabric [45]. Biochemical processing such as the use of enzymes is comparatively benign and does not adversely impact the UV protective ability of cotton fabric. Grifoni et al. [46] studied the UV protection properties of two fabrics made of natural fibers (flax and hemp) which were dyed with some of the most common natural dyes. UV transmittance of fabrics was measured by a spectrophotometer, and outdoor measurements were taken by a spectroradiometer. Experimental results revealed that natural dyes could confer good UV protection, depending mainly on their different UV-absorbing properties, provided that the fabric construction already guaranteed good cover. The authors also confirmed that UPFs calculated by in vitro measurements were generally lower than those based on outdoor data, indicating an underestimation of the actual level of protection of tested fabrics assessed by the in vitro test [46].

Sarkar [47] investigated the UV properties of natural fabrics dyed with natural colorants. Three cotton fabrics were dyed with three natural colorants. Fabrics were characterized with respect to fabric construction, weight, thickness, and thread count. A positive correlation between the weight of the fabric and their UPF values was observed [47]. Similarly, thicker fabrics offered more protection from UV rays. Thread count appears to negatively correlate with UPF. Dyeing with natural colorants dramatically increased the protective abilities of all three fabric constructions.

The fabric construction is a primary determinant of fabric porosity followed by fabric weight and thickness of the textile [43]. An increased density concerning the weave or knitting technique (smaller yarn-to-yarn spaces) leads to a decreased fabric's porosity – and consequently less UV radiation is transmitted. Spaces between the yarns are frequently larger in a knit than in a woven textile. Besides, plain-woven textiles have a lower porosity than textiles using other weaves [48].

Thickness is a useful parameter for understanding differences in UV protection between fabrics. Crews et al. [43] reported that thicker, denser fabrics transmitted less UV radiation. Therefore, they concluded that thickness is most useful in explaining differences in UV transmission when differences in percentage cover are also accounted for [49]. By contrast, Kan and Au [50] recently found that fabric weight is the most important factor to affect the UPF while thickness and stitch density were not the main parameters determining UV protection.

The color of the fabric may also influence the UPF since some dyes have an absorption spectrum extending into the UV spectrum. Enhanced UV protection of dyed textiles depends on the position and intensity of the absorption bands of the dyes within the UV wavelength and the concentration of the dye in the textile.

The absorbance of UV radiation can influence many substrate attributes, e.g., fluorescence, photodegradation, and UV protection. Generally, dark colors provide better UV protection due to increased UV absorption. This holds only true for the same UV absorbent dye provided that other characteristics of the textile, e.g., fabric type and construction, are the same [10]. However, dyes within particular hue types can vary considerably in the degree of UV protectiveness due to their individual transmission/absorption characteristics [51].

In order to improve UV protection, UV absorbers have been added recently with different techniques [50]. UV absorbers are colorless compounds that absorb in the wavelength range from 280 to 400 nm. Hilfiker et al. [52] found the cover factor to be useful in predicting the maximum UPF that could be achieved by treating the yarns with UV absorbers. Thus, fabrics could be made opaque to UV radiation with a sufficient level of UV absorber impregnation. The corresponding UPFs approached the theoretically predicted levels based on the cover factor. Osterwalder and Rohwer [53] demonstrated that a UV absorber can be brought into contact with a fabric during the wash or rinse cycle of a laundry operation. The high UV transmittance of 30 % of a thin, bleached cotton swatch in the dry state (UPF 3) can be reduced tenfold to about 3 % (UPF >30) in ten washing cycles.

Titanium dioxide is frequently used as a UV-blocking substance in fabrics. However, the absorptive and scattering properties of titanium dioxide particles in the UVA wavelength range are different and depend mainly on the particle size and geometry. Nevertheless, UV absorbers are suitable for significantly increasing UPF, especially that of nondyed lightweight summer fabrics such as cotton and viscose fabrics [10, 52, 54–56]. Recently, Wang et al. [57] presented a facile process to prepare uniform dumbbell-shaped ZnO crystallites. They discovered a unique morphological effect on the UV-blocking property. The as-prepared ZnO crystallites were characterized by different criteria including UV blocking and Raman scattering spectra. The as-prepared structural material demonstrated a significant advance in protective functional treatment and provided a potential commercialization [58]. Furthermore, Behler et al. [58] showed that the use of electro-spun nanofibers with a high load of nanodiamond can provide UV protection.

24.4 Fabric Use and Environmental Effects on the Ultraviolet Protection Factor

Moon and Pailthorpe [59] showed that stretching elastane-based garments about 10 %, in both the machine and the cross-machine directions, causes a dramatic decrease in the measured UPF of a textile. Their consumer survey also showed that, on average, about 15 % stretch is achieved when these textiles are worn. However, the 15 % stretch refers to power stretch, which is only a small segment of the clothing market. Elastane-based textiles for "tight fitting" should not be considered as defined UV protective clothing. Kimlin et al. [60] reported that the UPF of 50 denier stockings decreased 868 % when stretched 30 % of their original size.

Notably, the most popular type of stockings (15 denier) provides a UPF less than 2 [61]. The maximum stretch point on the body for tight-fitting garments is the upper back, where textiles can be stretched up to 15 %. However, realistically, the effect of stretch on the UPF of a textile may be of significance only for garments with a non-stretched UPF of less than 30, particularly leggings, women's stockings, and swimsuits [10].

When textiles become wet, by humidity in the air, perspiration, or water, UV transmission through the fabric can significantly change [62]. A marked reduction of the UPF was observed for textiles made from cotton and cotton blends. However, Wong et al. [63] recently reported that knitted fabrics with miss stitches retained good UV protection even when the fabrics were stretched by 20 % of its original dimensions. In a field-based study, it was shown that significant UV exposures may occur underneath garments, particularly white cotton fabrics in a wet state. Similar results were also observed in in vivo measurements of cotton and polyester blends [37, 64, 58]. In case of fabrics made of viscose or silk, or in fabrics that have been treated with broadband UV absorbers, the UPF frequently increases when the textile becomes wet. This was also observed in a recent study of modal fabrics treated with titan dioxide [37, 54]. Thus, UV protection of wet garments is not always poor. Most of the fabrics will undergo a combination of relaxation shrinkage and consolidation shrinkage when washed [65]. Therefore, the spaces between the yarns will decrease and UV protection increases. The effect of laundering on the UPF puts into perspective other fabric parameters and factors which decrease the UPF [10]. Stanford et al. [66] showed that UPFs of cotton T-shirts increased after the first washing and did not change significantly with subsequent washing. Wang et al. [67] observed only a moderate UPF increase of cotton fabrics after laundering. Adding UV-absorbing agents during laundering was found to substantially enhance UPF [67, 68]. Recently, Zhou and Crews [69] reported that UPF of cotton or cotton/polyester blended fabrics can be significantly enhanced by repeated laundering of the garment in a detergent containing optical brightening agent. This was not the case for fabrics comprised entirely of polyester or nylon [69]. Prolonged wear and tear beyond the "standard" lifetime of a garment may eventually cause thinning of the individual fibers and consequently alter the UPF. Photostability of a textile and its UV protectiveness is an important requirement for sun protective clothing [62]. Unfortunately, there are only limited data on the stability of the UV protectiveness of a textile against UV radiation or infrared [10].

24.5 Standardization of Sun Protective Garments

The first standard for sun protective clothing was published by the Australian Standardisation Institute in 1996. This standard, referred to as AS/NZS 4399, has set requirements for determining and labeling the UPF of sun protective fabrics and other items that are worn in close proximity to the skin [26]. Based on the standard, spectrophotometrically assessed UPF is for a specific type of fabric and does not address the degree of protection that is afforded by the design of a garment. The effects of stretch, wetness, wear, and use are not included in the AS/NZS 4399. According to the Australian/New Zealand standard, UPFs are classified in three categories: UPFs of 15–24 (ratings 15 and 20) offer good protection; UPFs of 25–39 (ratings 25, 30, and 35), very good protection; and UPFs of 40 and higher (ratings 40, 45, 50, and 50+), excellent protection. Fabrics with a UPF of less than 15 are not labeled. Three standard documents that pertain to the testing and labeling of UV protective textile products were also published by the American Society for Testing and Materials [70] and the American Association of Textile Chemists and Colorists [71]. More recently, the European Committee for Standardization (CEN) has developed a standard on requirements for test methods and labeling of sun protective garments. The first part of the standard (EN 13758-1 [72],) includes all details of test methods (e.g., spectrophotometric measurements) for textile materials, and part 2 (EN 13758-2 [73],) covers the classification and marking of apparel textiles [10]. UV protective clothing must fulfill all stringent instructions of testing, classification, and marking including a UPF larger than 40 (UPF 40+), average UVA transmission lower than 5 %, and design requirements as specified in part 2 of the standard to claim the European standard as described above. A pictogram, which is marked with the number of the standard EN 13758-2 and the UPF of 40+, shall be attached to the garment if it is in compliance with the standard [74]. Moreover, British, Canadian, South African, and multinational groups, including Commission on Illumination (CIE) and also the International Organization for Standardization (ISO), have been engaged in writing UV protective fabric standard documents [10].

24.6 Conclusions

Defined UV-blocking fabrics are important element not only in campaigns against skin cancer but also in prevention of photosensitive disorders and photoaging. The UPF of a garment depends on a variety of parameters, including fabric construction, type, color, weight, thickness, finishing processes, and presence of additives such as UV-absorbing substances (e.g., titan dioxide, brightening agents) (Table 24.2). Moreover, UV protection of a garment during use depends on wash and wear, including stretch and hydration [10]. Optimally, apparel textiles assigned for UV protective clothing should be therefore measured and labeled in accordance with a standard document (e.g., AATCC 183:1998; AS/NZS 4399:1996; EN 13758-1:2002). Sun protective clothing needs to be designed with special types of complex weaves allowing the passage of air to promote wearer comfort but to block the passage of sunlight through the textile. Fabrics may include UV absorbers of various types to increase UV protection [74]. It will of course be essential to select substances that have a low potential for irritation and sensitization. Moreover, stringent requirements for the design should be complied with garments assigned for sun protective clothing (EN 13758-2:2203). A recent German study indicated that more counseling on UV protective clothing is needed for young, male, and lower educated

Table 24.2 Collection of general recommendations and rules of the thumb for UV protective clothing

Labeled UV protective clothing with an UPF of at least 30 is preferred
The less the fabric's transparency to visible light, the better the UV protection
The darker the color of the fabric, the better the UV protection
Polyester or polyester blends usually offer better UV protection than other fabrics
Stretch and wetness[a] textiles significantly decrease the UPF of a garment
Looser fits are preferable; the garment should cover the skin as much as possible
New clothing, especially cotton fabrics, should be washed before wearing it
Despite of a high UPF, a significant amount of UVA can still be transmitted

[a]Especially cotton fabrics

individuals [42, 75]. The textile industry should be aware of the increasing demand for labeled sun protective clothing, in particular clothing segments such as baby wear, children wear, and leisure and outdoor worker wear [76, 77]. Light-weighted, breathable, natural fabrics made of cotton and linen are preferred textiles. The textile industry may consider such fabrics for the production of labeled sun protective clothing. Nevertheless, peoples' compliance of buying and wearing sun protective clothing may be impaired by several factors such as price, lack of knowledge, and desire to tan [10].

References

1. Lucas RM, McMichael AJ, Armstrong BK, Smith WT (2008) Estimating the global disease burden due to ultraviolet radiation exposure. Int J Epidemiol 37:654–667
2. Tucker MA (2009) Melanoma epidemiology. Hematol Oncol Clin North Am 23:383–395
3. Cho YR, Chiang MP (2010) Epidemiology, staging (new system), and prognosis of cutaneous melanoma. Clin Plast Surg 37:47–53
4. Holick MF, Jung EG (1999) Biologic effects of light 1998, proceedings of a symposium, Basel, Switzerland, November 1-3, 1998. Kluwer Academic Publishers, Norwell
5. Soehnge H, Ouhtit A, Ananthaswamy ON (1997) Mechanisms of induction of skin cancer by UV radiation. Front Biosci 2:D538–D551
6. Setlow RB, Grist E, Thompson K, Woodhead AD (1993) Wavelengths effective in induction of malignant melanoma. Proc Natl Acad Sci U S A 90:6666–6670
7. Boniol M, De Vries E, Coebergh JW, Dore JF (2005) Seasonal variation in the occurrence of cutaneous melanoma in Europe: influence of latitude. An analysis using the EUROCARE group of registries. Eur J Cancer 41:126–132
8. Moan J, Dahlback A, Setlow AB (1999) Epidemiological support for a hypothesis for melanoma induction indicating a role for UVA radiation. Photochem Photobiol 70:243–247
9. Rigel DS, Rigel EG, Rigel AC (1999) Effects of altitude and latitude on ambient UVB radiation. J Am Acad Dermatol 40:11411–11416

10. Gambichler T (2011) Ultraviolet protection of clothing. In: Functional textiles for improved performance, protection and health. Woodhead Publishing, Philadelphia, pp 45–63
11. Gies P (2007) Photoprotection by clothing. Photodermatol Photoimmunol Photomed 23:264–274
12. Hoffmann K, Lappere J, Avermaete A, Altmeyer P, Gambichler T (2001) Defined UV protection by apparel textiles. Arch Dermatol 137:1089–1094
13. Glanz K, Yaroch AL, Dancel M, Saraiya M, Crane LA, Buller DB, Manne S, O'Riordan DL, Heckman CJ, Hay J, Robinson JK (2008) Measures of sun exposure and sun protection practices for behavioral and epidemiologic research. Arch Dermatol 144:217–222
14. Hatch KL, Osterwalder U (2006) Garments as solar ultraviolet radiation screening materials. Dermatol Clin 24:85–100
15. Dobbinson S, Wakefield M, Hill D, Girgis A, Aitken JF, Beckmann K, Reeder AI, Herd N, Fairthorne A, Bowles KA (2008) Prevalence and determinants of Australian adolescents' and adults' weekend sun protection and sunburn, summer 2003-2004. J Am Acad Dermatol 59:602–614
16. Gambichler T, Rotterdam S, Altmeyer P, Hoffmann K (2001) Protection against ultraviolet radiation by commercial summer clothing: need for standardised testing and labelling. BMC Dermatol 1:6
17. Aguilera J, de Gálvez MV, Sánchez-Roldán C, Herrera-Ceballos E (2014) New advances in protection against solar ultraviolet radiation in textiles for summer clothing. Photochem Photobiol 90:1199–1206
18. Gambichler T, Laperre J, Altmeyer P, Hoffmann K (2002) UVA and UVB transmission of fabrics: critical wavelength based on absorbance and effective dose. Exog Dermatol 1:290–295
19. Gambichler T, Al-Muhammadi R, Boms S (2009) Immunologically mediated photodermatoses: diagnosis and treatment. Am J Clin Dermatol 10:169–180
20. O'Quinn RP, Wagner RF Jr (1998) Unusual patterns of chronic photodamage through clothing. Cutis 61:269–271
21. Roelandts R (2000) The diagnosis of photosensitivity. Arch Dermatol 136:1152–1157
22. Barankin B, Liu K, Howard J, Guenther L (2001) Effect of a sun protection program targeting elementary school children and their parents. J Cutan Med Surg 5:2–7
23. Robinson JK, Rigel DS, Amonette RA (2000) Summertime sun protection used by adults for their children. J Am Acad Dermatol 42:746–753
24. Laperre J, Gambichler T (2003) Sun protection offered by fabrics: on the relation between effective doses based on different action spectra. Photodermatol Photoimmunol Photomed 19:11–16
25. Diffey BL (1998) The CIE ultraviolet action spectrum for erythema. In: Mathes R, Sliney D (eds) Measurements of optical radiation hazards. Märkl-Druck, München, pp 63–67
26. Australian/New Zealand Standards AS/NZS (1996) Sun protective clothing – evaluation and classification. Homebush, NSW, Australia/Wellington, New Zealand, AS/NZS 4399
27. Gies HP, Roy CR, Elliott G, Zongli W (1994) Ultraviolet radiation protection factors for clothing. Health Phys 67:131–139
28. Hoffmann K, Kesners P, Bader A, Avermaete A, Altmeyer P, Gambichler T (2001) Repeatability of in vitro measurements of the ultraviolet protection factor (UPF) by spectrophotometry with automatic sampling. Skin Res Technol 7:223–226
29. Laperre J, Gambichler T, Böhringer B, Driscoll C, Varieras S, Gassan U (2001) Determination of the ultraviolet protection factor of textile materials: measurement reliability. Photodermatol Photoimmunol Photomed 17:223–229
30. Holman CDJ, Gibson IM, Stephanson M, Armstrong BK (1983) Ultraviolet irradiation of human body sites in relation to occupation and outdoor activity: field studies using personal UVR dosimeters. Clin Exp Dermatol 8:269–277
31. Moehrle M, Garbe C (2000) Solar UV-protective properties of textiles. Dermatology 201:82
32. Parisi AV, Kimlin MG, Mulheran L, Meldrum LR, Randall C (2000) Field-based measurements of personal erythemal ultraviolet exposure through a common summer garment. Photodermatol Photoimmunol Photomed 16:134–138

33. Ravishankar J, Diffey BL (1997) Laboratory testing of UV transmission through fabrics may underestimate protection. Photodermatol Photoimmunol Photomed 13:202–203
34. Quintern LE, Furusawa Y, Fukutsu K, Holtschmidt H (1997) Characterization and application of UV detector spore films: the sensitivity curve of a new detector system provides good similarity to the action spectrum for UV-induced erythema in human skin. J Photochem Photobiol B Biol 37:158–166
35. Gambichler T, Hatch KL, Avermaete A, Bader A, Herde M, Altmeyer P, Hoffmann K (2002) Ultraviolet protection factor of fabrics: comparison of laboratory and field-based measurements. Photodermatol Photoimmunol Photomed 18:135–140
36. Gambichler T, Avermaete A, Bader A, Altmeyer P, Hoffmann K (2001) Ultraviolet protection by summer textiles. Ultraviolet transmission measurements verified by determination of the minimal erythema dose with solar-simulated radiation. Br J Dermatol 144:484–489
37. Gambichler T, Hatch KL, Avermaete A, Altmeyer P, Hoffmann K (2002) The influence of wetness on the ultraviolet protection factor (UPF) of textiles: in vitro and in vivo measurements. Photodermatol Photoimmunol Photomed 18:29–35
38. Gies HP, Roy CR, Holmes G (2000) Ultraviolet radiation protection by clothing: comparison of in vivo and in vitro measurements. Radiat Prot Dosimetry 91:247–250
39. Greenoak GE, Pailthorpe M (1996) Skin protection by clothing from the damaging effects of sunlight. Australas Text 16:61
40. Lowe NJ, Bourget TD, Hughes SN, Sayre RM (1995) UV protection offered by clothing: an in vitro and in vivo assessment of clothing fabrics. Skin Cancer 10:89–96
41. Menzies SW, Lukins PB, Greenoak GE, Walker PJ, Pailthorpe M, Martin JM (1991) A comparative study of fabric protection against ultraviolet-induced erythema determined by spectrophotometric and human skin measurements. Photodermatol Photoimmunol Photomed 8:157–163
42. Gambichler T, Dissel M, Altmeyer P, Rotterdam S (2009) Evaluation of sun awareness with an emphasis on ultraviolet protection by clothing: a survey of adults in Western Germany. J Eur Acad Dermatol Venereol 24:155–162
43. Crews PC, Kachmann S, Beyer AG (1999) Influences on UVR transmission of undyed woven fabrics. Text Chemist Colorist 31:17–26
44. Davis S, Capjack L, Kerr N, Fedosejevs R (1997) Clothing as protection from ultraviolet radiation: which fabric is most effective? Int J Dermatol 36:374–379
45. Sarkar AK (2007) On the relationship between fabric processing and ultraviolet radiation transmission. Photodermatol Photoimmunol Photomed 23:191–196
46. Grifoni D, Bacci L, Zipoli G, Carreras G, Baronti S, Sabatini F (2009) Laboratory and outdoor assessment of UV protection offered by flax and hemp fabrics dyed with natural dyes. Photochem Photobiol 85:313–320
47. Sarkar AK (2004) An evaluation of UV protection imparted by cotton fabrics dyed with natural colorants. BMC Dermatol 4:15
48. Capjack L, Kerr N, Fedosejevs R, Hatch KL, Markee NL (1994) Protection of humans from ultraviolet radiation through the use of textiles: a review. Fam Consum Sci Res J 23:198–218
49. Pailthorpe M (1994) Textile and sun protection: the current situation. Australas Text 14:54–66
50. Kan CW, Au CH (2014) Effect of biopolishing and UV absorber treatment on the UV protection properties of cotton knitted fabrics. Carbohydr Polym 101:451–456
51. Srinivasan M, Gatewood BM (2000) Relationship of dye characteristics to UV protection provided by cotton fabric. Text Chemist Colorist 32:36–43
52. Hilfiker R, Kaufmann W, Reinert G, Schmidt E (1996) Improving sun protection factors of fabrics by applying UV-absorbers. Text Res J 66:61–70
53. Osterwalder U, Rohwer H (2002) Improving UV protection by clothing – recent developments. Recent results. Cancer Res 160:62–69
54. Hoffmann K, Hoffmann A, Hanke D, Böhringer B, Schindling G, Schön U (1998) Sun protected from optimally designed fabrics. Hautarzt 49:10–16
55. Hoffmann K (1998) UV protective clothing in Europe: recommendation of European working party. J Eur Acad Dermatol Venereol 11:198–199

56. Eckhardt C, Rohwer H (2000) UV protector for cotton fabrics. Text Chemist Colorist 32:21–23
57. Wang RH, Xin JH, Tao XM (2005) UV-blocking property of dumbbell-shaped ZnO crystallites on cotton fabrics. Inorg Chem 44:3926–3930
58. Behler KD, Stravato A, Mochalin V, Korneva G, Yushin G, Gogotsi Y (2009) Nanodiamond-polymer composite fibers and coatings. ACS Nano 3:363–369
59. Moon R, Pailthorpe M (1995) Effect of stretch and wetting on the UPF of elastane fabrics. Australas Text 15:39–42
60. Kimlin MG, Parisi AV, Meldrum LR (1999) Effect of stretch on the ultraviolet spectral transmission of one type of commonly used clothing. Photodermatol Photoimmunol Photomed 15:171–174
61. Sinclair SA, Diffey BL (1997) Sun protection provided by ladies stockings. Br J Dermatol 136:239–241
62. Khazova M, O'Hagan JB, Grainger KJ (2007) Radiation and chemical degradation of UVR protection characteristics of fabrics. Radiat Prot Dosimetry 123:369–377
63. Wong WY, Lam JK, Kan CW, Postle R (2014) In vitro assessment of ultraviolet protection of coloured cotton knitted fabrics with different structures under stretched and wet conditions. Radiat Prot Dosimetry ncu276 164(3):325–334
64. Jevtic AP (1990) The sun protective effect of clothing, including beachwear. Australas J Dermatol 31:5–7
65. Kaskel P, Rohwer H, Osterwalder U, Peter RU (2001) Improving textile sun protection by regular washing of clothing. Fortschr Med Orig 119(Suppl 2):91–94
66. Standford DG, Georgouras KE, Pailthorpe MT (1995) Sun protection by a summer-weight garment: the effect of washing and wearing. Med J Aust 162:422–425
67. Wang SQ, Kopf AW, Marx J, Bogdan A, Polsky D, Bart RS (2001) Reduction of ultraviolet transmission through cotton T-shirt fabrics with low ultraviolet protection by various laundering methods and dyeing: clinical implications. J Am Acad Dermatol 44:767–774
68. Osterwalder U, Schlenker W, Rohwer H, Martin E, Schuh S (2000) Facts and fiction on UV protection by clothing. Radiat Prot Dosimetry 91:255–260
69. Zhou Y, Crews PC (1998) Effect of OBAs and repeated launderings on UVR transmission through fabrics. Text Chemist Colorist 30:19–24
70. American Society for Testing and Materials. ASTM (2000) ASTM D 6544: standard practice for the preparation of textile prior to UV transmittance testing. ASTM, Conshohocken
71. American Association of Textile Chemists and Colorist. AATCC (2000) AATCC TM 183-1998 transmittance or blocking of erythemally weighted ultraviolet radiation through fabrics. AATC Tech Manual. AATCC, Research Park
72. EN 13758-1 (2002) Fabrics – solar UV protective properties – Method of test for apparel fabrics. Brussels, European Standard, CEN
73. EN 13758 -2 (2003) Fabrics –solar UV protective properties – classification and marking of apparel, Brussels, European Standard, CEN
74. Gambichler T, Laperre J, Hoffmann K (2006) The European standard for sun-protective clothing: EN 13758. J Eur Acad Dermatol Venereol 20:125–130
75. Eichhorn C, Seibold C, Loss J, Steinmann A, Nagel E (2008) Knowledge about UV-radiation and sun protection: survey of adolescents and young adults in Bavaria. Hautarzt 59:821–827
76. Turner D, Harrison SL (2014) Sun protection provided by regulation school uniforms in Australian Schools: an opportunity to improve personal sun protection during childhood. Photochem Photobiol 90(6):1439–1445
77. Wolska A, Owczarek G, Bartkowiak G (2010) UV protective textile clothing for workers exposed to natural and artificial UV radiation. Conf Proc IEEE Eng Med Biol Soc 2010:6260–6263

Chapter 25
Photoprotection by Glass

Manaf Shaban and Fahad Almutawa

Key Points

- Glass has the ability to block all ultraviolet-B (290–320 nm) and a variable amount of ultraviolet-A (320–400 nm). Factors affecting ultraviolet radiation transmission include glass type, thickness, color, and film coating.
- Glass, window films, and sunglasses play an important yet possibly under recognized role in our effort to decrease UVR damage.
- Sunglasses should meet one of the national lens safety standards, be of adequate circumference, wrap around the eye, and be as close to the forehead as possible.

25.1 Introduction

Many governmental educational strategies have been implemented to help increase the awareness of sun protection such as sunscreen use, avoiding sun between peak hours (10 am–2 pm), and wearing wide brimmed hats. These factors are essential, yet there appears to be a lack of education regarding physical sun protection, such as glass and sunglasses which shall be discussed.

Disclosures: No conflict of interest

M. Shaban, MD
Department of Dermatology, Asaad Al Hamad Center, Al Sabah, Safat, PO BOX 25252, Kuwait City 13113, Kuwait
e-mail: Manaf.shaban@gmail.com

F. Almutawa, MD (✉)
Department of Medicine, Kuwait University, Al-Jabriya, Safat, PO Box 24923, Kuwait City 13113, Kuwait
e-mail: fahad.almutawa@hsc.edu.kw

S.Q. Wang, H.W. Lim (eds.), *Principles and Practice of Photoprotection*,
DOI 10.1007/978-3-319-29382-0_25

25.2 Ultraviolet Radiation

Ultraviolet radiation (UVR) consists of UVC (100–290 nm), UVB (290–320 nm), and UVA (340–400 nm). Approximately 90 % of the UVB radiation and all of the UVC radiation are absorbed by the ozone layer. The remaining UVR that reaches the earth's surface consists mainly of UVA, with around 3.5 % UVB [1]. There are several biologic effects of UVR from sunlight. Acute cutaneous affects include erythema, edema, immediate pigment darkening, persistent pigment darkening, delayed tanning, epidermal hyperplasia, and vitamin D synthesis. The chronic effects include photoaging, photocarcinogenesis, and immunosuppression [2]. There are also several ocular effects that can occur to unprotected eyes. These include pterygium, photokeratitis, cortical cataracts, and climatic droplet keratopathy [3].

25.3 Photoprotection by Glass

Glass has chemical properties similar to that of a liquid with a melting point of around 1700 °C but at room temperature behaves as a solid [4]. Glass is mainly made of silica from sand, soda ash, and limestone which are melted together and mixed with various other chemical to change its properties and color. The float process is the classical method of creating smooth sheet glass. Melted glass is poured over a bath of molten tin leaving a perfectly smooth surface as it spreads and cools [5].

25.4 Main Types of Glass

Annealed glass is the most basic type of glass produced from the float process. It is usually the starting type of glass that can later be modified via lamination, toughening, etc. It is often used in double glazed windows; when broken, it results in large sharp pieces [6] (Table 25.1).

Tempered or toughened glass is created by gradual heating and sudden cooling of the glass. It breaks into small pieces that are less likely to cause injury and is four times stronger than annealed glass. It is commonly used in car side windows, glass sliding doors, and shower enclosures [6].

Laminated glass is created when two laminae are fused to a middle plastic PVB (polyvinyl butyral) layer. When this composite is broken, the pieces of glass adhere to the plastic preventing injury and maintaining the glass integrity. This is the main glass type used in front windshields of cars to prevent the passengers from being ejected from the vehicle; it is also increasingly being used for the side windows to increase passenger safety [7].

Table 25.1 Common types of glass

Types of glass	Comments
Annealed glass	Basic flat glass Breaks into large pieces
Toughened glass (tempered glass)	Breaks into small regular pieces Withstands higher compression than annealed glass
Laminated glass	Made of several layers of glass with a middle layer of plastic High protection from UVR Broken pieces are held together via the plastic layer
Coated glass	Coated with layers that can affect its properties, e.g., reflectivity, corrosion, or scratch resistance
Patterned glass	Flat glass with a regular pattern on its surface

Coated glass allows the glass to be modified, such as being scratch resistant, increased reflectivity or transmissibility, and corrosion resistance. It is created by allowing the coating vapor to bind to the surface of the glass often during the float process.

Patterned glass is created by making a pattern on the surface of the glass. This is usually done by passing the heated glass between rollers with an imprint on the rollers. The glass can take on any pattern and it is often used to allow in light but to prevent transparency [6].

25.5 UV Transmission Through Residential Glass

Glass in general has the ability to block all UVB (290–320 nm) and a variable amount of UVA (320–400 nm) depending on the type of glass [8]. The various factors that affect UVR transmission include glass type, thickness, color, and film coating.

In the glass film industry, UVA transmission is often measured up to 380 nm; in general, there is a sharp increase in the UVA transmission between 380 and 400 nm. According to a study performed using 40 different films on museum glass, the protection ranged from 86 to 99 %, only two products actually blocked 99 % of the UVR up to 400 nm [9].

A study by Duarte et al. measured the UVA and UVB penetration through different types of glass of varying colors at different distances from the UVA source [7]. They found that laminated glass blocked all the UVA regardless of distance from the UV source. At 0 cm from the UVA source, the greatest UVA transmission was through annealed glass (74 %), followed by tempered glass (71 %) and patterned glass (44 %).

The color of the glass also had an effect on the transmission of UVA. At 0 cm from the light source, the amount of transmission of UVA through green glass was 0 %, followed by yellow glass (1.3 %), wine glass (31.1 %), colorless glass (36.5 %), and blue glass (56.8 %).

The transmission of radiation was decreased with thicker glass but not significantly, showing that the color of the glass was a more important variable than glass thickness. Glass thickness of 0.2 cm allowed 75.7 % of UVA transmission, and the thickest glass of 1 cm allowed 51.4 % of UVA transmission at 0 cm from the UV source [7].

25.6 UV Exposure in Automobiles

A study by Ding et al. showed that the average driving time for Australians of 45 years of age or older in New South Wales was 84 mins/day [10]. This was similar to the result of a US study that shows that the average time in a car was 1–2 h per day in 169 individuals [11]. The clinical relevance of these findings was shown by the observation that patients with very severe polymorphic light eruption may be triggered by UVA doses of 5 J/cm^2 which can be achieved from 30 to 60 min of UV exposure through tempered glass [8].

In a study of UV exposure in cars, for a left-sided driver in a nonconvertible car with the windows rolled up, the maximal exposure was on the left arm (3–4 % of the ambient radiation) followed by left lateral head. With the windows rolled down, UV exposure was 25 % of the ambient UVR, and in a convertible car, this reached 61 % of the ambient UVR [12]. The size of the car also plays a role as a study by Kimlin et al. found that the average daily UVA exposure was 1.3 times higher in a large family sedan when compared to a small hatchback [13]. The annual UV exposure in people who drive as their primary occupation has been estimated to be around 35 MED which is approximately equivalent to a 1 week of skiing without UV protection [14].

In the USA, two retrospective studies showed that there was a slightly greater increase in basal cell carcinomas, squamous cell carcinomas, Merkel cell carcinomas, and melanomas on the left side corresponding to the driver's side [15, 16]. In Australia, where the driver's seat is on the right, two studies confirmed an increase in actinic keratosis and lentigo maligna on the right side [17, 18].

A recent meta-analysis reported higher risks for melanoma among pilots and cabin crew [19]. Another study showed an increase in mortality related to melanoma in pilots [20]. While these observations could be accounted for by the higher probability of intermittent, high-intensity UV exposure among pilots and cabin crew, the contributory factor of prolonged, intense UV exposure in the cockpit needs to be considered.

25.7 Automobile Glass/UV Transmission Through Automobile Glass

It has now been made compulsory to have laminated glass in the front windshield as the plastic layer prevents thc passenger from being ejected. In contrast, safety tempered glass is usually used in the side windows which shatter into small pieces. The factors that affect UV penetration include glass type, color, protective films, and thickness.

The transmission through a laminated windscreen of a Volvo S60 showed a 98 % blockage of the ambient UVA. Another study showed that a laminated 8 mm automobile glass completely blocked UVA at 0 cm from the UVA source [7]. Moehrle et al. studied blue-tinted, green-tinted, and infrared reflective laminated windscreens and found that they all completely blocked UVA up to 380 nm [12].

Tempered glass also blocks all UVB but allows more UVA penetrance than laminated glass. A study of a tempered side window transmitted 17.6 % of UVA at 0 cm from the source, and no UVA was detected at 25 and 50 cm from the source [7].

The most common color glass used in cars is green. However, it has been shown by Hampton et al. that gray is the most effective color at blocking the transmission of UVA, transmitting only 11.4 % of UVA. This is followed by dark green (22.9 %), light green (35.7 %), and clear (62.8 %) [8].

The thickness of glass decreased the UVA transmission but not in a statistically significant way compared to the other parameters such as color [7]. In contrast, a study by Moehrle et al. found that the average transmission of UVA was 0.8 % for insulative infrared reflective glass, 22.4 % for insulative blue glass, and 17.5 % for insulative green glass [12].

25.8 Window Films

The use of window films was started in the 1960s and was boosted during the 1970s with the energy crisis as a means to reduce heat loss to the external environment; films were also found to reflect infrared radiation back into the interior space [21]. In the USA, windshields have to maintain an American standard rating of 1(AS-1) which is the highest optical clarity allowing more than 70 % transmission of visible light [22]. The allowable side and back window tinting is highly variable according to state regulations [23].

Most films consist of several layers:

1. Protective release layer: This is polyester layer that is removed to expose the adhesive layer.
2. Adhesive layer: This is made of a transparent high-quality adhesive which does not distort and fixes the film to the glass.
3. A multilayered polyester film.
4. Metals, alloys, dyes, and UV inhibitors.
5. Scratch-resistant coating made from acrylic.

The metals, alloys, dyes, and filters work by either reflecting or absorbing the UVR. The most common method used is an individual film layer of UV-blocking material [24]. Bernstein et al. used fibroblast death from UVA exposure as an endpoint to correlate the protection of a UV film on a tempered side vehicle glass [25]. They found that before the film, the glass blocked 21 % of the UVR versus 99.6 % after the film application. Another study using a G50 sunlight control film and tempered 3 mm vehicle glass showed that in the presence of the film, 100 % of UVA transmission was blocked versus 82.4 % without the film [7].

25.9 Photoprotection with Sunglasses

25.9.1 UV Exposure to the Eye

The time of maximal exposure to UVR to the eyes is between 8 am to 10 am and 2 pm to 4 pm, which correlates to the sun's rays being almost parallel to the eye [14]. Almost 50 % of the UVR exposure to the eye occurs from scattering and cloud reflection. This is seen most with UVB as shorter wavelengths scatter the most. The scatter from grass is 2–5 %, water, 3–13 %; concrete buildings, 10 %; and snow, 94 % [26].

In general, the cornea absorbs more than 90 % of the UVB below 300 nm. Within the UVA range, most radiation is absorbed by the lens followed by the aqueous [3]. There is evidence to suggest a high correlation between UVR exposure and the development of pterygium, climactic droplet keratopathy, photokeratitis, keratopathy, and cortical cataract [3]. In the eye, UVB can cause similar effects of acute sunburn on the skin known as photokeratitis. UVB has also been associated with a 60 % increase in the formation of cortical cataract but not nuclear cataracts [27]. A meta-analysis by Sui et al. showed a clear correlation between increased sunlight exposure and the development of age-related macular degeneration [28]. Cumulative blue light exposure is now thought to be the cause of age-related macular degeneration (AMD), rather than UVA or UVB radiation [3].

25.9.2 Sunglasses Guidelines

There are currently three major national guidelines on sunglasses: (1) the Australian/New Zealand standards AS/NZS 1067:2003, (2) the American standard ANSI Z80.3 updated in 2010, and (3) the European standard EN 1836:2005, which will be replaced by the EN ISO 12312–1:2013 by March 2015. The new European standard will include transmittance and refractive changes, resistance to sweat and damage, temporal protection with highly tinted lenses, and increased coverage of the eye [29–31]. The Australian and European standards share the lens category definition but differ on the allowed UVB transmission (Table 25.2) [32, 33]. The American standard categorizes the lenses according to purpose, i.e., cosmetic versus professional use (Table 25.3).

A study performed in 2003 showed that 17 % of 646 sunglasses tested under the European standard failed to meet this standard, showing that self-regulation was insufficient. The Australian and EU standards are now mandatory for eyeglass producers, with the Australian requiring a third party for testing the lenses [34].

There is currently a proposal for the development of an eye-sun protection factor (E-SPF). It integrates the UV reflectance and transmission of the lens to act as an aid similar to skin SPF protection [26] (Table 25.4).

Table 25.2 Summary of the Australian standard (AS/NZ 1067:2003)

Lens category	Luminous transmittance (LT) (%)	UVB (% LT) 280–315 nm	UVA (% LT) 315–400 nm
0 (very light tint)	80–100	5	100 %
1 (light tint)	43–80	5	100 %
2 (medium tint)	18–43	5	100 %
3 (dark tint)	8–18	5	50 %
4 very dark tint)	3–8	5	50 %

Data from Australian Competition and Consumer Commission [29]
LT ratio of the transmitted luminous flux to the incident luminous flux. Luminous transmittance is usually specified with respect to one of the internationally accepted standard illuminants

Table 25.3 Summary of the US standard (ANSI Z80.3:2010)

			UVB (280–315 nm) (% LT)		UVA (315–380 nm)	
Lens color	Purpose	Luminous transmittance (LT) (%)	Normal use	Prolonged use	Normal use (% LT)	Prolonged use (% LT)
Light	Cosmetic	>40	12.5	1	100	50
Medium to dark	General purpose	8–40	12.5	1	100	50
Very dark	Special purpose	3–8	1	1	50	50
Strongly colored	Special purpose	>8	1	1	50	50

Data from American National Standards Institute. *Nonprescription sunglasses and fashion eyewear- requirements*. ANSI Z80.3:2010

Several factors affect the UV transmission of sunglasses. When sunglasses are worn near the forehead, almost 85 % of the UVR (290–350 nm) was blocked. This was reduced to almost 45 % when it was moved 6 mm away from the forehead [35]. There are also requirements in Australia for the minimum lens diameter: in adults, it is 28 mm and in children, 24 mm. The eye may be exposed to solar radiation when the sun is behind the individual between 133° and 155°. The light is reflected back into the eye particularly when the lens has an antireflective coating [36]. It was previously believed that wearing poor quality tinted lenses allowed the pupil to dilate and increase the risk of UVA exposure as the glasses would give the wearer a false sense of security and remain in the sun for longer. This was in contrast to a study analyzing 400 pairs of sunglasses which showed no significant dilation of the pupil when wearing sunglasses [35]. Many contact lens manufactures now offer UV protection incorporated within the lenses; these are usually at least 14 mm in diameter, thus providing protection to the limbus [26].

In general, sunglasses should comply with one of the national guidelines with regard to lens quality, should wrap around the eye with side shields, and should be kept as close to the forehead as possible to minimize harmful UVR reaching the eye.

Table 25.4 Examples of E-SPF based on transmittance and reflectance in the UV range

TUV (%)	RUV (%)	E-SPF
5	10	7
5	5	10
1.5	5	15
0	4	25
0	2	50

Data from Behar-Cohen et al. [26]

25.10 Summary

Glass, window films, and sunglasses play an important yet possibly under recognized role in our effort to decrease UVR damage. The most important factors in choosing glass with the highest UVA protection would be lamination, color, and possibly thickness. Sunglasses should meet one of the national lens safety standards, be of adequate circumference, wrap around the eye, and be as close to the forehead as possible.

References

1. Diffey BL (2002) What is light? Photodermatol Photoimmunol Photomed 18(2):68–74, PubMed
2. Jansen R, Wang SQ, Burnett M, Osterwalder U, Lim HW (2013) Photoprotection: part I. Photoprotection by naturally occurring, physical, and systemic agents. J Am Acad Dermatol 69(6):853 e1-12; quiz 65–6. PubMed
3. Yam JC, Kwok AK (2014) Ultraviolet light and ocular diseases. Int Ophthalmol 34(2):383–400, PubMed
4. British Glass (2014) Flat glass manufacture. Available from: http://www.britglass.org.uk/. Accessed 5 Oct 2014
5. Pilkington (2014) Step by step manufacturing of float glass. Available from: http://www.pilkington.com/. Accessed 12 Sept 2014
6. Glass for Europe (2014) The float process. Available from: http://www.glassforeurope.com/. Accessed 6 Nov 2014
7. Duarte I, Rotter A, Malvestiti A, Silva M (2009) The role of glass as a barrier against the transmission of ultraviolet radiation: an experimental study. Photodermatol Photoimmunol Photomed 25(4):181–184, PubMed
8. Hampton PJ, Farr PM, Diffey BL, Lloyd JJ (2004) Implication for photosensitive patients of ultraviolet A exposure in vehicles. Br J Dermatol 151(4):873–876, PubMed
9. Boye C, Preusser F, Schaeffer T (2010) UV-blocking window films for use in museums. WAAC Newslett 32(1):13–18
10. Ding D, Gebel K, Phongsavan P, Bauman AE, Merom D (2014) Driving: a road to unhealthy lifestyles and poor health outcomes. PLoS One 9(6):e94602, PubMed Pubmed Central PMCID: 4049576
11. McCurdy T, Graham SE (2003) Using human activity data in exposure models: analysis of discriminating factors. J Expo Anal Environ Epidemiol 13(4):294–317
12. Moehrle M, Soballa M, Korn M (2003) UV exposure in cars. Photodermatol Photoimmunol Photomed 19(4):175–181, PubMed
13. Kimlin MG, Parisi AV, Carter BD, Turnbull D (2002) Comparison of the solar spectral ultraviolet irradiance in motor vehicles with windows in an open and closed position. Int J Biometeorol 46(3):150–156, PubMed

14. Sasaki H, Sakamoto Y, Schnider C, Fujita N, Hatsusaka N, Sliney DH et al (2011) UV-B exposure to the eye depending on solar altitude. Eye Contact Lens 37(4):191–195, PubMed
15. Butler ST, Fosko SW (2010) Increased prevalence of left-sided skin cancers. J Am Acad Dermatol 63(6):1006–1010, PubMed
16. Paulson KG, Iyer JG, Nghiem P (2011) Asymmetric lateral distribution of melanoma and Merkel cell carcinoma in the United States. J Am Acad Dermatol 65(1):35–39, PubMed Pubmed Central PMCID: 3117975
17. Foley P, Lanzer D, Marks R (1986) Are solar keratoses more common on the driver's side? Br Med J 293(6538):18, PubMed Pubmed Central PMCID: 1340770
18. Foley PA, Marks R, Dorevitch AP (1993) Lentigo maligna is more common on the driver's side. Arch Dermatol 129(9):1211–1212, PubMed
19. Sanlorenzo M, Wehner MR, Linos E, Kornak J, Kainz W, Posch C et al (2015) The risk of melanoma in airline pilots and cabin crew: a meta-analysis. J Am Med Assoc 151(1):51–58
20. Yong LC, Pinkerton LE, Yiin JH, Anderson JL, Deddens JA (2014) Mortality among a cohort of U.S. commercial airline cockpit crew. Am J Ind Med 57(8):906–914
21. European Window Film Association (2014) Window film manufacturing process. Available from: http://www.ewfa.org/. Accessed 3 Nov 2014
22. Car windshields (2014) Car windshield markings. Available from: http://www.carwindshields.info/windshieldmarkings. Accessed 2 Dec 2014
23. International Window Film Association (2014) State window tinting rules & laws [updated January 2013]. Available from: http://www.iwfa.com/. Accessed 20 Oct 2014
24. Almutawa F, Vandal R, Wang SQ, Lim HW (2013) Current status of photoprotection by window glass, automobile glass, window films, and sunglasses. Photodermatol Photoimmunol Photomed 29(2):65–72, PubMed
25. Bernstein EF, Schwartz M, Viehmeyer R, Arocena MS, Sambuco CP, Ksenzenko SM (2006) Measurement of protection afforded by ultraviolet-absorbing window film using an in vitro model of photodamage. Lasers Surg Med 38:337–342
26. Behar-Cohen F, Baillet G, de Ayguavives T, Garcia PO, Krutmann J, Pena-Garcia P et al (2014) Ultraviolet damage to the eye revisited: eye-sun protection factor (E-SPF(R)), a new ultraviolet protection label for eyewear. Clinical Ophthalmol 8:87–104, PubMed Pubmed Central PMCID: 3872277
27. Taylor HR, West S, Munoz B, Rosenthal FS, Bressler SB, Bressler NM (1992) The long-term effects of visible light on the eye. Arch Ophthalmol 110(1):99–104, PubMed
28. Sui GY, Liu GC, Liu GY, Gao YY, Deng Y, Wang WY et al (2013) Is sunlight exposure a risk factor for age-related macular degeneration? A systematic review and meta-analysis. Br J Ophthalmol 97(4):389–394, PubMed
29. Australian Competition & Consumer Commission (2003) Sunglasses & fashion spectacles. Available from: http://www.productsafety.gov.au. Accessed 3 Dec 2014
30. American National Standards Institute (2010) Nonprescription sunglass and fashion eyewear requirements. Available from: http://www.ansi.org. Accessed 3 Dec 2014
31. Bureau Veritas Consumer Product Services (2013) Withdrawal of the EN 1836 sunglasses standard and its replacements by two new EN ISO standards. Available from: http://www.bureauveritas.com. Accessed 7 Dec 2014
32. Dain SJ (2003) Sunglasses and sunglass standards. Clin Exp Optom 86(2):77–90, PubMed
33. Wang SQ, Balagula Y, Osterwalder U (2010) Photoprotection: a review of the current and future technologies. Dermatol Ther 23(1):31–47, PubMed
34. Dain SJ, Ngo TP, Cheng BB, Hu A, Teh AG, Tseng J et al (2010) Sunglasses, the European directive and the European standard. Ophthalmic Physiol Opt 30(3):253–256, PubMed
35. Rosenthal FS, Bakalian AE, Lou CQ, Taylor HR (1988) The effect of sunglasses on ocular exposure to ultraviolet radiation. Am J Public Health 78(1):72–74, PubMed Pubmed Central PMCID: 1349214
36. Krutmann J, Behar-Cohen F, Baillet G, de Ayguavives T, Ortega Garcia P, Pena-Garcia P et al (2014) Towards standardization of UV eye protection: what can be learned from photodermatology? Photodermatol Photoimmunol Photomed 30(2–3):128–136, PubMed

Chapter 26
Augmenting Skin Photoprotection Beyond Sunscreens

Thomas Meyer, Donathan Beasley, and Kerry Hanson

Key Points

- Sun exposure generates an abundance of reactive oxygen species (ROS) within skin, which overwhelm skin's natural defenses (leading to oxidative stress) and which over the course of our lives exact a toll on skin's health and appearance (especially photoaging).
- Recent research establishes that generation of sun-induced ROS within skin occurs from exposure not only to the ultraviolet (UV) but also to the visible and infrared spectral regions; these results prompt thinking of new strategies for photoprotection that go beyond the UV attenuation capacities of sunscreen filters.
- In addition to sunscreen filters, antioxidants (AOX) and quenchers of photoexcited states (QPES) represent promising, complimentary intervention strategies for topical products that can suppress or scavenge ROS and thereby optimize skin's protection against the harmful effects of sun-induced ROS formation.
- Selection of AOX and QPES for use in sunscreens needs to be conducted judiciously, since they have potential to function as pro-oxidants (i.e., photosensitizers) when applied to skin and exposed to the sun, which would exacerbate the burden of excess ROS formation within skin.
- Addition of appropriate AOX to sunscreens can significantly improve protection against ROS formation within skin over a broad range of low to high SPFs.

T. Meyer (✉) • D. Beasley
Design Innovation, Bayer Consumer Health, Memphis, TN, USA
e-mail: thomas.meyer3@bayer.com

K. Hanson
Department of Chemistry, University of California, Riverside, CA, USA
e-mail: kerry.hanson@ucr.edu

S.Q. Wang, H.W. Lim (eds.), *Principles and Practice of Photoprotection*,
DOI 10.1007/978-3-319-29382-0_26

26.1 Introduction

Skin is under constant assault by a strong oxidizing environment, including pollutants, ozone, smoke, and solar radiation, which stimulates the formation of reactive oxygen species (ROS). While skin possesses a full complement of its own antioxidant defenses, research has shown that these defenses can be overwhelmed easily when exposed to ultraviolet radiation (UVR) [1–3]. When this occurs, oxidative stress sets in leaving ROS free to attack biomolecules (DNA, lipids, proteins, carbohydrates) or to influence signal transduction pathways and gene expression [4, 5]. Excess ROS are strongly linked to photoaging and are detrimental to skin's overall health [6–8].

Until recently, it was believed that ROS induced in skin by terrestrial solar radiation (including UV, visible, infrared radiation) originated predominantly from the UV portion of the solar spectrum. However, newer research suggests that this traditional view needs to be amended based on findings that significant levels of ROS formation are stimulated by radiation well outside the UV region. Beginning in the mid-1990s, research began to show that, in addition to UVR, visible radiation can generate ROS within skin [9–11]. In addition, and most recently, Zastrow *et al.* determined the free radical effectiveness spectrum in *ex vivo* human skin exposed to sun over 280–700 nm, and while they observed a maximum peak of ROS formation in the UVA region, they also found unexpectedly that as much as 50 % of the total ROS measured was induced by visible wavelengths [12]. In agreement with these results, Liebel *et al.* recently reported that exposures to solar relevant doses of visible radiation were as effective as UVR in generating ROS within human epidermal equivalents [13]. Moreover, others have also discovered that even longer wavelengths of radiation in the near-infrared region (IRA – 770–1400 nm) appear capable of inducing ROS formation in human skin and more specifically in dermal mitochondria, which have important implications for photoaging of human skin [14–16]. These recent publications provide mounting evidence that radiation outside the UV spectrum contributes significantly to ROS generation within skin with strong links to photoaging, which prompt thinking of new strategies for photoprotection that go beyond the UV attenuation capacities of sunscreen filters.

In recognition of the growing importance of ROS in mediating skin responses to solar radiation, we open this chapter with a brief review of the chemistry and formation of ROS followed by an overview of the main intervention strategies to help suppress or scavenge ROS within skin. We then focus on the use of antioxidants (AOX) as an obvious strategy to help skin cope with the burden of excess ROS formation induced by UVR exposure. While we provide a brief survey of the main experimental techniques to assess effectiveness of AOX, we also share some simple methods we have both developed and reported that are useful to select and confirm that AOX are indeed appropriate for use in sunscreen products. Lastly, we demonstrate the utility of AOX in low to high SPF sunscreens to improve their ability to attenuate ROS formation in UVR-exposed skin.

Table 26.1 Common ROS in skin

ROS molecule	Symbol
Singlet oxygen	$^1O_2$
Hydrogen peroxide	H_2O_2
Superoxide anion	$O_2{\cdot}^-$
Hydroxyl radical	$\cdot OH$
Alkoxy radical	$RO\cdot$
Alkyl peroxy radical	$RCOO\cdot$

26.2 Basics of ROS Chemistry and Formation

Reactive oxygen species (ROS) are a class of oxygen derivatives which have the potential to initiate radical reactions, and nowhere is this potential more evident than in a cell, where ROS can exhibit a duality in behavior. They occur naturally to maintain healthy cell function, most clearly represented by their integral role in mitochondrial respiration and participation in cellular signaling, and are typically inhibited from undergoing uncontrolled radical reactions through an endogenous network of both enzymatic and small-molecule antioxidants [17, 18]. However, when the AOX network fails, oxidative stress ensues from ROS, initiating chain radical reactions on cellular targets such as polyunsaturated fatty lipids, proteins, and both mitochondrial and nuclear DNA [19–22]. Failure of the AOX network in the skin can result from a depletion in AOX as well as an increase in the concentration of pro-oxidant ROS that overwhelms the skin's intrinsic AOX network [1, 22, 23]. The end result is the same – an increase in oxidative stress in the skin through ROS-initiated radical reactions [1, 2].

ROS include both free radical and non-radical species (Table 26.1). In general free radicals, like hydroxyl radical ($\cdot OH$), superoxide anion ($O_2{\cdot}^-$), and peroxide radical ($ROO\cdot$), have an unpaired electron centered on the oxygen, in contrast to non-radical species like hydrogen peroxide (H_2O_2), which have full electron shells on all atoms. Oxygen is a particularly unique ROS because of its diradical nature and ground-state triplet character, making it a highly reactive molecule, and of particular importance in biological systems. Its reactivity can be more fully understood through a diagram of the distribution of its valence electrons. Recalling that electrons in molecules are contained in molecular orbitals (MO), where each MO can hold two electrons with opposite spins denoted by an up or down arrow, we can see that most molecules fill their MOs with paired spins, such that no net spin exists, and the molecule would be considered to be in a "singlet" state. The exception to this rule is molecular oxygen, which, because of Hund's rule, has two electrons with the same spin in two different molecular orbitals of equal energy (Fig. 26.1) yielding a net ± spin such that the molecule exists in a "triplet" state ($^3O_2$). This is an important characteristic of oxygen because, as a triplet, it can participate in triplet-state reactions (Fig. 26.1), which can lead to the formation of the highly reactive singlet oxygen ($^1O_2$) as well as the superoxide anion ($O_2{\cdot}^-$). Both are highly destructive ROS, but $^1O_2$ warrants a particular focus because in its short lifetime (2 μs in H_2O), it has the ability to act in signal transduction as well as in more destructive reactions with saturated bonds of cellular molecules like lipids and proteins forming derivatives of hydroperoxides, endoperoxides, and cycloaddition products. Its highly reactive nature can be more fully understood, again, by looking at its valence electrons (Fig. 26.1), which show that upon energy transfer by another triplet-state molecule (i.e., triplet sensitization), one electron flips spin and joins its pair in one of two available π MOs such that there is no net spin and the molecule is considered a "singlet" state. Unlike most singlet states, $^1O_2$ is highly unstable compared to its $^3O_2$ ground state and thus is highly reactive.

In order to interact with skin photochemically to induce ROS formation, solar radiation must be absorbed by chromophores resident in skin cells and extracellular matrix. Table 26.2 lists common chromophores in the skin and the ROS that they have been found to sensitize. Each reaction that leads to ROS generation is unique to the energetics and kinetics of the chromophore involved; however, in general, understanding how these molecules can generate ROS can be gained through a Jablonski diagram (Fig. 26.2), which shows that following absorption of a photon,

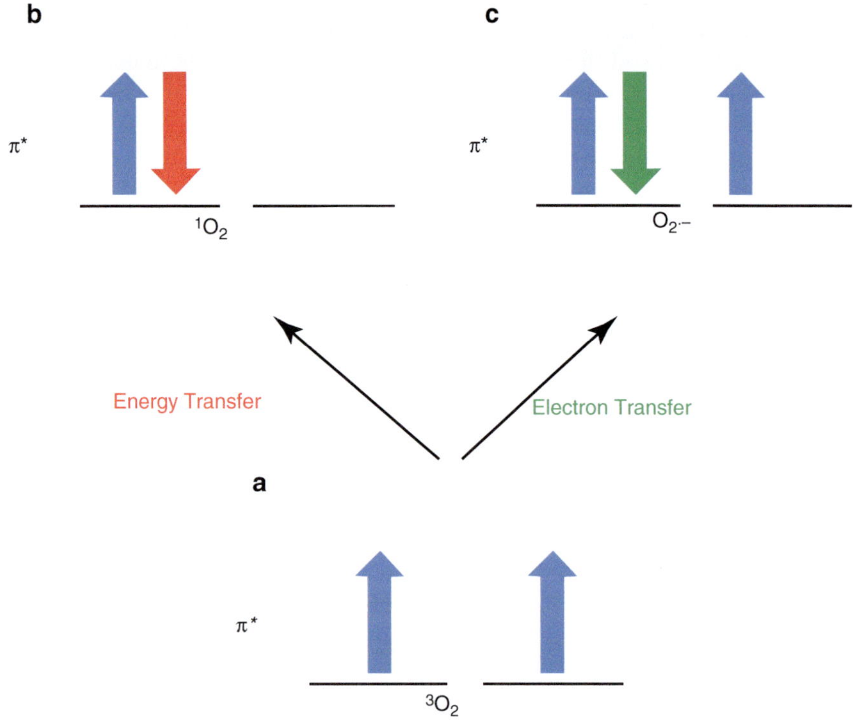

Fig. 26.1 Abbreviated molecular orbitals for ground state oxygen (**a**), the lowest excited state of oxygen (**b**), and superoxide anion (**c**). In its ground state, because of Hund's rule, the outermost electrons of the molecule have parallel spins in the two p^* orbitals, indicating a triplet state. When excited, the one of these electrons flips a spin and can pair with the other electron in one p orbital, thus forming an unstable and thus highly reactive singlet state. Superoxide anion forms (**c**) when an extra electron is donated to $^3O_2$ from another molecule

Table 26.2 Common chromophores in skin

Chromophore	Wavelength of excitation (nm)	ROS sensitized
Bilirubin [24, 25]	400–600	H_2O_2
Collagen: Pentosidine in advanced glycation end products (AGEs) [26–28]	320–400	$O_2\cdot^-$, H_2O_2, OH
Collagen/elastin [29]	320–400	H_2O_2
Copper -cytochrome C complex IV [14, 15, 30]	770–1400	ROS unidentified
Melanin [31, 32]	230–600	H_2O_2
NADH, NADPH [33–35]	290–405	$O_2\cdot^-$, $^1O_2$
Nucleosides (2-thiouracil, 4-thiouridine) [34, 35]	290–405	$O_2\cdot^-$, $^1O_2$
Porphyrins [24–27, 36–38]	290–700	$O_2\cdot^-$, H_2O_2, $^1O_2$
Riboflavin [21, 23, 27, 28, 39]	290–465	$O_2\cdot^-$, $^1O_2$
Tryptophan [40, 41]	300–400	$O_2\cdot^-$, H_2O_2, $^1O_2$
Urocanic acid [31, 42]	310	$^1O_2$

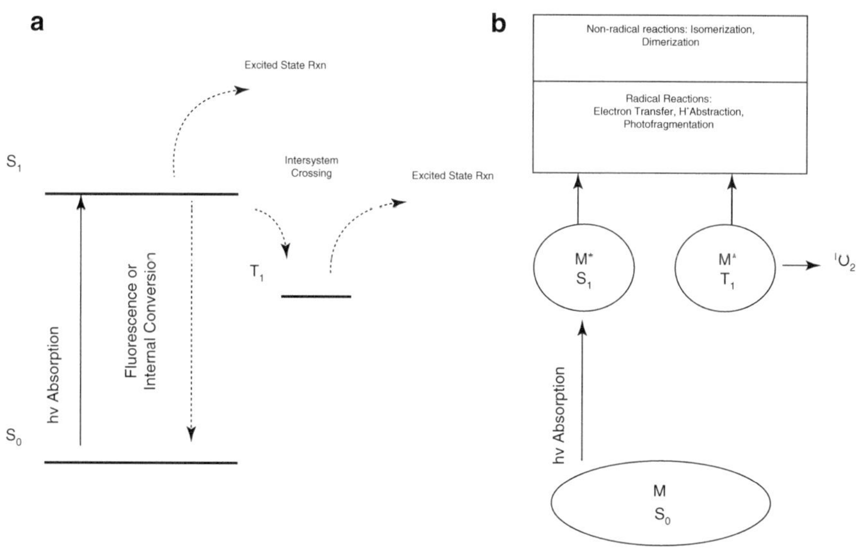

Fig. 26.2 (**a**) A Jablonski diagram showing the possible energy levels and reaction pathways of a skin chromophore M, where S_0 is the ground state, S_1 is the first excited singlet state, and T_1 is the first triplet state. (**b**) A more detailed description of the potential excited state reactions that may occur from S_1 or T_1. ROS can be formed through energy transfer through the triplet manifold to form singlet oxygen, or other radical reactions can occur with proteins, lipids, DNA, sugars. Non-radical reactions can lead to the formation of photoproducts

a molecule (M) is excited from the ground (S_0) to, most often, the excited singlet state (S_1) (the exception being molecular oxygen as discussed above). From S_1 a molecule can dissipate the excess energy via innocuous mechanisms of internal conversion (heat) or fluorescence (light). However, as described in Fig. 26.2b, for

ROS sensitization we become concerned when two pathways are favored: (1) intersystem crossing to the excited state triplet manifold (T_1) or (2) excited state reactions from S_1 or T_1. If the molecule forms a triplet, then sensitization of singlet oxygen ($^1O_2$) can occur through the triplet manifold with ground-state molecular oxygen $^3O_2$. Additionally, if the energetics and kinetics are favorable, the excited molecule (M*) in S_1 or T_1 may undergo both non-radical reactions (isomerization, dimerization) and radical reactions with proteins, lipids, nucleic acids, and sugars (R) to form a radicalized R. Multiple radical reactions are possible, including peroxidation. Figure 26.2 is a simplified drawing to illustrate some of the potential pathways by which a chromophore may sensitize ROS. It is important to emphasize that any chromophore, either endogenous in the skin or exogenously applied to the skin if it is energetically and kinetically allowed, may sensitize ROS formation.

The information in Table 26.2 also raises the general recognition that skin contains many different types of chromophores that may serve to sensitize ROS formation over a broad range of wavelengths, including UV (290–400 nm), visible (400–770 nm), and IRA (770–1400 nm) radiation. The different wavelength regions comprise vastly different energies and have different capacities to penetrate skin. Owing to these factors, Grether-Beck *et al.* emphasized that the three different wavelength bands likely interact with different chromophores in different cellular compartments to exert their biological effects [15]. A good example is ROS overproduction by IRA radiation where the main chromophore has been identified as the copper complex of intramitochondrial cytochrome-C complex IV of dermal fibroblasts. The resulting increase in intracellular ROS correlates with the upregulation of the matrix metalloproteinase-1 (MMP-1) enzyme, which degrades collagen in the extracellular matrix in a process that is associated with many of the hallmark signs of photoaging, including coarse wrinkles and skin laxity. While the specific ROS generated by IRA radiation have not been elucidated to date as the research is so new, this example among others listed in Table 26.2 stresses the need for additional skin photoprotective strategies that go beyond the traditional protection afforded by UV filters in sunscreen products.

26.3 Topical Intervention Strategies to Reduce ROS Induced by Solar Radiation

Topical formulations containing three unique classes of ingredients have emerged in the scientific literature to reduce the burden of sun-induced formation of ROS within skin, including:

- Sunscreens
- Quenchers of photoexcited states (QPES)
- Antioxidants (AOX)

As illustrated in Fig. 26.3, the striking feature of these three ingredient is how well they appear to complement one another to suppress formation or scavenge

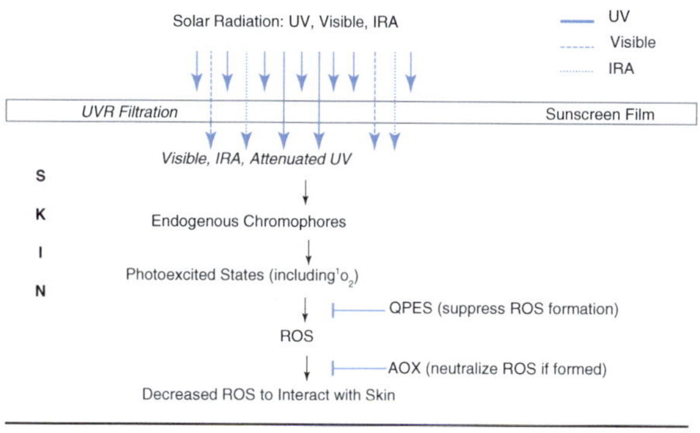

Fig. 26.3 Schematic illustrating the complimentary action of sunscreens, quenchers of photoexcited states (*QPES*), and antioxidants (*AOX*) to prevent, suppress, or neutralize ROS within skin. Sunscreens attenuate UV before it can interact with skin's endogenous chromophores, while QPES relax photoexcited states before they can sensitize ROS formation and AOX neutralize ROS if formed. The action of all three ingredients functions to decrease the extra burden of ROS formed within skin during exposure to solar radiation

ROS within skin. Sunscreens filter sun's UV radiation at skin's surface to attenuate levels of UVR that can reach and interact with endogenous chromophores in the underlying skin, whereas QPES and AOX each work within skin below the protective sunscreen film. QPES function upstream of ROS formation by relaxing photoexcited states via electron transfer or energy transfer pathways before they can sensitize the formation of ROS. Antioxidants, on the other hand, scavenge ROS once formed before they can initiate damaging radical interactions with skin.

Sunscreens represent the first line of defense against ROS formation from UVR when skin is exposed to the sun. While exposure to UVB and UVA both induce ROS formation, research has firmly established that filtration of UVA rays plays a more important role in reducing ROS formation within skin, in agreement with the free radical effectiveness spectrum [12, 43–45]. Indeed, sunscreens containing combinations of UVB, UVA, and broadband UVA/UVB sunscreen actives can be highly effective at reducing ROS generation within skin. For example, Flober-Muller *et al.* reported a radical skin/sun protection factor (RSF) as high as 51 was achieved for a lotion formulation containing a combination of the UVA sunscreen diethylamino hydroxybenzoyl hexyl benzoate (5 %) with the UVB sunscreen actives octocrylene (5 %) and octinoxate (5 %) [45]. As RSF represents the ratio of the number of free radicals generated in unprotected skin to the number of free radicals generated in protected skin, a value of 51 means that the broad-spectrum sunscreen lotion reduced free radical generation caused by UVR exposure within skin by about 98 %.

While their ability to protect against UVR damage associated with both acute and chronic skin damage is undisputed, sunscreens lack ability to neutralize ROS, and they cannot prevent ROS formation stimulated by wavelengths outside their UV attenuation capacities (290–400 nm). This latter point is important since it is now appreciated (a) that as much as 50 % of ROS formed in human skin exposed to solar radiation may be caused by visible radiation (400–700 nm) and (b) that near-infrared radiation (IRA, 770–1400 nm) can also generate ROS in dermal fibroblasts through mitochondrial interactions that appear to have clinical relevance for photoaging of human skin [12, 15].

As depicted in Fig. 26.3, the protective action of sunscreens against sun-induced ROS formation can be augmented by the inclusion of QPES or AOX along with sunscreens. QPES is a term coined by Wondrak *et al.* to describe agents that can assist excited states of skin's endogenous chromophores (including singlet oxygen) by dissipating their excess energies acquired from absorption through alternative pathways (energy or charge-transfer reactions) that are harmless to skin [46]. QPES neither absorb radiation directly nor become consumed during the process, so they can continue to catalyze relaxation of skin's endogenous excited states as long as skin is exposed to the sun. In separate publications, Wondrak *et al.* outlined the various mechanisms by which QPES can inactivate photoexcited states and described a battery of test methods to identify QPES, including use of reconstructed human skin exposed to solar-simulated UVR [46, 47]. Wondrak lists several effective QPES agents from his and other research groups, including molecules that incorporate secondary cyclic amines (L-proline methyl ester, ectoine, mycosporine amino acids) or plant-derived polyphenols (genticaulein) [48]. Most recently, Jockusch *et al.* identified that cyanoacrylates with fused aromatic rings effectively quenched excited states of porphyrins to suppress formation of singlet oxygen [49]. Porphyrins cause photosensitivity skin disorders called porphyrias, which are caused by an abnormality in the heme metabolic pathway leading to an accumulation of porphyrins in the skin and other body tissues. Exposure to visible radiation (400–410 nm) triggers the disease, which manifests clinically with vesicles, bullae, and hyper- or hypopigmentation [50].

AOX, on the other hand, help neutralize ROS once formed in skin before they can oxidize biomolecules or influence signal transduction pathways. Classic AOX typically function by one-electron or hydrogen atom donation to neutralize free radicals and help terminate chain reactions. As indicated earlier, while skin has a full complement of enzymatic (superoxide dismutase, catalase, peroxidases) and nonenzymatic (vitamin E, ascorbic acid, glutathione) antioxidants to cope with excess ROS formation, exposure to sun produces such an abundance of ROS that skin's own defenses become easily overwhelmed [1, 2]. Supplementation of topical products with AOX can bolster skin's natural antioxidant defenses and help prevent UV-induced oxidative damages [18, 51, 52]. However, as will be shown below, selection of AOX for use in sunscreens needs to be conducted judiciously. For example, care must be taken to ensure that AOX themselves do not become strong pro-oxidants (i.e., photosensitizers) when applied to skin and subsequently exposed to UVR.

Thus, sunscreens with high UVA protection factors combined with QPES or AOX represent promising complimentary intervention strategies to optimize protection of skin against the harmful effects of sun-induced ROS formation. It must be emphasized, however, that both QPES and AOX must be present at the right levels and must be within close physical proximity to their intended targets within skin in order to perform their functions successfully. Formulations must be designed to release AOX and QPES so they become bioavailable. Many *in vivo* human studies now document the ability of various combinations of AOX from topical applications to exert protective effects within epidermis and dermis from ROS induced by UVR, visible, or IRA radiation [12, 14, 50]. Especially significant is the finding that topical AOX can reduce expression of MMP-1 within skin. MMP-1 is the main matrix metalloproteinase enzyme responsible for degradation of collagen from exposure to solar radiation and is now accepted as a major biomarker of photoaging in human skin [53].

26.4 Methods to Select and Monitor AOX Performance

There are many *in vitro* assays based on transfer of a single electron or hydrogen atom that have been used to assess the relative performance of AOX to quench free radicals in solution [54]. While these methods are useful to measure antioxidant capacities in various biological matrices (plasma, saliva, food extracts) or even track AOX integrity and stability in finished product formulations, they have limited utility to predict AOX efficacy in skin exposed to solar radiation. These assays neither provide any indication of AOX bioavailability within different cellular compartments of skin nor take into account possible photochemical reactions of AOX when they are applied to skin and exposed to solar radiation. The importance of using methods that include exposures to solar radiation to qualify AOX for use in sunscreen products is critical, since AOX can become powerful photosensitizers when exposed to solar radiation. Under these circumstances, AOX can significantly increase rather than decrease ROS formation within skin, which is exactly opposite of the intended effect. As reported below, this is especially true for some botanical AOX.

26.4.1 Main Experimental Techniques to Monitor AOX Performance in Skin

The ability of AOX to neutralize ROS within skin is typically assessed by employing either spectroscopic techniques to measure changes in ROS levels or biological assays to track various biomarkers that result from ROS damage. A summary of the experimental methods appears in Table 26.3. All of these methods involve exposure to UVR and interestingly comprise a mixture of *in vitro* and *in vivo* methods plus invasive and noninvasive *in vivo* techniques. While it is beyond the scope of this chapter to review all these different techniques, in the remaining sections below, we provide more complete descriptions of the methods we have used to screen AOX and to confirm AOX compatibility for use in sunscreen products.

Table 26.3 Spectroscopic and biological assays of ROS detection

Method	Characteristics
Chemiluminescence of $^1O_2$ [13, 55]	Direct noninvasive *in vivo* measure of human skin Measures $^1O_2$ emission at 1296 nm Measures signal from total skin
Electron spin resonance in vivo [56]	Direct noninvasive *in vivo* measure of human skin Measures decrease in applied stable free radical (TEMPO) Measures signal from total skin
Electron spin resonance ex vivo [43–45]	Indirect *in vitro* measure of ROS ROS trapped by spin traps Measures signal from total skin
Two-photon fluorescence microscopy [11, 56–58]	Indirect *in vitro* measure of ROS Fluorescent probes to detect ROS Quantification with 1 μm resolution up to 100 μm
Biological assays (in vitro *or* in vivo)	Detection of oxidation products of lipids, proteins, DNA [3, 18, 21, 60] Depletion of enzymatic and nonenzymatic AOX (catalase, vitamin E, glutathione, ascorbic acid) [1–3] Detection of MMPs, inflammatory mediators (IL-a, PGE_2, TNF), AGE [15, 18, 51, 61, 62]

AOX antioxidant, *IL-1a* interleukin-1α, *PGE_2* prostaglandin E 2, *TNF_α* tumor necrosis factor α, *AGE* advanced glycation end products

26.4.2 ROS Detection: Quantification by Two-Photon Fluorescence Imaging Spectroscopy

Advances in two-photon fluorescence imaging microscopy (TPM) and fluorescence probe technologies in the early 2000s led to the development of methodologies to image ROS generation as a function of skin depth on a <1 um scale. The result is a visualization of the density of ROS throughout a skin layer and/or a cell in a skin layer following a perturbation like UV irradiation, which provides support to the adage "a picture is worth a thousand words." TPM monitors the fluorescence intensity or fluorescence lifetime of endogenous chromophores or exogenous fluorescence probes. TPM has been used to study the structure of the skin as well as biochemical processes including pH, barrier homeostasis, as well as UV-induced ROS [11, 57, 59, 79–81]. Herein, we focus upon the latter.

Using TPM for ROS detection in skin requires tissue, an ROS fluorescence probe, and a two-photon fluorescence microscope. In general, a skin tissue sample is incubated with an ROS fluorescence probe like dihydrorhodamine (DHR) that is non-fluorescent until reacted with ROS, whereupon the probe becomes highly fluorescent upon two-photon excitation. For example, DHR is converted to rhodamine 123 (R123) upon reaction with different ROS including $^1O_2$, H_2O_2, and $ONOO^-$ [11, 63–66]. TPM works by the simultaneous interaction of two ultrafast (10^{-15} s) infrared photons in an $\chi^{(3)}$ process with the converted ROS probe, which then emits photons from its excited singlet state through the fluorescence pathway.

The fluorescence can be detected using a photomultiplier detector on the microscope, with an increase in fluorescence intensity, compared to a pre-UV irradiated control, primarily representing an increase in ROS. Scanning mirrors can be used to image throughout the *xyz* dimensions.

Figure 26.4 shows a typical series of two-photon fluorescence images of different epidermal cell layers pre- and post-UV (solar-simulated) radiation. A rainbow scale reflects the fluorescence intensity of the ROS probe either before UVR (DHR) or after UVR (R123). The pre-UVR images are predominately blue-black, which indicates as expected that R123 has not been formed through reaction of DHR with ROS and that background autofluorescence is minimal. Post-UVR, however, the intensity dramatically increases. All images show a large increase in fluorescence indicating the generation of ROS. Because of the anucleated lipid-rich nature of the stratum corneum, images of this layer appear inhomogeneous and lack apparent cell structure. We believe that this results from the inhomogeneous labeling of the ROS probe throughout the layer. In contrast, TPM images of the nucleated epidermal layers show obvious cell structure, with nuclei, cytoplasm, and its organelles, as well as intercellular spaces clearly differentiated. The images show that ROS are generated predominately in the cytoplasm, which may result in an inability of the ROS probe to label the cell membranes, intercellular space, and/or nuclei. Other fluorescence ROS probes may label the keratinocytes differently than DHR.

As the images show, compared to one-photon confocal methods, TPM is intrinsically three dimensional with <1 μm spatial resolution. In addition, because the near-IR light (>800 nm) that is used in TPM is non-resonant with endogenous skin chromophores (Table 26.2), the excitation is localized only in the focal region such that photodamage to the tissue sample as well as background fluorescence are minimized, with the concomitant benefit of an increased penetration depth up to the dermis [67–69].

More specific details of how TPM is used to image skin can be found in several references, but two points are worth mentioning here [67–69]. First, both *ex vivo* and living skin equivalents like MatTek EpiDerm™ have been successfully used to detect UV-induced ROS in epidermis and yield similar results. Second, many ROS probes like DHR have limitations: they are unspecific, reacting with multiple ROS like $^1O_2$, hydroxyl radical, or $ONOO^-$; they may undergo autoxidation, although this pathway is considered minor compared to the direct DHR + ROS pathway; and they distribute heterogeneously throughout a cell and/or cell layer. As such, the fluorescence signal from a converted ROS probe in an experiment can represent a lower limit to the ROS density that is generated under UVR.

To determine the effect of an ingredient, like UV filters or antioxidants (AOX) on UV-induced ROS levels in our skin models, the fluorescence intensity of each TPM image, or in the case of nucleated layers, the fluorescence intensity of each cell throughout an image, is recorded. Comparisons between tissues with different ingredients can then be made to a control tissue sample to determine the effect an ingredient has upon the ROS level. This value is typically reported as a fraction of the control (*f*ROS) where *f*ROS > 1 indicates the ingredient sensitized ROS above the control and *f*ROS < 1 indicates the ingredient neutralized ROS relative to the control [11, 58, 57, 59]. A % reduction in ROS can be calculated by Eq. 26.1.

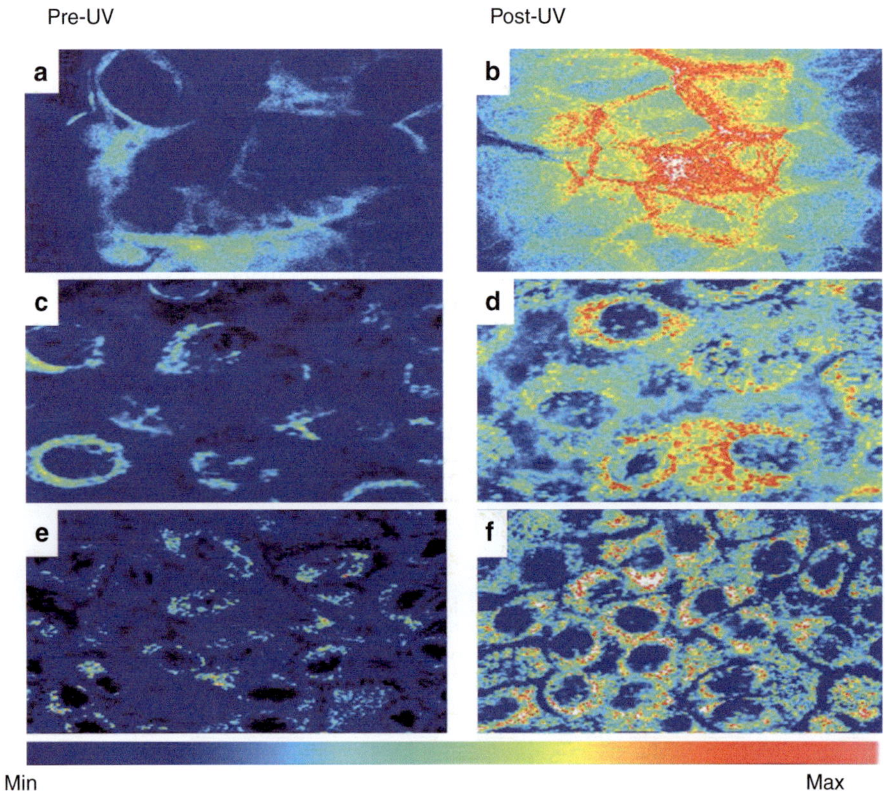

Fig. 26.4 Two-photon fluorescence images of skin tissue incubated with the ROS probe DHR both before (**a**, **c**, **e**) and after (**b**, **d**, **f**) solar-simulated UV irradiation (22 mJ cm^{-2} UVB, 660 mJ cm^{-2} UVA) at *ca.* 5 μm (**a**, **b**), 20 μm, (**c**, **d**) and 70 μm (**e**, **f**)

$$\%\ \text{ROS Reduction} = 100 - 100\left(f\text{ROS}\right) \tag{26.1}$$

26.4.3 Biomarker Assessment: Lipid Hydroperoxides

It is firmly established that exposure of skin to UVR mediates peroxidation of lipids through ROS and that lipid hydroperoxides (LOOH) represent a useful biomarker to monitor effectiveness of AOX within skin [60]. LOOH have been linked to immune suppression, photoaging, and solar elastosis through breakdown of LOOH to form small reactive carbonyl compounds and singlet oxygen [61, 70–72]. Intriguingly, LOOH has also been linked to development of a characteristic cross-hatched pattern of fine lines in skin of hairless mice following one daily application of squalene monohydroperoxide for 15 weeks, which contrasted starkly with the pattern of deeper wrinkles and furrows that formed in hairless mice exposed to UVB only in the same study [73].

We developed a straightforward, noninvasive *ex vivo* method that measures the ability of AOX to prevent oxidation of physiologically relevant stratum corneum lipids that are removed from human skin and subsequently exposed to solar-simulated UVR [74]. The method utilizes a simple lotion base as a placebo into which AOX can be added. Lotions are then applied (2 mg cm^{-2}) to rectangular areas outlined on the inner forearms of human subjects, with placebo lotion applied to one site and with placebo + AOX lotions applied to other forearm sites. After the lotions dry for at least 30 min, surface skin layers inside the application sites are removed with tape, which are subsequently irradiated with solar-simulated UVR (2 MED), extracted into isopropanol, and assayed for total lipid hydroperoxide content using an assay kit from Kamiya Biomedical (Thousand Oaks, CA). The percent reduction in LOOH formation for the AOX lotion is then calculated relative to the maximum LOOH formed from placebo lotion without any AOX. Figure 26.5 summarizes the results for several different types and combinations of AOX. The results showcase several interesting features:

- The method is capable of differentiating between AOX that reduce (antioxidative) versus increase (pro-oxidative) LOOH formation.
- Most of the pro-oxidants tested comprise botanical extracts.
- Pro-oxidant behaviors of botanical extracts can be negated by adding vitamin E.
- Vitamin E, green tea extract, and tetrahydrocurcuminoids have strong ability to protect lipids in skin's outer layers from UVR-induced oxidation.

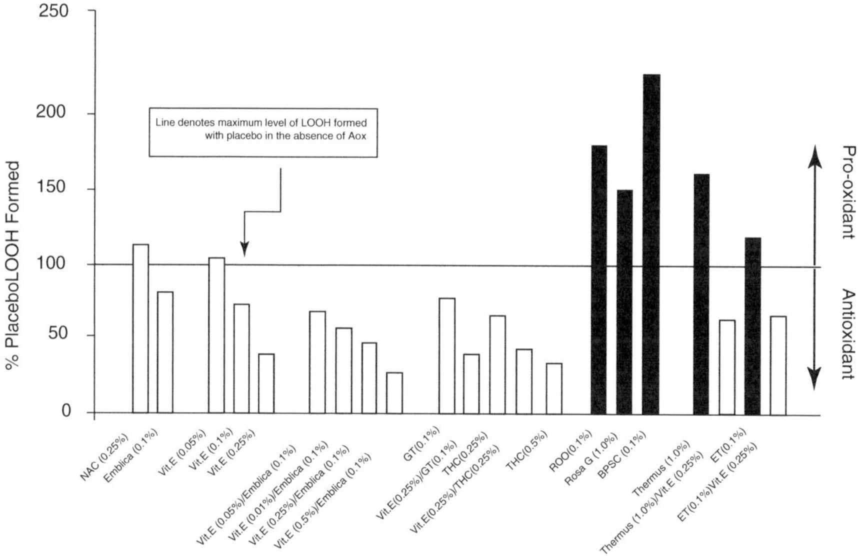

Fig. 26.5 Examples of antioxidants (*AOX*) showing their ability to inhibit or enhance UVR-induced formation of lipid hydroperoxides (*LOOH*) in an *ex vivo* study using tape strips to collect lipids from human skin in the absence or presence of different types and levels of AOX. The results highlight the need to qualify AOX for use in sunscreen products. *NAC* n-Acetyl cysteine, *Emblica Phyllanthus emblica* fruit extract, *Vit.E* vitamin E, *GT* green tea extract, *THC* tetrahydrocurcuminoids, *ROO Rosmarinus officinalis* oleoresin, *Rose G Rose gallica* extract, *BPSC* bioactive photosynthetic complex from green tea, *Thermus Thermus thermophilus* ferment, *ET* ergothiotaine

The experimental design provides additional advantages in that (a) each subject serves as their own control; (b) the tape strips fix the lipids, AOX, and squames to its surface in a similar spatial arrangement as existed on the skin; and (c) the method eliminates the need to irradiate skin of human subjects.

26.4.4 The Need to Confirm That AOX Do Not Act as Photosensitizers

As reported above, during the assessment of AOX to protect lipids removed from human skin against UVR- induced peroxidation, we observed that many botanical AOX behaved as strong pro-oxidants to increase LOOH levels significantly above the maximum levels formed in unprotected skin in the absence of AOX (Fig. 26.5). This result was also confirmed for Rosa G extract using two-photon fluorescence imaging of the nucleated epidermis, which shows that application of Rosa G extract (1 %) increases the ROS probe fluorescence significantly compared to the control (Fig. 26.6). Similar results using TPM were also obtained for other botanical AOX, including chardonnay grape extract, vitamin C complex, and fennel seed extract (Fig. 26.6).

Botanical AOX typically comprise complex mixtures of polyphenols. Many plant polyphenols have been shown to exert strong photoprotective effects in skin, including catechins from green tea, proanthocyanidins from grape seeds, and anthocyanidins from berries, among others [75, 76]. Indeed, we also observed that green tea, tetrahydrocurcumoids, and *Phyllanthus emblica* fruit extract conferred significant protection against UVR-induced lipid peroxidation (Fig. 26.5). However, plant polyphenols can also be potent sensitizers of ROS formation when exposed to UVR, as recently reported for verbascoside, isoverbascoside, and tyrosol or silibinin [77, 78].

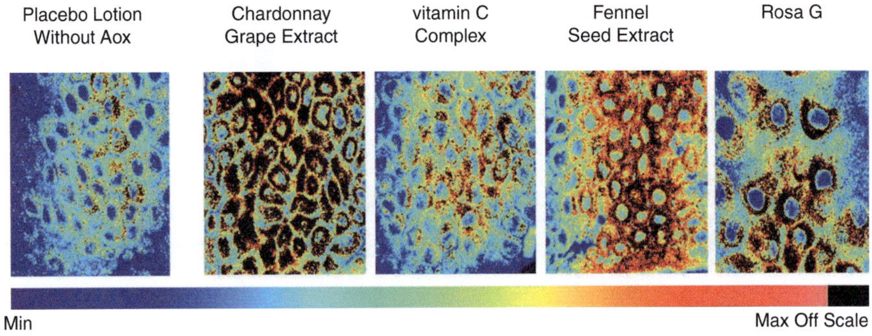

Fig. 26.6 Two-photon fluorescence images (z=30–50 mm) of skin applied with or without botanical extracts and obtained post-solar-simulated UVB/UVA irradiation. The images show that each "AOX" becomes pro-oxidative in nucleated epidermis under UV radiation. These data are confirmed by the LOOH test for Rosa G (Fig. 26.5) and dramatically show how under UVR some botanical AOX become pro-oxidants

Interestingly, of the seven natural extracts tested by us in Fig. 26.5, four were found to be strong pro-oxidants.

These data illustrate the point made in the Jablonski diagram of Fig. 26.2 depicting how a molecule including an AOX can undergo radical reactions once it reaches its excited state following absorption of a photon and indicate that not all AOX may be equally effective at quenching light-induced ROS. These results also underscore the need to qualify AOX selected for use in sunscreen products using appropriate methods to ensure that when applied to skin, they help reduce rather than exacerbate the burden of excess ROS formation induced by sun exposure.

26.4.5 Monitoring AOX Stability in Sunscreen Formulations

Use of AOX in finished sunscreen products necessitates that AOX remain physically and chemically stable from their point of manufacture until the product has been used up for all practical purposes by consumers. By virtue of their ability to scavenge ROS, AOX themselves are reactive molecules. Hence, during formulation development, it is important to ensure that AOX are chemically compatible with all the ingredients comprising a formulation and that once incorporated into a formulation, the AOX remain stable and can continue to scavenge ROS effectively.

An easy way to monitor AOX activity in finished formulations is by using one of the routine *in vitro* techniques that measures the capacity of an AOX to quench a free radical in solution. One such test is based on use of α,α-diphenyl-β-picrylhydrazyl (DPPH), which is a stable organic free radical with an intense purple coloration ($\lambda_{max}=515$ nm). When dissolved in methanol (or other appropriate solvent) and exposed to AOX, the purple color fades as DPPH is reduced. The extent to which the color fades can be readily measured using a spectrophotometer, and the color change can be used to construct a scale of relative effectiveness to rank AOX or to track AOX stability within a given formulation. Either hydrophilic or hydrophobic AOX can be assessed using DPPH provided the AOX are soluble in the solvent selected to conduct the assay.

An example to illustrate the usefulness of DPPH to monitor the stability of AOX in a finished sunscreen formulation appears in Fig. 26.7. The extent to which an aliquot of the lotion caused the purple color of DPPH in methanol to fade (referred to as antioxidant reducing units) was measured at regular intervals using a defined protocol after the lotion was stored either at room temperature or 50 °C for 30 days. In this case, the results show that AOX in the formulation was stable and maintained its activity over the entire period of the stability test. Advantages of the method are that few formulation ingredients, including sunscreens, interfere with the absorbance readings at 515 nm, it is simple and fast to perform, and it provides a measurement on whether the AOX capacity of the formulation remains intact or has degraded.

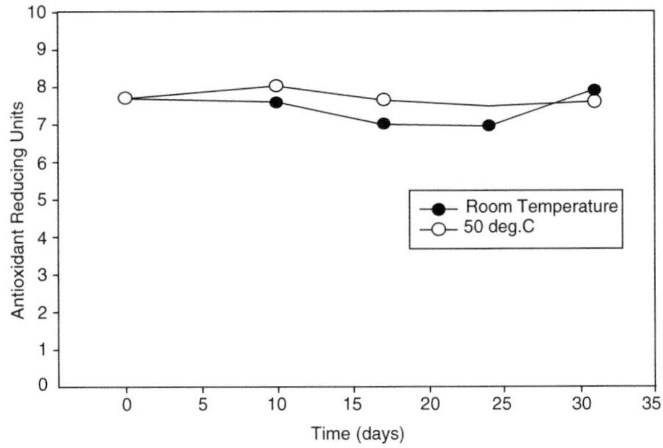

Fig. 26.7 A plot illustrating the usefulness of DPPH to monitor the stability of AOX in a finished sunscreen product stored at room temperature or 50 °C for 30 days

26.5 Benefits of AOX to Reduce ROS as a Function of SPF

TPM has proven highly effective in probing how sunscreens and AOX affect UV-induced ROS density in the epidermis and in redefining what constitutes efficacious photoprotection. Sunscreens at any SPF yield some protection against the generation of UV-induced ROS in the lower stratum corneum, from their inherent ability to absorb UV photons at the skin surface before they penetrate deeper into the skin; however, they afford incomplete photoprotection against ROS. For example, Fig. 26.8 shows a series of TPM images of *ex vivo* skin applied with a broad-spectrum SPF 30 sunscreen that have been irradiated with UVB-UVA radiation from a solar simulator fitted with WG 320 and UG 11 filters (4 MED, 88 mJ cm^{-2} UVB; 2.6 kJ cm^{-2} UVA (Solar Light Company); note that the output from this lamp contained negligible visible light). The control image (Fig. 26.8a) of unprotected skin shows the maximum fluorescence detected, and by comparison, we see that a broad-spectrum SPF 30 sunscreen affords some protection against UV-induced ROS with a 39 % decrease ($f\text{ROS}_{\text{SPF30}}=0.61$) compared to unprotected skin (Fig. 26.8b). In terms of photoprotection against ROS, there is room for improvement, which we see with the addition of two antioxidants to the SPF 30 formulation 0.5 % vitamin E and 0.1 % *Phyllanthus emblica* fruit extract (Fig. 26.8c). These data show that skin applied with the SPF30+AOX formulation yields a dramatic decrease in fluorescence intensity of the ROS probe, corresponding to a 73 % decrease ($f\text{ROS}_{\text{SPF30+AOX}}=0.27$) in UV-induced ROS compared to unprotected skin and a twofold increase in ROS photoprotection compared to the SPF 30-AOX formulation itself .

To gain a better understanding of the effect that SPF with and without AOX has on ROS generation in the skin, we performed TPM experiments on a series of formulations in a common placebo base with increasing SPF and either with or without AOX. A comparison of the sunscreen actives and AOX appears in Table 26.4.

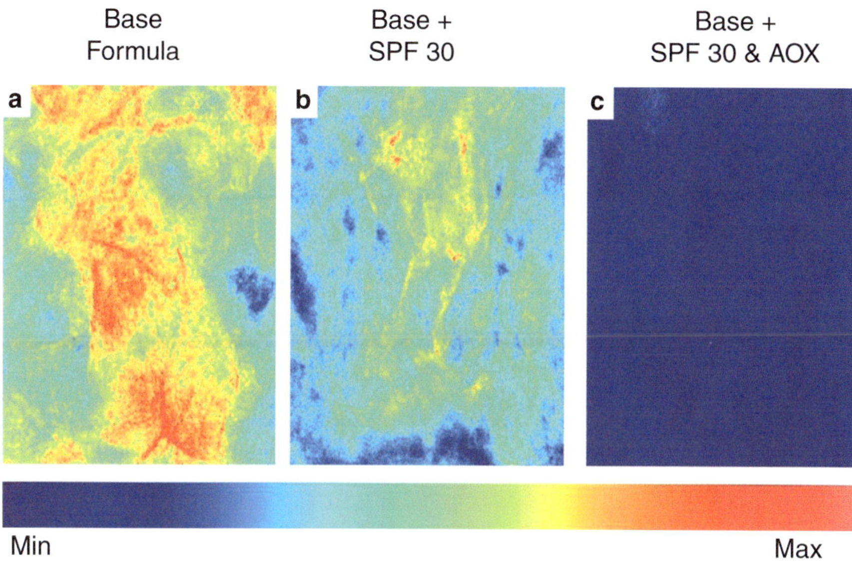

Fig. 26.8 Two-photon fluorescence images of skin ($z=5$ μm) incubated with DHR and a base formula (**a**), the based + a broad-spectrum SPF 30 sunscreen (**b**), or the base + sunscreen + 0.5 % vitamin E and 0.1 % Emblica fruit extract (**c**). All images are post-solar-simulated UV irradiation (88 mJ cm^{-2}, 2.6 kJ cm^{-2} UVA). fROS of the SPF 30 only is 0.61 (39 % reduction in ROS), and fROS of the SPF 30 + AOX is 0.27 (71 % reduction in ROS)

Table 26.4 Sunscreen actives, antioxidant combinations, and broad-spectrum indications for the formulas created to investigate the role of AOX to attenuate UV-induced levels of ROS in sunscreens with increasing levels of SPF

	Placebo	SPF 4	SPF 15	SPF 50	SPF 70
Oxybenzone	–	–	3.0	5.0	6.0
Octinoxate	–	2.0	–	–	–
Homosalate	–	–	5.0	10.0	15.0
Octisalate	–	–	5.0	5.0	5.0
Octocrylene	–	3.0	2.0	10.0	10.0
Avobenzone	–	–	2.0	3.0	3.0
Tocopherol (vitamin E)	–	0.5	0.5	0.5	0.5
Diethylhexyl syringlidene malonate (DESM)	–	0.9	0.9	0.9	0.9
Broad spectrum ($\lambda_c \geq 370$ nm) ?	N/A	No	Yes	Yes	Yes

Just as increasing SPF correlates with greater erythemal protection, so does increasing the SPF correlate with greater UV-induced ROS protection because of the increasing optical density provided by the UV filters at the skin surface. This effect can be seen in Fig. 26.9 where the fraction of UV-induced ROS detected in the lower stratum corneum decreases with increasing SPF. The data also show that the same formulations can yield significantly improved ROS photoprotection through the

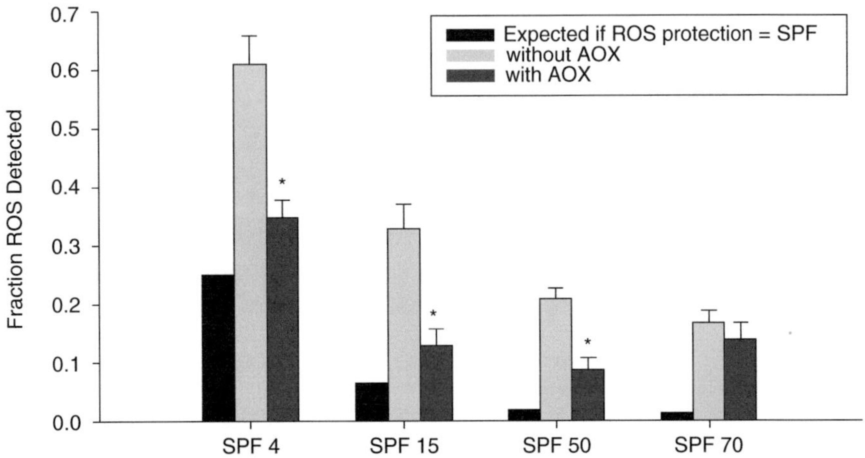

Fig. 26.9 The fraction of ROS detected in the lower stratum corneum based upon two-photon images and at different SPF values. The addition of AOX improves ROS protection for each SPF, although much less than what is predicted if ROS protection was equivalent to the SPF. Each SPF formula without AOX was compared to the same SPF formula with AOX using an unpaired *t*-test (*denotes $p<0.5$)

addition of the antioxidants vitamin E and diethylhexylsyringlidene malonate (DESM). Three additional interesting observations were detected with these data. First, a higher SPF without AOX may provide less photoprotection against UV-induced ROS than a formulation of lower SPF with AOX. For example, SPF 15 with AOX yields fewer ROS (12 % ROS) compared to SPF 50 without AOX (21 % ROS). Second, although the addition of these AOX to the highest SPF tested (SPF 70) did lead to a decrease in the ROS density, these data were not statistically significant which may illustrate that the effect was small and outside the signal-to-noise detection limits of the experiment. The data do indicate that at most 93 % of ROS are quenched by AOX (SPF 50). Further research might identify whether or not greater concentrations of AOX could improve protection against UV-induced ROS.

26.6 Conclusions

Exposure to solar radiation induces abundant levels of ROS within skin. Biologically relevant levels of ROS originate not only from the UV but also from the visible and IRA regions of the solar spectrum. ROS stimulated by the different portions of solar spectrum likely provoke biological responses within different epidermal and dermal compartments and are strongly associated with photoaging of skin. Sunscreens containing high levels of UVA filters combined with QPES and AOX represent promising intervention strategies to optimize protection of skin against the harmful effects of solar-induced ROS formation. Inclusion of AOX in sunscreen products can significantly improve protection against ROS over a broad range of SPFs. However, AOX need to be selected judiciously for use in sunscreens as some AOX can behave as pro-oxidants as opposed to antioxidants when applied to skin and exposed to the sun.

References

1. Rhie G, Shin MH, Seo JY, Choi WW, Cho KH, Kim KH, Park KC, Eun HC, CHung JH (2001) Aging-and photoaging-dependent changes of enzymic and non-enzymic antioxidants in the epidermis and dermis of human skin in vivo. J Invest Dermatol 117:1212–1217
2. Thiele JJ, Traber MG, Packer L (1998) Depletion of human stratum corneum vitamin E: an early and sensitive in vivo marker of UV induced photo-oxidation. J Invest Dermatol 110:756–791
3. Hellemans L, Corstjens H, Neven A, Declrq L, Maes D (2003) Antioxidant enzyme activity in human stratum corneum shows seasonal variation with an age-dependent recovery. J Invest Dermatol 120:434–439
4. Xu F, Fisher GJ (2002) Ultraviolet (UV) light irradiation induced signal transduction in skin photoaging. Arch Dermatol 138:1462–1470
5. Gutteridge JMC (1987) Thiobarbituric acid-reactivity following iron-dependent free-radical damage to amino acids and carbohydrates. FEBS Lett 128:343–346
6. Bickers DR, Athar M (2006) Oxidative stress in the pathogenesis of skin disease. J Invest Dermatol 126:2565–2575
7. Biniek K, Levi K, Dauskardt RH (2012) Solar UV radiation reduces the barrier function of human skin. Proc Natl Acad Sci U S A 109:1–6
8. Fisher JF (2002) Mechanisms of photoaging and chronological skin aging. Arch Dermatol Res 138:1462–1470
9. Pathak MA, Stratton K (1968) Free radicals in human skin before and after exposure to light. Arch Biochem Biophys 123:468–476
10. Jurkiewicz BA, Buettner GR (1996) EPR detection of free radicals in UV-irradiated skin: mouse versus human. Photochem Photobiol 64:918–922
11. Hanson KM, Clegg RM (2002) Observation and quantification of UV-induced ROS generation in ex vivo human skin. Photochem Photobiol 76:57–63
12. Zastrow L, Groth N, Klein F, Kockott D, Lademann J, Renneberg R, Ferrero L (2009) The missing link-light induced (280 Nm – 1600 Nm) free radical formation in human skin. Ski Pharmacol Physiol 22:31–44
13. Liebel F, Kaur S, Ruvolo E, Kollias N, Southall MD (2012) Irradiation of skin with visible light induces reactive oxygen species and matrix-degrading enzymes. J Invest Dermatol 132:1901–1907
14. Grether-Beck S, Marini A, Jaenicke T, Krutmann J (2015) Effective photoprotection of human skin against infrared a radiation by topically applied antioxidants: results from a vehicle controlled, randomized study. Photochem Photobiol 91(1):248–250
15. Grether-Beck S, Marini A, Jaenicke T, Krutmann J (2014) Photoprotection of human skin beyond ultraviolet radiation. Photodermatol Photoimmunol Photomed 30:167–174
16. Darvin ME, Haag S, Meinke M, Zastrow L, Sterry W, Lademann J (2001) Radical production by infrared a irradiation in human tissue. Skin Pharmacol Physiol 23:40–46
17. Droge W (2002) Free radicals in the physiological control of cell function. Physiol Rev 82:47–95
18. Chen L, Hu JY, Wang SQ (2012) The role of antioxidants in photoprotection: a critical review. J Am Acad Dermatol 67:1013–1024

19. Pryor WA (1986) Oxy-radicals and related species: their formation, lifetimes, and reactions. Annu Rev Physiol 48:657–667
20. Rubbo H, Radi R, Trujillo M, Telleri R, Kalyanaraman B, Barnes S, Kirk M, Freeman BA (1994) Nitric oxide regulation of superoxide and peroxynitrite-dependent lipid peroxidation. Formation of novel nitrogen-containing oxidized lipid derivatives. J Biol Chem 269:26066–26075
21. Sanders CS, Chang H, Salzmann S, Muller SL, Ekanayake-Mudiyanselage S, Elsner P, Thiele JJ (2002) Photoaging is associated with protein oxidation in human skin in vivo. J Invest Dermatol 118:618–625
22. Richter C, Park JW, Ames BN (1988) Normal oxidative damage to mitochondrial and nuclear DNA is extensive. Proc Natl Acad Sci U S A 85:6465–6467
23. Thiele JJ, Schroeter C, Hsieh SN, Podda M, Packer L (2001) The antioxidant network of the stratum corneum. In: Thiele J, Elsner P (eds) Current problems in dermatology: oxidants and antioxidants in cutaneous biology. Karger, Basel, pp 26–42
24. Rosenstein BS, Ducore JM, Cummings SW (1983) The mechanism of bilirubin-photosensitized D N a strand breakage in human cells exposed to phototherapy light. Mutat Res 112:397–406
25. Christensen T, Roll EB, Jaworska A, Kinn G (2000) Bilirubin- and light induced cell death in a murine lymphoma cell line. J Photochem Photobiol B 58:170–174
26. Wondrak GT, Jacobson EL, Jacobson MK (2002) Photosensitization of DNA damage by glycated proteins. Photochem Photobiol Sci 1:355–363
27. Masaki H (1999) Generation of active oxygen species from advanced glycation End-products (AGEs) during ultraviolet light a (UVA) irradiation and a possible mechanism for cell damaging. Biochim Biophys Acta 1428:45–56
28. Wondrak GT, Roberts MJ, Jacobson MK, Jacobson EL (2002) Photosensitized growth inhibition of cultured human skin cells: mechanism and suppression of oxidative stress from solar irradiation of glycated proteins. J Invest Dermatol 119:489–498
29. Wondrak GT, Roberts MJ, Cervantes-laurean D, Jacobson MK, Jacobson EL (2003) Proteins of the extracellular matrix are sensitizers of photo-oxidative stress in human skin cells. J Invest Dermatol 121:578–586
30. Karu TI (2008) Mitochondrial signaling in mammalian cells activated by red and near-IR radiation. Photochem Photobiol 84:1091–1099
31. Simon JD (2000) Spectroscopic and dynamic studies of the epidermal chromophores trans -urocanic acid and eumelanin. Acc Chem Res 33:307–313
32. Sarna T, Sealy RC (1984) Free radicals from eumelanins: quantum yields and wavelength dependence. Arch Biochem Biophys 232:574–578
33. Cunningham ML, Johnson JS, Giovanazzi SM, Peak MJ (1985) Photosensitized production of superoxide anion by monochromatic (290–405 Nm) ultraviolet irradiation of NADH and NADPH coenzymes. Photochem Photobiol 42:125–128
34. Cunningham ML, Krinsky N, Giovanazzi SM (1985) Superoxide anion is generated from cellular metabolites by solar radiation and its components. J Free Radic Biol Med 1:381–385
35. Peak JG, Peak MJ, MacCoss M (1984) DNA breakage caused by 334 Nm ultraviolet light is enhanced by naturally occurring nucleic acid components and nucleotide coenzymes. Photochem Photobiol 39:713–716
36. Menon IA, Becker MAC, Persad SD, Haberman HF (1989) Quantitation of hydrogen peroxide formed during UV-visible irradiation of protoporphyrin, coproporphyrin and uroporphyrin. Clin Chim Acta 186:375–381
37. Moan J, Berge K (1991) The photodegradation of porphyrins in cells can be used to estimate the lifetime of singlet oxygen. Photochem Photobiol 53:549–553
38. Reddi E, Jori G, Rodgers MAJ, Spikes JD (1983) Flash photolysis studies of hemato- and copro-porphyrins in homogeneous and microheterogeneous aqueous dispersions. Photochem Photobiol 38:639–645
39. Speck WT, Rosenkranz S, Rosenkranz HS (1976) Further observations on the photooxidation of DNA in the presence of riboflavin. Biochim Biophys Acta 435:39–44

40. Smith GJ (1992) Singlet oxygen produced by UV irradiation of wool keratin. J Photochem Photobiol B 2:173–178
41. Craggs J, Kirk SH, Ahmad SI (1994) Synergistic action of near-UV and phenylalanine, tyrosine or tryptophan on the inactivation of phage T7 : role of superoxide radicals and hydrogen peroxide. J Photochem Photobiol B 24:123–128
42. Hanson KM, Simon JD (1998) Epidermal trans-UA and the UVA-induced photoaging of the skin. Proc Natl Acad Sci U S A 95:10576–10578
43. Herrling T, Jung K, Chatelain E, Langenquer M (2006) Radical skin/sun protection factor RSF-protection against UV-induced free radicals. SOFW J 132:24–29
44. Osterwalder U, Jung K, Seifert M, Herrling T (2009) Importance of UVA sun protection: a comparative analysis of different quality control methods. SOFW J 135:2–13
45. Flober-Muller H, Champ S, Kandzia C, Jung K, Siefert M, Herrling T (2008) Strategy for efficient prevention of photo-ageing. SOFW J 134:23–29
46. Wondrak GT, Jacobson MK, Jacobson EL (2005) Identification of quenchers of photoexcited states as novel agents for skin photoprotection. J Pharmacol Exp Ther 312:482–491
47. Wondrak GT, Jacobson MK, Jacobson EL (2006) Endogenous UVA-photosensitizers: mediators of skin photodamage and novel targets for skin photoprotection. Photochem Photobiol Sci 5:215–237
48. Wondrak GT (2007) Let the sun shine in: mechanisms and potential for therapeutics in photodamage. Curr Opin Investing Drugs 8:390–400
49. Jockusch S, Bonda C, Hu S (2014) Photostabilization of endogenous porphyrins: excited state quenching by fused ring cyanoacrylates. Photochem Photobiol Sci 13:1180–1184
50. Lowe NJ (2006) An overview of ultraviolet radiation, sunscreens, and photo-induced dermatoses. In: Thiers BH, Draelos ZD (eds) Dermatologic clinics. Saunders, Philadelphia, pp 9–17
51. Oresajo C, Yatskayer M, Galdi A, Foltis P, Pillai S (2010) Complementary effects of antioxidants and sunscreens in reducing UV-induced skin damage as demonstrated by biomarker expression. J Cosmet Laser Ther 12:157–162
52. Matsui MS, Hsia A, Miller JD, Hanneman K, Scull H, Cooper KD, Baron E (2009) Non-sunscreen photoprotection: antioxidants add value to a sunscreen. J Invest Dermatol 14:56–59
53. Brenna M, Bhatti H, Nerusu KC, Bhagavathula N, Kang S, Fisher GJ (2003) Matrix metalloproteinase-1 is the major collagenolytic enzyme responsible for collagen damage in UV-irradiated human skin. Photochem Photobiol 78:43–48
54. Serafini M (2008) Role of the antioxidant network in the prevention of age-related disease. In: Miwa S, Beckman KB, Muller FL (eds) Aging medicine: oxidative stress in aging: from model systems to human diseases. Humana Press, Totowa, pp 269–289
55. Baier J, Maisch T, Maier M, Landthaler M, Baumler W (2007) Direct detection of singlet oxygen generated by UVA irradiation in human cells and skin. J Invest Dermatol 127:1498–1506
56. Lauer A, Groth N, Haag SF, Darvin ME, Lademann J, Meinke MC (2013) Radical scavenging capacity in human skin before and after vitamin C uptake: an in vivo feasibility study using EPR spectroscopy. J Invest Dermatol 133:1102–1104
57. Hanson KM, Beasley DG, Meyer TA, Bardeen CJ (2001) Antioxidants in sunscreen for improved ROS photoprotection. Cosm Toil 126:712–716
58. Hanson KM, Bardeen CJ (2009) Applications of nonlinear optical microscopy for imaging skin. Photochem Photobiol 85:33–44
59. Hanson KM, Gratton E, Bardeen CJ (2006) Sunscreen enhancement of UV-induced reactive oxygen species in the skin. Free Radic Biol Med 41:1205–1212
60. Mudiyanselage SE, Hamburger M, Elsner P, Thiele JJ (2003) Ultraviolet a induces generation of squalene monohydroperoxide isomers in human sebum and skin surface lipids in vitro and in vivo. J Invest Dermatol 120:915–922
61. Jeanmaire C, Danoux L, Pauly G (2001) Glycation during human dermal intrinsic and actinic aging: an in vivo and in vitro model study. Br J Dermatol 145:10–18

62. Halliday GM (2010) Common links among pathways leading to UV-induced immunosuppression. J Invest Dermatol 130:1209–1212
63. Crow JP, Beckman JS, McCord JM (1995) Sensitivity of the essential zinc-thiolate moiety of yeast alcohol dehydrogenase to hypochlorite and peroxynitrite. Biochemistry 34:3544–3552
64. Kooy NW, Royall JA, Ischiropoulos H, Bekman JS (1994) Peroxynitrite-mediated oxidation of dihydrorhodamine 123. Free Radic Biol Med 16:149–156
65. Royall JA, Ischiropoulos H (1993) Evaluation of 2',7'-dichlorofluorescin and dihydrorhodamine 123 as fluorescent probes for intracellular H2O2 in cultured endothelial cells. Arch Biochem Biophys 302:348–355
66. Henderson LM, Chappell JB (1993) Dihydrorhodamine 123: a fluorescent probe for superoxide generation? Eur J Biochem 217:973
67. Master BR, So PTC (1999) Multiphoton excitation microscopy and confocal imaging of in vivo human skin: a comparison. Mircosc Microanal 5:282–289
68. Ragan TR, Huang H, So PTC (2003) In vivo and ex vivo tissue applications of two-photon microscopy. Methods Enzymol 361:481–506
69. Master BR, So PTC, Gratton E (1997) Multiphoton excitation fluorescence microscopy and spectroscopy of in vivo human skin. Biophys J 72:2405–2412
70. Yuen KS, Halliday GM (1997) A-tocopherol, an inhibitor of epidermal lipid peroxidation, prevents ultraviolet radiation from suppressing the skin immune system. Photochem Photobiol 65:587–592
71. Tanaka N, Tajima S, Ishibashi A, Uchida K, Shigemastsu T (2001) Immunohistochemical detection of lipid peroxidation products, protein-bound acrolein and 4-hydroxynonenal protein adducts in actinic elastosis of photodamaged skin. Arch Dermatol Res 293:363–367
72. Miyamoto S, Matinez GR, Medeiros MHG, Mascio PD (2003) Singlet molecular oxygen generated from lipid hydroperoxides by the russell mechanism: studies using 18O-labelled linoleic acid hydroperoxide and monomol light emission. J Am Chem Soc 125:6172–6179
73. Chiba K, Kawakami K, Sone T, Onoue M (2003) characteristics of skin wrinkling and dermal changes induced by repeated application of squalene monohydroperoxide to hairless mouse skinitle. Skin Pharmacol Appl Skin Physiol 16:242–251
74. Meyer TA, Hanson KM, Beasley DG (2008) Judicious Use of antioxidants in broad spectrum sunscreens enhances protection beyond that afforded by sunscreens alone. J Am Acad Dermatol Suppl 58:112
75. Vayalil P, Mittal A, Hara Y, Elmets CA, Katiyar SK (2004) Green tea polyphenols prevent ultraviolet light-induced oxidative damage and matrix metalloproteinases expression in mouse skin. J Invest Dermatol 122:1480–1487
76. Nichols JA, Katiyar SK (2010) Skin photoprotection by natural polyphenols: anti-inflammatory, antioxidant and DNA repair mechanisms. Arch Dermatol Res 302:71–83
77. Narayanapillai S, Agarwal C, Tilley C, Agarwal R (2012) Silibinin is a potent sensitizer of UVA radiation-induced oxidative stress and apoptosis in human keratinocyte HaCaT cells. Photochem Photobiol 88:1135–1140
78. Lecci RM, Logrieco A, Leone A (2014) Pro-oxidative action of polyphenols as action mechanism for their pro-apoptotic activity. Anticancer Agents Med Chem 14:1–13
79. Hanson K, Behne M, Barry N, Mauro T, Gratton E, Clegg R (2002) Two-photon fluorescence lifetime imaging of the skin stratum corneum pH gradient. Biophys J 83:1682–1690
80. Behne M, Meyer J, Hanson K, Barry N, Murata s, Crumrine D, Clegg R, Gratton E, Holleran W, Elia P, Mauro T (2002) NHE1 regulates the stratum corneum permeability barrier homeostasis J Biol Chem 277: 47399–47406
81. Plasencia I, Norlen L, Bagatolli L (2007) Direct visulation of lipid domains in human skin stratum corneum lipid membranes: effect of pH and temperature 93: 3142–3155

Part IV

Chapter 27
Education, Motivation, and Compliance

Brian P. Hibler and Steven Q. Wang

Key Points
- Nearly five million people are treated annually for skin cancer in the United States, with an estimated cost of over $8 billion.
- While knowledge that photoprotection from ultraviolet radiation can reduce the incidence of skin cancer which is high, meaningful behavioral changes have not yet been achieved.
- A multifaceted approach to improve compliance is required, combining ongoing public education as primary prevention, stricter indoor tanning legislation, a change in social norms regarding tanned skin, and community-level interventions at schools and the workplace.
- Increased research, surveillance, and monitoring can measure the effects of our prevention efforts and assist in designing future efforts to motivate behavioral change and reduce the incidence of skin cancer.

27.1 Introduction

Skin cancer is the most common form of cancer in the United States and is a major public health concern [1–3]. Nearly five million people in the United States are treated for skin cancer every year, and the incidence and associated healthcare expenditures of skin cancer continue to rise, currently with an estimated annual cost of over $8 billion [4–6]. The vast majority of skin cancers are nonmelanoma skin cancer (NMSC), which can be treated with topical medications, radiation, or surgery with good prognosis. Although the risk of metastasis is low, NMSC is locally destructive and can impair quality of life. While cutaneous melanoma makes up

B.P. Hibler, BS • S.Q. Wang, MD (✉)
Division of Dermatology, Memorial Sloan-Kettering Cancer Center, Basking Ridge, NJ, USA
e-mail: wants@mskcc.org

S.Q. Wang, H.W. Lim (eds.), *Principles and Practice of Photoprotection*,
DOI 10.1007/978-3-319-29382-0_27

only about 5 % of the total number of skin cancers, it is more deadly [3, 5]. In the United States in 2014, it is estimated that there would be over 76,000 new cases of invasive melanoma and 9710 melanoma-related deaths [7].

It is well established that ultraviolet (UV) radiation plays a major role in the development of skin cancer [1, 8, 9]. Comprehensive photoprotective strategies have been shown to reduce the incidence of skin cancer [10]. While the general knowledge regarding the harmful effects of UV radiation and safe sun behaviors in Western countries is high [11, 12], this knowledge has not always translated into meaningful change of behavior. Studies continue to show significant levels of sun exposure in children and adults with inadequate protection from UV radiation [13–19]. Only 3 in 10 adults routinely practice sun protection behaviors in the United States [20]. Surveys found the majority (83 %) of teenagers, and nearly half (37 %) of all adults experienced at least one sunburn in the previous year [21, 22]. Furthermore, approximately 30 million people in the United States use tanning beds each year, including 2.3 million adolescents [23]. Among adolescents aged 13–19, 11 % of males and 37 % of females report ever using indoor tanning [24]. These numbers increase to 38 % of males and over 73 % of females by age 40 [23].

As highlighted by these statistics, there is a dramatic need for further public education and new motivational strategies to effectively change sun-protective behaviors. This chapter will discuss the major participants in the public health campaign, the current disconnect between knowledge and behaviors among the general population, and provide suggestions for improving motivation and compliance when it comes to skin cancer prevention.

27.2 Current Education in Photoprotection

27.2.1 The Messengers and Participants: A Collaborative Effort

27.2.1.1 Medical Community

The medical community plays a key role in educating the public regarding proper photoprotection. When it comes to skin cancer prevention and education, dermatologists are the most experienced and have led the way. As skin specialists, they are able to appeal to both health- and appearance-based motivations to change behaviors. For example, for patients with a history of skin cancer, the annual skin exam is the perfect time to reinforce the importance of proper photoprotection to prevent further malignancies. Similarly, clinic visits for patients presenting for cosmetic procedures can also be an ideal time to remind the patient that photoprotection slows the signs of aging. In addition, the American Academy of Dermatology (AAD), along with other organizations, has launched health campaigns to educate the public about the need for photoprotection.

Aside from dermatologists, primary care physicians are in the unique position to provide counseling to patients. In 2011, a systematic review for the US Preventive Services Task Force (USPSTF) found that counseling in the primary care setting can increase photoprotective behaviors and decrease intentional indoor and outdoor tanning [25]. As a result, the USPSTF recommends physicians counsel fair-skinned patients aged 10–24 years to minimize their UV exposure and effectively reduce their risk of skin cancer [26]. By incorporating together a total skin examination and photoprotection counseling, primary care providers can efficiently combine both primary and secondary prevention strategies into their visits.

Physicians from other specialties, such as pediatricians, obstetricians, and gynecologists, can also deliver education guidelines. For pediatricians in particular, evidence has shown that education to adolescents can be especially effective in reducing UV exposure [26, 27]. Additionally, pediatric checkups are generally oriented toward anticipatory guidance and serve as an ideal platform to integrate cancer prevention education into the visit for both the child and parent [28]. As individuals age, annual physical exams are a good time to plant the seed and keep encouraging proper skin care with a consistent and clear message.

While nearly all physicians agree that education regarding photoprotection is important, only a small percentage actually counsels their patients in practice. In a review of over 18 billion total patient visits between 1989 and 2010, sunscreen was mentioned at only 0.9 % of patient visits associated with a diagnosis of skin disease [29]. Commonly cited reasons include not remembering and lack of knowledge. Other major barriers include lack of time and lack of monetary incentive, as procedures, diagnostics, and other interventions are favored over preventive care [30, 31].

27.2.1.2 Educational Programs

School-based educational programs teach children at a young age to foster lifelong habits regarding sun protection [32, 33]. Two such programs are the SunWise School Program started by the US Environmental Protection Agency (EPA) and the SunSafe programs based on research funded by the National Cancer Institute, both of which are aimed at providing a national educational program regarding sun safety to children in primary schools [34–38]. Children who were part of the SunSafe program practice better sun safety techniques, including better sunscreen habits, than children who did not participate [35]. A systematic review showed these health educational programs are effective [39], and it is estimated that the SunWise program alone can prevent nearly 11,000 skin cancer cases among students who participated in the program [34].

27.2.1.3 Government Agencies and Organizations

The US government has played a role in educating the public about skin cancer prevention. For most areas of the United States, the National Weather Service provides UV index measurements that the EPA publishes with suggested UV protective measures. This set of information is useful to reduce overexposure to UV radiation when planning outdoor activities. A study evaluating the public's response to the UV index found that nearly 64 % of people had heard of the UV index and almost 40 % reported changing their sun practices as a result of it [40]. Another movement includes designation of May as "Melanoma/Skin Cancer Detection and Prevention Month." This initiative, sponsored by the AAD and endorsed by the US Department of Health and Human Services, serves as a timely opportunity each year to remind the public about safe sun practices as the summer approaches.

27.2.1.4 Media and Social Marketing

The traditional media, such as magazines, newspaper, radio, and television, have played an important role in disseminating information related to the skin cancer prevention message. Although members of the medical community are most trusted, the media channels are the primary source where large segments of public learn about UV risks and photoprotection [41]. In the past decades, the Internet and social media have overtaken traditional media. In addition to distributing information, social media can also play a role in influencing behavioral change by opening a forum for interaction with peers and family who also engage in certain behaviors [42]. As technologies advances, novel media approaches have been introduced to reach larger and targeted demographics. A recent example is the development of a short messaging service (SMS)-based sun safety intervention which improved skin cancer prevention behaviors and knowledge among adolescents [43].

In summary, members of the medical community, educational organizations, government agencies, and media and social marketing groups all play a collective role in educating the public about photoprotection. Through their combined efforts, they are able to reach a significant proportion of the public in a myriad of ways to increase skin cancer prevention awareness.

27.2.2 Their Message: Reaching the Public

27.2.2.1 Motivating Factors

In the public health campaign, there is a health-based approach and an appearance-based approach. In the health-based approach, an emphasis is placed on the risk of developing skin cancer from increased UV exposure. Specifically, this approach focuses on the disfiguration, functional limitations, and overall morbidity and mortality associated with skin cancer. This approach typically resonates with those with a personal or family history of skin cancer.

Alternatively, an appearance-based approach focuses on the effects of UV exposure on premature skin aging. In studies of young adults, appearance-based messages were more influential than health-based messages mainly because the risk of skin cancers is too distant [44, 45]. In view of the continual interest in cosmetic procedures and antiaging therapies, sunscreen marketed as a cosmeceutical with focus on its "antiaging" properties may increase use and compliance in the younger population and ultimately have an effect on future skin cancer rates.

27.2.2.2 Current Instructions: Overview of Guidelines for Photoprotection

In order of importance, the photoprotective strategies include sun avoidance; seeking shade; wearing protective clothing, hat, and sunglasses; and using sunscreens. A list of the major skin cancer prevention recommendations from major organizations is outlined in Table 27.1. Sun avoidance, especially during the peak hours of UV intensity (10 a.m.–4 p.m.), is the best strategy to limit unnecessary UV exposure. However, this is not easy for most individuals to comply with, as these are the optimal hours for working, exercising, and completing outdoor activities. Additionally, sunlight improves psychological and emotional well-being and generates vitamin D. In sum, total abstinence from sunlight is neither achievable nor desirable for a large proportion of the population. Practice of proper photoprotection should allow all of us to participate in outdoor activities, while at the same time protecting our skin.

Seeking shade and wearing protective clothing are viable options for those who enjoy the outdoors. Trees and shade structures may be placed strategically at schools, parks, and public pools to provide protection in the community. In the United States, however, local and national governments do not fund these endeavors, and it is up to private beneficiaries and nonprofit organizations to support these initiatives. In terms of protective clothing, tightly weaved fabrics and wide brim hats are important to maximize coverage over all anatomic sites predisposed to UV exposure. Compared with sunscreens, the benefits of protective clothing include more balanced protection from both UVA and UVB rays, and there is no need for reapplication as seen with sunscreen use. Proper photoprotection of the eyes using sunglasses is equally important. The use of clothing for UV protection has become more popular, especially for kids and adolescents.

Although sunscreen is less effective in preventing UV exposure compared to sun avoidance and physical barriers, it is the most frequently used protection by the public. The popularity of sunscreens over other measures is due to marketing by the sunscreen and cosmetic industry and recommendation by physicians. Nevertheless, sunscreen use has its own limitations impairing its photoprotective capabilities, namely, poor compliance and inappropriate application. Studies have shown that many individuals do not apply sunscreen adequately in terms of the amount, timing, and reapplication, and they frequently use sunscreens that are not broad-spectrum [49]. SPF values are determined by applying a 2.0 mg/cm^2 concentration of sunscreen; when in reality, most people use approximately 0.5–1.0 mg/cm^2 [50]. Consequently, the in-use effectiveness of the sunscreen protection is significantly

Table 27.1 Key photoprotective strategies from major organizations

Resource	Strategies
American Academy of Dermatology [46]	Apply broad-spectrum, water-resistant sunscreen of at least SPF 30 every 2 h Seek shade, especially during peak hours Wear protective clothing (long-sleeved shirt, wide brim hat, pants, sunglasses) Use extra caution around water, sand, and snow which may reflect UV rays Eat foods rich in vitamin D or take vitamin D supplements To achieve a tanned appearance, consider a self-tanning product and continue to use sunscreen Avoid tanning beds Check your skin annually for signs of skin cancer
Centers for Disease Control and Prevention [47]	Seek shade, especially during midday hours Wear clothing that covers exposed skin Wear a wide brim hat to shade your face, head, ears, and neck Wear sunglasses that provide UVA and UVB protection Use broad-spectrum sunscreen of SPF 15 or greater Avoid indoor tanning
American Cancer Society [48]	Avoid being outdoors in direct sunlight between 10 am and 4 pm Be careful in areas with sand, water, and snow Wear clothing with tightly woven fabrics to protect as much skin as possible Wear a hat with at least a 2–3 in. brim all around Wear sunglasses that block UV rays Use broad-spectrum, water-resistant sunscreen with SPF values of 30 or higher Be sure to apply sunscreen properly and reapply at least every 2 h Avoid tanning beds and sunlamps Protect children from the sun Get vitamin D from your diet and supplements rather than from sun exposure

less [50]. Moreover, to achieve the desired protection, sunscreens must be applied 30 min prior to exposure and reapplied every 2 h when outdoor. Lastly, SPF is measured based on protection against erythema or burning as an indicator of photodamage, which is mainly produced by UVB. Thus, the SPF rating does not indicate the level of protection from UVA, which is known to cause reactive oxygen species-mediated damage to cells [51, 52]. As a result, individuals must be cognizant to choose a sunscreen that also contains UVA active ingredients affording broad-spectrum protection. In the United States and many other countries, these are specific testing guidelines mandated by regulatory agencies for sunscreen product to be labeled as "broad-spectrum" [53].

27.3 Barriers to Behavior Change

As stated above, despite the evidence showing most people understand the harmful effects of UV radiation, this knowledge has not translated into meaningful behavioral change [54]. A number of barriers to making these changes have been identified. First, in the Western societies, tanned skin is viewed as attractive, healthy, and affluent. As a result, many individuals, especially young women, are influenced by their peers and trends in the media to purposefully receive high doses of UV exposure to achieve a darker and tanned appearance [12]. Second, there are health benefits associated with UV and sunlight exposure. UV radiation, specifically UVB, is needed to synthesize vitamin D, which is important for bone health [55]. Sunlight regulates the circadian rhythm and natural sunlight is effective to ameliorate seasonal affective disorder [56]. Being outdoors and living an active lifestyle is important to combat the obesity epidemic and other public health concerns, including diabetes and heart disease [49]. Third, changing behavior for preventive health actions is intrinsically challenging as seen in weight loss and smoking cessation programs. It is difficult to persuade individuals to make these behavioral changes when there is a lack of immediate rewards. Furthermore, for young individuals, the future risk of skin cancer is too distant to motivate and compel individuals to change. Lastly, maintaining these improved health habits requires sustained commitment. Far too often, the change on the part of individuals may be disruptive and inconvenient. For example, wearing protective clothing and applying sunscreens may be considered as hassles in one's busy daily routine.

27.4 A Multifaceted Approach: Instilling Motivation and Compliance

The need to bridge the gap between knowledge and behavior is clear. Attempts at further increasing public awareness regarding the association between sun exposure and skin cancer risk may have diminished effects on influencing behaviors, as most people are already aware of this connection [57]. As a result, it is necessary to understand the key concepts behind behavior modification in order to develop an effective marketing campaign that targets specific demographics and to take a collaborative approach to improve compliance among the population.

27.4.1 Improving Compliance

A comprehensive effort is required to influence and maintain sun protection behaviors at the population level. Ongoing public education represents the primary prevention measure to improve photoprotection and reduce the incidence of skin cancer. However, our endeavors must continue to build upon increasing knowledge and move toward focusing on behavior-based interventions to encourage change.

27.4.2 Ongoing Public Education as Primary Prevention Measure

Behavior change requires lifelong education and intervention; however, many interventions are complex, expensive, and difficult to implement. While education alone is not an effective way to change behavior, it is the first and foremost approach to change behaviors, especially during the early stages of behavior modification. These stages include the pre-contemplation and contemplation stages, in which individuals have either a favorable attitude toward sun-seeking behaviors or considerable ambivalence, as is common in the case of photoprotection. These individuals place more weight on the benefits of UV exposure, either its physiological effects or the cosmetic appeal of having tanned skin, rather than the harmful effects of sunbathing. For example, healthy teenagers are not concerned with the far-off thought of skin cancer, which inhibits their progression to making sustainable behavior change.

Education also needs to be taken into account for individuals in the other stages of behavior modification. Those who are in the later stages of behavior modification understand that the benefits of photoprotection outweigh the risks of unprotected UV exposure. In those cases, education needs to be focused more on the interventional side, with an emphasis placed on learning habits and methods to maintain healthy lifestyle adjustments. Furthermore, photoprotection messages should offer a comprehensive approach, including seeking shade; wearing protective clothing, hat, and sunglasses; and applying sunscreen appropriately.

27.4.3 Moving Beyond Education to Change Behaviors

A substantial portion of US adults do not perceive cancer as preventable and are less likely to engage in sun protection behaviors. Avoiding sunbathing and indoor tanning is one key component of education that must be emphasized. Indoor tanners may incorrectly believe that tanning indoors is safer and has health benefits compared to outdoor tanning. In actuality, indoor tanning is responsible for an estimated 450,000 NMSC and more than 10,000 melanoma cases in Europe, Australia, and the United States each year [58]. In order to reduce the harms from indoor tanning, it is necessary to further evaluate the attitudes and behaviors of indoor tanners. Targeted messages should be developed that resonate with the different groups who participate in indoor tanning and sunbathing. Additionally, the medical professionals need to assist the Federal Communications Commission in identifying and correcting the deceptive and misleading advertisements.

As seen in the movement to decrease the prevalence of smoking, many times legislation is more effective than education alone. Increasing taxes on indoor tanning salons may have similar effects as the tax increase on the cigarette industry. Under the Patient Protection and Affordable Care Act, a 10 % excise tax on indoor tanning services went into effect on July 1, 2010. Additionally, the FDA recently reclassified sunlamps to moderate-risk (Class II) devices, up from Class I, requiring premarket notification to the FDA for new tanning devices, and black box warning label displayed on the UV tanning devices [59, 60]. Further laws or regulations have been placed on indoor tanning in 44 states and the District of Columbia [4]. The three types or regulations include (1) harm-reduction regulation including use of eye protection or a time limit, (2) required parental consent or parental accompaniment, and (3) absolute age restriction (ban) for minors under a certain age, ranging from 14 to 18 years [4]. In 2011, California became the first state to enact an outright ban on tanning for individuals younger than 18, and since then, a number of other states have followed suit [61, 62]. These legislations have already made an impact on reducing the number of tanning bed users [61, 63–65]. After implementation of legislative restrictions in Utah, there was a 36 % decrease in indoor tanning among teens [64]. Nationwide, estimates show a 42 % decrease in states with stricter legislative policies [63]. Additionally, the increased legislation has led to a significant increase in news coverage throughout the entire year regarding skin protection and the risks of indoor tanning [66]. Nationwide adoption of such legislation in banning tanning for minors under age of 18 would have a significant impact on reducing this avoidable UV exposure.

As we continue to advocate for additional government policy to take hold, there must be a change in social norms regarding tanned skin to support the message of UV avoidance. The idealization of tanned skin representing health and attractiveness is a powerful social pressure for individuals to conform to this beauty standard. In the Western societies, pale skin was once considered beautiful and a sign of wealth, and currently tanned skin has become associated with a life of leisure and outdoor activities and a sign of health, fitness, and youth. This association has been further perpetuated in the media. For many individuals, the cosmetic appeal of having tan skin competes against the health-related concern of developing skin cancer. A shift is needed in the way our society portrays beauty, and the fashion and entertainment industries should be encouraged to head these efforts. The media have initiated limited campaigns by portraying natural skin as being healthy and beautiful. The cosmetic industry can further support this movement through promoting that beauty is the color of the skin one was born with. In sum, sociocultural influences motivate behaviors, and we need to realign and redefine the definition of beauty with the assistance of the media and beauty and entertainment industries. An appearance-based message can be more impactful than health-based message to change sun protection behaviors.

Additional widespread strategies and programs are needed at the community-level that facilitate both education and behavioral changes. Schools and the workplace represent enticing opportunities to improve sun protection knowledge and compliance. Schools can reinforce the photoprotective message introduced by curricular changes by allowing students to wear sun-protective clothing or by adopting the Australian "no hat, no play" policy that restricts children from playing outdoors without proper protective clothing. Children receiving interactive didactic sessions and completing take-home activities about sun protection have improved behaviors [67, 68]. In addition to school instruction, education for outdoor employees can increase sun protection in working professionals [69]. Environmental approaches encouraging sun protection, such as shaded areas and workplace policies supporting sun protection practices, are effective [4]. The ideal goal is for a domino effect whereby these workers will disseminate this public health information to other coworkers and clients to propagate the message. Strides should be made to increase sun protection availability, including sunscreens, in recreational and tourism settings. When adopting these photoprotective strategies, efforts should be made to reach out to various ethnic communities, with educational messages and campaigns tailored accordingly to the target demographic. Overall, multicomponent interventions in a variety of settings are our greatest chance to effectively change behavior and reduce skin cancer risk.

27.5 Conclusion

Despite ongoing public health campaigns to raise awareness of the skin cancer epidemic and need for improved photoprotection, there exists a disconnect between knowledge and behavior. The development of successful interventions relies heavily on a thorough understanding of the attitudes and beliefs that influence specific behaviors. The best strategy is to align efforts in a variety of settings that target different demographics with a coordinated approach. Enhanced sun protection knowledge and awareness is crucial for initiating behavioral change, and the public needs information required to make informed choices. We should continue to support and reinforce these efforts through community-level interventions, along with increased research, surveillance, and monitoring to determine the utility of these approaches and measure the effect of our prevention efforts. With this comprehensive approach, we can potentially motivate behavioral change and reverse the trend of increasing skin cancer.

References

1. Armstrong BK, Kricker A (2001) The epidemiology of UV induced skin cancer. J Photochem Photobiol B 63(1–3):8–18
2. Rogers HW et al (2010) Incidence estimate of nonmelanoma skin cancer in the United States, 2006. Arch Dermatol 146(3):283–287
3. Wang SQ, Halpern AC (2008) Public education in photoprotection. In: Clinical guide to sunscreens and photoprotection. New York: Informa Healthcare, pp 281–291

4. U. S. Department of Health and Human Services (2014) Reports of the surgeon general. In: The surgeon general's call to action to prevent skin cancer. Office of the Surgeon General (US), Washington (DC)
5. Jemal A et al (2011) Recent trends in cutaneous melanoma incidence and death rates in the United States, 1992–2006. J Am Acad Dermatol 65(5 Suppl 1):S17–25.e1–3
6. Lazovich D, Choi K, Vogel RI (2012) Time to get serious about skin cancer prevention. Cancer Epidemiol Biomarkers Prev 21(11):1893–1901
7. Siegel R et al (2014) Cancer statistics, 2014. CA Cancer J Clin 64(1):9–29
8. Saraiya M et al (2003) Preventing skin cancer: findings of the task force on community preventive services on reducing exposure to ultraviolet light. MMWR Recomm Rep 52(Rr-15):1–12
9. Berwick M, Pestak C, Thomas N (2014) Solar ultraviolet exposure and mortality from skin tumors. Adv Exp Med Biol 810:342–358
10. Simard EP et al (2012) Cancers with increasing incidence trends in the United States: 1999 through 2008. CA Cancer J Clin 62(2):118–128
11. MacKie RM (2004) Awareness, knowledge and attitudes to basal cell carcinoma and actinic keratoses among the general public within Europe. J Eur Acad Dermatol Venereol 18(5):552–555
12. Spradlin K et al (2010) Skin cancer: knowledge, behaviors, and attitudes of college students. South Med J 103(10):999–1003
13. Lovato CY et al (1998) Canadian national survey on sun exposure & protective behaviours: youth at leisure. Cancer Prev Control 2(3):117–122
14. Shoveller JA et al (1998) Canadian national survey on sun exposure & protective behaviours: adults at leisure. Cancer Prev Control 2(3):111–116
15. Hall HI et al (1997) Sun protection behaviors of the U.S. white population. Prev Med 26(4):401–407
16. Robinson JK et al (1997) Summer sun exposure: knowledge, attitudes, and behaviors of Midwest adolescents. Prev Med 26(3):364–372
17. Jones SE et al (2012) Trends in sunscreen use among U.S. high school students: 1999–2009. J Adolesc Health 50(3):304–307
18. Basch CH et al (2012) Improving understanding about tanning behaviors in college students: a pilot study. J Am Coll Health 60(3):250–256
19. Ellis RM et al (2012) Sunscreen use in student athletes: a survey study. J Am Acad Dermatol 67(1):159–160
20. Buller DB et al (2011) Prevalence of sunburn, sun protection, and indoor tanning behaviors among Americans: review from national surveys and case studies of 3 states. J Am Acad Dermatol 65(5 Suppl 1):S114–S123
21. Holman DM et al (2014) The association between demographic and behavioral characteristics and sunburn among U.S. adults – National Health Interview Survey, 2010. Prev Med 63:6–12
22. Geller AC et al (2002) Use of sunscreen, sunburning rates, and tanning bed use among more than 10 000 US children and adolescents. Pediatrics 109(6):1009–1014
23. Levine JA et al (2005) The indoor UV tanning industry: a review of skin cancer risk, health benefit claims, and regulation. J Am Acad Dermatol 53(6):1038–1044
24. Demko CA et al (2003) Use of indoor tanning facilities by white adolescents in the United States. Arch Pediatr Adolesc Med 157(9):854–860
25. Lin JS, Eder M, Weinmann S (2011) Behavioral counseling to prevent skin cancer: a systematic review for the U.S. Preventive Services Task Force. Ann Intern Med 154(3):190–201
26. Moyer VA (2012) Behavioral counseling to prevent skin cancer: U.S. Preventive Services Task Force recommendation statement. Ann Intern Med 157(1):59–65
27. Balk SJ (2011) Ultraviolet radiation: a hazard to children and adolescents. Pediatrics 127(3):e791–e817
28. Crane LA et al (2006) A randomized intervention study of sun protection promotion in well-child care. Prev Med 42(3):162–170

29. Akamine KL et al (2014) Trends in sunscreen recommendation among US physicians. JAMA Dermatol 150(1):51–55
30. Nutting PA (1986) Health promotion in primary medical care: problems and potential. Prev Med 15(5):537–548
31. Wechsler H et al (1983) The physician's role in health promotion–a survey of primary-care practitioners. N Engl J Med 308(2):97–100
32. Buller DB et al (2006) Evaluation of the sunny days, healthy ways sun safety curriculum for children in kindergarten through fifth grade. Pediatr Dermatol 23(4):321–329
33. Banks BA et al (1992) Attitudes of teenagers toward sun exposure and sunscreen use. Pediatrics 89(1):40–42
34. Kyle JW et al (2008) Economic evaluation of the US Environmental Protection Agency's SunWise program: sun protection education for young children. Pediatrics 121(5):e1074–e1084
35. Olson AL et al (2007) SunSafe in the Middle School Years: a community-wide intervention to change early-adolescent sun protection. Pediatrics 119(1):e247–e256
36. Dietrich AJ et al (1998) A community-based randomized trial encouraging sun protection for children. Pediatrics 102(6):E64
37. Grant-Petersson J et al (1999) Promoting sun protection in elementary schools and child care settings: the SunSafe Project. J Sch Health 69(3):100–106
38. Dietrich AJ et al (2000) Sun protection counseling for children: primary care practice patterns and effect of an intervention on clinicians. Arch Fam Med 9(2):155–159
39. Saraiya M et al (2004) Interventions to prevent skin cancer by reducing exposure to ultraviolet radiation: a systematic review. Am J Prev Med 27(5):422–466
40. Geller AC et al (1997) Evaluation of the Ultraviolet Index: media reactions and public response. J Am Acad Dermatol 37(6):935–941
41. Polster AM et al (1998) Reports by patients and dermatologists of skin cancer preventive services provided in dermatology offices. Arch Dermatol 134(9):1095–1098
42. Centola D (2013) Social media and the science of health behavior. Circulation 127(21):2135–2144
43. Hingle MD et al (2014) Effects of a short messaging service-based skin cancer prevention campaign in adolescents. Am J Prev Med 47(5):617–623
44. Jones JL, Leary MR (1994) Effects of appearance-based admonitions against sun exposure on tanning intentions in young adults. Health Psychol 13(1):86–90
45. Tuong W, Armstrong AW (2014) Effect of appearance-based education compared with health-based education on sunscreen use and knowledge: a randomized controlled trial. J Am Acad Dermatol 70(4):665–669
46. American Academy of Dermatology Prevent skin cancer. 2015. Available from: https://www.aad.org/spot-skin-cancer/learn-about-skin-cancer/prevent-skin-cancer
47. Centers for Disease Control and Prevention (2014) What can I do to reduce my risk of skin cancer? Available from: http://www.cdc.gov/cancer/skin/basic_info/prevention.htm
48. American Cancer Society (2014) Skin cancer prevention and early detection: how do I protect myself from UV rays? Available from: http://www.cancer.org/cancer/cancercauses/sunanduvexposure/skin-cancerpreventionandearlydetection/skin-cancer-prevention-and-early-detection-u-v-protection
49. Eide MJ, Weinstock MA (2006) Public health challenges in sun protection. Dermatol Clin 24(1):119–124
50. Faurschou A, Wulf HC (2007) The relation between sun protection factor and amount of sunscreen applied in vivo. Br J Dermatol 156(4):716–719
51. Jansen R et al (2013) Photoprotection: part II. Sunscreen: development, efficacy, and controversies. J Am Acad Dermatol 69(6):867.e1–867.e14
52. Baumler W et al (2012) UVA and endogenous photosensitizers–the detection of singlet oxygen by its luminescence. Photochem Photobiol Sci 11(1):107–117
53. Wang SQ, Lim HW (2011) Current status of the sunscreen regulation in the United States: 2011 Food and Drug Administration's final rule on labeling and effectiveness testing. J Am Acad Dermatol 65(4):863–869

54. Kristjansson S, Ullen H, Helgason AR (2004) The importance of assessing the readiness to change sun-protection behaviours: a population-based study. Eur J Cancer 40(18):2773–2780
55. O'Leary RE, Diehl J, Levins PC (2014) Update on tanning: more risks, fewer benefits. J Am Acad Dermatol 70(3):562–568
56. Wirz-Justice A et al (1996) 'Natural' light treatment of seasonal affective disorder. J Affect Disord 37(2-3):109–120
57. Peacey V et al (2006) Ten-year changes in sun protection behaviors and beliefs of young adults in 13 European countries. Prev Med 43(6):460–465
58. Wehner MR et al (2014) International prevalence of indoor tanning: a systematic review and meta-analysis. JAMA Dermatol 150(4):390–400
59. US Food and Drug Administration (2014) FDA to require warnings on sunlamp products. FDA News Release. 2014 May 29. Available from: http://www.fda.gov/NewsEvents/Newsroom/PressAnnouncements/ucm399222.htm
60. Ernst A, Grimm A, Lim HW (2015) Tanning lamps: health effects and reclassification by the Food and Drug Administration. J Am Acad Dermatol 72(1):175–180
61. Chen LL, Wang SQ (2012) Post-California tanning ban: a brief update on current youth access laws. Arch Dermatol 148(9):1071–1072
62. Grewal SK et al (2013) Compliance by California tanning facilities with the nation's first statewide ban on use before the age of 18 years. J Am Acad Dermatol 69(6):883–889.e4
63. Guy GP Jr et al (2014) State indoor tanning laws and adolescent indoor tanning. Am J Public Health 104(4):e69–e74
64. Simmons RG, Smith K, Balough M (2014) Decrease in self-reported tanning frequency among Utah teens following the passage of Utah senate bill 41: an analysis of the effects of youth-access restriction laws on tanning behaviors. J Skin Cancer 2014:839601. http://www.ncbi.nlm.nih.gov/pubmed/25215240
65. Hester EJ et al (2005) Compliance with youth access regulations for indoor UV tanning. Arch Dermatol 141(8):959–962
66. Mayer JE et al (2015) The impact of indoor tanning legislation: newspaper coverage of the risks of indoor tanning before and after the California indoor tanning Ban for minors. J Cancer Educ 30(1):124–129. http://www.ncbi.nlm.nih.gov/pubmed/24882438
67. Geller AC et al (2002) The environmental protection Agency's national SunWise school program: sun protection education in US schools (1999–2000). J Am Acad Dermatol 46(5):683–689
68. Glanz K, Halpern AC, Saraiya M (2006) Behavioral and community interventions to prevent skin cancer: what works? Arch Dermatol 142(3):356–360
69. Horsham C et al (2014) Interventions to decrease skin cancer risk in outdoor workers: update to a 2007 systematic review. BMC Res Notes 7:10

Index

S.Q. Wang, H.W. Lim (eds.), *Principles and Practice of Photoprotection*,
DOI 10.1007/978-3-319-29382-0

P